Transcultural Concepts in Nursing Care

Transcultural Concepts in Nursing Care

Third Edition

Margaret M. Andrews, Ph.D., R.N., C.T.N.

Chairperson and Professor
Department of Nursing
Nazareth College of Rochester
Rochester, New York

Joyceen S. Boyle, Ph.D., R.N., F.A.A.N., C.T.N.

Professor and Chair
Department of Community Nursing
School of Nursing
Medical College of Georgia
Augusta, Georgia

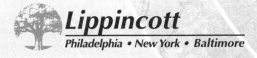
Lippincott
Philadelphia • New York • Baltimore

Acquisitions Editor: Margaret Zuccarini
Sponsoring Editor: Sara Lauber
Production Editor: Jahmae Harris
Senior Production Manager: Helen Ewan
Production Coordinator: Mike Carcel
Designer: Doug Smock

Third Edition

Library of Congress Cataloging in Publications Data

Andrews, Margaret M.
    Transcultural concepts in nursing care / Margaret M. Andrews,
Joyceen S. Boyle.—3rd ed.
        p.   cm.
    Includes bibliographical references and index.
    ISBN 0-7817-1038-3
    1. Transcultural nursing.   2. Nursing—Social aspects.
3. Nursing—Cross-cultural studies.   I. Boyle, Joyceen S.
II. Title.
    [DNLM: 1. Transcultural Nursing.   WY 107 A568t 1998]
RT86.54.A53   1998
362.1′73—dc21
DNLM/DLC
for Library of Congress   98-3026
                                                                CIP

Care has been taken to confirm the accuracy of the information presented and to describe generally accepted practices. However, the authors, editors, and publisher are not responsible for errors or omissions or for any consequences from application of the information in this book and make no warranty, express or implied, with respect to the contents of the publication.

The authors, editors and publisher have exerted every effort to ensure that drug selection and dosage set forth in this text are in accordance with current recommendations and practice at the time of publication. However, in view of ongoing research, changes in government regulations, and the constant flow of information relating to drug therapy and drug reactions, the reader is urged to check the package insert for each drug for any change in indications and dosage and for added warnings and precautions. This is particularly important when the recommended agent is a new or infrequently employed drug.

Some drugs and medical devices presented in this publication have Food and Drug Administration (FDA) clearance for limited use in restricted research settings. It is the responsibility of the health care provider to ascertain the FDA status of each drug or device planned for use in their clinical practice.

9   8   7   6   5   4   3   2   1

Preface

Initially published in 1989, this text began as a collegial effort among faculty and doctoral students at the University of Utah College of Nursing to help us expand and clarify our view of transcultural nursing. Because many of the contributors had strong clinical backgrounds and an interest in solving practice problems, we wanted a book that would apply transcultural nursing concepts to clinical practice. At the same time, many of us were teaching in baccalaureate and masters' programs in nursing. We accepted the challenge to teach our students the application of transcultural concepts to practice. And, because we recognized that the practice of nursing is theory-based, we worked to develop a research based theoretical framework relevant to transcultural nursing practice.

In light of the development of this book through three editions, it is not surprising to discover that the third edition of *Transcultural Concepts in Nursing Care* strongly reflects the current challenges faced by nurses who are practicing in a changing clinical environment. Although we have gone our different ways, each of the original authors has retained a strong tie to nursing practice and to transcultural nursing education. Overall, we share a commitment to:

- Foster the development and maintenance of a disciplinary knowledge base and expertise in culturally competent care.
- Synthesize existing theoretical and research knowledge regarding nursing care of different ethnic/minority, marginalized and disenfranchised populations.
- Create an interdisciplinary knowledge base that reflects heterogeneous health care practices within various cultural groups.
- Identify, describe, and examine methods, theories and frameworks appropriate for developing knowledge that will improve health and nursing care to minority, marginalized and disenfranchised populations.

The National League for Nursing, most state boards of nursing and other accrediting or certification bodies require or strongly encourage inclusion of cultural aspects of client care in the nursing curriculum. This underscores the importance of the purpose, goals, and objectives for publishing the third edition of **Transcultural Concepts of Nursing Care.**

Purpose: To contribute to the development of theoretically based transcultural nursing and the advancement of transcultural nursing practice.

Goal: to increase the delivery of culturally competent client care.

Objectives:

1. To expand the theoretical basis for using concepts from the natural and behavioral sciences for nursing practice.
2. To apply a transcultural nursing framework to guide nursing practice in diverse health care settings.
3. To analyze major concerns and issues encountered by nurses in providing transcultural nursing care to clients—individuals, families, groups, communities, and institutions.

Recognizing Individual Differences and Acculturation

When considering transcultural issues, nurses and other health care professionals are, with increasing frequency, referring to the federally defined population categories, i.e., white, black, Hispanic, Asian/Pacific Islander, and American Indian/Alaska Native. The creation of these defined population categories by our government has had a tremendous impact on our conceptualization of the various groups that constitute our society. The unique characteristics and individual differences of the five cultural groups have often been ignored, along with the impact acculturation has had on these groups. The outcome is reminiscent of the melting pot metaphor, only now we have five pots instead of one!

We believe that it is tremendously important to recognize the myriad of health-related beliefs and practices that exist within the population categories. For example, the differences are rarely recognized among people who identify themselves as Hispanic/Latino: this group includes people from Puerto Rico, Mexico, Spain, Guatemala, or "Little Havana" in Miami, who may have some similarities but who also may have distinct cultural differences.

We would like to comment briefly on the terms *minority* and *ethnic minorities*. These terms are perceived to be offensive by some because they connote inferiority and marginalization. Although we have used these terms occasionally, we prefer to make reference to a specific subculture or culture whenever possible. We refer to categorizations according to race, ethnicity, religion, or a combination, such as ethno-religion (e.g., Amish), but we make every effort to avoid using any label in a pejorative way. We do believe, however, that the concepts or terms *minority* or *ethnicity* are limiting not only for those to whom the label may be applied, but also for nursing theory and practice.

Critical Thinking Linked to Delivering Culturally Competent Care

We believe that cultural assessment skills, combined with the nurse's critical thinking ability, will provide the necessary knowledge on which to base transcultural nursing care. Using this approach, we are convinced that nurses will be able to provide culturally competent and contextually meaningful care for clients from a wide variety of cultural backgrounds, rather than simply memorizing the esoteric health beliefs and practices of any specific cultural group. We believe that nurses must acquire the skills needed to assess clients from virtually any and all groups that they encounter throughout their professional careers. We have also attempted to address transcultural nursing from a Canadian perspective when it seemed appropriate to do so.

New to the Third Edition

All content in this edition has been reviewed and updated to capture the nature of the changing health care delivery system and to explain how nurses and other health care providers can use culturally competent skills to improve the care of clients, families, groups and communities.

Emphasis on Clinical Application

Clinical Application has been emphasized by integrating current research throughout the text and expanding content related to cultural assessment.

New Chapters

At the request of colleagues who are using this text, *Chapter 8: Trends in Health Care Delivery and Contributions of Transcultural Nursing, Chapter 13: Ethics and Culture: Contemporary Challenges, and Chapter 14: Cultural Diversity in the Health-care Workforce* have been added. In addition, *Chapter 11: Culture and Nutrition,* a topic that was included in the first edition, has been revised and included in this edition.

Chapter Pedagogy

Learning Activities

All of the chapters include review questions as well as learning activities to promote critical thinking. In addition, each chapter includes chapter objectives and key terms to help readers understand the purpose and intent of the content they will be reading.

Research Applications

Current research studies related to the content of the chapter are presented as Research Applications. We have added a section to each Research Box describing appropriate clinical applications derived from the research findings.

Case Studies Based on Actual Experiences

Case studies based on the authors' actual clinical experiences and research findings are presented to make conceptual linkages and to illustrate how concepts are applied in health care settings. (*Authors' note:* The case studies use pseudonyms to protect the confidentiality and anonymity of the authors' clients and research subjects.)

Text Organization

Part One: Foundations of Transcultural Nursing Care

The first section focuses on the historical and theoretical aspects of transcultural nursing. The development of a transcultural nursing framework that includes concepts from the natural and behavioral sciences is described as it applies to nursing practice. Because nursing perspectives are used to organize the content of this book, the reader will not find a chapter purporting to describe the nursing care of a specific cultural group. Instead, the nursing needs of culturally diverse groups are used to illustrate cultural concepts used in nursing care. For example, Chapter 2 discusses domains of cultural knowledge that are important in cultural assessment and describes how this cultural information can be incorporated into all aspects of nursing care.

Part Two: A Developmental Approach to Transcultural Nursing

Chapters 3–6 use a developmental framework to discuss transcultural concepts across the life span. The care of childbearing women and their families, children, adolescents, middle-aged adults, and the elderly is examined, and information about various cultural groups is used to illustrate common transcultural nursing issues, trends, and problems.

Part Three: Application of Transcultural Concepts in Nursing Care Delivery

In the third section of the text, Chapters 7 to 10, selected clinical topics and issues are used to illustrate the application of cultural concepts in nursing practice. The clinical application of concepts throughout this section uses situations commonly encountered by nurses and describes how transcultural nursing principles can be applied in diverse settings. The chapters in this section are intended to illustrate the application of transcultural nursing knowledge to nursing practice. In this section, transcultural nursing care in mental illness, as well as the transcultural aspects of pain, are examined. Community-based transcultural care is highlighted throughout this section and a chapter is included that examines cultural aspects of families and communities.

Part Four: Contemporary Challenges in Transcultural Nursing

In the fourth section of the text, Chapters 11 to 15, transcultural nursing care in specific settings such as critical care in a changing health care environment is described and the importance of transcultural nursing concepts in selected practice settings is examined. The selection of clinical topics varies widely and reflects the interests and diversity of the contributing authors as well as the changing health care systems in both the United States and Canada. The interrelationship between religion and culture is the focus of Chapter 12. This section includes new chapter additions on culture and nutrition, ethical issues in transcultural nursing practice and transcultural issues in a multicultural workforce. In Chapter 15, the nurse is introduced to global health issues and concerns and to the roles of nurses in international practice settings.

A Final Note

We are pleased several members of the original group who wrote the 1st edition are still with us and that colleagues who helped us with the 2nd edition are continuing. New contributors have been welcomed. Their significant contributions have enriched this 3rd edition, both in scope and content, and have assisted all who have worked on this text to achieve our stated purpose of contribution to the development of transcultural nursing theory and practice.

MMA
JSB

Acknowledgments

We gratefully acknowledge the assistance of our families, friends, and colleagues in making this book possible. We also appreciate the help of many nursing faculty, practitioners, and students who have offered their comments and suggestions.

A number of colleagues reviewed specific sections of the text and offered invaluable constructive criticism and suggestions. Special thanks to Dr. M. Katherine Maeve, Medical College of Georgia, for her reviews. She also shared selected chapters with students and passed their comments along to us.

We are indebted to the many individuals who allowed us to take photographs of them, including members of our families and friends. Particular appreciation is extended to Dr. Patti Ludwig-Beymer, Dr. Margaret A. McKenna, Dr. Kathleen Kavanagh and again to Dr. M. Katherine Maeve, all of whom took special photographs for us.

A special word of thanks to Margaret Zuccarini, Nursing Editor, Helen Ewan, Production Manager, and Sara Lauber, Sponsoring Editor, at Lippincott-Raven Publishers who have supported and encouraged us throughout this project. We are grateful to Jahmae Harris, Production Editor, and Doug Smock, Designer, for assistance with editing and design and for their careful attention to details during the final stages of production.

We acknowledge and thank our secretaries, Marilyn S. Brulé and Lisa M. Carrier, for their help in preparing this manuscript. It is their 2nd edition too and their contributions increased and were invaluable. Without their expertise and skill, this project would not have been possible.

We wish to express gratitude to our mothers, Virginia Andrews and Joyce Spencer, and to our fathers (now deceased), Henry Andrews and Harold Spencer, for teaching us to respect and value differences in people. Thanks also to Henry, Marilyn, Michael, Peter, and Suzanne Andrews and John Boyle for their interest and support over the years. We are also grateful for the support of our friends, too numerous to list by name, who often stopped by our offices or called to express their interest.

Lastly, once again we would like to thank each other for a friendship that has withstood the test of time (and now *three* editions of this book). We started with sharpened pencils and yellow legal pads with our 1st edition and have progressed to email, computers and fax machines. Throughout it all, we have found our professional endeavors in transcultural nursing and the friends we have made to be both satisfying and rewarding.

Contributing Authors

Margaret M. Andrews, Ph.D., R.N., C.T.N.
Chairperson and Professor
Department of Nursing
Nazareth College of Rochester
Rochester, New York

Joyceen S. Boyle, Ph.D., R.N., F.A.A.N., C.T.N.
Professor and Chair
Department of Community Nursing
School of Nursing
Medical College of Georgia
Augusta, Georgia

Patricia A. Hanson, Ph.D., R.N., C.S.
Associate Professor
Department of Nursing
Nazareth College of Rochester
Rochester, New York

Paula Herberg, Ph.D., R.N., F.N.P.
Associate Dean (Nursing) and Director
The Aga Khan University
Karachi, Pakistan

Kathryn Hopkins Kavanagh, Ph.D., R.N.
Associate Professor
Psychiatric Community Health and Adult Primary
    Care
University of Maryland at Baltimore
Baltimore, Maryland

Jana Lauderdale, Ph.D., R.N.
Assistant Professor
Vanderbilt School of Nursing
Nashville, Tennessee

Patti A. Ludwig-Beymer, Ph.D., R.N., C.T.N.
Director, Clinical Quality
Advocate Health Care
Oak Brook, Illinois

Mary E. Norton, Ed.D., C.N.S.
Associate Professor
Department of Professional Nursing
Felician College
Lodi, New Jersey

Margaret A. McKenna, Ph.D., M.N., M.P.H.
Principal
ConTEXT Sociocultural Research & Analysis
Seattle, Washington

REVIEWERS

Sara Aronson, R.N., B.S., M.P.H.
Director RN Pathway Program
Hunter-Bellevue School of Nursing
New York, New York

Mary Ellen Echelbarger, Ph.D., R.N.
Assistant Professor
Ohio State University
Columbus, Ohio

Linda M. Hartley, R.N., M.S.
Professor of Nursing
Elgin Community College
Elgin, Illinois

Mary E. Leavell Malone, R.N., B.S.N., M.A., M.S.
Professor of Nursing
University of Kentucky—Jefferson Community
    College
Louisville, Kentucky

Marilyn Stoner, R.N., M.S.N.
Assistant Professor of Nursing
California State University, San Bernardino
San Bernardino, California
Adjunct Faculty
Department of Health Services
University of Washington
Seattle, Washington

Foreword

More than forty years have passed since transcultural nursing was conceived and began to be developed as an essential area of study and practice within the nursing profession. While the evolutionary process of establishing transcultural nursing as an integral part of the nursing discipline has appeared slow, a core of committed transcultural nurses have made consistent headway in its development. The past dominant emphasis on medical diseases and treatment regimes, along with the lack of knowledge about cultures and culture-specific care, has delayed this process and has impeded the process of changing nurses' thinking and action modalities. Nonetheless, transcultural nursing is now of growing importance to professional nurses and consumers of healthcare services.

As the founder and central leader of transcultural nursing and a leader in promoting human caring as the essence of nursing, I have been most encouraged to see transcultural nursing knowledge, theory, research, and practice valued by nursing students, teachers and practitioners. One of the most rewarding developments, however, has been to see students that I have taught or mentored take active leadership in advancing the discipline of transcultural nursing. The authors of the third edition of **Transcultural Concepts in Nursing Care** reflect such leadership. Dr. Joyceen S. Boyle was at the University of Utah when I served as Dean and Professor of Nursing and established the first courses and Ph.D. program in transcultural nursing. Dr. Margaret M. Andrews came to the University a short time later. Both Dr. Boyle and Dr. Andrews completed the doctoral program with a focus in transcultural nursing.

In many places in the world, it has been the nursing students who have experienced competent transcultural teachers and who have been strong advocates of working to incorporate transcultural nursing content into nursing curricula and clinical practices. Many of these nursing students have been leaders in urging faculty, administrators, and nurses in clinical practice settings to incorporate transcultural nursing into their work.

Today, there are several transcultural nursing books, chapters, and articles available to nurses. Some of these publications contain accurate and reliable content about cultures while others are of a lesser quality. **Transcultural Concepts in Nursing Care** provides sound, credible and important content and learning experiences to guide nursing students, faculty, and clinical staff who are beginning to study and practice transcultural nursing. Among the several distinctive features in this book is an emphasis on the concepts of culture, health, and nursing in clinical and community contexts. The authors demonstrate how these concepts and related principles can be used to provide culturally congruent and responsible care, which is the ultimate goal of transcultural nursing. Still another important feature of this book is the emphasis on transcultural nursing throughout the life cycle, with attention to ethical issues, nutrition, and religious needs of clients in diverse health care systems.

Most encouragingly, the authors draw upon foundational and early knowledge, established in the first transcultural nursing text, *Nursing and Anthropology* (Leininger, 1970) and *Transcultural Nursing: Concepts, Theory, and Practice* (Leininger, 1978), along with current substantive articles in the Journal of Transcultural Nursing (1984 to present). Accordingly, this book contains many rich sources to study and understand both early and current transcultural nursing.

As the 21st Century approaches, nursing must become transculturally based and practiced to care for the growing number of immigrants and others from many diverse cultures in the world. There are great opportunities today for students to express their transcultural insights in creative and rewarding ways. This book is an important stepping stone toward this pathway. The third edition of **Transcultural Concepts in Nursing Care** offers nursing students valuable information, focussing on the clinical application of cultural and health concepts and principles. The authors are to be applauded for their seminal work in disseminating transcultural nursing knowledge in meaningful and creative ways.

Madeline M. Leininger, Ph.D., L.H.D., D.S., C.T.N., F.A.A.N., R.N.
Founder and Leader of Transcultural Nursing and Human Care Theory and Research
Professor Emeritus of Nursing
Wayne State University and University of Nebraska
Transcultural Global Nursing Consultant
Residing in Omaha, Nebraska

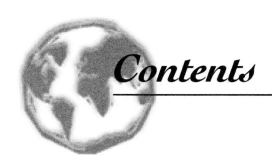

Contents

One

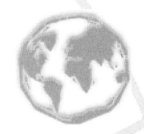

Transcultural Nursing: Theoretical Perspectives

Chapter 1

Theoretical Foundations of Transcultural Nursing

Margaret M. Andrews

KEY TERMS

Culture
Transcultural nursing
Anthropology
Population groups
Culture-specific nursing care
Culture-universal nursing care
Ethnocentrism

Cultural imposition
Culturally competent nursing care
Culturally congruent care
Subculture
Ethnic group
Panethnic group

Ethnic minority
Diversity
Population trends
Paradigm
Nursing paradigm
Nursing theories

OBJECTIVES

1. Critically analyze the need for transcultural nursing in contemporary society.
2. Examine the historical origins of transcultural nursing with special emphasis on its roots in anthropology.
3. Analyze the complex integration of knowledge, attitudes, and skills needed for cultural competence.
4. Explore population trends for cultural groups in the U.S. and Canada.
5. Critically analyze prevailing nursing paradigms and nursing theories from a transcultural nursing perspective.
6. Identify resources available in transcultural nursing and health care.

The first record of the term *culture* as it is used today is credited to Sir Edward Tylor, a British anthropologist who wrote in 1871 that culture refers to the complex whole including knowledge, belief, art, morals, law, custom, and any other capabilities and habits acquired by people as members of society. According to Mead (1955), culture refers "not only to the arts and sciences, religions and philosophies, to which the world culture has historically applied, but also the system of technology, the political practices, the small intimate habits of daily life, such as the ways of preparing or eating food, or of hushing a child to sleep. . . ." p. 5. Culture represents a way of perceiving, behaving, and evaluating the world. It provides a blueprint or guide for determining people's values, beliefs, and practices, including those pertaining to health and illness.

The term *transcultural nursing* is sometimes used interchangeably with *cross cultural, intercultural,* or *multicultural* nursing. In analyzing the Latin derivations of the prefixes associated with these terms, you will notice that *trans-* means *across, inter-* means *between,* and *multi-* means *many.* Given these derivations, it is understandable that various words have been used with similar connotative meaning. Some have used the term *ethnic nursing care* (Orque, Bloch, & Monrroy, 1983) or referred to caring for *people of color* (Branch & Paxton, 1976).

We have chosen to use *transcultural nursing* in this book in recognition of the historical and theoretical contributions of Dr. Madeleine M. Leininger, a nurse-anthropologist who in the mid-1950s envisioned transcultural nursing as a formal area of study and practice for nurses and coined the term *transcultural nursing* (Leininger, 1995). In her classic work, *Nursing and Anthropology: Two Worlds to Blend,* Dr. Leininger notes that "the fields of anthropology and nursing must be interdigitated so that each field will profit from the contribution of the other. . . . It is apparent that if these two fields were sharing their special knowledge and experiences, both would undoubtedly see new pathways in thinking and research" (Leininger, 1970, p. x).

As the name implies, transcultural nursing goes across cultural boundaries seeking to find the essence of nursing. Transcultural nursing is the blending of nursing and anthropology in both theory and practice. Recognizing that nursing is an art and a science, transcultural nursing enables us to view our profession from a cultural perspective. Transcultural nursing is not just for immigrants, people of color, or members of the federally defined panethnic minority groups.

Transcultural nursing is a specialty within nursing focused on the comparative study and analysis of different cultures and subcultures. These groups are examined with respect to their caring behavior, nursing care, and health-illness values, beliefs, and patterns of behavior. The goal of transcultural nursing is to develop a scientific and humanistic body of knowledge in order to provide *culture-specific* and *culture-universal* nursing care practices. *Culture-specific* refers to particular values, beliefs, and patterning of behavior that tend to be special or unique to a group and which do not tend to be shared with members of other cultures. *Culture-universal* refers to the commonly shared values, norms of behavior, and life patterns that are similarly held among cultures about human behavior and lifestyles (Leininger, 1978, 1995).

Transcultural nursing requires sophisticated assessment and analytic skills and the ability to plan, design, implement and evaluate nursing care for individuals, families, groups, and communities representing various cultures. You must also be able to apply knowledge related to the culture of organizations, institutions, and agencies, especially those concerned with health and nursing.

Why is Transcultural Nursing Needed?

Anthropologists tell us that every human being is *ethnocentric,* which means that we subconsciously tend to view other people by using our own group or our own customs as the standard for all judgments. Although we consider our own way of life to be natural and good, we subconsciously tend to view others' ways as inferior to our own. As a professional nurse, you will need to be aware of your ethnocentric tendencies and develop strategies for avoiding *cultural imposition,* i.e., imposing on your patients and clients your own cultural beliefs and practices while disregarding or trivializing theirs.

Lack of cultural competence by health care providers wastes millions of dollars annually and sometimes results in misdiagnoses, often with tragic and dangerous consequences. In extreme cases, health care providers' ethnocentrism and cultural imposition have resulted in the institutionalization of people from diverse cultures who have been incorrectly diagnosed with schizophrenia and other mental disorders, failure to provide adequate pain relief due to a lack of understanding about the cultural expression of discomfort, the arrest of parents for child abuse because culturally based childrearing practices were poorly understood, and many other adverse consequences (Andrews, 1992).

Transcultural nursing is needed today more than ever because of the growing *diversity* that characterizes our national and global populations. In its broadest sense, *diversity* refers to differences in race, ethnicity, national origin, religion, age, gender, sexual orientation, ability/disability, social and economic status or class, education, and related attributes of groups of people in society. Throughout this book, we will examine various types of diversity, but we also will explore the universal attributes that we have in common with other members of the human race, e.g., the need for food, sleep, shelter, safety, human interaction and so forth. Let us begin our discussion by examining some key developments in transcultural nursing from a historical perspective.

History of Transcultural Nursing

In the 1950s, Dr. Madeleine M. Leininger noted cultural differences between patients and nurses when working with emotionally disturbed children. This clinical experience led her to study cultural differences in the perceptions of care in 1954, and in 1965 she earned a doctorate in cultural anthropology from the University of Washington (Reynolds & Leininger, 1993; Leininger, 1995). Leininger recognized that one of anthropology's most important contributions to nursing was the realization that health and illness states are strongly influenced by culture. See Table 1-1 for a summary of four decades of contributions to the development of transcultural nursing by Dr. Madeleine Leininger.

Transcultural Perspectives on Conceptual Frameworks and Theories

In order to help develop, test, and organize the emerging body of knowledge in transcultural nursing, it is necessary to have a specific conceptual framework from which various theoretical statements can emerge. Leininger's Sunrise model (Figure 1-1) is based on the concept of cultural care and presents three major nursing modalities that guide nursing judgments and activities to provide *culturally congruent care,* that is, care that is beneficial and meaningful to the people being served.

Leininger's theory of culture care diversity and universality focuses on describing, explaining, and predicting nursing similarities and differences focused primarily on human care and caring in human cultures. Leininger uses world view, social structure, language, ethnohistory, environmental context, and the generic (folk) and professional

TABLE 1-1
Contributions of Madeleine Leininger to the Development of Transcultural Nursing

Date	Achievement and Contribution
1954	Dr. Madeleine Leininger noticed and studied the cultural differences in the perception of care
1965	Leininger earned a doctorate in cultural anthropology [U of Washington]
1965–69	Leininger offered first courses and telelectures offered in transcultural nursing [U of Colorado School of Nursing]
	Established first PhD nurse–scientist program combining anthropology and nursing [U Colo School of Nursing]
1973	First Academic Department in Transcultural Nursing Established [U of Washington School of Nursing]
1974	*Transcultural Nursing Society* established as the official organization of transcultural nursing
1978	First Advanced Degree Programs [Master's and Doctoral] established [U of Utah School of Nursing]
1988	*Transcultural Nursing Society*–initiated certification examinations: Certified Transcultural Nurse [CTN]
1989	*Journal of Transcultural Nursing* [JTN] first published as official publication of the Transcultural Nursing Society; Dr. Madeleine Leininger is founding editor. The goal of the JTN is to disseminate transcultural ideas, theories, research findings, and/or practice experiences.
1991	Dr. Leininger published **Culture Care Diversity and Universality: A Theory of Nursing** in which she outlines her theory [Culture Care Diversity and Universality and the Sunrise Model] and its research applications

systems to provide a comprehensive and holistic view of influences in culture care and well-being. The three modes of nursing decisions and actions—culture care preservation and/or maintenance, culture care accommodation and/or negotiation, and culture care repatterning and/or restructuring—are presented to demonstrate ways to provide culturally congruent nursing care (Leininger, 1991, 1995). Among the strengths of Leininger's theory is its flexibility for use with individuals, families, groups, communities, and institutions in diverse health systems. Leininger's Sunrise Model depicts components of the theory of cultural care diversity and universality, and provides a visual schematic representation of the key components of the theory and the interrelationships among the parts of the theory. As the world of nursing and health care has become increasingly multicultural, the theory's relevance has increased as well.

Although Leininger's Sunrise Model and her theory of Culture Care Diversity and Universality are the best known, other nurses have made significant contributions to advancing our knowledge of transcultural nursing and concepts related to it. You might find it useful to compare and contrast Leininger's work with Purnell's Model for Cultural Competence (Purnell & Paulanka, 1998), Spector's (1996) Model of Heritage Consistency, and Giger and Davidhizar's Transcultural Assessment Model (Giger & Davidhizar, 1995). Brink (1990) has provided a book of readings on transcul-

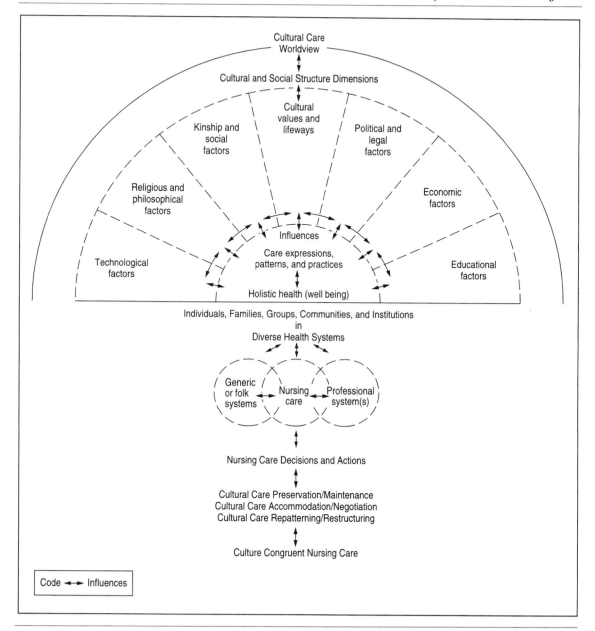

FIGURE 1-1. Leininger's sunrise model to depict theory of cultural care diversity and universality. (Leininger, M. M. [1991]. Culture Care Diversity and Universality: A Theory of Nursing [p. 43]. New York: National League for Nursing Press. Reprinted by permission.)

tural nursing. Kavanagh and Kennedy (1992) have contributed significantly to our knowledge of cultural diversity and have suggested strategies for health care professionals in promoting diversity. The relevance of anthropology to nursing practice has been noted extensively in the literature (DeSantis, 1994; Dougherty & Tripp-Reimer, 1985; Henderson & Primeaux, 1981; Lipson & Bauwens, 1988; McKenna, 1984; Omeri & Cameron-Traub, 1996; Osborne, 1969; Spector, 1996). Recognizing that *clinical practice* is an integral component of professional and technical nursing, in Chapter 2 we have presented a conceptual framework for transcultural nursing that is intended to guide your application of transcultural concepts in *clinical practice*. The *Andrews/Boyle Transcultural Nursing Assessment Guide* in Appendix A has been developed as a companion instrument to assist you in gathering culturally relevant health assessment data.

Cultural Competence

Some nurses use the term *cultural competence* when referring to the complex integration of knowledge, attitudes, and skills that enhance cross-cultural communication and appropriate/effective interactions with others (American Academy of Nursing, 1992, 1993). Cultural competence also has been defined as a process, as opposed to an end point, in which the nurse continuously strives to effectively work within the cultural context of an individual, family, or community from a diverse cultural background (Campinha-Bacote, 1995; Campinha-Bacote, et al., 1996). Campinha-Bacote (1991, 1995) identifies four components to developing cultural competence: cultural awareness, cultural knowledge, cultural skill, and cultural encounter.

Although strategies for developing cultural competence, or perhaps more accurately cultural competenc*ies,* will be integrated throughout the book, it should be noted that the term is problematic. *Competence* is derived from the Latin root, *competere,* meaning to fit or to be suitable. The nursing behaviors or actions needed for cultural competence are often stated in vague terms that are subject to multiple interpretations. Furthermore, if cultural competence is accepted as the goal, does that mean you are providing *incompetent* care every time you fail in effective cross-cultural communication or overlook a client's subtle cultural cues? Because you may encounter clients from literally hundreds of different cultures in your professional career and those of mixed cultural heritage, it is virtually impossible to know about the culturally based, health-related beliefs and practices of them all. It is, however, possible to master the knowledge and skills associated with cultural assessment and learn about *some* of the cultural dimensions of care for clients representing the groups most frequently encountered. In-depth knowledge of several cultures is often a reasonable goal if you are living in a large urban center characterized by a high degree of diversity.

The development of cultural competencies requires learning in the affective (attitudes, values, feelings, beliefs), cognitive or intellectual, and psychomotor or behavioral domains and assumes your skill in critical thinking. The affective or attitudinal aspects of providing culturally competent care are difficult to learn because they require that you engage in a cultural self-assessment and overcome your ethnocentric tendencies You also must struggle against cultural stereotypes that perpetuate prejudice and discrimination against members of certain groups.

We will examine culture values, cultural self-assessment, and specific areas in which knowledge about one's own and others' cultural values, beliefs, attitudes, and practices affect health, illness, and health-seeking behaviors of individuals, families, groups, and communities in diverse health care systems. Some of the cultural competencies may be useful when you practice, teach, research, or administer in multicultural settings (Andrews, 1995b; Andrews & Boyle, 1997; McFarland, 1996). When appropriate, the psychomotor or behavioral skills (see Box 1-1) necessary to provide culturally competent care will be presented. It should be noted that the mastery of some skills, such as the assessment of cyanosis in people with darkly pigmented skin, may be critical for a patient's survival. Other skills may be helpful in promoting hygiene or comfort, but do not have such dire consequences.

Box 1-1 *Selected Examples of Psychomotor Skills Useful in Transcultural Nursing*

Assessment

- Techniques for assessing biocultural variations in health and illness, e.g., assessing cyanosis, jaundice, anemia and related clinical manifestations of disease in darkly pigmented clients; differentiating between mongolians spots and ecchymoses (bruises).
- Measurement of head circumference and fontanelles in infants using techniques not in violation of taboos for selected cultural groups
- Growth and development monitoring for children of Asian heritage, using culturally appropriate growth grids
- Cultural modification of the Denver II and other developmental tests used for children
- Conducting culturally appropriate obstetric and gynecologic examinations of women from various cultural backgrounds

Communication

- Speaking and writing the language(s) used by clients
- Using alternative methods of communicating with non-English speaking clients and families when no interpreter is available (e.g., pantomime)

Hygiene

- Skin care for clients of various racial/ethnic backgrounds
- Hair care for clients of various ethnic/racial backgrounds, e.g., care of African American hair

Activities of Daily Living

- Assisting Chinese American clients to regain use of chopsticks as part of rehabilitation regimen following a stroke
- Assisting paralyzed Amish client with dressing when buttons and pins are used
- Assisting West African client who uses "chewing stick" with oral hygiene

Religion

- Emergency baptism and anointing of the sick for Catholics
- Care before and after ritual circumcision by *mohel* (performed 8 days after the birth of a male Jewish infant)

Population Groups

Let us examine some key terms used to describe population groups. *Subculture* refers to a large group of people who, although members of a larger cultural group (or in transition from one cultural identification to another), have shared characteristics that are not common to all members of the larger cultural group and that enable them to be thought of as a subgroup with distinct traits. Subcultures can be categorized by geographic region, religion, age, gender, social class, political party, ethnic, racial or cultural identify, occupational role, or isolation from the dominant society by choice, discrimination, or locale. Subcultural groups are distinguished from one another and from the dominant culture by such characteristics as speech patterns, dress, gestures, etiquette, forms of worship, foods, eating habits, and lifestyles.

An *ethnic group* refers to people within a larger social system whose members have common ancestral, racial, physical or national characteristics and who share cultural symbols such as language, lifestyle, religion, and other characteristics that are not fully understood or shared by outsiders. The term *minority* or *ethnic minority* refers to a group of people who, because of physical or cultural characteristics, receive different and unequal treatment from others in the society. Minority group members frequently see themselves as recipients of collective discrimination. It should be noted that the term *minority* is considered offensive to some as it connotes inferiority and marginalization.

Panethnic Population Groups

In the U.S., there are five *panethnic* population groups that are federally defined and recognized: white, black, Hispanic, Asian/Pacific Islander and American Indian/Alaska Native. Currently, in North America whites are referred to as the *majority,* whereas the others are called *ethnic minorities.* Data about each of these groups are gathered every 10 years by the U.S. Bureau of the Census, in years ending with zero—1980, 1990, 2000, 2010, and so forth.

Historically, the federal panethnic classification was initiated so that demographic data about traditionally under-represented populations could be gathered in a systematic manner. Among the rationale for establishing this panethnic population classification was that group-specific statistical information could be systematically gathered and used to help government officials make equitable decisions about public policies and allocation of resources for these five population groups. The use of panethnic population groups has gained widespread acceptance and has been embraced by many people as a convenient way to refer to the hundreds of cultures and subcultures in the U.S.

The creation of these five panethnic groups has had a tremendous influence on our thinking about ethnic groups and has affected the health care services people in certain population categories receive (Andrews, 1995b). In addition to establishing specific ethnic minority groups, the unique characteristics of each group's culture and subculture have become hopelessly enmeshed with others in the same category. One serious disadvantage of the use of panethnic groups is that each panethnic group is treated homogeneously and seldom is consideration given to the myriad health-related beliefs and practices that exist within each group. For example, there are hundreds of cultures and subcultures that are subsumed under the broad category known as *whites*, i.e., those whose origins traditionally are traced to Europe. Those of Italian, Irish, German, or Polish (for example) ancestry are categorized in the same group despite vast differences. Similarly, there may be no recognition given to the differences among the dozens of cultures representing those who identify themselves as *Hispanic* or *Latino/a*, a group that includes Spanish-speaking individuals from Spain, Central America and South America. *Blacks* may trace their ancestry to literally thousands of different African tribes on a vast continent, or in more recent history, to Central or South America. The *Asian/Pacific Islander* panethnic group includes people from more than 60 countries and Native Hawaiians from dozens of subcultural groups. Although there are more than 550 *American Indian* and *Alaska Native* groups, all are treated homogeneously with the federal panethnic classification system despite significant inter-tribal differences.

Developing Sensitivity to Differences Within a Panethnic Group

Rather than embracing the prevailing panethnic classification system, you should ask clients and patients, "With what cultural group or groups do you identify?" Listen attentively to the response and use the same language they do. You are encouraged to be as specific as you can. Rather than calling a person American Indian, for example, identify the *specific tribe* with which the individual identifies. Why is this important? Let us consider the manner in which diabetes mellitus is reported. With 55 percent of the population over age 35 being affected, the Pima Indians of Arizona have the highest non–insulin-dependent diabetes mellitus prevalence rates in the world (Office of Minority Health, 1995). Yet when diabetes rates for all American Indians/Alaska Natives are reported for panethnic category, the prevalence is reported at 20.5 percent (Indian Health Service, 1996). Thus, generalization of data about diabetes among the Pima Indians to all American Indians would be inaccurate (Andrews & Krouse, 1995).

Population Trends

The current population statistics for selected U.S. and Canadian cultural groups are summarized in Table 1-2. Cultural diversity in North America continues to increase. Demographers project that by the year 2080, 51.1 percent of the total U.S. population will be comprised of members of the federal panethnic minority groups: Hispanics, 23.4 percent; blacks, 14.7 percent; Asians and others, 12 percent (U.S. Bureau of the Census, 1990). Table 1-3 summarizes how the U.S. racial and ethnic mix will look in the next three decades.

The total U.S. population is now close to 269 million. By 2020, the total population is expected to reach 323 million, 60 percent of that increase the result of more births than deaths and 40 percent from immigration. According to the U.S. Immigration and Naturalization Service (1997), immigrants and their children will account for close to one half of the growth in the U.S. population. By 2005 the Hispanic population will be the largest of the panethnic minority groups, and by 2025 their number will double. Two-thirds of all Hispanics will be immigrants or children of immigrants. The place of birth for immigrants to the U.S. (Table 1-4) and Canada (Table 1-5) are identified in order of prevalence.

TABLE 1-2
Selected U.S. and Canadian Populations by Cultural Group

Cultural Group	United States	Canada
Amish	160,000	N/A
Arab	3,000,000	144,050
Black	33,000,000	224,620
Brazilian	3,000,000	2,525
Chinese	1,500,000	586,645
Cuban	860,000	660
Dutch	6,227,000	358,180
Egyptian	1,000,000	18,950
English	32,652,000	3,958,405
Filipino	1,450,000	157,250
French	10,321,000	6,129,680
German	57,946,000	911,560
Greek	1,400,000	151,150
Haitian	365,000	22,805
Hungarian	1,582,000	100,725
India	570,000	324,840
Iranian	1,000,000	38,915
Irish	38,736,000	725,660
Italian	14,665,000	750,055
Japanese	1,004,645	48,595
Korean	626,000	44,095
Mexican	11,587,000	8,015
North American Indian	4,300,000	365,375
Polish	9,366,000	272,810
Portugese	1,153,000	246,890
Puerto Rican	2,400,000	N/A
Russian	2,953,000	N/A
Scottish	5,394,000	893,125
Turkish	85,000	8,525
Ukranian	741,000	406,645

Table created, in part, using data from the following sources:
Statistical Abstract of the United States 1996. Washington, D.C.: U.S.
  Government Printing Office.

Statistics Canada. (1997). Catalogue no. 93-315.

Multiple Nursing Paradigms from a Transcultural Perspective

A *paradigm*, like any general perspective, is a way of viewing the world and the phenomena in it. A paradigm includes the assumptions, premises, and interrelationships that hold together a prevailing interpretation of reality. Although paradigms may shift, they usually are slow to change and do so only if and when their explanatory power is exhausted. In some instances, the nursing care of clients from culturally

TABLE 1-3

U.S. Racial and Ethnic Population Projections for the 21st Century

	White	Black	Hispanic	Asian/Pacific Islander	Native American
1998	72.9%	12.1%	10.7%	3.5%	0.7%
2005	69.9%	12.4%	12.6%	4.4%	0.8%
2010	68.0%	12.6%	13.8%	4.8%	0.8%
2015	66.1%	12.7%	15.1%	5.3%	0.8%
2020	64.3%	12.9%	16.3%	5.7%	0.8%
2030	60.5%	13.1%	18.9%	6.6%	0.8%

Source: U.S. Bureau of the Census (1997). *Current Population Reports.* P25-1130. Washington, D.C.: U.S. government Printing Office.

diverse backgrounds fails to "fit" or be congruent with the prevailing nursing paradigms. Metaphors such as a *spider web*, *salad bowl*, *mosaic* or a multicolored *woven rug* can be used to demonstrate the intricate and complex interweaving of the threads that together comprise a person's culture. The process used by the spider or weaver is a dynamic one that requires a constant revisiting of the steps in the problem-solving or nursing process to assess, diagnose, plan, intervene and evaluate clients' care. For example, in considering the sociocultural dimensions of nursing care, you may find yourself evaluating the effectiveness of the interventions administered by a highly skilled folk healer before planning or implementing nursing interventions, which are

TABLE 1-4

Highest Ranking Countries of Birth of U.S. Foreign-born Population, 1995

Country	Number
Mexico	6,719,000
Philippines	1,200,000
China/Taiwan	816,000
Cuba	797,000
Canada	695,000
El Salvador	650,000
Great Britain	617,000
Germany	598,000
Poland	538,000
Jamaica	531,000
Dominican Republic	509,000

Table based on data from Bureau of the Census. U.S. Department of Commerce. 1994.

TABLE 1-5
Canadian Immigrant Population by Place of Birth

	Population	Percent Migrated Before 1961
All places of birth	4,342,900	100
United Kingdom	717,700	26.5
Southern Europe	711,600	20.7
Western Europe	431,500	21.4
Eastern Europe	420,500	17.7
Eastern Asia	377,200	1.8
South East Asia	312,000	0.2
United States	249,100	5.0
Caribbean & Bermuda	232,500	0.7
Southern Asia	228,800	0.4
Africa	166,200	0.5
South America	150,600	0.4
Western Asia and Middle East	146,800	0.4
Other Norther European	83,400	3.8
Central America	68,800	0.2
Oceania and other countries	46,300	0.5

Table based on data from *Statistics Canada* (1997). Catalogue no. 93-316.

usually biomedical and Western in nature. Thus, evaluation precedes the other steps of the nursing process and necessitates that this be reordered.

As Leininger (1995) notes, the interconnections among the cultural and social structure dimensions—cultural values and lifeways, kinship, and social, religious, philosophical, technological, political, legal, economic, educational, historical, environmental, and language factors—are embedded and interwoven in such an intricate manner that it is often impossible to sort or separate them from one another. Similarly, all these factors are integral to transcultural nursing care—whether referring to the process by which information is gathered or its content.

Critical Analysis of Transcultural Nursing

Transcultural nursing has been criticized for its definitional, theoretical, and practical limitations. Let us begin by examining the criticism that transcultural nursing contains ambiguous terminology and lacks clarity in describing key concepts. For example, nurses have struggled to achieve clarity in concepts such as *cultural awareness, cultural sensitivity, cultural competence,* and *cultural congruence* (American Academy of Nursing, 1992, 1993; Andrews & Boyle, 1997; Campinha-Bacote, 1995, Campinha-Bacote, et al. 1996; Talabere, 1996). In a review of the nursing literature, Habayeb (1995) examined eight themes related to *cultural diversity:* immigrant status, noncompliant patient behavior, different population susceptibility to disease, differences among population groups, demographic changes, urban and rural contexts, workforce diversity, and methodological issues faced when conducting research on individuals from diverse backgrounds. Color, religion, and geographic location are most often used to narrowly define culture and highlight cultural diversity, which is often portrayed as a minority/majority issue. Discrepancies in definition arise when you fail to recognize that every person has a cultural heritage. Talabere (1996) suggests that *cultural diversity* is itself an ethnocentric term because it focuses on how different the other person is *from me* rather than *how different I am* from the other. In using the term cultural diversity, the white panethnic group is frequently viewed as the norm against which the differences in everyone else (ethnocentrically referred to as *nonwhites*) are measured or compared.

According to Mulholland (1995), a fundamental limitation of transcultural nursing models is their inadequate theorization of power. The failure of nurses to confront power as a feature of their relations with each other, with those who employ them, and with their clients is closely related to their failure to recognize the relationship between knowledge and power. This constitutes a substantial limitation for the analysis of prejudice and discrimination. Although Leininger and other transcultural nurses address the need to consider the political, economic and social dimensions in their theoretical formulations, there is criticism that transcultural nursing has done too little to encourage nurses to be actively involved in setting political, economic and social policy agendas.

Culley (1996) criticizes transcultural nursing for failing to recognize the power relations that exist between groups. When clients from traditionally underrepresented groups fail to behave as you expect, the behavior is sometimes referred to as *noncompliant,* a term with a negative connotation that is sometimes used synonymously with different, deviant, abnormal or pathologic. Problems are thought to be generated by customs or traditions deemed by the nurse to be *inappropriate,* a judgment that may be the result of personal bias, lack of knowledge concerning the cultural context in which they are practiced, the nurse's inexperience, or other factors. As a result, complex sociocultural phenomena are often reduced to overgeneralized stereotypes. For example, some North American nurses are critical of the role of women in traditional African and Middle Eastern cultures. In concentrating on culturally determined gender issues, you may ignore or minimize the significance of power, inequality, and racism as embedded in structures or institutions, factors that fundamentally affect the health of cultural groups and their members' access to quality health care. The same criticism might be applied to nursing's failure to address other forms of bias, prejudice, discrimination and social injustice.

Finally, transcultural nursing has been criticized for embracing models based on the assumption that understanding one's own culture and the culture of others creates tolerance and respect for people from diverse backgrounds. It has become apparent that the mere awareness of one's own culture and that of others is insufficient for the alleviation and potential eradication of prejudice, bigotry, racial, ethnic or cultural conflicts, discrimination or ethnoviolence. Rather, nursing students, nurses, and other health care providers must have positive experiences with members of other cultures and learn to value genuinely the contributions all cultures make to our multicultural society.

In the remainder of this book, the authors will attempt to address these criticisms of transcultural nursing through our approach to topics. It should be noted, however, that many of the issues raised by critics have deeply rooted historical, socioeconomic, religious, cultural and political origins. Because the nursing profession is a microcosm of society, it mirrors the biases and prejudices found in the larger social order. It is unrealistic to expect that transcultural nursing can reverse all of the inequalities cited by the critics. It is realistic, however, to expect more definitional, conceptual, and theoretical clarity as transcultural nursing prepares for the 21st century. It also is realistic to expect nurses to become increasingly active in setting political, economic and social policy agendas at the local, state/provincial, national and international levels.

For example, you can empower yourself and your profession by running for elected offices; supporting candidates with health-related agendas congruent with your own; voting for candidates from diverse cultural backgrounds; using print, broadcast and electronic media to influence public opinion; and joining professional organizations or unions that employ professional lobbyists to represent them. You have the power to confront prejudice and discrimination by refusing to tolerate ethnic jokes and other expressions of prejudice in the health care or educational settings, using peer pressure to change culturally insensitive or offensive behaviors by others, and ensuring that medical and surgical procedures, health-related appointments, and schedules are congruent with the religious and cultural calendars of clients, staff, and students.

Nurse educators can examine admissions and recruitment policies, curricula, pedagogy, academic calendars, and teaching strategies from a transcultural nursing perspective. Nurse researchers need to ensure that there is diversity represented in the population studied, that appropriate translation and interpretation has been used for non-English speaking informants or subjects, and that research instruments are appropriate for use with diverse populations. Finally, nurses in key administrative positions can critically assess the organizational climate and culture for its encouragement of diversity, examine the organization's administrative hierarchy for the presence of diversity in leadership positions, evaluate its commitment to culturally sensitive and appropriate personnel policies, and foster an openness to different perspectives on leadership and management. The examples cited are intended to be illustrative, not exhaustive.

Transcultural Perspectives on Nursing Theories

More than a dozen nurse-scholars have developed conceptual models, theoretical frameworks or theories of nursing. Although we intend to communicate no value judgments concerning the nursing theories developed to date, Leininger's (1991, 1995) theory of culture care diversity and universality emphasizes the cultural dimensions of human care and caring.

Although it is beyond the scope of this chapter to review all the recognized nursing theories from a transcultural perspective, you are encouraged to evaluate critically the cultural relevance of a theory before using it with clients from culturally diverse backgrounds. Several nursing theories have been examined to see if they can contribute to culturally sensitive research-based theory building (Geissler & Morgan, 1997), including Roy's Adaptation Model (Morgan, 1997), Leininger's Theory of Cultural Care Diversity and Universality (Rosenbaum, 1997), Rogers' Science of Unitary

Human Beings (Hardin, 1997), King's Theory of Goal Attainment (Husting, 1997), and Watson's Theory of Human Caring (Eddins & Riley-Eddins, 1997). It is especially important to analyze the assumptions of the theory from a transcultural vantage point. For example, let us consider theoretical pespectives on self-care (Orem, 1980). As defined by Orem, *self-care* is "the practice of activities that individuals initiate and perform on their own behalf in maintaining life, health, and well-being" (Orem, 1980, p. 35). The concept of self-care with a central focus on the individual, self-control, and autonomy may be counter to the cultural beliefs, values, and norms found in some cultures, especially in non-Western cultures. As evident in Anglo-American and European cultures, the dominant Western values of individualism, autonomy, independence, self-reliance, self-control, self-regulation, and self-management may be the source of cultural conflict with non-Western cultures that have almost the opposite values. In many non-Western cultures, individuals promote and maintain the caring role of others reflecting values such as interdependence, interconnectedness, understanding, presence (being with), and responsibility for others. In contrast, the idea of self-care "deficits" or mobilizing clients to become self-sufficient, independent, or self-reliant is often an enigma because their world view and cultural values are different, especially if they are not acculturated to Western norms (Leininger, 1992). Furthermore, the consequences of promoting self-care among people who value group interdependence, cooperation, and responsibility for others need to be examined critically (cf., Lipson & Steiger, 1996). Leininger (1992) poses the question, what are the short- and long-term consequences of mobilizing people to be self-carers when their culture values "other-care" norms? (Leininger, 1992). Research Application 1-1 summarizes a theory-testing study using Orem's Self-Care Deficit Theory of Nursing with Mexican Americans.

Research Application 1-1

Testing Orem's Theory with Mexican Americans

Villarruel, A.M., & Denyes, M.J. (1997). **Testing Orem's theory with Mexican Americans.** *Image: Journal of Nursing Scholarship, 29(3)*, 283–288.

Using 10 theory-verification criteria for inductive methods of inquiry, the investigators examined an ethnographic study of Mexican Americans experiencing pain conceptualized within Orem's self-care deficit theory of nursing. The study sample consisted of 20 Mexican American key informants from 13 families. Primary data sources were focused observations and a series of ethnographic interviews. The study purposes, methods, selected findings, confirmability and credibility of study findings, and relevance to Orem's Theory were presented in the context of each of the ten theory-verification criteria.

Although the researchers identified some components of Orem's Theory as relevant for Mexican Americans, the findings revealed the need for clearer articulation of dependent-care agency (abilities to care for others) with self-care agency (abilities to care for self). The dynamic and highly interrelated nature of care of self and others evident in the findings suggest that a single "agency" construct would provide a more appropriate way of understanding and caring for Mexican Americans.

Clinical Application

Among the stated purposes of nursing theory is the notion that theory ought to guide clinical practice, for clients from *all* cultures. Because theory-testing research with diverse ethnic and racial populations has been limited, there has been little examination of assumptions, concepts and propositions as they relate to diverse populations. In this study the researchers identified some strengths of Orem's Theory with a Mexican American population experiencing pain, but they also discovered limitations which require modification of the theory for culture relevance. In other words, the theory had limitations when applied to the care of Mexican Americans and raised questions about its relevance for other cultural groups, necessitating further study. Although Orem's concepts and proposed relationships were adequate to guide the study, elements of the theory judged to be highly relevant to Mexican Americans were not well developed. These concepts included dependent care agency and its relationship to self-care agency. If nurses use Orem's Theory with clients from culturally diverse backgrounds, they should be aware that modifications may be needed if culture congruent or culturally competent care is to be provided. Alternatively, nurses may choose to use other theories (e.g., Leininger's Theory of Culture Care Diversity and Universality) that have been shown to be relevant when caring for clients from diverse cultures.

Professional Resources

There is a variety of organizations, professional publications, and electronic resources (Andrews, 1995a) that support the development of transcultural nursing and health. Table 1-6 provides some basic information on selected resources.

Appendix B provides the names, addresses, and phone numbers for selected professional organizations that are concerned with the cultural aspects of care or with the issues of nurses from particular cultural groups. It is possible to contact some of these groups electronically by e-mail or internet (visit www.ajn.org, then search for a listing of professional organizations with web sites).

TABLE 1-6
Selected Resources for Transcultural Nursing

Professional Resources	Description	Description and Purpose
Professional Organizations	Council on Nursing and Anthropology Association (CONAA) (1968)	Organization for nurse-anthropologists, transcultural nurses, and anthropologists Purpose: promotes interdisciplinary research exchange
	Transcultural Nursing Society (TNS) (1974)	Organization of transcultural nurses Purpose: to promote transcultural nursing knowledge and competencies globally through education, research, consultation, and clinical services
	Council on Cultural Diversity of the American Nurses' Association (1978)	ANA Council of transcultural nurses Purpose: to focus on diversity issues in clinical practice

TABLE 1-6 *(Continued)*

Professional Resources	Description	Description and Purpose
	International Association of Human Caring (1987)	Organization of qualitative researchers, some of whom are nurses Purpose: to explore the cultural similarities and differences in expressions of human care.
	Committee on Cultural diversity	Committee established by the American Academy of Nursing Purpose: to develop guidelines for 'culturally competent nursing'.
	**see Appendix B for information on additional groups	
Refereed Printed Materials on Transcultural Nursing and Health	Journal of Transcultural Nursing	Only publication focused on transcultural nursing theory, research methods, consultation, teaching and clinical community practices.
	Journal of Multicultural Nursing & Health (MNCNH)	Interdisciplinary; Addresses multi culturalism in nursing education and/or health.
	Journal of Cultural Diversity	Focuses on cultural diversity theory & principles from a variety of perspectives
	Association of Black Nursing Faculty Journal (ABNF)	Documents the distinct nature and health-care needs of the Black patient
	International Nursing Review International Journal of Nursing Studies	Both published by the International Council of Nurses
Nonrefereed Print Materials	Minority Nurse Newsletter	Examines minority issues affecting patient care and nursing education
	Closing the Gap (newsletter)	Published by the (federal) Office of Minority Health; focuses on federal interventions aimed at improving the health of panethnic groups
	IHS Primary Care Provider (newsletter)	Published by the (federal) Indian Health Service; free to nursing and medical students and health care providers.
Electronic Resources	Asian and Pacific Islander American Health forum (Institute for Global Communications) Web Site: http://www.apiahf.org/apiahf	Offers updates on HIV programs, rates of tobacco use, and developments in welfare and health
	American Journal of Nursing Web Site: htt://www.ajn.org	Enables nurses worldwide to electronically access experts in a variety of specialties, including transcultural nursing (http://www.ajn.org/ajnnet/nrsorgs/tcn)

Summary

In this introductory chapter, we have examined the historical origins of transcultural nursing as a blending of two fields, anthropology and nursing. Founded by the nurse-anthropologist Dr. Madeleine M. Leininger, transcultural nursing has provided a theoretical foundation to guide nurses in the provision of culturally congruent and competent care for individual clients and patients of all ages, families, groups, and communities. Transcultural nursing also enables nurses to examine the cultural dimensions of health and nursing organizations, institutions, and agencies. Leininger's theory of culture care diversity and universality and her sunrise model were introduced. After critically analyzing the prevailing nursing paradigm and transcultural nursing itself, the potential cultural contributions of selected conceptual models and nursing theories were examined. Finally, selected resources in transcultural nursing and health care were identified.

Review Questions

1. Conceived in the early 1950s by the nurse-anthropologist Dr. Madeleine M. Leininger, the term transcultural nursing was coined in 1970 with her seminal work titled, *Nursing and Anthropology: Two Worlds to Blend.* Define transcultural nursing in your own words.
2. Summarize the historical development of transcultural nursing during its four decades of development.
3. Review the limitations of transcultural nursing cited by critics. What can be done to address the criticisms?
4. Identify electronic and print resources in transcultural nursing and health.

Learning Activities to Promote Critical Thinking

1. Using a search engine such as *Yahoo* enter the keyword *alternative medicine.* Visit at least five web sites for *alternative medicine.*
   a. Briefly summarize the information you found at each web site.
   b. Identify the source of the information, i.e., what individual or group is responsible for maintaining the web site? How reliable is the source? How confident are you that the information is accurate and current?
   c. Critically evaluate the strengths and limitations of the information source and data available at each web site.
   d. What clinical relevance does the electronic information on alternative medicine have for you as a nurse?
2. Using the Cumulative Index to Nursing and Allied Health Literature (CINAHL), enter the words *transcultural nursing* and search for references cited during the past year. How many references are identified? What are the subcategories under which you can narrow your search? If you want information about a specific cultural, ethnic or minority group, what key words will help you to narrow the search? Consult a reference librarian for assistance if you need help.

References

American Academy of Nursing (1993). Promoting cultural competence in and through nursing education. Draft, Subpanel on Cultural Competence in Nursing Education, American Academy of Nursing: New York.

American Academy of Nursing (1992). AAN expert panel report: Culturally competent health care. *Nursing Outlook, 40,* 277–283.

Andrews, M. M. (1992). Cultural perspectives on nursing in the 21st century. *Journal of Professional Nursing, 8(1),* 1–9.

Andrews, M. M. (1995a). Guide to searching on-line for information on transcultural nursing and health. *Journal of Transcultural Nursing, 7(1),* 36–40.

Andrews, M. M. (1995b). Transcultural nursing: Transforming the curriculum. *Journal of Transcultural Nursing 6(2),* 4–9.

Andrews, M. M., & Boyle, J. S. (1997). Competence in transcultural nursing care. *American Journal of Nursing, 97(8),* 16AAA–16DDD.

Andrews, M. M., & Krouse, S. A. (1995). Research on excess deaths among American Indians and Alaska Natives: A critical review. *Journal of Cultural Diversity, 2(1),* 8–13.

Brink, P. J. (1990). *Transcultural Nursing: A Book of Readings.* Prospect Heights, IL: Waveland Press, Inc.

Branch, M. F., & Paxton, P. P. (Eds.). (1976). *Providing Safe Nursing Care for Ethnic People of Color.* New York: Appleton-Century-Crofts.

Campinha-Bacote, J. (1991). *The Process of Cultural Competence: A Cultural Competent Model of Care.* Wyoming, OH: Transcultural C.A.R.E. Associates.

Campinha-Bacote, J. (1995). Cultural competence: A critical factor in nursing research. In J. Campinha-Bacote. *Readings in Transcultural Health Care.* pp. 117–121.

Campinha-Bacote, J., Yahle, T., & Langenkamp, M. (1996). The challenge of cultural diversity for nurse educators. *The Journal of Continuing Education in Nursing, 27(2),* 59–64.

Culley, L. (1996). A critique of multiculturalism in health care: The challenge for nursing education. *Journal of Advanced Nursing, 23,* 564–570.

DeSantis, L. (1994). Making anthropology clinically relevant to nursing care. *Journal of Advanced Nursing, 20,* 707–715.

Dougherty, M. C., & Tripp-Reimer, T. (1985). The interface of nursing and anthropology. *Annual Review of Anthropology, 14,* 219–241.

Eddins, B. B., & Riley-Eddins, E. A. (1997). Watson's theory of human caring: The twentieth century and beyond. *Journal of Multicultural Nursing & Health 3(3),* 30–36.

Geissler, E., & Morgan, M. G. (1997). Editorial: Nursing theories and culture. *Journal of Multicultural Nursing & Health, 3(3),* 5.

Habayeb, G. L. (1995). Cultural diversity: A nursing concept not yet reliably defined. *Nursing Outlook, 43(5),* 224–227.

Hardin, S. R. (1997). Culture: A manifestation of pattern. *Journal of Multicultural Nursing & Health, 3(3),* 21–23.

Henderson, G., & Primeaux, M. (1981). *Transcultural Health Care.* Menlo Park, CA: Addison-Wesley Publishing Company.

Husting, P. M. (1997). A transcultural critique of Imogene King's theory of goal attainment. *Journal of Multicultural Nursing & Health, 3(3),* 15–20.

Kavanaugh, K., & Kennedy, P. (1992). *Promoting Cultural Diversity.* Newbury Park, NJ: Sage.

Leininger, M. (1970). *Nursing and Anthropology: Two Worlds to Blend.* New York: John Wiley & Sons.

Leininger, M. (1978). *Transcultural Nursing: Concepts, Theories and Practices.* New York: John Wiley & Sons.

Leininger, M. (1991). *Culture Care Diversity and Universality: A Theory of Nursing.* New York: National League for Nursing.

Leininger, M. (1992). Self-care ideology and cultural incongruities: Some critical issues. *Journal of Transcultural Nursing, 4(1),* 2–4.

Leininger, M. (1995). *Transcultural Nursing: Concepts, Theories, Research and Practices.* New York: McGraw-Hill, Inc.

Leininger, M. M. (1997). Future directions in transcultural nursing in the 21st century. *International Nursing Review, 44(1),* 19–23.

Lipson, J., & Bauwens, E. (1988). Uses of anthropology in nursing. *Practicing Anthropology, 10,* 4–5.

Lipson, J. G., & Steiger, N. J. (1996). *Self-care Nursing in a Multicultural Context.* Thousand Oaks, CA: Sage Publications.

Macgregor, F. C. (1967). Uncooperative patients: Some cultural interpretations. *American Journal of Nursing, 67,* 88–91.

McKenna, M. (1984). Anthropology and nursing—The interaction between two fields of inquiry. *Western Journal of Nursing Research, 6(4),* 423–431.

McFarland, M. R. (1996). A focus on the implementation of transcultural nursing practice. *Journal of Transcultural Nursing, 7(2),* 2.

Mead, M. (1955). *Cultural Patterns and Technical Change.* UNESCO, New York: A Mentor Book, The New American Library.

Morgan, M. G. (1997). The Roy adaptation model and multicultural nursing. *Journal of Multicultural Nursing & Health, 3(3),* 10–14.

Mulholland, J. (1995). Nursing humanism and transcultural theory: the "bracketing out" of reality. *Journal of Advanced Nursing, 22,* 442–449.

Office of Minority Health (1995, January). Wellness camp for Indian youth: Understanding diabetes. *Closing the Gap,* 2,5.

Omeri, A., & Cameron-Traub, E. (1996). *Transcultural Nursing in Multicultural Australia.* Deaken, Australian Capital Territory: Royal College of Nursing, Australia.

Orem, D. E. (1980). *Nursing: Concepts of Practice.* Second edition. New York: McGraw Hill Book Company.

Orque, M. S., Bloch, B., & Monrroy, L. S. (1983). *Ethnic Nursing Care.* St. Louis: C. V. Mosby.

Osborne, O. (1969). Anthropology and nursing: Some common traditions and interests. *Nursing Research, 18(3),* 251–255.

Purnell, L. D., & Paulanka, B. J. (1998). *Transcultural Health Care: A Culturally Competent Approach.* Philadelphia: F.A. Davis Company.

Reynolds, C. L., & Leininger, M. (1993). *Madeleine Leininger: Cultural Care Diversity and Universality Theory*. Newbury Park: Sage Publications.

Rosenbaum, J. N. (1997). Leininger's theory of cultural care diversity and universality: A transcultural critique. *Journal of Multicultural Nursing & Health, 3*(3), 24–29, 36.

Roessler, G. (1990). Transcultural nursing certification. *Journal of Transcultural Nursing, 1*, 59.

Spector, R. (1996). *Cultural Diversity in Health and Illness* (4th ed.) Stamford, CT: Appleton & Lange.

Talabere, L. R. (1996). Meeting the challenge of culture care in nursing: Diversity, sensitivity, and congruence. *Journal of Cultural Diversity, 3*(2), 53–61.

Tylor, E. B. (1871). *Primitive Culture* (Vols. 1 and 2.) London: Murray.

U.S. Bureau of the Census (1990). *General Population Characteristics*. Washington, D.C.: U.S. Government Printing Office.

U.S. Immigration and Naturalization Service (1997). *Statistical Abstracts of the United States 1996*. Washington, D.C.: U.S. Government Printing Office.

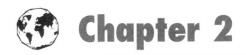
Chapter 2

Transcultural Nursing Care

Margaret M. Andrews
Paula Herberg

KEY TERMS

Cultural assessment
Culture values
Culture care meanings
Cultural lifeways
Communication
Cross-cultural communication
Technology
Language
Space
Distance

Time
Folk healer
Culture-bound syndrome
Biocultural variation
Mongolian spot
Keloids
Vitiligo
Cyanosis
Jaundice

Pallor
Erythema
Petechiae
Leukoedema
Oral hyperpigmentation
Ethnopharmacology
Traditional Chinese medicine
Clinical decision making
Cultural empathy

OBJECTIVES

1. Explore the process and content needed for the comprehensive cultural assessment of individuals, families, and groups from diverse cultures.
2. Conduct a cultural self-assessment to increase awareness of attitudes, values, beliefs, and practices that influence your ability to provide culturally competent and congruent nursing care.
3. Identify biocultural variations in health and illness for individuals, families, and groups from diverse cultures.
4. Explore cross-cultural communication as an integral component of transcultural nursing.
5. Use a conceptual model for transcultural nursing when assessing, planning, implementing and evaluating care for individuals, families, and groups from diverse cultures.
6. Critically examine the role of cultural empathy in transcultural nursing.

aving been introduced to the theoretical and historical foundations of transcultural nursing in Chapter 1, we will now examine the clinical use of transcultural nursing in the provision of culturally competent and congruent nursing care. Experienced transcultural nurses synthesize culturally relevant data about clients and apply their knowledge and skills when caring for people from various cultures. For the purpose of clarity, the components that comprise transcultural nursing care will be introduced as if they existed separately from each other. You are likely to find that in clinical nursing practice, the process may not follow the linear, sequential order presented in this chapter. The chapter will conclude with remarks about cultural empathy in nurse-client interactions and the evaluation of care from a transcultural perspective.

Cultural Assessment

Cultural or *culturologic nursing assessment* refers to a "systematic appraisal or examination of individuals, groups, and communities as to their cultural beliefs, values, and practices to determine explicit nursing needs and intervention practices within the cultural context of the people being evaluated" (Leininger, 1978, pp. 85–86). Because they deal with cultural values, belief systems, and lifeways, cultural assessments tend to be broad and comprehensive, although it is possible to focus on a smaller segment. Cultural assessment consists of both *process* and *content*. *Process* refers to your approach to the client, consideration of verbal and nonverbal communication, and the sequence/order in which data are gathered. The *content* of the cultural assessment consists of the actual data categories in which information about clients is gathered.

Although there are several cultural assessment instruments or tools available, **Appendix A** contains the **Andrews/Boyle Transcultural Nursing Assessment Guide**. The major categories in this guide include cultural affiliation(s), values orientation, cultural sanctions and restrictions, communication, health-related beliefs and practices, nutrition, socioeconomic considerations, organizations providing cultural support, education, religion, cultural aspects of disease incidence, biocultural variations and developmental considerations across the life span. You might find it useful to compare this assessment guide with Leininger's Acculturation Health Care Assessment Tool for Cultural Patterns in Traditional and Non-Traditional Lifeways (Leininger, 1991) and Bloch's Assessment Guide for Ethnic/Cultural Variation (Orque, Bloch, & Monrroy, 1983).

Cultural Values

Cultural values refer to the powerful, persistent, and directive forces that give meaning, order, and direction to the individual's, group's, family's, or community's actions, decisions, and lifeways, usually over a span of time (Leininger, 1995). Between cultures and even within one culture, values vary along a continuum. Many Asian, Islamic, and tribal societies make loyalty to the group their highest value. In these cultural groups, individual values are subservient to whatever is best for the group. In most parts of North America, however, individuality is emphasized. Individual rights are protected, sometimes even to the detriment of others or of the whole group. This stimulates individual creativity but weakens social stability.

The European American obsession for bodily cleanliness and the compulsion to eliminate body odors is reflected in a multimillion dollar business for the manufacturers of mouthwashes, deodorants, perfumes, aftershave lotions, douches and similar products. In other cultures, the natural odor of the body is valued, and little effort is made to disguise it. Ironically, some colognes and perfumes such as those with musk oil are marketed to U.S. and Canadian people for their more *natural* odor, which is alleged to give its wearer more sex appeal.

All cultures emphasize the importance of telling the truth and view deception as wrong. They differ widely, however, in their definitions of the terms *truth* and *deception*. One culture believes that truth is what corresponds most closely with reality regardless of the consequences. Another culture may hold a pragmatic view of truth as being that which brings the greatest benefit to the person or the group. Consider the implications of truth as a cultural value when deciding whether or not to inform a client about his or her impending death.

When interacting with clients from various cultural backgrounds, you must be aware of your own cultural values, attitudes, beliefs, and practices. To gain insight into the way you relate to various groups of people in society, describe your level of response to the groups identified in Box 2-1.

Box 2-1 *How Do You Relate to Various Groups of People in the Society?*

Described below are different levels of response you might have toward a person.

Levels of Response

1. *Greet:* I feel I can *greet* this person warmly and welcome him or her sincerely.
2. *Accept:* I feel I can honestly *accept* this person as he or she is and be comfortable enough to listen to his or her problems.
3. *Help:* I feel I would genuinely try to *help* this person with his or her problems as they might relate to or arise from the label-stereotype given to him or her.
4. *Background:* I feel I have the *background* of knowledge and/or experience to be able to help this person.
5. *Advocate:* I feel I could honestly be an *advocate* for this person.

The following is a list of individuals. Read down the list and place a checkmark next to anyone you would *not* "greet" or would hesitate to "greet." Then move to response level 2, "accept," and follow the same procedure. Try to respond honestly, not as you think might be socially or professionally desirable. Your answers are only for your personal use in clarifying your initial reactions to different people.

	Level of Response				
	1	2	3	4	5
Individual	Greet	Accept	Help	Background	Advocate
Ethnic/racial					
1. Haitian American	☐	☐	☐	☐	☐
6. Mexican American	☐	☐	☐	☐	☐
11. Native American	☐	☐	☐	☐	☐
16. Vietnamese American	☐	☐	☐	☐	☐
21. Black American	☐	☐	☐	☐	☐
26. White Anglo-Saxon	☐	☐	☐	☐	☐

(continued)

Box 2-1 *(Continued)*

Individual	1 Greet	2 Accept	3 Help	4 Background	5 Advocate
Social issues/problems					
2. Child abuser	☐	☐	☐	☐	☐
7. IV drug user	☐	☐	☐	☐	☐
12. Prostitute	☐	☐	☐	☐	☐
17. Gay/lesbian	☐	☐	☐	☐	☐
22. Unmarried expectant teenager	☐	☐	☐	☐	☐
27. Alcoholic	☐	☐	☐	☐	☐
Religious					
3. Jew	☐	☐	☐	☐	☐
8. Catholic	☐	☐	☐	☐	☐
13. Jehovah's Witness	☐	☐	☐	☐	☐
18. Atheist	☐	☐	☐	☐	☐
23. Protestant	☐	☐	☐	☐	☐
28. Amish person	☐	☐	☐	☐	☐
Physically/mentally handicapped					
4. Person with hemophilia	☐	☐	☐	☐	☐
9. Senile elderly person	☐	☐	☐	☐	☐
14. Cerebral palsied person	☐	☐	☐	☐	☐
19. Person with AIDS	☐	☐	☐	☐	☐
24. Amputee	☐	☐	☐	☐	☐
29. Person with cancer	☐	☐	☐	☐	☐
Political					
5. Neo-Nazi	☐	☐	☐	☐	☐
10. Teamster Union member	☐	☐	☐	☐	☐
15. ERA proponent	☐	☐	☐	☐	☐
20. Communist	☐	☐	☐	☐	☐
25. Ku Klux Klansman	☐	☐	☐	☐	☐
30. Nuclear armament proponent	☐	☐	☐	☐	☐

Reproduced with permission of the Association for the Care of Children's Health, 7910 Woodmont Avenue, Suite 300, Bethesda, MD 20814, from E. Randall-David (1989). *Strategies for Working with Culturally Diverse Communities and Clients*, pp. 7–9.

	Level of Response				
Individual	1 Greet	2 Accept	3 Help	4 Background	5 Advocate
1. Haitian	☐	☐	☐	☐	☐
2. Child abuser	☐	☐	☐	☐	☐
3. Jew	☐	☐	☐	☐	☐
4. Person with hemophilia	☐	☐	☐	☐	☐
5. Neo-Nazi	☐	☐	☐	☐	☐
6. Mexican American	☐	☐	☐	☐	☐
7. IV drug user	☐	☐	☐	☐	☐
8. Catholic	☐	☐	☐	☐	☐

Box 2-1 *(Continued)*

			Level of Response		
	1	2	3	4	5
Individual	Greet	Accept	Help	Background	Advocate
9. Senile, elderly person	☐	☐	☐	☐	☐
10. Teamster Union member	☐	☐	☐	☐	☐
11. Native American	☐	☐	☐	☐	☐
12. Prostitute	☐	☐	☐	☐	☐
13. Jehovah's Witness	☐	☐	☐	☐	☐
14. Cerebral palsied person	☐	☐	☐	☐	☐
15. ERA proponent	☐	☐	☐	☐	☐
16. Vietnamese American	☐	☐	☐	☐	☐
17. Gay/lesbian	☐	☐	☐	☐	☐
18. Atheist	☐	☐	☐	☐	☐
19. Person with AIDS	☐	☐	☐	☐	☐
20. Communist	☐	☐	☐	☐	☐
21. Black American	☐	☐	☐	☐	☐
22. Unmarried expectant teenager	☐	☐	☐	☐	☐
23. Protestant	☐	☐	☐	☐	☐
24. Amputee	☐	☐	☐	☐	☐
25. Ku Klux Klansman	☐	☐	☐	☐	☐
26. White Anglo-Saxon	☐	☐	☐	☐	☐
27. Alcoholic	☐	☐	☐	☐	☐
28. Amish person	☐	☐	☐	☐	☐
29. Person with cancer	☐	☐	☐	☐	☐
30. Nuclear armament proponent	☐	☐	☐	☐	☐

Scoring Guide: The previous activity may help you anticipate difficulty in working with some clients at various levels. The 30 types of individuals can be grouped into 5 categories: ethnic/racial, social issues/problems, religious, physically/mentally handicapped, and political. Transfer your checkmarks to the following form. If you have a concentration of checks within a specific category of individuals or at specific levels, this may indicate a conflict that could hinder you from rendering effective professional help.

Cultural Values and Cultural Care Meanings

Among the greatest challenges you face is providing care that is congruent with the client's values and care meanings. Cultural values and care meanings influence nurse-client interactions, provide useful information about the client's expectations of care, and influence the client's sense of appropriate sick role behaviors, choice of healers, views toward technology and other health-related beliefs and practices. Table 2-1 summarizes the human care expressions and patterns of cultures for selected groups that have been studied by transcultural nurse researchers.

TABLE 2-1
Cultural Values and Culture Care Meanings and Action Modes for Selected Groups

Cultural Values Are:	Culture Care Meanings and Action Modes Are:

Anglo American Culture (Mainly U.S. Middle and Upper Classes)

1. Individualism—focus on a self-reliant person	1. Stress alleviation by
2. Independence and freedom	—Physical means
3. Competition and achievement	—Emotional means
4. Materialism (things and money)	2. Personalized acts
5. Technology dependent	—Doing special things
6. Instant time and actions	—Giving individual attention
7. Youth and beauty	3. Self-reliance (individualism) by
8. Equal sex rights	—Reliance on self
9. Leisure time highly valued possible	—Reliance on self (self-care)
10. Reliance on scientific facts and numbers	—Becoming as independent as
11. Less respect for authority and the elderly	—Reliance on technology
12. Generosity in time of crisis	4. Health instruction
	—Teach us how "to do" this care for self
	—give us the "medical" facts

Mexican American Culture*

1. Extended family valued	1. Succorance (direct family aid)
2. Interdependence with kin and social activities	2. Involvement with extended family ("other care")
3. Patriarchal (machismo)	3. Filial love/loving
4. Exact time less valued	4. Respect for authority
5. High respect for authority and the elderly	5. Mother as care decision maker
6. Religion valued (many Roman Catholics)	6. Protective (external) male care
7. Native foods for well-being	7. Acceptance of God's will
8. Traditional folk-care healers for folk illnesses	8. Use of folk-care practices
9. Belief in hot-cold theory	9. Healing with foods
	10. Touching

Haitian American Culture**

1. Extended family as support system	1. Involve family for support (other care)
2. Religion—God's will must prevail	2. Respect
3. Reliance on folk foods and treatments	3. Trust
4. Belief in hot-cold theory	4. Succorance
5. Male decision maker and direct caregivers	5. Touching (body closeness)
6. Reliance on native language	6. Reassurance
	7. Spiritual healing
	8. Use of folk food, care rituals
	9. Avoid evil eye and witches
	10. Speak the language

African American Culture†

1. Extended family networks	1. Concern for my "brothers and sisters"
2. Religion valued (many are Baptists)	2. Being involved
3. Interdependence with "blacks"	3. Giving presence (physical)
4. Daily survival	4. Family support and "get togethers"
5. Technology valued, e.g., radio, car	5. Touching appropriately
6. Folk (soul) foods	6. Reliance on folk home remedies

TABLE 2-1 *(Continued)*

Cultural Values Are:	Culture Care Meanings and Action Modes Are:
7. Folk healing modes 8. Music and physical activities	7. Rely on "Jesus to save us" with prayers and songs

North-American Indian Culture‡

1. Harmony between land, people, and environment 2. Reciprocity with "Mother Earth" 3. Spiritual inspiration (spirit guidance) 4. Folk healers (shamans) (the circle and four directions) 5. Practice culture rituals and taboos 6. Rhythmicity of life with nature 7. Authority of tribal elders 8. Pride in cultural heritage and "nations" 9. Respect and value for children	1. Establishing harmony between people and environment with reciprocity 2. Actively listening 3. Using periods of silence ("Great Spirit" guidance) 4. Rhythmic timing (nature, land and people) in harmony 5. Respect for native folk healers, carers, and curers (use of circle) 6. Maintaining reciprocity (replenish what is taken from Mother Earth) 7. Preserving cultural rituals and taboos 8. Respect for elders and children

*These findings were from the author's transcultural nurse studies (1970, 1984) and other transcultural nurse studies in the United States during the past two decades.

**These data were from Haitians living in the United States during the past decade (1981–1991).

†These findings were from the author's study of two southern U.S. villages (1980–1981) and from a study of one large northern urban city (1982–1991) along with other studies by transcultural nurses.

‡These findings were collected by the author and other contributors in the United States and Canada during the past three decades. Cultural variations among all nations exist, and so these data are some general commonalities about values, care meanings, and actions.

From M. M. Leininger (1991). *Culture Care Diversity and Universality: A Theory of Nursing* (pp. 355–357). New York: National League for Nursing Press. Reprinted by permission.

Conceptual Model for Determining Cultural Influences on the Nurse-Client Interaction

Figure 2-1 identifies the cultural components of a conceptual model of the nurse-client interaction. Whenever you interact with clients in an environmental context (e.g., hospital, ambulatory care, home, community or other health care setting) , there is a complex web of interrelated factors that influence your relationship. Because each person is a cultural being, all nurse-client interactions are inherently transcultural. Both you and your clients are influenced by cultural identity, ethnohistory, cultural values, family, kinship and other social factors. Religious and spiritual beliefs, philosophical point of view, and moral and ethical perspectives also influence the nurse-client interaction.

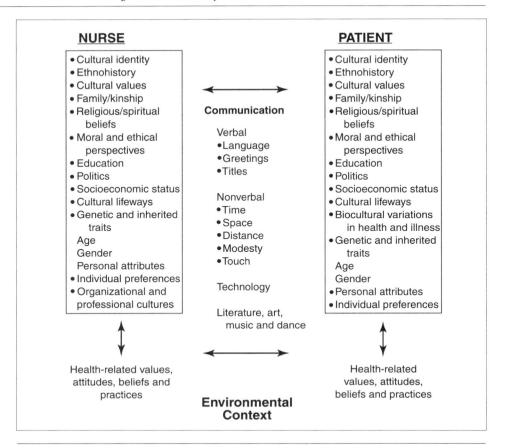

FIGURE 2-1.   Conceptual model for understanding cultural influences on nurse-patient interactions.

The learning style, informal learning and highest level of formal education achieved, and the type of schools (e.g., public, private, church-related) attended are factors in the interaction. The local, state/provincial, national and global politics must be considered as well as each person's past experience with political organizations. Those who migrated to the U.S. or Canada to escape violence in their homeland, Native Americans who have developed a mistrust for the government due to a long-standing history of broken treaties, and other groups who have been victimized by political forces bring their recollection of these experiences to the nurse-client interaction. In some instances, you may be perceived as a representative of the oppressor, particularly nurses affiliated with government agencies such as the U.S. Public Health Service, the military, state/provincial or county health departments or similar organizations. Undocumented immigrants and others residing in the U.S. or Canada without the legally mandated authorization may fear that you will report them to the immigration authorities.

The *cultural lifeways* (e.g., beliefs about dress, diet, and other activities of daily living), genetic and inherited traits (e.g., gender, race, age, and personal attributes such as height, size, personality), and individual preferences influence the nurse-client interaction. You are influenced by your professional culture and the organizational culture of the health care setting in which the nurse-client interaction occurs (e.g., hospital, nursing home, mental health center, community health agency, birthing center, and so forth). Although clients are affected by the organizational culture, it is usually in a manner different from that of the nurse, who is frequently the employee of the organization. For example, an African American client is affected by the mission, nursing philosophy, and staffing demographics of a hospital. If all of the professional staff and administrators are white, whereas the housekeeping and other auxiliary staff are African American, this influences the nurse-client interaction because the client may reason that African Americans are unwelcome as professional staff or patients. Throughout this book the influence of these factors on the health-related beliefs and practices of both the nurse and client will be examined.

Communication is an organized, patterned system of behavior that regulates and makes possible all nurse-client interactions. It is the exchange of messages and the creation of meaning. Because they are acquired simultaneously, communication and culture are integrally linked. In effective communication there is mutual understanding of the meaning attached to the messages. Barriers to communication include differences in language, worldview, and values.

Cross-Cultural Communication

To begin the discussion on cross-cultural communication, it is necessary to examine the ways in which people from various cultural backgrounds communicate with each other. In addition to oral and written communication, messages are conveyed nonverbally through gestures, body movements, posture, tone of voice, and facial expressions. Frequently overlooked is the context in which communication occurs. The *environmental context* imparts its own message, and is influenced by the setting, purposes of the communication, and perception of the nurse and client concerning time, space, distance, touch, modesty, and other factors. For example, let us imagine you know that a Mexican American patient is extremely anxious about having a mammogram. Following the procedure, you intend to send an empathetic, caring message by remarking, "It's all over, *Señora* Garcia." *Señora* Garcia bursts into tears because she believes she has been diagnosed with terminal breast cancer. Needless to say, communication between individuals having the same cultural background may be fraught with pitfalls. When you communicate with others from cultural backgrounds unlike your own and with those for whom English is a second language, the probability of miscommunication increases significantly. In promoting effective cross-cultural communication, you should avoid technical jargon, slang, colloquial expressions, abbreviations, and excessive use of medical terminology.

Lipson and Steiger (1996) suggest affective, cognitive and behavioral strategies for effective cross-cultural communication. In the affective domain, they suggest respect for, appreciation of, and comfort with cultural differences, enjoyment of learning through cultural exchange, ability to observe behavior without judging, awareness of one's own cultural values and biases, and belief in cultural relativity, i.e., there are many acceptable cultural ways.

In the cognitive domain, they emphasize knowledge about different cultures, ability to recognize when there is a cultural explanation for an interpersonal problem, understanding that meanings can differ for others, and understanding the sociopolitical system with respect to its treatment of minorities. In the behavioral domain (communication skills), they advocate flexibility in verbal and nonverbal communication style, ability to speak slowly and clearly without excessive slang, ability to encourage to others to express themselves, ability to communicate sincere interest and empathy, patience, and ability to observe and intervene when there is misunderstanding.

Communication with Family Members and Significant Others

Knowledge of a client's family and kinship structure helps you to ascertain the values, decision-making pattern, and overall communication within the household. It is necessary to identify those significant others whom clients perceive to be important in their care and who may be responsible for decision making that affects their health care. For example, for many clients, *familism*—which emphasizes interdependence over independence, affiliation over confrontation, and cooperation over competition—may dictate that important decisions affecting the client be made by the family, not the individual alone. When you work with clients from cultural groups that value cohesion, interdependence, and collectivism, you may perceive the family as being overly involved and usurping the autonomy of the client. Clients are likely to perceive the involvement with family as a source of mutual support, security and fulfillment.

The family is the basic social unit in which children are raised and learn culturally based values, beliefs, and practices about health and illnesses. The essence of *family* consists of living together as a unit. Relationships that may seem apparent sometimes warrant further exploration when the nurse interacts with clients from culturally diverse backgrounds. For example, most European Americans define siblings as two persons with either the same mother, the same father, the same mother and father, or the same adoptive parents. In some Asian cultures, a sibling relationship is defined as any infants breast-fed by the same woman. In other cultures, certain kinship patterns, such as maternal first cousins, are defined as sibling relationships. In some African cultures, anyone from the same village may be called brother or sister.

Members of some ethnoreligious groups (e.g., the Roman Catholics of Italian, Polish, Spanish, or Mexican descent), recognize relationships such as *godmother* or *godfather* in which an individual who is not the biologic parent promises to assist with the moral or spiritual development of an infant and agrees to care for the child in the event of parental death. The godparent makes these promises during the religious ceremony of baptism.

When communicating with the parent or parent surrogate of infants and children, it is important to identify the primary provider of care and the key decision maker who acts on behalf of the child. In some instances this person may not be the biologic parent. Among some Hispanic groups, for example, female members of the nuclear or extended family such as sisters and aunts are primary providers of care for infants and children. In some African American families, the grandmother may be the decision maker and primary caretaker of children. In many Asian cultures, it is the obligation and duty of the eldest son to assume primary responsibility for his aging parents and to make health care decisions for them. In order to provide culturally congruent care, you must be certain that you are effectively communicating with the appropriate decision maker(s).

When making health-related decisions, some members of culturally diverse backgrounds in which *lineal relationships* predominate may seek assistance from other members of the family. It is sometimes culturally expected that a relative (e.g., parent, grandparent, or elder brother) will make decisions about important health-related matters. If *collateral relationships* are valued, decisions about the client may be interrelated with the impact of illness on the entire family or group. For example, among the Amish, the entire community is affected by the illness of a member because the community pays for health care from a common fund, members join together to meet the needs of both the sick person and his or her family throughout the illness, and the roles of dozens of people in the community are likely to be affected by the illness of a single member. The *individual values orientation* concerning relationships is predominant among the dominant cultural majority in America. Although members of the nuclear family may participate to varying degrees, decision making about health and illness is often an individual matter.

Because initial impressions are so important in all human relationships, cross-cultural considerations concerning introductions warrant a few brief remarks. In order to ensure that a mutually respectful relationship is established, you should introduce yourself and indicate to the client how you prefer to be called, i.e., by first name, last name, and/or title. You should elicit the same information from the client because this enables you to address the person in a manner that is culturally appropriate. See Chapter 5 for further discussion of the use of titles and names for selected cultural groups.

Space, Distance, and Intimacy

The concepts of space and distance are significant in cross-cultural communication, with the perception of appropriate distance zones varying widely among cultural groups. Although there are individual variations in spatial requirements, people of the same culture tend to act in similar ways. For example, if you are of European American heritage, you may find yourself backing away from clients of Hispanic, East Indian, or Middle Eastern origins who seem to invade your personal space with annoying regularity. This behavior by the client is probably an attempt to bring you closer into the space that is comfortable to them. Although you may be uncomfortable with the close physical proximity of these clients, the clients are perplexed by *your* distancing behaviors and may perceive you as aloof and unfriendly.

Because individuals are usually not consciously aware of their personal space requirements, they frequently have difficulty understanding a different cultural pattern. For example, sitting in close proximity to another person may be perceived by one client as an expression of warmth and friendliness but by another as a threatening invasion of personal space. According to Watson (1980), Americans, Canadians, and British require the most personal space, whereas Latin American, Japanese, and Arabs need the least.

In the early 1960s Edward T. Hall pioneered the study of *proxemics*, which focuses on how people in various cultures relate to their physical space. Although there are intercultural variations, the intimate distance in interpersonal interactions ranges from 0 to 18 inches. At this distance, people experience visual detail and each other's smell, heat, and touch. Personal distance varies from 1.5 to 4 feet, the usual space within which communication between friends and acquaintances occurs. Nurses frequently interact with clients in the intimate or personal distance zones. Social distance refers to 4 to 12 feet, whereas anything greater than 12 is considered public distance (Hall, 1963).

Interactions between you and your client are influenced by the degree of intimacy desired—which may range from very formal interactions to close personal relationships. For example, some Asian American clients expect you and other health care providers to be authoritarian, directive, and detached. In seeking health care, some clients of Chinese decent may expect you to intuitively know what is wrong with them, and you may actually lose some credibility by asking a fairly standard interview question such as, "What brings you here?" The Asian American patient may be thinking, "Don't you know why I'm here? You're supposed to be the one with all the answers." Reserved interpersonal behavior characteristics of many Asian-Americans may leave you with the impression that the client agrees with or understands your explanation. Nodding or smiling by Asians may simply reflect their cultural value for interpersonal harmony, not agreement with what you have said. The emphasis on social harmony among Asian American clients may prevent the full expression of concerns or feelings.

In Thai culture there is a high value placed on *kreengcaj*, or awareness and anticipation of the feelings of others by kindness and avoidance of interpersonal conflict. You may distinguish between socially compliant client responses aimed at maintaining harmony and genuine concurrence by obtaining validation of assumptions. This may be accomplished by inviting the client to respond frankly to suggestions or by giving the client "permission" to disagree.

In contrast, Appalachian clients often have close family interaction patterns that lead them to expect close personal relationships with health care providers. The Appalachian client may evaluate your effectiveness on the basis of interpersonal skills rather than professional competencies. Some Appalachian clients may be uncomfortable with the impersonal, orientation of most health care institutions.

In cultures in which kissing is a form of greeting, you should determine how and where to kiss. Kissing in traditional Asian cultures is considered to be an intimate sexual act, not permissible in public, whereas kissing in most Western cultures has the meaning of friendship and is considered a form of social greeting.

Among some Hispanic groups such as Mexican Americans and Cuban Americans, *simpatia* and *personalismo* should be considered. *Simpatia* refers to the need for smooth or harmonious interpersonal relationships, characterized by courtesy, respect, and the absence of critical or confrontational behavior. The concept of *personalismo* emphasizes intimate, personal relationships. Those of Latin American or Mediterranean origins often expect a high degree of intimacy and may attempt to involve you in their family system by expecting you to participate in personal activities and social functions. These individuals may come to expect personal favors that extend beyond the scope of what you believe to be professional practice, and they may feel it is their privilege to contact you at home during any time of the day or night for care. If your cultural value system emphasizes a high level of personal privacy, you may choose to give clients the agency's phone number and address rather than disclose information about your personal residence.

Overcoming Communication Barriers

If you find yourself feeling uncomfortable because a client is asking too many questions, assuming a defensive posture, or otherwise experiencing discomfort, it might be appropriate to pause for a moment to examine the source of the conflict from a transcultural perspective. During illness, culturally acceptable *sick role behavior* may range from aggressive, demanding behavior to silent passivity. Researchers have found that complaining, demanding behavior during illness is often rewarded with attention among American Jewish and Italian groups. Because Asian and Native American patients are likely to be quiet and compliant during illness, they may not receive the attention they need. Children are socialized into culturally acceptable sick role behaviors at an early age.

Many Asian clients may provide you with the answers they think are expected, behavior consistent with the dominant cultural value for harmonious relationships with others. Thus you should attempt to phrase questions or statements in a neutral manner that avoids foreshadowing an expected response.

Nonverbal Communication

There are five types of nonverbal behaviors that convey information about the client: vocal cues, such as pitch, tone, and quality of voice, including moaning and groaning; action cues, such as posture, facial expression, and gestures; object cues, such as clothes, jewelry, and hair styles; use of personal and territorial space in interpersonal transactions and care of belongings; and touch, which involves the use of personal space and action (Lapierre & Padgett, 1991).

Unless you make an effort to understand the client's nonverbal behavior, you may overlook important information such as that which is conveyed by facial expressions, silence, eye contact, touch, and other body language. Communication patterns vary widely transculturally even for such conventional social behaviors as smiling and handshaking. Among many Hispanic clients, for example, smiling and handshaking are considered an integral part of sincere interactions and essential to establishing trust, whereas a Russian American client might perceive the same behavior to be inappropriate.

Wide cultural variation exists when interpreting *silence*. Some individuals find silence extremely uncomfortable and make every effort to fill conversational lags with words. Conversely, many Native Americans consider silence essential to understanding and respecting the other person. A pause following your question signifies that what has been asked is important enough to be given thoughtful consideration. In traditional Chinese and Japanese cultures, silence may mean that the speaker wishes the listener to consider the content of what has been said before continuing. Other cultural meanings of silence may be found. The English and Arabs may use silence out of respect for another's privacy, whereas the French, Spanish, and Russians may interpret it as a sign of agreement. Asian cultures often use silence to demonstrate respect for elders. Among some African Americans, silence is used in response to what is perceived as an inappropriate question.

The use of *eye contact* is among the most culturally variable nonverbal behaviors that clients use to communicate with you. Although most nurses have been taught to maintain eye contact when speaking with clients, individuals from culturally diverse backgrounds may attribute other culturally based meanings to this behavior. Asian, Native American, Indochinese, Arab, and Appalachian clients may consider direct eye contact impolite or aggressive, and they may avert their own eyes when talking with you. Native Americans often stare at the floor during conversations, a culturally appropriate behavior indicating that the listener is paying close attention to the speaker. Some African Americans use *oculistics* (eye rolling) in response to what is perceived to be an inappropriate question. Among Hispanic clients, respect dictates appropriate deferential behavior in the form of downcast eyes toward others on the basis of age, sex, social position, economic status, and position of authority. Elders expect respect from younger individuals, adults from children, men from women, teachers from students, and employers from employees. In the nurse-client relationship with Hispanic clients, eye contact is expected of you but will not necessarily be reciprocated by the client.

In some cultures, including Arab, Hispanic, and African American groups, *modesty for both women and men* is interrelated with eye contact. For Muslim-Arab women, modesty is, in part, achieved by avoiding eye contact with males (except for one's husband) and keeping the eyes downcast when encountering members of the opposite sex in public situations. In many cultures, the only woman who smiles and establishes eye contact with men in public is a prostitute. Hasidic Jewish males also have culturally based norms concerning eye contact with females. You may observe the male avoiding direct eye contact and turning his head in the opposite direction when walking past or speaking to a woman. The preceding examples are intended to be illustrative, not exhaustive.

Touch

You are urged to give careful consideration to issues concerning *touch*. While recognizing the benefits reported by many in establishing rapport with clients through touch, including the promotion of healing through therapeutic touch, physical contact with clients conveys various meanings cross-culturally. In many Arab and Hispanic cultures, male health care providers may be prohibited from touching or examining part, or all, of the female body. Adolescent girls may prefer female health care providers or refuse to be examined by a male. You should be aware that the client's significant others also may exert pressure by enforcing these culturally meaningful norms in the health care setting.

In some cultures, there are strict norms related to touching children. Many Asians believe that touching the head is a sign of disrespect because it is thought to be the source of a person's strength. You need to be aware that patting a child on the head or examining the fontanelles of a Southeast Asian infant should be avoided or done only with parental permission. Whenever possible, you should explore alternative ways to express affection or to obtain information necessary for assessment of the client's condition (e.g., hold the child on the lap, observe for other manifestations of increased intracranial pressure or signs of premature fontanelle closure, or place one's hand over the mother's while asking for a description of what she feels). Approximately 80 percent of the world's people believe in *mal ojo*, or evil eye. In this culture-bound syndrome, the child is believed to become ill as a result of excessive admiration by another person.

Sex and Gender Considerations

Nonverbal behaviors are culturally very significant, and failure to adhere to the *cultural code* (set of rules or norms of behavior used by a cultural group to guide their behavior and to interpret situations) is viewed as a serious transgression. When in doubt, the best approach is to ask the client about culturally relevant aspects of male-female relationships, preferably at the time of admission or early in your relationship.

Violating norms related to appropriate male-female relationships among various cultures may jeopardize your therapeutic relationship with clients and their families. Among Arab Americans, you may find that adult males avoid being alone with members of the opposite sex (except for their wives) and are generally accompanied by one or more male companions when interacting with females. The presence of the companion(s) conveys that the purpose of the interaction is honorable and that no sexual impropriety will occur. Some women of Middle Eastern origin do not shake hands with men, nor do men and women touch each other outside the marital relationship. Given that clients who have recently immigrated are in various stages of assimilation, traditional customs such as these may or may not be practiced. If in doubt, you should ask the client or observe the client's behaviors.

A brief comment about same-sex relationships is warranted. In some cultures, it is considered an acceptable expression of friendship and affection to openly and publicly hold hands with or embrace members of the same sex without any sexual connotation being associated with the behavior. For example, you may note that although a Nigerian American woman may not demonstrate overt affection for her husband or other male family members, she will hold hands with female relatives and friends while walking or talking with them. You may find that clients display similar behaviors toward you and should feel free to discuss cultural differences and similarities openly with the client. The discussion should include how each person feels about the cultural practice and exploration of mutually acceptable—and unacceptable—avenues for communicating.

Language

Nearly 32 million people in the United States speak a language other than English at home. Summarized in Table 2-2 are the number and age group of Americans who speak other languages and the percent who report that they have difficulty speaking English well. One of the greatest challenges in cross-cultural communication occurs when you and your client speak different languages. After assessing the language skills of non-English-speaking clients, you may find yourself in one of two situations—either struggling to communicate effectively through an interpreter or communicating effectively when there is no interpreter.

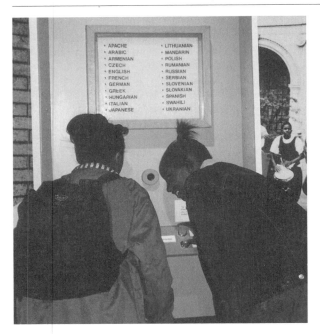

Children on a field trip to a popular Cleveland museum learn about the most common languages spoken in the culturally diverse urban area.

Non-English–Speaking Clients

Interviewing the non-English–speaking person requires a bilingual interpreter for full communication. Even the person from another culture or country who has a basic command of English (those for whom English is a second language) may need an interpreter when faced with the anxiety-provoking situation of entering a hospital, encountering a strange symptom, or discussing a sensitive topic such as birth control or gynecologic or urologic concerns. Ideally, a trained medical interpreter should be used. This person knows interpreting techniques, has a health care background, and understands patients' rights. The trained interpreter also is knowledgeable about cultural beliefs and health practices. This person can help you to bridge the cultural gap and can give advice concerning the cultural appropriateness of your recommendations.

Although you will be in charge of the focus and flow of the interview, the interpreter should be viewed as an important member of the health care team. It is tempting to ask a relative, friend, or even another client to interpret because this person is readily available and likely is anxious to help. This violates confidentiality for the client, however, who may not want personal information shared. Furthermore, the friend or relative, though fluent in ordinary language usage, is likely to be unfamiliar with medical terminology, hospital or clinic procedures, and health care ethics.

Whenever possible, work with a bilingual member of the health care team. In ideal circumstances, you should ask the interpreter to meet the client beforehand to establish rapport and to obtain basic descriptive information about the client such as age, occupation, educational level, and attitude toward health care. This eases the interpreter into the relationship and allows the client to talk about aspects of his or her life that are relatively nonthreatening.

TABLE 2-2

Persons Speaking a Language Other Than English at Home, by Age and Language

Age Group and Language Spoken at Home	Persons Who Speak Language (1,000)	Percent Who Speak English Less Than "Very Well"	Language	Persons, 5 Years Old and Over Who Speak Language (1,000)
Persons 5 years old and over	230,446	(X)	Speak only English	198,601
Speak only English	198,601	(X)	Spanish	17,339
Speak other language	31,845	43,9	French	1,702
Speak Spanish or Spanish Creole	17,345	47.9	German	1,547
Speak Asian or Pacific Island language	4,472	54.1	Italian	1,309
Speak other language	10,028	32.4	Chinese	1,249
			Tagalog	843
Persons 5 to 17 years old	45,342	(X)	Polish	723
Speak only English	39,020	(X)	Korean	626
Speak other language	6,323	37.8	Vietnamese	507
Speak Spanish or Spanish Creole	4,168	39.3	Portuguese	430
Speak Asian or Pacific Island language	816	44.2	Japanese	428
Speak other language	1,340	29.2	Greek	388
			Arabic	355
Persons 18 to 64 years old	153,908	(X)	Hindi (Urdu)	331
Speak only English	132,200	(X)	Russian	242
Speak other language	21,708	45.1	Yiddish	213
Speak Spanish or Spanish Creole	12,121	49.6	Thai (Laotian)	206
Speak Asian or Pacific Island language	3,301	54.7	Persian	202
Speak other language	6,286	31.4	French Creole	188
			Armenian	150
Persons 65 years old and over	31,195	(X)	Navaho	149
Speak only English	27,381	(X)	Hungarian	148
Speak other language	3,814	47.2	Hebrew	144
Speak Spanish or Spanish Creole	1,057	62.3	Dutch	143
Speak Asian or Pacific Island language	355	72.0	Mon-Khmer (Cambodian)	127
Speak other language	2,402	36.9	Gujarathi	102

X Not applicable

Source: U.S. Bureau of the Census, *1990 Census of Population and Housing Data Paper Listing* (CPH-L-133), and Summary Tape File 3C.

When using an interpreter, you should expect that the interaction with the client will require more time than caring for English-speaking clients. It will be necessary to organize nursing care so that the most important interactions or procedures are accomplished first before any of the parties (including yourself) become fatigued.

Both you and the client should speak only a sentence or two and then allow the interpreter time. You should use simple language, not medical jargon that the interpreter must simplify before it can be translated. Summary translation goes faster and is useful for teaching relatively simple health techniques with which the interpreter is already familiar. Be alert for nonverbal cues as the client talks. This can give valuable data. A skilled interpreter also will note nonverbal messages and pass them on to you.

Summarized in **Box 2-2** are suggestions for the selection and use of an interpreter and for overcoming language barriers when an interpreter is unavailable. Although

---

Box 2-2 *Overcoming Language Barriers*

Use of an Interpreter

- Before locating an interpreter, be sure that the language the client speaks at home is known, since it may be different from the language spoken publicly (e.g., French is sometimes spoken by well-educated and upper-class members of certain Asian or Middle Eastern cultures).
- Avoid interpreters from a rival tribe, state, region, or nation (e.g., a Palestinian who knows Hebrew may not be the best interpreter for a Jewish client).
- Be aware of gender differences between interpreter and client. In general, same gender is preferred.
- Be aware of age differences between interpreter and client. In general, an older, more mature interpreter is preferred to a younger, less experienced one.
- Be aware of socioeconomic differences between interpreter and client.
- Ask the interpreter to translate as closely to verbatim as possible.
- An interpreter who is a nonrelative may seek compensation for services rendered.

Recommendations for Institutions

- Maintain a computerized list of interpreters who may be contacted as needed.
- Network with area hospitals, colleges, universities, and other organizations that may serve as resources.
- Utilize the translation services provided by telephone companies (e.g., American Telephone and Telegraph Company).

What to Do When There Is No Interpreter

- Be polite and formal.
- Greet the person using the last or complete name. Gesture to yourself and say your name. Offer a handshake or nod. Smile.
- Proceed in an unhurried manner. Pay attention to any effort by the patient or family to communicate.
- Speak in a low, moderate voice, Avoid talking loudly. Remember that there is a tendency to raise the volume and pitch of your voice when the listener appears not to understand. The listener may perceive that the nurse is shouting and/or angry.
- Use any words known in the patient's language. This indicates that the nurse is aware of and respects the client's culture.
- Use simple words, such as *pain* instead of *discomfort.* Avoid medical jargon, idioms, and slang. Avoid using contractions. Use nouns repeatedly instead of pronouns. Example: Do *not* say, "He has been taking his medicine, hasn't he?" Do say, "Does Juan take medicine?"
- Pantomime words and simple actions while verbalizing them.

Box 2-2 *(Continued)*

- Give instructions in the proper sequence. Example: Do *not* say, "Before you rinse the bottle, sterilize it." do say, "First, wash the bottle. Second, rinse the bottle."
- Discuss one topic at a time. Avoid using conjunctions. Example: Do *not* say, "Are you cold and in pain?" Do say, "Are you cold [while pantomiming]?" Are you in pain?"
- Validate if the client understands by having him or her repeat instructions, demonstrate the procedure, or act out the meaning.
- Write out several short sentences in English, and determine the person's ability to read them.
- Try a third language. Many Indo-Chinese speak French. Europeans often know three or four languages. Try Latin words or phrases, if the nurse is familiar with the language.
- Ask who among the client's family and friends could serve as an interpreter.
- Obtain phrase books from a library or bookstore, make or purchase flash cards, contact hospitals for a list of interpreters, and use both formal and informal networking to locate a suitable interpreter.

Adapted from M. Andrews (1995). Transcultural considerations: in health assessment. In C. Jarvis, *Physical Examination and Health Assessment* (p. 75). Philadelphia: W.B. Saunders. Reprinted by permission.

use of an interpreter is the ideal, you will need a strategy for promoting effective communication when none is present.

Folk, Indigenous and Traditional Healers

Most cultures have traditional (sometimes referred to as folk, indigenous or generic) healers, most of whom speak the native tongue of the client, sometimes make house calls, and may cost significantly less than healers practicing in the biomedical/scientific health care system (cf., Leininger, 1997). In addition, many cultures have lay midwives (e.g., *parteras* for Hispanic women), *doulas* (support women for new mothers and babies), or other health care providers available for meeting the needs of clients. **Table 2-3** identifies indigenous or folk healers for selected groups.

Traditional healers should be an integral part of the health care team and should be included in as many aspects of the client's care as possible. For example, you might include the traditional healer in obtaining a health history and in determining what treatments already have been used in an effort to bring about healing. When discussing traditional remedies, it is important to be respectful and to listen attentively to healers who effectively combine spiritual and herbal remedies for a wide variety of illnesses, both physical and psychological in origin. Chapter 12 provides detailed information about the religious beliefs and spiritual healers for major religious groups.

TABLE 2-3
Healers and Their Scope of Practice

Culture/Folk Practitioner	Preparation	Scope of Practice
Hispanic		
Family member	Possesses knowledge of folk medicine	Common illnesses of a mild nature that may or may not be recognized by modern medicine.
Curandero	May receive training in an apprenticeship. May receive a "gift from God" that enables her/him to cure. Knowledgeable in use of herbs, diet, massage, and rituals.	Treats almost all of the traditional illnesses. Some may not treat illness caused by witchcraft for fear of being accused of possessing evil powers. Usually admired by members of the community.
Espiritualista or spiritualist	Born with the special gifts of being able to analyze dreams and foretell future events. May serve apprenticeship with an older practitioner.	Emphasis on prevention of illness or bewitchment through use of medals, prayers, amulets. May also be sought for cure of existing illness.
Yerbero	No formal training. Knowledgeable in growing and prescribing herbs.	Consulted for preventive and curative use of herbs for both traditional and Western illnesses.
Sabador	Knowledgeable in massage and manipulation of bones and muscles.*	Treats many traditional illnesses, particularly those affecting the musculoskeletal system. May also treat nontraditional illnesses.
Black		
"Old Lady"	Usually an older woman who has successfully raised her own family. Knowledgeable in child care and folk remedies.	Consulted about common ailments and for advice on child care. Found in rural and urban communities.
Spiritualist	Called by God to help others. No formal training. Usually associated with a fundamentalist Christian church.	Assists with problems that are financial, personal, spiritual or physical. Predominantly found in urban communities.
Voodoo priest or priestess or *Hougan*	May be trained by other priests(esses). In the U.S. the eldest son of a priest becomes a priest. A daughter of a priest(ess) becomes a priestess if she is born with a veil (amniotic sac) over her face.	Knowledgeable about properties of herbs; interpretation of signs and omens. Able to cure illness caused by voodoo. Uses communication techniques to establish a therapeutic milieu like a psychiatrist. Treats blacks, Mexican Americans, and Native Americans.
Chinese		
Herbalist	Knowledgeable in diagnosis of illness and herbal remedies.	Both diagnostic and therapeutic. Diagnostic techniques include interviewing, inspection, auscultation, and assessment of pulses.

TABLE 2-3 *(Continued)*

Culture/Folk Practitioner	Preparation	Scope of Practice
Acupuncturist	3 1/2 to 4 1/2 years (1,500 to 1,800 hours of courses on acupuncture, Western anatomy & physiology, & Chinese herbs. Usually requires a period of apprenticeship learning from someone else who is licensed or certified. Licensure is required in North America.	Diagnosis and treatment of yin/yang disorders by inserting needles into *meridians,* pathways through which life energy flows. When heat is applied to the acupuncture needle, the term *moxibustion* is used. May combine acupuncture with herbal remedies and/or dietary recommendations. Acupuncture is sometimes used as a surgical anesthetic.

Amish

Braucher or baruch-doktor	Apprenticeship	Men or women who use a combination of modalities including physical manipulation, massage, herbs, teas, reflexology, and *brauche,* folk-healing art with origins in 18th and 19th century Europe. Especially effective in the treatment of bedwetting, nervousness, and women's health problems. May be generalist or specialist in practice. Some set up treatment rooms. Some see non-Amish as well as Amish patients.
Lay midwives	Apprenticeship	Care for women before, during, and after delivery.

Greek

Magissa "magician"	Apprenticeship	Woman who cures *matiasma* or evil eye May be referred to as doctor
Bonesetters	Apprenticeship	Specialize in treating uncomplicated fractures
Priest (Orthodox)	Ordained clergy Formal theological study	May be called on for advice, blessings, exorcisms, or direct healing.

Native Americans

shaman	Spiritually chosen Apprenticeship	Uses incantations, prayers and herbs to cure a wide range of physical, psychological and spiritual illnesses
Crystal gazer hand trembler (Navajo)	Spiritually chosen Apprenticeship	Diviner diagnostician who can identify the cause of a problem, either by using crystals or placing hand over the sick person. Does not implement treatment.

Culture and Symptoms

All symptoms are believed to have cultural meanings. The tendency to interpret symptoms only as manifestations of a biologic reality should be questioned. According to Wenger (1993), you should not assume that the perceived symptoms or complaints of clients are equivalent to the names of recognized diseases or syndromes familiar to you or other professional healers. **Symptoms** are defined as phenomena experienced by individuals that signify a departure from normal function, sensation, or appearance and may include physical aberrations. As individuals experience symptoms, they interpret them and react in ways that are congruent with their cultural norms. Symptoms cannot be attributed to another person; rather, individuals experience symptoms from their knowledge of bodily function and sociocultural interactions. When people experience symptoms, they are perceived, recognized, labeled, reacted to, ritualized, and articulated in ways that make sense within the cultural world view of the person experiencing the symptoms (Good & Good, 1980; Wenger, 1993).

Symptoms are defined according to the client's perception of the meaning attributed to the event. This perception must be considered in relation to other sociocultural factors and biologic knowledge. People develop culturally based explanatory models to explain how their illnesses work and what their symptoms mean (Kleinman, Eisenberg, & Good, 1978).

The search for cultural meaning in understanding symptoms involves a translation process that includes both your world view and your client's. You need to assess the symptoms within the sociocultural and ethnohistorical context of the client. You should learn the terms clients use for symptoms and the meanings attributed to the specific symptoms. Simultaneously, you must translate the scientific meaning generally attributed to physiologic and psychological data and therapeutic intervention. Through negotiation and analysis, the cultural meanings of the symptoms are restructured in a manner that is congruent with your professional knowledge. Your knowledge of the cultural expression of symptoms will influence the decisions you make and facilitate your ability to provide culture-congruent or culturally competent nursing care (Wenger, 1993).

Culture-Bound Syndromes

Although all illness may be culturally defined, ethnopsychiatrists and psychological anthropologists have used the term **culture-bound syndromes** when referring to disorders restricted to a particular culture or group of cultures because of certain psychosocial characteristics of those cultures. For example, anorexia nervosa is believed to be a Western culture-bound syndrome because the condition is largely confined to Western cultures or those non-Western cultures undergoing the process of Westernization, such as Japan. Culture-bound syndromes are thought to be illnesses created by personal, social, and cultural reactions to malfunctioning biologic or psychological processes and can be understood only within defined contexts of meaning and social relationships (Kleinman, 1980). **Table 2-4** summarizes selected culture-bound syndromes found in specific cultural groups.

TABLE 2-4
Selected Culture-Bound Syndromes

Group	Disorder	Remarks
Whites	Anorexia nervosa	Excessive preoccupation with thinness; self-imposed starvation
	Bulimia	Gross overeating and then vomiting or fasting
African Americans : Haitians	Blackout	Collapse, dizziness, inability to move
	Low blood	Not enough blood or weakness of the blood that is often treated with diet
	High blood	Blood that is too rich in certain things due to ingestion of too much red meat or rich foods
	Thin blood	Occurs in women, children, and old people; renders the individual more susceptible to illness in general
	Diseases of hex, witchcraft, or conjuring	Sense of being doomed by spell; gastrointestinal symptoms, e.g., vomiting; hallucinations; part of voodoo beliefs
Chinese/Southeast Asian	Koro	Intense anxiety that penis is retracting into body
Greeks	Hysteria	Bizarre complaints and behavior because the uterus leaves the pelvis for another part of the body
Hispanics	Empacho	Food forms into a ball and clings to the stomach or intestines causing pain and cramping
	Fatigue	Asthma-like symptoms
	Mal ojo, "evil eye"	Fitful sleep, crying, diarrhea in children caused by a stranger's attention; sudden onset
	Pasmo	Paralysis-like symptoms of face or limbs; prevented or relieved by massage
	Susto	Anxiety, trembling, phobias from sudden fright
Native Americans	Ghost	Terror, hallucinations, sense of danger
North India Indians	Ghost	Death from fever and illness in children; convulsions, delirious speech (or incessant crying in infants); choking, difficulty breathing; based on Hindu religious beliefs and curing practices
Japanese	Wagamama	Apathetic childish behavior with emotional outbursts
Korean	Hwa-byung	Multiple somatic and psychological symptoms; "pushing up" sensation of chest; palpitations, flushing, headache, "epigastric mass," dysphoria, anxiety, irritability, and difficulty concentrating; mostly afflicts married women

Biocultural Variations in Health and Illness

The purpose of this discussion is to identify selected biocultural variations that sometimes are found in clients from various cultural backgrounds. The distribution of selected genetic traits and disorders prevalent among children from some cultural groups is presented in Chapter 4. **Table 2-5** provides an alphabetical listing of selected

TABLE 2-5
Biocultural Aspects of Disease

Disease	Remarks
Alcoholism	Indians have double the rate of whites; lower tolerance to alcohol among Chinese and Japanese Americans
Anemia	High incidence among Vietnamese due to presence of infestations among immigrants and low iron diets; low hemoglobin and malnutrition found among 18.2 percent of Native Americans, 32.7 percent of blacks, 14.6 percent of Hispanics, and 10.4 percent of white children under 5 years of age
Arthritis	Increased incidence among Native Americans Blackfoot 1.4 percent Pima 1.8 percent Chippewa 6.8 percent
Asthma	Six times greater for Native American infants <1 year; same as general population for Native Americans, ages 1–44 years
Bronchitis	Six times greater for Native American infants <1 year; same as general population for Native Americans, ages 1–44 years
Cancer	Nasopharyngeal: High among Chinese Americans and Native Americans Breast: Black women 1½ times more likely than white Esophageal: No. 2 cause of death for black males aged 35–54 years *Incidence:* White males 3.5/100,000 Black males 13.3/100,000 Liver: Highest among all ethnic groups are Filipino Hawaiians Stomach: black males twice as likely as white males; low among Filipinos Cervical: 120% higher in black females than in white females Uterine: 53% lower in black females than white females Prostate: Black males have highest incidence of all groups Most prevalent cancer among Native Americans: biliary, nasopharyngeal, testicular, cervical, renal, and thyroid (females) cancer Lung cancer among Navajo uranium miners 85 times higher than among white miners Most prevalent cancer among Japanese Americans: esophageal, stomach, liver, and biliary cancer Among Chinese Americans, there is a higher incidence of nasopharyngeal and liver cancer than among the general population
Cholecystitis	*Incidence:* Whites 0.3 percent Puerto Ricans 2.1 percent Native Americans 2.2 percent Chinese 2.6 percent
Colitis	High incidence among Japanese Americans

TABLE 2-5 *(Continued)*

Disease	Remarks
Diabetes mellitus	Three times as prevalent among Filipino Americans as whites; higher among Hispanics than blacks or whites Death rate is 3–4 times as high among Native Americans aged 25–34 years, especially those in the West such as Utes, Pimas, and Papagos *Complications* Amputations: Twice as high among Native Americans vs. General U.S. population Renal failure: 20 times as high as general U.S. population, with tribal variation, e.g., Utes have 43 times higher incidence
G6PD	Present among 30 percent of black males
Influenza	Increased death rate among Native Americans ages 45+
Ischemic heart disease	Responsible for 32 percent of heart-related causes of death among Native Americans; blacks have higher mortality rates than all other groups
Lactose intolerance	Present among 66 percent of Hispanic women; increased incidence among blacks and Chinese
Myocardial infarction	Leading cause of heart disease in Native Americans, accounting for 43 percent of death from heart disease; low incidence among Japanese Americans
Otitis media	7.9 percent incidence among school-aged Navajo children versus 0.5 percent in whites Up to ⅓ of Eskimo children <2 yrs have chronic otitis media Increased incidence among bottle-fed Native Americans and Eskimo infants
Pneumonia	Increased death rate among Native Americans ages 45+
Psoriasis	Affects 2–5 percent of whites, but <1 percent of blacks; high among Japanese Americans
Renal disease	Lower incidence among Japanese Americans
Sickle cell anemia	Increased incidence among blacks
Trachoma	Increased incidence among Native Americans and Eskimo children (3 to 8 times greater than general population)
Tuberculosis	Increased Incidence among Native Americans Apache 2.0 percent Sioux 3.2 percent Navajo 4.6 percent
Ulcers	Decreased incidence among Japanese Americans

Based on data reported in T. Overfield (1995). *Biologic Variation in Health and Illness: Race, Age, and Sex Differences.* NY: CRC Press; and Office of Minority Health (Aug. 1995). Cancer in minority communities. *Closing the Gap,* Washington, DC: U.S. Govt. Printing Office.

diseases and their increased or decreased prevalence among members of certain cultural groups. Accurate assessment and evaluation of clients require knowledge of normal biocultural variations that are found among healthy members of selected populations. You must also possess assessment skills that will enable you to recognize variations that occur in illness. The following remarks are intended to be illustrative, not exhaustive. As more research on biocultural variations is conducted, undoubtedly there will be additions and perhaps some modifications.

Measurements

Body Proportions, Height, and Weight

Summarized in **Box 2-3** are average heights for men and women from selected cultural groups that have been studied. For all groups, *height* increases up to 1.5 inches as socioeconomic status improves. First-generation immigrants may be up to 1.5 inches taller than counterparts in their country of origin owing to (1) better nutrition; and (2) decreased interference with growth by infectious diseases. It is interesting to note that during the past decade, the overall height of men increased by 0.7 inches, whereas women grew an average of 0.5 inches taller (Overfield, 1995).

Box 2-3 *Biocultural Variations in Height for Selected Groups*

Height (in inches) for All Groups

All Groups of Men	Whites American	African American	Mexican American	Asian
69.1	69.1	69.2	67.2	65.7
All Groups of Women				
63.7	63.8	63.8	61.8	60.3

Table developed using data from: Overfield, T. (1995). *Biologic Variation in Health and Illness.* New York: CRC Press.

Biocultural variations are found in the *body proportions* of individuals, largely due to differences in bone length. In examining sitting/standing height ratios, you will notice that African Americans of both genders have longer legs and shorter trunks than whites. Because proportionately most of the weight is in the trunk, white men appear more obese than African American counterparts. The reverse is true for women. Clients of Asian heritage are markedly shorter, weigh less, and have smaller body frames (Overfield, 1995).

Biocultural differences exist in the amount of body fat and the distribution of fat throughout the body. As a general rule, people from the lower socioeconomic class are more obese than those from the middle class, who are more obese than members of the upper class. On average, African American men weigh less than their white counterparts throughout adulthood (166.1 lbs versus 170.6 lbs). The opposite is true for women. Despite their longer legs, African American women are consistently heavier than white women at every age (149.6 lbs versus 137 lbs). Between the ages of 35 to 64 years, African American women weigh on average 20 lb more than white women. Mexican Americans weigh more per height than non-Hispanic whites due to differences in truncal fat patterns. Most differences in the amount of body fat are related to socioeononomic factors which in turn influence nutrition and exposure to communicable diseases. People around the world tend to have more body fat in cold climates whereas those residing in warmer areas have less. African Americans have smaller skinfold thicknesses on their trunks and arms than white counterparts. Although their length is similar, bottle-fed infants are heavier on average than those who are breast-fed (Overfield, 1995).

Clinical Measures

Although the average pulse rate is comparable across cultures, there are racial and gender differences in *blood pressure*. African American men have lower systolic blood pressures than their white counterparts from ages 18 to 34, but between the ages of 35 and 64 it reverses with African Americans having an average 5-mm Hg higher systolic blood pressure. After age 65 there is no difference between the two races. African American women have a higher average systolic blood pressure than their white counterparts at every age. After age 45, African American women's average blood pressure reading may be as much as 16 mm Hg higher than white women in the same age group (Overfield, 1995).

Biocultural Differences in the Physical Examination

General Appearance

In assessing the general appearance, you should survey the person's entire body. You will want to note the general health state and any obvious physical characteristics and readily apparent biologic features unique to the individual. In assessing the client's general appearance, you should consider four areas: physical appearance, body structure, mobility, and behavior. The *physical appearance* includes age, gender, level of consciousness, facial features, and skin color (evenness of color tone, pigmentation, intactness, presence of lesions or other abnormalities). *Body structure* includes stature, nutrition, symmetry, posture, position, and the overall body build or contour. *Assessment of mobility* includes gait and range of motion. *Behavior* includes facial expression, mood and affect, fluency of speech, ability to communicate ideas, appropriateness of word choice, grooming and attire or dress (Jarvis, 1996).

If you notice that someone from an ethnoreligious group is wearing characteristic clothing, you might find it useful to gather further data related to religious and cultural beliefs, values, and practices. You will readily recognize the outward appearance of ethnic and/or religious affiliation by the client's dress for the following groups: Amish wear characteristic clothing similar to that worn during the 19th century (solid colors, use of snaps or pins instead of buttons, bonnets cover the heads of women); some women from India wear saris; some Muslim-Arab men wear kafias (cloth headdress) and long robes (*note:* the same individual may alternate between traditional and Western-style clothing); and members of the Church of Jesus Christ of Latter-Day Saints (Mormons) may wear special white underwear called temple garments. Although dress or clothing suggests a particular ethnic and/or religious affiliation, you should avoid stereotyping individual clients and you need to explore the meaning of the dress, ethnoreligious beliefs and health-related practices with the client and/or significant others.

Skin

An accurate and comprehensive examination of the skin of clients from culturally diverse backgrounds requires that you possess knowledge of biocultural variations and skill in recognizing color changes, some of which may be very subtle. Awareness of normal biocultural differences and the ability to recognize the unique clinical manifestations of disease are developed over time as you gain experience with clients having various skin colors.

The assessment of a client's skin is subjective and highly dependent on your observational skill, ability to recognize subtle color changes, and repeated exposure to individuals having various gradations of skin color. *Melanin* is responsible for the various colors and tones of skin observed among people. Melanin protects the skin against harmful ultraviolet rays, a genetic advantage accounting for the lower incidence of skin cancer among darkly pigmented African American and Native American clients.

Normal skin color ranges widely, and there are health care practitioners who have made attempts to describe the variations seen by labeling observations with some of the following adjectives—*copper, olive, tan*, and various shades of *brown* (*light, medium*, and *dark*). In observing pallor in clients, the term *ashen* is sometimes used. Of most clinical significance, particularly for clients whose health condition may be linked to changes in the skin color, is your ability to establish a reliable description of a baseline color and subsequently to recognize when variations occur in the same individual.

Mongolian spots, irregular areas of deep-blue pigmentation, are usually located in the sacral and gluteal areas but sometimes occur on the abdomen, thighs, shoulders, or arms. During embryonic development, the melanocytes originate near the embryonic nervous system in the neural crest. They then migrate into the fetal epidermis. Mongolian spots consist of embryonic pigment that has been left behind in the epidermal layer during fetal development. The result looks like a bluish discoloration of the skin.

Mongolian spots are a normal variation in children of African, Asian, or Latin descent. By adulthood, these spots become lighter but usually remain visible. Mongolian spots are present in 90 percent of African Americans, 80 percent of Asian and Native Americans, and 9 percent of whites (Overfield, 1995). If you are unfamiliar with Mongolian spots, it is important to exercise caution so that you do not confuse them with bruises. Recognition of this normal variation is particularly important when dealing with children who might be erroneously identified as victims of child abuse, causing much anguish to the parents or guardians.

Vitiligo, a condition in which the melanocytes become nonfunctional in some areas of the skin, is characterized by unpigmented skin patches. Vitiligo affects more than 2 million Americans, primarily dark-skinned individuals. Clients with vitiligo also have a statistically higher than normal chance of developing pernicious anemia, diabetes mellitus, and hyperthyroidism. These factors are believed to reflect an underlying genetic abnormality (Overfield, 1995).

Other areas of the skin affected by hormones and, in some cases, differing for people from certain ethnic backgrounds are the sexual skin areas, such as the nipples, areola, scrotum, and labia majora. In general, these areas are darker than other parts of the skin in both adults and children, especially among African American and Asian clients. When assessing these skin surfaces on dark-skinned clients, you must observe carefully for erythema, rashes, and other abnormalities because the darker color may mask their presence.

Cyanosis is the most difficult clinical sign to observe in darkly pigmented persons. Because peripheral vasoconstriction can prevent cyanosis, you need to be attentive to environmental conditions such as air conditioning, mist tents, and other factors that may lower the room temperature and thus cause vasoconstriction. In order for the client to manifest clinical evidence of cyanosis, the blood must contain 5 g of reduced hemoglobin in 1.5 g of methemoglobin per 100 ml of blood (Overfield, 1995).

Given that most conditions causing cyanosis also cause decreased oxygenation of the brain, other clinical symptoms, such as changes in the level of consciousness, will be evident. Cyanosis usually is accompanied by increased respiratory rate, use of accessory muscles of respiration, nasal flaring, and other manifestations of respiratory distress. You must exercise caution when assessing persons of Mediterranean descent for cyanosis because their circumoral region is normally dark blue.

Jaundice

In both light- and dark-skinned clients, *jaundice* is best observed in the sclera. When examining culturally diverse individuals, caution must be exercised to avoid confusing other forms of pigmentation with jaundice. Many darkly pigmented people, e.g., African Americans, Filipino Americans, and others, have heavy deposits of subconjunctival fat that contains high levels of carotene in sufficient quantities to mimic jaundice. The fatty deposits become more dense as the distance from the cornea increases. The portion of the sclera that is revealed naturally by the palpebral fissure is the best place to accurately assess color. If the palate does not have heavy melanin pigmentation, jaundice can be detected there in the early stages (i.e., when the serum bilirubin level is 2–4 mg/100 ml). The absence of a yellowish tint of the palate when the sclerae are yellow indicates carotene pigmentation of the sclerae rather than jaundice. Light- or clay-colored stools and dark golden urine often accompany jaundice in both light- and dark-skinned clients. If you are to distinguish between carotenemia and jaundice, it will be necessary to inspect the posterior portion of the hard palate using bright daylight or good artificial lighting (Overfield, 1995).

Pallor

When assessing for *pallor* in darkly pigmented clients, you may experience difficulty because the underlying red tones are absent. This is significant because these red tones are responsible for giving brown or black skin its luster. The brown-skinned individual will manifest pallor with a more yellowish brown color, and the black-skinned person will appear ashen or gray. Generalized pallor can be observed in the mucous membranes, lips, and nail beds. The palpebrae, conjunctivae, and nail beds are preferred sites for assessing the pallor of anemia. When inspecting the conjunctiva, you should lower the lid sufficiently so you can see the conjunctiva near the inner and outer canthi. The coloration is often lighter near the inner canthus.

In addition to skin assessment, the pallor of impending shock is accompanied by other clinical manifestations, such as increasing pulse rate, oliguria, apprehension, and restlessness. Anemias, particularly chronic iron-deficiency anemia, may be manifest by the characteristic "spoon" nails, which have a concave shape. A lemon-yellow tint of the face and slightly yellow sclerae accompany pernicious anemia, which is also manifested by neurologic deficits and a red, painful tongue. You also will note that fatigue, exertional dyspnea, rapid pulse, dizziness, and impaired mental function accompany most severe anemias (Overfield, 1995).

Erythema

You may find that it is difficult to assess *erythema* (redness) in darkly pigmented clients. Erythema is frequently associated with localized inflammation and is characterized by increased skin temperature. The degree of redness is determined by the quantity of blood present in the subpapillary plexus, whereas the warmth of the skin is related to the rate of blood flow through the blood vessels. When assessing inflammation in dark-skinned clients, it is often necessary to palpate the skin for increased warmth, tautness or tightly pulled surfaces that may be indicative of edema, and hardening of deep tissues or blood vessels. You will find that the dorsal surfaces of your fingers will be the most sensitive to temperature sensations. The erythema associated with rashes is not always accompanied by noticeable increases in skin temperature. Macular, papular, and vesicular skin lesions are identified by a combination of palpation and inspection. In addition, it is important that you listen to the client's description of symptoms. For example, persons with macular rashes usually will complain of itching, and evidence of scratching will be apparent. When the skin is only moderately pigmented, a macular rash may become recognizable if the skin is gently stretched. Stretching the skin decreases the normal red tone, thus providing more contrast and making the macules appear brighter. In some skin disorders with generalized rash, you will observe that the hard and soft palates are the locations where the rash is most readily visible (Overfield, 1995).

The increased redness that accompanies carbon monoxide poisoning and the blood disorders collectively known as the *polycythemias* can be observed in the lips of dark-skinned clients. Because lipstick masks the actual color of the lips, you should ask the client to remove it prior to inspection.

Petechiae

In dark-skinned clients, *petechiae* are best visualized in the areas of lighter melanization, such as the abdomen, buttocks, and volar surface of the forearm. When the skin is black or very dark brown, petechiae cannot be seen in the skin. Most of the diseases that cause bleeding and the formation of microscopic emboli, such as thrombocytopenia, subacute bacterial endocarditis, and other septicemias, are characterized by petechiae in the mucous membranes and skin. You will find that petechiae are most easily seen in the mouth, particularly the buccal mucosa, and in the conjunctiva of the eye (Overfield, 1995).

In assessing *ecchymotic lesions* caused by systemic disorders, you will note that they are found in the same locations as petechiae, although their larger size makes them more apparent on dark-skinned individuals. When differentiating petechiae and ecchymoses from erythema in the mucous membrane, pressure on the tissue will momentarily blanch erythema but not petechiae or ecchymoses.

Skin Changes and Normal Aging

Although aging is accompanied by the growing presence of wrinkles in all cultures, African Americans, Asian Americans, American Indians and Eskimos wrinkle later in life than their Anglo American counterparts. Light skin shows the effects of sun damage more than dark skin, regardless of race or ethnicity. The area of the skin that is exposed to the sun shows aging effects more than protected skin such as those parts covered by clothing. Regardless of climate, dry skin is inevitable in individuals 70+ years of age. In part, dry skin is caused by transepidermal water loss, which decreases in older adults. African-Americans have a significantly higher transepidermal water loss than Whites, which correlates with the water content of the stratum corneum layer of the skin. Because the number of *moles* increases with age, they are thought to be the result of long-term exposure to the sun. People with lighter skin have more *moles* than those with darkly pigmented skin. Whites have more moles than Asian Americans or African Americans (Overfield, 1995).

Nurses and other health care providers often over- or underestimate the age when dealing with clients whose cultural heritage is different from their own. Whites tend to underestimate the age of African American, Asian American, and American Indian clients, whereas African Americans, Asian American, and American Indians tend to overestimate the age of white clients (Overfield, 1995).

Secretions

The *apocrine* and *eccrine sweat glands* are important for fluid balance and for thermoregulation. Approximately 2 to 3 million glands open onto the skin surface through pores and are responsible for the presence of sweat. When they are contaminated by normal skin flora, odor results. Most Asians and Native Americans have a mild to absent body odor, whereas whites and African Americans tend to have strong body odor.

Eskimos have made an environmental adaptation whereby they sweat less than whites on their trunks and extremities but more on their faces. This adaptation allows for temperature regulation without causing perspiration and dampness of their clothes, which would decrease their ability to insulate against severe weather and would pose a serious threat to their survival.

The amount of chloride excreted by sweat glands varies widely, and African Americans have lower salt concentrations in their sweat than do whites. A study of Ashkenazi Jews (European descent) and Sephardic Jews (North African and Middle Eastern descent) revealed that those of European origin had a lower percentage of sweat chlorides (Levin, 1966). This variation may be significant when caring for clients with renal or cardiac conditions or with children having cystic fibrosis (Overfield, 1995).

Head, Eyes, Ears, Mouth

Hair

Perhaps one of the most obvious and widely variable cultural differences occurs with assessment of the hair. African Americans' hair varies widely in texture. It is very fragile and ranges from long and straight to short, spiraled, thick, and kinky. The hair and scalp have a natural tendency to be dry and require daily combing, gentle brushing, and the application of oil. By comparison, clients of Asian backgrounds generally have straight, silky hair.

Obtaining a baseline hair assessment is significant in diagnosing and treating certain disease states. For example, hair texture is known to become dry, brittle, and lusterless with inadequate nutrition. The hair of African American children with severe malnutrition, as in the case of marasmus, frequently changes not only in texture but also in color. The child's hair often becomes straighter and turns a reddish copper color. Certain endocrine disorders are also known to affect the texture of hair.

Although gray hair correlates with age for both men and women, there are cultural differences in the rate of hair graying. Whites gray significantly faster than any other group. Sixty-six percent of fair-haired individuals are fully white by age 60, whereas 37 percent of dark-haired persons are totally white by the same age (Overfield, 1995). Among Asian Americans, graying may be delayed significantly, with some in their 8th or 9th decade of life showing little or no graying.

Eyes

Biocultural differences in both the structure and color of the eyes are readily apparent among clients from various cultural backgrounds. Racial differences are evident when examining the palpebral fissures. Persons of Asian background are often identified by their characteristic epicanthal eye folds, whereas the presence of narrowed palpebral fissures in non-Asian individuals may be diagnostic of a serious congenital anomaly known as *Down syndrome* or *trisomy 21*.

There is culturally based variability in the color of the iris and in retinal pigmentation, with darker irises being correlated with darker retinas. Clients with light retinas generally have better night vision but can suffer pain in an environment that is too light. The majority of African Americans and Asians have brown eyes, whereas many individuals of Scandinavian descent have blue eyes (Overfield, 1995).

It is clinically relevant that differences in visual acuity occur among people from different cultures. African Americans have poorer corrected visual acuity than Whites. The visual acuity of Hispanic Americans is between that of blacks and whites. American Indians are comparable to Whites, whereas Japanese and Chinese Americans have poorest corrected visual acuity, due to a high incidence of myopia (Overfield, 1995).

Ears

It does not take long to notice that ears come in a variety of sizes and shapes. Earlobes can be free-standing or attached to the face. Ceruminous glands are located in the external ear canal and are functional at birth. Cerumen is genetically determined and comes in two major types: (1) dry cerumen, which is gray, flaky, and frequently forms a thin mass in the ear canal, and (2) wet cerumen, which is dark brown and moist. Asians and Native Americans (including Eskimos) have an 84 percent frequency of dry cerumen, whereas African Americans have a 99 percent and whites have a 97 percent frequency of wet cerumen (Overfield, 1995). The clinical significance of this occurs when examining or irrigating the ears. You should be aware that the presence and composition of cerumen are not related to poor hygiene, and caution should be exercised to avoid mistaking the flaky, dry cerumen for the dry lesions of eczema.

Hearing gradually declines with age, especially in the high frequencies. After age 40, men have poorer hearing than women. African Americans have better hearing at high and low frequencies, whereas whites have better hearing at middle frequencies. African Americans are less susceptible to noise-induced hearing loss (Overfield, 1995).

Mouth

Oral hyperpigmentation also shows variation by race. Usually absent at birth, hyperpigmentation increases with age. By age 50 years, 10 percent of whites and 50 to 90 percent of African Americans will show oral hyperpigmentation, a condition that is believed to be caused by a lifetime of accumulation of postinflammatory oral changes (Overfield, 1995).

Cleft uvula, a condition in which the uvula is split either completely or partially, occurs in 18 percent of some Native American groups and 10 percent of Asians. The occurrence in whites and African Americans is rare. *Cleft lip* and *cleft palate* are most common in Asians and Native Americans and is least common in African Americans (Overfield, 1995).

Leukoedema, a grayish white benign lesion occurring on the buccal mucosa, is present in 68 to 90 percent of blacks but only 43 percent of whites. Care should be taken to avoid mistaking leukoedema for oral thrush or related infections that require treatment with medication (Overfield, 1995).

Teeth

Because teeth are often used as indicators of developmental, hygienic, and nutritional adequacy, you should be aware of biocultural differences. Although it is rare for a white baby to be born with teeth (1 in 3000), the incidence rises to 1 in 11 among Tlingit Indians and to 1 or 2 in 100 among Canadian Eskimo infants. Although congenital teeth are usually not problematic, extraction is necessary for some breast-fed infants (Overfield, 1995).

The size of teeth varies widely, with the teeth of whites being the smallest, followed by blacks and then Asians and Native Americans. The largest teeth are found among Eskimos and Australian Aborigines. Larger teeth cause some groups to have prognathic, or protruding, jaws, a condition that is seen more frequently in African and Asian Americans. The condition is normal and does not reflect a serious orthodontic problem.

Agenesis or absence of teeth varies by race, with missing third molars occurring in 18 to 35 percent of Asians, 9 to 25 percent of whites, and 1 to 11 percent of African Americans. Throughout life, whites have more tooth decay than African Americans, which may be related to a combination of socioeconomic factors and biocultural variation. Complete tooth loss occurs more often in whites than in African Americans despite the higher incidence of periodontal disease in African Americans. Approximately one-third of whites 45 years or older have lost all their teeth, compared with 25 percent of African Americans in the same age group (Overfield, 1995).

The differences in tooth decay between African Americans and whites can be explained by the fact that African Americans have harder and denser tooth enamel, which makes their teeth less susceptible to the organisms that cause caries. The increase in periodontal disease among African Americans is believed to be caused by poor oral hygiene. When obvious signs of periodontal disease are present, such as bleeding and edematous gums, a dental referral should be initiated (Overfield, 1995).

Chest

Mammary Venous Plexus

Regardless of gender, the superficial veins of the chest form a network over the entire chest that flows in either a transverse or a longitudinal pattern. In the transverse pattern, the veins radiate laterally and toward the axillae. In the longitudinal pattern, the veins radiate downward and laterally like a fan. These two patterns occur with different frequencies in the two populations that have been studied. White women have the recessive longitudinal pattern 6 to 10 percent of the time, whereas this pattern occurs 30 percent of the time in Navajos. The only known alteration of either pattern is produced by breast tumor. Although this variation has no clinical significance, it is mentioned so that if nurses note its presence during physical assessment, they will recognize it as a nonsignificant finding (Overfield, 1995).

Musculoskeletal System

You will note that many normal biocultural variations are found in clients' musculoskeletal systems. The long bones of African Americans are significantly longer, narrower, and denser than those of whites. Bone density measured by race and sex show that African American males have the densest bones, thus accounting for the relatively low incidence of osteoporosis in this population. Bone density in the Chinese, Japanese, and Eskimos is below that of white Americans (Overfield, 1995).

Curvature of the body's long bones varies widely among culturally diverse groups. Native Americans have anteriorly convex femurs, whereas African Americans have markedly straight femurs, and whites are intermediate. This characteristic is related to both genetics and body weight. Thin African Americans and whites have less curvature than average, whereas obese African Americans and whites display increased curvatures. It is possible that the heavier density of the bones of African Americans helps to protect them from increased curvature due to obesity (Overfield, 1995). **Table 2-6** summarizes biocultural variations occurring in the musculoskeletal system

---

TABLE 2-6
Biocultural Variations in the Musculoskeletal System

Component	Remarks	
Bone		
Frontal	Thicker in African-American males than in white males	
Parietal occiput	Thicker in white males than in African-American males	
Palate	Tori (protuberances) along the suture line of the hard palate Problematic for denture wearers *Incidence:*	
	African Americans	20 percent
	Whites	24 percent
	Asians	Up to 50 percent
	Native Americans	Up to 50 percent

TABLE 2-6 *(Continued)*

Component	Remarks
Mandible	Tori (protuberances) on the lingual surface of the mandible near the canine and premolar teeth
	Problematic for denture wearers
	Most common in Asians and Native Americans; exceeds 50 percent in some Eskimo groups
Humerus	Torsion or rotation of proximal end with muscle pull
	Whites > African Americans
	Torsion in African Americans is symmetric; torsion in whites tends to be greater on right than left side
Radius	Length at the wrist variable
Ulna	Ulna or radius may be longer
	Equal length
	Swedes 61 percent
	Chinese 16 percent
	Ulna longer than radius
	Swedes 16 percent
	Chinese 48 percent
	Radius longer than ulna
	Swedes 23 percent
	Chinese 10 percent
Vertebrae	Twenty-four vertebrae are found in 85 to 93 percent of all people; racial and sex differences reveal 23 or 25 vertebrae in select groups
	Vertebrae Population
	23 11 percent of African-American females
	25 12 percent of Eskimo and Native American males
	Related to lower back pain and lordosis
Pelvis	Hip width is 1.6 cm (0.6 in) smaller in African-American women than in white women; Asian women have significantly smaller pelvises
Femur	Convex anterior Native American
	Straight African American
	Intermediate White
Second tarsal	Second toe longer than the great toe
	Incidence:
	Whites 8–34 percent
	African Americans 8–12 percent
	Vietnamese 31 percent
	Melanesians 21–57 percent
	Clinical significance for joggers and athletes
Height	White males are 1.27 cm (0.5 in) taller than African American males and 7.6 cm (2.9 in) taller than Asian males
	White females = African American females
	Asian females are 4.14 cm (1.6 in) shorter than white or African American females

(continued)

TABLE 2-6 (Continued)

Component	Remarks
Composition of long bones	Longer, narrower, and denser in African Americans than in whites; bone density in whites > Chinese, Japanese, and Eskimos
	Osteoporosis lowest in African American males; highest in white females

Muscle

Peroneus tertius	Responsible for dorsiflexion of foot
	Muscle absent:
	Asians, Native Americans, and whites 3–10 percent
	African Americans 10–15 percent
	Berbers (Sahara desert) 24 percent
	No clinical significance because the tibialis anterior also dorsiflexes the foot
Palmaris longus	Responsible for wrist flexion
	Muscle absent:
	Whites 12–20 percent
	Native Americans 2–12 percent
	African Americans 5 percent
	Asians 3 percent
	No clinical significance because three other muscles are also responsible for flexion

Based on data reported by T. Overfield (1995). *Biologic Variation in Health and Illness: Race, Age, and Sex Differences.* NY: CRC Press.

that have been identified through observation and study of people from various cultures and subcultures.

Laboratory Tests

You should be aware that biocultural variations occur with some laboratory test results, such as measurement of *hemoglobin/hematocrit, cholesterol, serum transferrin* and *blood glucose.* You also will want to consider cultural differences in the results of tests conducted during pregnancy. The *multiple-marker screening* test and two tests of *amniotic fluid constituents* are used to screen pregnant women for potential fetal problems. Although the reasons for these differences are unknown, genetic, environmental, dietary, socioconomic, cultural and lifestyle factors are being studied determine the extent to which they contribute to the differences in test results. **Table 2-7** identifies biocultural variations and clinical significance for selected laboratory tests.

TABLE 2-7
Biocultural Variations and Clinical Significance for Selected Laboratory Tests

Test	Remarks
Hemoglobin/Hematocrit	1 g lower for African Americans than other groups African Americans < counterparts in other groups
Serum transferrin	Biocultural variation in children ages 1 to 3 1/2 years Mean for African Americans 22 mg/100 ml > whites Note: May be due to lowered hemoglobin and hematocrit levels found in African Americans. *Clinical significance:* Transferrin levels increase in the presence of anemia, thus influencing the diagnosis, treatment and nursing care of children with anemia.
Serum Cholesterol	Biocultural variation across the life span Birth African Americans = whites Childhood African Americans 5 mg/100 ml > whites Pima Indians 20–30 mg/100 ml < whites Adulthood African Americans < whites Pima Indians 50–60 ml/100 ml < whites *Clinical significance:* Prevention, treatment and nursing care of clients with cardiovascular disease
High Density Lipoproteins (HDL)	Biocultural variation in adults African Americans > whites Asian Americans ≥ whites Mexican Americans < whites
Ratio of HDL to total cholesterol	African Americans < whites
Low Density Lipoproteins (LDL)	Biocultural variation in adults African Americans < whites *Clinical significance:* Prevention, treatment and nursing care of clients with cardiovascular disease
Blood glucose	Biocultural variation in adults American Indians, Hispanic Americans, Japanese Americans > whites African Americans = whites (for equivalent socioeconomic groups) *Clinical significance:* Diagnosis, treatment and nursing care of adults with hypoglycemia and diabetes mellitus
Multiple-marker screening	Biocultural variations in blood levels for protein and hormones in pregnant women Alphafetoprotein (AFP), hCG and estriol levels in African American and Asian American women > whites *Clinical significance:* High AFP levels signal that the woman is at increased risk for delivering an infant with spina bifida and neural tube defects whereas low levels may signal Down Syndrome. Down Syndrome also is associated with low levels of estriol and high levels of hCG. African American and Asian American women have higher average levels of AFP, hCG and estriol than white counterparts.

(continued)

TABLE 2-7 *(Continued)*

Test	Remarks
	Using a single median for women of all cultures: *Causes African American and Asian American women to be *falsely* identified as being *at risk* for having infants with spina bifida and neural tube defects. By being classified as *high risk*, women are more likely to be subjected to invasive and expensive procedures such as amniocentesis. Some may elect to abort the pregnancy based on screening test results. **Inappropriately lowers* the identified Down Syndrome risk for African American and Asian American women
Lecithin/sphingomyelin ratio	Biocultural variations in amniotic fluid measures of fetal pulmonary maturity African Americans have higher ratios than whites from 23 to 42 weeks gestation *Clinical significance:* the ratio is used to calculate the risk of respiratory distress in premature infants. Lung maturity in African Americans is reached 1 week earlier than in whites (34 versus 35 weeks). Racial differences should be considered in making decisions about inducing labor or delivering by Cesarean Section.

Table based on data from:

Allanson, A., Michie, S., & Matreau, T.M. (1997). Presentation of screen negative results on serum screening for Down's Syndrome. *Journal of Medical Screening, 4(1),* 21–22.

Chapman, S.J., Brumfield, C.G., Wenstrom, K.D., & DuBard, M.B. (1997). Pregnancy outcomes following false-positive multiple marker screening test. *American Journal of Perinatology, 14(8),* 475–478.

O'Brien, J.E., Dvorin, E., Drugan, A., Johnson, M.P., Yaron, Y., & Evans, M.I. (1997). Race-ethnicity-specific variation in multiple-marker biochemical screening: alpha-fetoprotein, hCG, and estriol. *Obstetrics and Gynecology, 89(3),* 355–358.

Overfield, T. (1995). *Biologic Variation in Health and Illness: Race, Age, and Sex Differences.* New York: CRC Press.

Ethnopharmacology and Cultural Differences in Drug Response

The term *ethnopharmacology* was first used to describe the study of medicinal plants used by indigenous cultures. In more recent years, it is being used as a general reference to the *pharmacokinetics* and *pharmacodynamics* of drugs in people from diverse racial, ethnic and cultural backgrounds. *Phamacokinetics* refers to the study of the metabolism and action of drugs with particular emphasis on the time required for absorption, duration of action, distribution in the body, and method of excretion. *Pharmacodynamics* addresses how drugs affect the body, commonly by interacting with receptors that bind with endogenous and exogenous substances. Although largely neglected and rarely the focus of research, nonbiologic factors also exert significant influences on how an individual responds to medications. These include "compliance," placebo effects, stress, social support, personality and the prescription styles of physicians, nurse practitioners, and others with prescriptive privileges.

Since prehistoric times, people have attempted to discover plants, marine organisms, arthropods, animals and minerals with healing properties. According the World Health Organization, 80 percent of the people residing in less developed countries use traditional medicine, including medicinal plants, for their major primary health care needs. Of the 119 plant-derived drugs currently used in the U.S. and Canada, 74 percent were discovered as a result of chemical studies designed to isolate the active ingredients responsible for the use of the plants in traditional medicine. These drugs are derived from approximately 90 of the 250,000 known species of flowering plants on this planet (Farnsworth, 1993).

In North America, there is a high level of interest in studying the medicinal uses of plants and validating scientifically their effects and side effects. It is reasonable to assume that if a plant has been used by indigenous cultures over a long period of time, there must be valid drug potential in the plant. According to Farnsworth (1993), it has been estimated that to develop a new synthetic drug from discovery to approval by the U.S. Federal Drug Administration (FDA) requires 12 years of work at a cost of $12 million. For every 10,000 compounds synthesized and evaluated *in vitro*, 20 will be tested in animals, half of these in humans, and one will receive FDA approval to be marketed. Thus, it makes sense to learn from the experience of folk and indigenous healers in identifying plants with healing potential rather than relying on randomly screened synthetic compounds in large and costly drug trials.

Historically, most clinical drug trials were conducted on white middle class males, many of whom were students in colleges, medical schools, and similar settings, where they were readily available as volunteer subjects for investigators. The majority of studies providing evidence for differences in *pharmacokinetic* and *pharmacodynamic* properties of various drugs have compared individuals from the federal panethnic groups—blacks, Hispanics, Asian/Pacific Islanders, and American Indians/Alaska Natives—with Whites. Although it is problematic to view Whites as the norm, there is insufficient data from investigations involving people from diverse backgrounds to provide valid and reliable data on the ethnic-specific responses to all drugs. As indicated in **Table 2-8** for some drugs, there is growing research-based evidence to suggest that modifications in dosages be made for some members of racial and ethnic groups. Due to intermarriage, individual differences (e.g., weight, body fat index) and related factors, it may be difficult to develop ethnic-specific norms for drug dosages. It is possible, however, to alert nurses and other health care providers to the variations that occur in side effects, adverse reactions, and toxicity so clients from diverse cultural backgrounds can be monitored for possible untoward symptoms.

Mechanisms Affecting Drug Responses

Drug metabolism is a complex process governed by various enzymatic reactions, which in turn are genetically influenced. Because most drugs are metabolized in more than one pathway, the following may occur. There may be (1) a direct impact on the total clearance of the parent drug (resulting in the need for an increased dosages)

TABLE 2-8
Cultural Differences in Response to Drugs

Drug Category	Remarks

African-Americans

Analgesics	Despite decreased sensitivity to pain-relieving therapeutic action of drugs, there are increased gastrointestinal side effects, especially with acetominaphen.
Antihypertensives	Respond best to treatment with a single drug (versus combined antihypertensive therapy) Research suggests favorable response to diuretics, calcium antagonists, and alpha-blockers Less responsive to beta-blockers (e.g., propranalol) and angiotensin-converting enzyme (ACE) inhibitors (e.g., enalapril, imidapril) Increased side effects such as mood response (e.g., depression) to thiazides (e.g., hydrochlorothiazide), which may explain reluctance to take drug as prescribed There is little justification to use racial profiling to avoid drug classes. Current research is focusing on differences in the etiology of hypertension in blacks to explain differences in drug responses.
Mydriatics	Less dilation occurs with dark colored eyes
Psychotropics	Increased extrapyramidal side effects with tricyclic antidepressants (TCAs) such as haloperidol.
Steroids	When methylprednisolone is used for immunosuppression in renal transplant patients, there is increased toxicity such as steroid-associated diabetes. Although Blacks are four times as likely to develop End-stage renal disease as whites, they have the poorest long-term graft survival of any ethnic group.
Tranquilizers	15–20 percent are poor metabolizers of Valium (diazepam)

Arab Americans

Antiarrhythmics	Some may need lower dosage
Antihypertensives	Some may need lower dosage
Neuroleptics	Some may need lower dosage
Opioids	Some may require higher dosage due to diminished ability to metabolize codeine to morphine
Psychotropics	Some may need lower dosage

Asian/Pacific Islanders

Be aware that drugs are part of the yin/yang belief system embraced by some Asian Americans and that herbal remedies may be used in addition to prescription drugs.
Be sure to consider lower body weight and mass when calculating doses.

Narcotic Analgesics	Chinese may be less sensitive to the respiratory depressant and hypotensive effects of morphine but more likely to experience nausea. Chinese have a significantly higher clearance of morphine.
Antihypertensives	Respond best to calcium antagonists
Neuroleptics	Require lower dose
Psychotropics	Require lower dose, sometimes as little as one-half the normal dose for TCAs and lithium.

TABLE 2-8 *(Continued)*

Drug Category	Remarks
Fat-soluble drugs	On average, Asian Americans have a lower percentage of body fat so dosage adjustments must be made for fat-soluble vitamins and other drugs, e.g., Vitamin K used to reverse the anticoagulant effect of Coumadin (warfarin). Consider dietary intake of vitamins when calculating doses.

Hispanics

Psychotropics	May require lower dosage and experience higher incidence of side effects with TCAs.

Greeks, Italians and others of Mediterranean Descent with G-6-PD Deficiency

Oxidating Drugs	The following drugs may precipitate a hemolytic crisis: primaquine quinidine, thiazolsulfone, furzolidone, nitrofural, naphthalene, toluidine blue, phenylhydrazine, chloramphenicol. Aspirin

Jewish Americans (Ashkenazi)

Psychotropics	20 percent develop agranulocytosis when clozapine is used to treat schizophrenia; thus, the granulocyte count should be checked before administering the drug.

Native Americans

Muscle Relaxants	Alaskan Eskimos may suffer prolonged muscle paralysis and an inability to breathe without mechanical ventilation for several hours post-op when succinylcholine has been administered in surgery.

Table based partially on data from:

Caraco, Y., Langerstrom, P.O., & Wood, A.J. (1996). Ethnic and genetic determinants of omeprazole and effect. *Clinical Pharmacology and Therapeutics, 60(2)*, 157–167.

Lawson, W.B. (1996). Clinical issues in the pharmacotherapy of African-Americans. *Psychopharmacology Bulletin, 32(2)*, 275–281.

Lin, K., Anderson, D., & Poland, R. (1995). Ethnicity and psychopharmacology: Bridging the gap. *Psychiatric Clinics of North America, 18(3)*, 635–647.

Rudorfer, M. (1993). Pharmacokinetics of psychotropic drugs in special populations. *Journal of Psychiatry, 54(4) supplement*, 50–54.

Tornatore, K.M., Biocevich, D.M., Reed, K., Tousley, K., Singh, J.P., & Venuto, R.C. (1995). *Transplantation, 59(5)*, 729–736.

Zhou, H.H., Sheller, J.R., Nu, H., Wood, M., & Wood, A.J.J. (1993). Ethnic differences in response to morphine. *Clinical Pharmacology and Therapeutics, 54(3)*, 507–513.

and/or (2) an effect on the ratio of active and inactive metabolites present in the bloodstream (resulting in slower metabolism). Slow metabolizers require decreased dosages to reduce side effects and toxicity.

Differences in pharmacokinetics may be genetic or may be due to environmental influences. According to Lin et al. (1995), up to one-third of African Americans and 19 to 32 percent of Asian Americans may be poor debrisoquine metabolizers compared with 2.9 to 10 percent of whites. In contrast, 18 to 22 percent of African Americans and Asians are poor mephenytoin metabolizers compared with 3 percent of whites. There also is evidence of variability in protein binding based on ethnicity. Habits such as smoking and drinking alcohol are known to speed drug metabolism, whereas a low-protein, high-carbohydrate diet is known to slow metabolism. The fact that whites and African Americans drink significantly more alcohol than Asians and eat differently may provide an environmental explanation for the greater drug impact experienced by Asian clients. Furthermore, the expense of developing racial or ethnic norms could become prohibitive for pharmaceutical companies, a group that already is required to meet stringent clinical testing standards before it can legally manufacture and sell new drugs.

Because African Americans are more likely to be overdiagnosed as having a psychotic illness, psychotropic medication may be overprescribed. Poorer adherence to recommended regimens, delays in seeking treatment, higher prescribed dosages, and more PRN use of medication by providers add to ethnic differences in treatment outcomes. African Americans also are at greater risk for medication side effects and adverse reactions. These problems may be exacerbated by ethnic differences in pharmacokinetics. Some of the more recently developed drugs may be more helpful for nonwhites because they are better tolerated, produce fewer side effects, and have better efficacy.

African American clients are significantly misdiagnosed as psychotic, viewed as more violent by staff, and spend more time in seclusion than whites, Hispanics, or Asians. Thus the actual dose of medication prescribed for African American clients may be more a function of staff perception than a decision based on serum levels or clinical observations (Keltner & Folks, 1992; Lawson, 1996).

Perception of Side Effects

Research indicates that there are wide variations in the perception of side effects by clients from diverse cultural backgrounds. The reason for the variation may be due to metabolic differences that result in higher or lower levels of the drug circulating in the system, to individual differences such as amount of body fat, and/or cultural differences in the way individuals from diverse backgrounds interpret the meaning of clinical manifestations related to side effects and toxicity.

Cultural Influences on Patient Behavior

It should be noted that terms such as *compliance* and *noncompliance* have a negative connotation, and their use is problematic. The underlying assumption in labeling a client *noncompliant* is that the health care provider knows what is best for client, has effectively communicated his/her advice. It also assumes that the client understood the advice and agrees that the drug will be efficacious. When clients fail to do what you suggest, recommend or order, you may be tempted to label the behavior as *noncompliant*. When clients seem to disregard our advice, perhaps it would be useful to examine our communication and other aspects of the nurse-client interaction critically for an explanation. We might ask ourselves, Why *should* the client comply? Have I clearly explained *why* the person should follow my recommendations to achieve his/her health-related goals? Are cultural factors, personal preferences, mental/ cognitive status, or other variables contributing to the person's refusal to follow my advice? Are there more culturally appropriate alternative approaches that will accomplish the same goal? A less empirical but real consideration is the issue of the client's confidence and trust in the health care provider. Based on a combination of historical fact and myth, some African American, Hispanic, and Southeast Asian clients have little confidence or trust in white health care providers. This may be the result of cross-cultural differences in values, communication, and health related practices or a more generalized mistrust of authority figures, especially for immigrants from war-ravaged nations.

If the medication prescribed, its route of administration, or the substances given with it conflict with clients' yin/yang, hot/cold or other belief system, it is unlikely that they will follow our advice concerning the medication. You should be aware that some clients of Hispanic, Middle Eastern and Asian heritage believe that it is important to take medicine with certain beverages or foods in order to provide the necessary balance for health. If the client gives cues that he/she is uncomfortable with the beverage or food being used in the health care setting, you should discuss alternatives. For example, in most health care facilities, medications are given with cold water, but they could be given with hot water, tea, coffee or similars drink if the client believes his/her healing would be promoted. Some Mexican Americans believe that grapefruit juice has healing properties, so you might contact the dietary department to assure that this type of juice is available when medications are administered. If the cultural healing beliefs and practices of the client are incorporated into the medication administration, there is a higher probability that the client will believe in the healing properties of the drugs and will continue to take them as prescribed after discharge.

When planning for a patient's discharge or reviewing a home care patient's medications, you should provide clients with verbal and written information about their medications including the reasons for them, dosage, route of administration, side effects, toxicity, and the length of time they will need to take the drugs. For antibiotics, antihypertensives and other drugs that must be taken regardless of the presence of obvious symptoms, you must be sure that the patient (and significant others involved in the person's care) understand the rationale for continuing the medicine. This is especially important for clients such as some Chinese Americans whose traditional health beliefs consider medicine necessary only as long as the symptom persists.

Anxiety, cross-cultural miscommunication, and language differences may prevent clients from understanding your instructions about medications. After discussing medications, you should verify that clients have understood the instructions by asking them to repeat or demonstrate them. A return demonstration is essential for medicines given by injection. Ask the client about significant others who may be responsible for his/her injections at home or who may share the responsibility with the client. Be sure to include these individuals when teaching the client about medications. Although many clients will express reluctance or anxiety when drugs are administered by vaginal or rectal routes, those from Hispanic, Middle Eastern, and Asian cultures may have additional cultural reasons. For example, discussion of the reproductive anatomy and physiology may not be considered an appropriate topic for discussion or cultural norms for modesty may be affronted. Non-English–speaking clients may be unfamiliar with the genitourinary terminology, which usually is not among the first vocabulary words taught in English language courses! In requesting a return demonstration for medications administered vaginally or rectally or those applied topically to the genitalia, you should be aware of the gender sensitivities discussed previously. In some instances, it may be advisable to have a health care provider of the same gender for instructional purposes.

Complementary or Alternative Health Care Systems

Some clients rely on more than one health care system to promote health, prevent disease, and convalesce from acute and chronic illnesses. According to Micozzi (1996), a *health care system* must include a developed theory of the body-person that includes the causes and treatments of malfunction, education of new practitioners, a subsystem that delivers care to the needy, a means of producing substances or technologies necessary to deliver care and educate practitioners, a legal mandate that provides for the official recognition of practitioners and maintains minimum practice standards, and a social mandate that reveals levels of community acceptance as evidenced by frequency of use, willingness to pay, and so forth. In recent years there has been a growing awareness among professional health care providers that *complementary* or *alternative* health care systems co-exist with Western biomedicine. Chinese and Ayurvedic medicine, curanderismo, homeopathic, osteopathic, chiropractic and naturopathic medicine, aromatherapy, reflexology, light therapy, and herbalism are a few of the many systems that clients may use. Due to its long-standing history, widespread global influence and large number of followers, we will examine traditional Chinese medicine as one example of a complementary or alternative health care system.

Traditional Chinese Medicine

Traditional Chinese medicine includes herbal remedies, diet therapy, acupuncture, moxibustion (application of heat), therapeutic massage, skin scraping or coining (rubbing a wet, blunt object over the skin to reinforce body points and channels), cupping (placing a small bottle or cup on the skin to create a gentle suction), use of animal secretions and organs, and other interventions aimed at treating the symptoms of disease.

The notion of balancing the two opposing energies of *yin* and *yang* is derived from the ancient Tao philosophy that posits that *harmony* is necessary for the body to function properly. Chinese herbal medicine has been used for centuries. Its continued popularity is evident in neighborhood stores such as those found in the Chinatowns of large cities and in the proliferation of internet sites that provide information on the more prevalent herbs including ways to order them electronically or by mail.

Many of the active ingredients in the herbs are unknown and remain largely unregulated by government agencies, except for customs officials who make efforts to control the flow of illegal drugs. There are five categories of Chinese medicines based on their taste: sour, bitter, sweet, peppery, or salty. There are eight functions or uses for these medicines: perspiration inducing, emetic, purgatory, neutralizing,

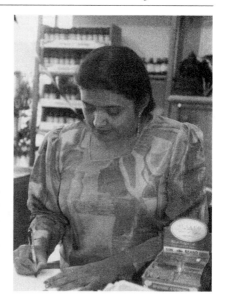

Shopkeeper of Indian ancestry sells herbal remedies used in Ayurvedic healing in a neighborhood
store that attracts recent immigrants from India.
People from diverse backgrounds who embrace
Ayurvedic medicine also patronize the store which
sells pre-packaged herbal remedies or dried herbs
used when brewing teas.

stimulating, heat clearing, deflecting (to correct stagnation or dissolve clots and
phlegm), and yin and yang stimulating (tonic method drugs). Fresh or dried herbs
are usually brewed into a tea, with the dosage adjusted according to the chronicity
or acuteness of illness, age, and size of the patient. Traditional Chinese medicine
usually is used only as long as symptoms persist. Some patients extend the same logic
to Western biomedicine. For example, they may stop taking an antibiotic as soon as
the symptoms subside rather than completing the course of treatment for the prescribed length of time.

Although not all drug properties of each herb are known, some are more popularly
used and known in the U.S. and Canada (see **Table 2-9**). When known, their potential
interaction with Western medicines should be considered. The root of the shrub
ginseng, for example, is widely used for the treatment of arthritis, back and leg pains,
and sores. Because ginseng is known to potentiate the action of some antihypertensive
drugs, you must ask if the patient if he/she is experiencing side effects or toxicity
and monitor blood pressure frequently. It may be necessary to withhold doses of the
Western antihypertensive medicine if the blood pressure is low or ask the client to
discontinue or reduce the strength of the ginseng. When assessing the patient's use
of traditional Chinese medicine, you should be aware that some Chinese Americans
who use herbs topically do not consider them to be drugs. For further information
about the herbs, the nurse should ask the patient and family, consult with an herbalist,
search for reputable sources on the internet, or check reference books such as *The
Barefoot Doctor's Manual* (distributed by the U. S. Department of Health and Human
Services—see **Appendix B**—for address and phone number). Many pharmacists are
familiar with the active ingredients of herbal remedies, their uses, side effects, toxicity

TABLE 2-9
Herbal Remedies

Aloe Vera
Aloe vera

Source:	Leaf of *Aloe barbadensis* Mill. (family Liliaceae)
Action:	topical analgesic, anti-inflammatory, antibacterial, and antifungal agent
Traditional Uses:	Applied topically for treatment of inflammation, minor burns, sunburn, cuts, bruises and abrasions.
	Orally, aloe juice was used for gastrointestinal upset, arthritis, diabetes mellitus and gastric ulcers
Current Uses:	Promotes wound healing in soft tissue injuries
	Prevents wound pain by inhibiting the action of the pain-producing agent bradykinin
	May prevent progression of skin damage from electrical burns and frostbite
	Prevention of wound infection due to antibacterial and antifungal properties
	Used in a wide variety of ointments, creams, lotions and shampoos
Dosage:	Apply topically PRN
Warnings:	Rarely, skin rash follows topical application
	May cause burning if applied after removal of acne scars
	To avoid deterioration of active ingredients, use the fresh gel and avoid diluted extracts.
	When taken internally as *aloe latex*, it causes intestinal cramping, and may lead to ulcers and bowel irritation.

Dong-Quai (Chinese Angelica)
Angelica sinensis

Source:	Dried root of a member of the parsley family.
Action:	Smooth muscle relaxant; antispasmodic
Traditional Uses:	A highly regarded herb in Chinese medicine, Dong-Quai means "proper order." Used to suppress menstruation, cleanse the blood and promote harmony in the body.
	In the West, used to regulate menstrual periods, symptoms of menopause and premenstrual syndrome (PMS).
Current Uses:	Relaxes uterine muscle and improves circulation to the uterus.
	Improves circulation and lowers blood pressure. Reduces inflammation, pains and spasm; increases number of RBCs and platelets.
	Protects liver from toxins.
Dosage:	5–12 g (1 to 3 teaspoons) daily
Warnings:	Contraindicated for pregnant and breastfeeding women and persons with abdominal distention or diarrhea.
	Large doses may cause contact dermatitis and photodermatitis.

Echinacea
Echinacea angustifolia, E. pallida, E. pururea

Source:	Member of the daisy family. Also known as purple cone flower.
Action:	Reduces cold symptoms
Traditional Uses:	Used by Native Americans in poultices, mouthwashes and teas for colds, cancer and other disorders.
	Some herbalists consider it a blood purifier and an aid to fighting infections
Current Uses:	Enhances the immune system by stimulating the production of WBCs needed to fight infection or cancer
Dosage:	Follow directions on label. Needed at onset of symptoms. Usually taken for no longer than 2 weeks

TABLE 2-9 (Continued)

Warnings:	Contraindicated for pregnant or breast-feeding v
	to ragweed
	Not recommended for people with severely co
	with HIV/AIDS, tuberculosis or multiple scler
	Look for reputable suppliers as a high percent
	adulterated with less expensive inactive sul

70   Part One—Transcultural   TABLE 2-9 (Continue   Ginseng (Ameri   Panax quinquefol   Panax gingeng   Source: Action: Tradit

Evening Primrose Oil
Oenothera biennis

Source:	Seeds of the wildflower Evening Primrose
Action:	Antihypertensive, immunostimulant, weight
Traditional Uses:	Used by Native Americans for food. In East
	hemorrhoids. New settlers to North Ame...
	and sore throats.
Current Uses:	Used as a dietary supplement for essential fatty acids. Believed to help asthma, ...g
	headaches, inflammations, premenstrual syndrome (PMS), diabetes mellitus, and arthritis.
	Also believed to lower blood pressure and lower cholesterol; slow the progression of
	multiple sclerosis; promote weight loss without dieting; alleviate hangovers; and
	moisturize dry eyes, brittle hair and fingernails.
Dosage:	Follow directions on label. Will take at least one month to experience benefits.
Warnings:	Side effects include occasional reports of headache, nausea and abdominal discomfort. Not
	recommended for children.
	Some capsules may be altered with other types of oil such as soy or safflower.

Ginger

Current Uses:	Effective in reducing morning sickness and post-operative nausea for some people. Used in
	China to treat first and second degree burns.
Dosage:	Boil 1 ounce dried ginger root in 1 cup water for 15 to 20 minutes
	Follow label directions on ginger supplements
Warning:	Large doses may cause CNS depression and cardiac arrythmias
	Side effects include heartburn
	Contraindicated in the presence of gall bladder disease

Gingko
Gingko biloba

Source:	Extract from leaves of the gingko tree, a living fossil, believed to be more than 200 million
	years old
Action:	Antioxidant; improves blood circulation
Traditional Uses:	Used in China since the 15th century for cough, asthma, diarrhea, skin lesions and removal
	of freckles
Current Uses:	Promotes vasodilation and improves circulation of blood
	May be an effective free radical scavenger or antioxidant
	Improves short-term memory, attention span and mood in early stages of Alzheimer's
	disease by improving oxygen metabolism in the brain
Dosage:	Range: 120–160 mg t.i.d.
	May take 6–8 weeks before results are evident
Warnings:	Large doses may cause irritability, restlessness, diarrhea, nausea and vomiting.
	Some people (who are also sensitive to poison ivy) are unable to tolerate even low doses
	Contraindicated for women who are pregnant or breast-feeding.
	Contraindicated for persons with clotting disorders
	Not recommended for children

(continued)

d)

an and Asian)
us (American)
(Asian)

Dried root of several species of the genus *Panax* of the family Aralaceae.
Tonic

onal Uses: Treatment of anemia, atherosclerosis, edema, ulcers, hypertension, influenza, colds, inflammation, and disorders of the immune system (American)

In traditional China, used for treatment of shock, diaphoresis, dyspnea, fever, thirst, irritability, diarrhea, vomiting abdominal distention, anorexia, and impotence. Considered a "heat raising" tonic for the blood and circulatory system (Asian)

Current Uses: Used to enhance sexual experience and treat impotence, though there is no current research to support this claim (American)

In Germany may be labeled as a tonic to treat fatigue, reduced work capacity, lack of concentration and for convalescence (Asian)

Improved sense of well-being (Asian)

Dosage: American: Follow directions on label
Asian: 100 mg B.I.D.

Warnings: American: May cause headaches, insomnia, anxiety, breast tenderness, rashes, asthma attacks, hypertension, cardiac arrhythmias, and post-menopausal uterine hemorrhage.

Should be used with caution for the following conditions: pregnancy, insomnia, hay fever, fibrocystic breasts, asthma, emphysema, hypertension, clotting disorders, and diabetes mellitus.

Asian: Same as American

Gotu-Kola
Centella asiatica

Source: Dried and powdered leaves of a member of the parsley family
Action: Improves memory
Traditional Uses: In ancient India, considered a rejuvenating herb that increases intelligence, longevity, and memory while slowing the aging process

In China, used as a tea for colds, lung and urinary tract infections and topically for snakebite, wounds and shingles

Recommended for treatment of mental disorders, hypertension, abscesses, rheumatism, fever,ulcers, skin lesions, and jaundice.

Current Uses: Acceleration of wound healing
Diuretic
Treatment of phlebitis

Dosage: Follow directions on label. Lower dose needed for children and older adults.
Warnings: Side effects include headaches and skin rash
Contraindicated for pregnant or breast-feeding women and children under 2 years.
Contraindicated when using tranquilizers or sedatives

Saint John's Wort
Hypericum perforatum

Source: Tea made from the leaves and flowering tops of the perennial *Hypericum perforatum*, which is particularly abundant on June 24th, the feast of St. John the Baptist.
Action: Antidepressant

TABLE 2-9 *(Continued)*

Traditional uses:	Used in 1st century Greece for wound healing, menstrual disorders, and as a diuretic
	In 19th century North America, used its astringent, wound healing, diuretic, and mild sedative effects.
Current Uses:	Treatment of mild to moderate depression. Effects are linked to various substances that act as monoamine oxidase (MAO) inhibitors
Dosage:	300 mg daily
Warnings:	Fair-skinned people may develop urticaria or vesicular skin lesions upon exposure to sunlight.
	Clinical manifestations of depression should be considered seriously.
	Encourage client to see a mental health care provider.

Valerian
Valeriana officianalis

Source:	Dried rhizome and roots of the tall perennial, *Valeriana officinalis.*
Action:	Mild tranquilizer and sedative
Traditional Uses:	Used by the ancient Greeks for the treatment of epilepsy and menstrual disorders, and as a diuretic.
	Used by 17th and 18th century Europeans as an antispasmodic and sedative.
	Listed as an official remedy in the U.S. Pharmacopoeia from 1820–1936
Current Uses:	Used as a mild tranquilizer and sedative. Relieves muscle spasms.
	Especially effective for insomniacs and older adults.
Dosage:	300–400 mg daily. Take 1 hour before bedtime as a sleeping aid.
Warnings:	Reported side effects include headache, gastrointestinal upset, and excitability.
	Signs of overdose include severe headache, restlessness, nausea, morning grogginess, or blurred vision.
	Must not be taken in combination with other tranquilizers or sedatives.
	Client should be cautioned against operating a motor vehicle after ingesting.

Table developed using data from:
Bremness, L. (1994). *Herbs.* New York: Dorling Kindersley.

Foster, S. (1996). *Herbs for you health.* Loveland, CO: Interweave Press.

Monte, T. (1997). *The complete guide to natural healing.* New York: Berkeley Publishing Group.

Tyler, V.E. (1994). *Herbs of choice: The therapeutic use of phytomedicinals.* New York: Pharmaceutical Products Press.

and interactions with Western prescription or over-the-counter drugs, or they can refer the nurse to reliable sources of information.

Analysis of Cultural Data

Your analysis should include identification of daily activities the client can perform (1) without your assistance; (2) with the assistance of a family member or significant other; (3) with the assistance of a folk, indigenous or traditional healer; (4) with the assistance of a paid but unlicensed health care provider; (5) with the assistance of a nurse or other licensed health care provider; and (6) with assistance from a combination of these.

Clinical Decision Making and Nursing Actions

After you have completed a comprehensive cultural assessment, you are ready to analyze your subjective and objective data, set mutual goals with the client, develop a plan of care, make referrals as needed, and implement a plan of care, either alone or with others. Before making clinical decisions or taking an action, you should identify the client's strengths and limitations, including his or her social support network—family, friends, clergy and other health visitors from the client's place of worship, ethnic or cultural organizations, or other sources that can be mobilized to assist the client. Next, you will want to determine if there are client goals or needs for which professional nursing care is required.

Leininger (1991) suggests three major modalities to guide nursing judgments, decisions, and actions for the purpose of providing culturally congruent care that is beneficial, satisfying, and meaningful to the people nurses serve. The three modes are *cultural preservation and/or maintenance, cultural care accommodation and/or negotiation*, and *cultural care repatterning and/or restructuring*. Let us briefly examine each of these modes.

Cultural preservation and/or maintenance refers to "those assistive, supporting, facilitative, or enabling professional actions and decisions that help people of a particular culture to retain and/or preserve relevant care values so that they can maintain their well-being, recover from illness, or face handicaps and/or death" (Leininger, 1991a, p. 48; see also Jackson, 1993).

Cultural care accommodation and/or negotiation refers to "those assistive, supporting, facilitative, or enabling creative professional actions and decisions that help people of a designated culture to adapt to, or to negotiate with, others for beneficial or satisfying health outcome with professional careproviders" (Leininger, 1991, p. 48). Cultural negotiation is sometimes referred to as *culture brokering* (Chalanda, 1995; DeSantis, 1994; Jackson, 1993; Jezewski, 1990, 1993).

Cultural care repatterning and/or restructuring refers to "those assistive, supporting, facilitative, or enabling professional actions and decisions that help a client(s) reorder, change, or greatly modify their lifeways for new, different, and beneficial health care pattern while respecting the client(s) cultural values and beliefs and still providing a beneficial or healthier lifeway than before the changes were coestablished with the client(s)" (Leininger, 1991, p. 49).

These modes are care-centered and based on use of the client's care knowledge. Negotiation increases understanding between the client and the nurse and promotes culturally congruent nursing care.

Cultural Empathy

As indicated in **Figure 2-2** sociocultural factors, ethnocentrism, cultural biases, prejudice, and cultural stereotypes combine with attitudes, values, beliefs, and practices about health, healing, illness and role expectations held by the nurse and client.

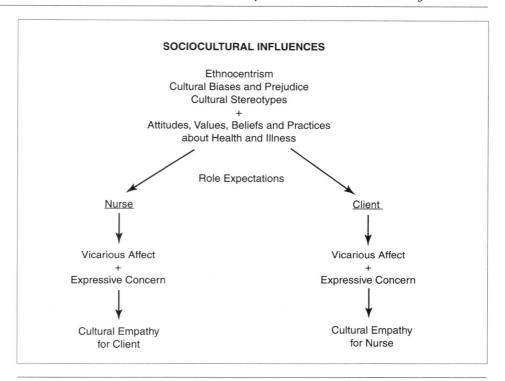

FIGURE 2-2. Framework for understanding empathy in the cultural context of nurse-client interactions.

According to Pedersen, et al. (1996), two affective processes are involved in *cultural empathy*: *vicarious affect* and *expressive concern*. Beyond our universal desire to understand one another is a desire to communicate to others our understanding of them. The challenge of transcultural nurse-client interactions is for individuals of different traditions to express their empathy in ways that each one recognizes.

Vicarious affect refers to your ability to experience "as" clients experience instead of "how" they experience themselves. Regardless of race or culture, nobody can ever feel exactly as another does. You can, however, use your own subjective experience as a reference for empathizing. You can explore possible feelings, thoughts, behaviors, sensations, beliefs and the links joining them, some of which the client may experience below conscious awareness. These vicarious experiences should be verified with the client to assure their validity. You should be careful to avoid indicating that you understand. Rather, you should encourage the client to continue expressing his/her feelings.

Expressive concern refers to your ability to emote feelings that indicate genuine interest in the struggles, challenges, and conflicts surrounding the client's health-related problems. You also express affirmation at the achievements and successes of your clients. Unless you express an attitude of genuine concern, clients are unlikely to perceive that you care.

Evaluation

Evaluation of the effectiveness of clinical decisions and nursing actions should occur in collaboration with the client and his or her significant others—which may include members of the extended family, traditional healers, those with culturally determined, nonsanguine relationships, and friends. A careful evaluation of each component of the transcultural nursing interaction should be undertaken in collaboration with the client. It may be necessary to gather further data, reinterpret existing findings, redefine mutual nurse-client goals, or renegotiate roles and responsibilities of nurses, clients and members of their support system.

The previous discussion has focused, to large extent, on the individual during the period of hospitalization or when being cared for by nurses in the home or community environment. Next, we will look at the issue of evaluation after discharge. In the current managed care environment, there is growing emphasis on patient or client *outcomes* and reported satisfaction with the care provided by nurses and other health care providers. You need to participate in the establishment of *quality assurance*, *total quality management*, and/or *continuous quality improvement* initiatives aimed at gathering information from clients/patients about their overall satisfaction with care. You also need to assure that the process and instruments are culturally appropriate. For example, how are the needs of linguistically diverse clients met? Is translation or interpretation available? Are the questions asked in a culturally appropriate manner? It is imperative that nurses be included in all aspects of the evaluation and that they use feedback to improve their nursing care in the future.

Summary

In this chapter the knowledge and skill needed to develop cultural competencies have been examined. All nursing care is transcultural because people are cultural beings. Culture values, cross-cultural communication, cultural assessment, traditional healers, cultural perceptions of symptoms, biocultural variations in health and illness, clinical decision making and nursing actions, cultural empathy and evaluation of care were explored.

Review Questions

1. Identify the key components in the process and content of a cultural assessment.
2. Analyze the differences in body proportions, height, and weight among clients from diverse cultural backgrounds and indicate the reasons for differences among the groups.
3. Compare and contrast your approach to the assessment of light- and dark-skinned clients for cyanosis, jaundice, pallor, erythema, and petechiae.
4. Review the biocultural variations in laboratory tests for hemoglobin, hematocrit, serum cholesterol, serum transferrin, multiple-marker screeing, and amniotic fluid constituents.

5. Critically analyze the reasons for the current interest in ethnopharmacology by nurses, physicians, pharmacists, and other health care providers. How does knowledge of ethnopharmacology and cultural differences in response to medications facilitate the your ability to provide culturally competent and congruent nursing care?

6. Critically examine the strategies for promoting effective cross-cultural communication between nurses and clients in overcoming communication barriers. What can you do to communicate effectively with non-English–speaking clients?

Learning Activities to Promote Critical Thinking

1. Critically analyze the instrument, tool or form used by nurses when conducting an initial patient or resident *admission assessment* at a hospital, extended care facility, or other health care agency in terms of its relevance to the health and nursing needs of persons from diverse cultures. From a transcultural nursing perspective, identify the *strengths* and *limitations* of the admission assessment instrument. What suggestions would you make to enhance the effectiveness of the instrument in assessing the cultural needs of newly admitted patients or residents? Be sure to consider the *practical* constraints that nurses face in the current managed care environment, such as time limitations, external forces that require us care for increasingly large numbers of patients, and so forth before suggesting modifications.

2. In order to provide culturally competent nursing care, you should engage in a cultural self-assessment. Answer the questions in **Box 2-1**, *How Do You Relate to Various Groups of People in Society?* and score your answers using the guide provided. What did you learn about yourself? How would you learn more about the background of those groups mentioned, including information about their health-related beliefs and practices? What resources might you use in your search for information?

3. Using the **Andrews/Boyle Transcultural Nursing Assessment Guide** (Appendix A), answer the questions in each data category as they apply to *yourself*. As you write your responses to the questions, critically reflect on your own health-related cultural values, attitudes, beliefs and practices.

4. Using the **Andrews/Boyle Transcultural Nursing Assessment Guide** (Appendix A), interview someone from a cultural background different from your own to assess his/her health-related cultural values, attitudes, beliefs and practices. After you have completed the interview, compare and contrast these responses with your own responses in Question #3. Identify the ways in which you are *alike*. Critically analyze the *differences* as potential sources of cross-cultural conflict and explore ways in which they might influence the nurse-client interaction.

5. Conduct a head-to-toe physical examination of a person from a racial background different from your own. Summarize your findings in writing. In a constructively self-critical manner, reflect on what aspects of the exam

were (a) easiest and (b) most difficult for you. Try to determine the reason(s) why some aspects were relatively easy or difficult for you. What further information or skill development would assist you in gaining confidence in your ability to conduct physical examinations on people from diverse racial backgrounds?

6. The internet is a valuable resource for learning more about the culturally based health-related beliefs and practices of people from diverse backgrounds. During your assessment of a Chinese American patient, you discover that he/she has been seeing an acupuncturist for low back pain. Although you have a general knowledge of acupuncture, you would like to search the internet for further information.

a. How will you go about searching for information on this subject? What search engines and key words are likely to lead you to the appropriate sites?

b. Once you have visited an internet site, what criteria will you use to evaluate it? For example, how will you determine the accuracy of the information, credibility of the source, biases, and so forth?

c. If you encountered any technical difficulties using the internet (e.g., unable to login, print, or download files), examine the reasons for them.

d. After you have completed the exercise, critically examine the results of your search. Did you obtain the amount and quality of information that you desired on the topic? As a professional nurse, were you satisfied with the level at which the information was presented and its depth? What unanswered questions remain? What other sources of information might you use to answer them?

References

Chalanda, M. (1995). Brokerage in multicultural nursing. *International Nursing Review, 42(1)*, 19–22.

DeSantis, L. (1994). Making anthropology clinically relevant to nursing care. *Journal of Advanced Nursing, 23*, 564–570.

Farnsworth, N. R. (1993). Ethnopharmacology and future drug development: the North American experience. *Journal of Ethnopharmacology, 38*, 145–152.

Good, B. J., & Good, M. J. (1980). The meaning of symptoms: A cultural hermeneutic model for clinical practice. In L. Eisenberg & A. Kleinman (Eds.). *The Relevance of Social Science for Medicine*. Boston: D. Reidel.

Hall, E. (1963). Proxemics: The study of man's spatial relationships. In I. Gladstone (Ed.). *Man's Image in Medicine and Anthropology*, pp. 109–120. New York: International University Press.

Jackson, L. E. (1993). Understanding, eliciting and negotiating clients' multicultural beliefs. *Nurse Practitioner, 18(4)*, 30–43.

Jarvis, C. (1996). *Physical Examination and Health Assessment*. Philadelphia: W. B. Saunders, Co.

Jezewski, M. A. (1993). Culture brokering as a model for advocacy. *Nursing and Health Care, 14(2)*, 78–85.

Jezewski, M. A. (1990). Culture brokering in migrant farmworker health care. *Western Journal of Nursing Research, 12(4)*, 497–513.

Keltner, N. L., & Folks, D. G. (1992). Psychopharmacology update: Culture as a variable in drug therapy. *Perspectives in Psychiatric Care, 28(1)*, 33–36.

Kleinman, A. (1980). *Patients and Healers in the Context of Culture*. Berkeley, CA: University of California Press.

Kleinman, A., Eisenberg, L., & Good, B. (1978). Culture, illness and care: Clinical lessons from anthropologic and cross-cultural research. *Annals of Internal Medicine, 88*, 251–258.

Lapierre, E. D., & Padgett, J. (1991). How can we become more aware of culturally specific body language and use this awareness therapeutically? *Journal of Psychosocial Nursing, 29(11)*, 38–41.

Lawson, W. B. (1996). Clinical issues in the pharmacotherapy of African-Americans. *Pharmacology Bulletin, 32(2)*, 275–81.

Leininger, M. M. (1978). *Transcultural Nursing: Concepts, Theories, and Practices*. New York: John Wiley & Sons.

Leininger, M. M. (1990). Issues, questions, and concerns related to the nursing diagnosis cultural movement from a transcultural nursing perspective. *Journal of Transcultural Nursing, 2(1)*, 23–32.

Leininger, M. M. (1991). *Culture Care Diversity and Universality: A Theory of Nursing*. New York: National League for Nursing Press.

Leininger, M. M. (1994). Time to celebrate and reflect on progress with transcultural nursing. *Journal of Transcultural Nursing, 6(1),* 2–4.

Leininger, M. M. (1995). *Transcultural Nursing: Concepts, Theories, Research and Practices.* New York: McGraw-Hill, Inc.

Leininger, M. M. (1997). Founder's focus flternative to what? Generic vs. professional caring, treatments and healing modes. *Journal of Transcultural Nursing, 91(1),* 37.

Levin, S. (1966). Effect of age, ethnic background and disease on sweat chloride. *Israeli Journal of Medical Science, 2(3),* 333–337.

Lin, K., Anderson, D., & Poland, R. E. (1995). Ethnicity and pharmacology. *Psychiatric Clinics of North America, 18(3),* 635–646.

Lipson, J. G., & Steiger, N. J. (1996). *Self-care Nursing in a Multicultural Context.* Thousand Oaks, CA: Sage Publications.

Meleis, A. L., Lipson, J. G., & Paul, S. M. (1992). Ethnicity and health among five Middle Eastern immigrant groups. *Nursing Research, 41(2),* 98–103.

Micozzi, M.S. (1996). *Fundamentals of Complementary and Alternative Medicine.* New York: Churchill Livingstone.

Orque, M. S., Bloch, B., & Monrroy, L. A. (1983). *Ethnic Nursing Care.* St. Louis: C. V. Mosby.

Overfield, T. (1995). *Biologic Variation in Health and Illness.* New York: CRC Press.

Pedersen, P. B., Draguns, J. G., Lonner, W. J., & Trimble, J. E. (Eds.). (1996). *Counseling Across Cultures.* (4th ed.) Thousand Oaks, CA: Sage Publications.

United States Department of Health and Human Services, Public Health Service. (1992). *Health People 2000.* Boston: Jones and Bartlett Publishers.

Watson, O. M. (1980). *Proxemic Behavior: A Cross Cultural Study.* The Hague, Netherlands: Mouton Press.

Wenger, A. F. (1993). Cultural meaning of symptoms. *Holistic Nursing Practice, 7(2),* 22–35.

Two

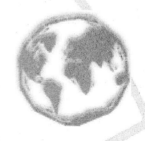

A Developmental Approach to Transcultural Nursing

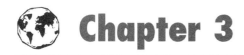

Chapter 3

Childbearing and Transcultural Nursing Care Issues

Jana Lauderdale RN, PhD

OBJECTIVES

1. Analyze how culturally related issues influence behavior of the childbearing woman and her family during pregnancy.
2. Understand one's own cultural values and norms toward members of special populations of childbearing women.
3. Develop an understanding of the care and support necessary for women choosing to experience pregnancy but relinquish their newborns.
4. Examine the needs of the childbearing lesbian couple.
5. Explore the health care and psychological needs of the pregnant incarcerated woman.
6. Increase awareness of the influence cultural beliefs and customs may have on a woman's response to abuse and/or domestic violence during pregnancy.

This chapter will explore the cultural patterns, rituals, and beliefs that may influence the experience of childbirth and childbearing. The experience of the woman as well as of her significant other during pregnancy, birth, and the postpartum are discussed. Recommendations for practice are outlined for nurses caring for childbearing women and their families in each section. Also included are discussions related to culturally specific circumstances and behaviors that can impose risk to the childbearing woman and her family.

Childbearing and Culturally Appropriate Nursing Care

Childbirth is a time of transition and social celebration of central importance in any society, signaling a realignment of existing cultural roles and responsibilities, psychological and biologic states, and social relationships. For some time, these rites of passage have been described as *matrescence* (mother-becoming) and *patrescence* (father-becoming) (Raphael, 1976). The different ways in which a particular society views this transitional period and manages childbirth are dependent on the culture's consensus regarding health, medical care, reproduction, and the role and status of women (Dickason, Silverman & Schult, 1994).

The dominant cultural view of pregnancy and childbirth in the United States is that of pregnancy as a disease or incipient disease state (Johnston, 1980). Health care focuses on the pregnant woman and fetus while the father and other family members or significant others, if they are included at all, are relegated to observer rather than participant status. Dominant cultural practices or rituals in the United States include formal prenatal care (including childbirth classes), ultrasound to view the fetus, and hospital delivery. Monitoring fetal status, inducing labor, providing anesthesia for labor and delivery, and placing the woman in the lithotomy position during the birth are all part of routine hospital care provided in the United States today. A highly specialized group of nurses, obstetricians, perinatologists, and pediatricians actively monitors the mother's physiologic status, delivers the infant, and provides newborn care. However, because there is not total cultural agreement in this country about the value of these practices, some health care providers elect to offer their pregnant clients alternative health care services. These alternatives include in-hospital and free-standing birth centers and care by nurse practitioners and nurse midwives who promote family centered care and emphasize pregnancy as a normal process requiring minimal technologic intervention.

Additionally, there are subcultural groups within the U.S. that have very different practices, values, and beliefs about childbirth and the roles of women, men, social support networks, and health practitioners. These include proponents of the "back to nature" movement, who are often vegetarian, use lay midwives for home deliveries, and practice herbal or naturopathic medicine. Other groups that may have distinct cultural practices include African Americans, Native Americans, Hispanics, Middle Eastern groups, and Asians among others. Additionally, religious background, regional variations, age, urban or rural background, sexual preferences, and other individual characteristics all may contribute to cultural differences in the experience of childbirth.

Great variations exist in the social class, ethnic origin, family structure, and social support networks of women, men, and families in the United States. Despite these differences, many health care providers assume that the changes in status and rites of passage associated with pregnancy and birth are experienced similarly by all people. In addition, it has long been a concern that the individual or cultural experiences of mother-becoming or father-becoming are frequently disrupted by the emphasis of Western medicine on obstetric technology (Milinaire, 1974; Arms, 1975; Wertz & Wertz, 1977). In addition, many of the traditional cultural beliefs, values, and practices related to childbirth have been viewed by some professional nurses as "old fashioned" or "old wives' tales." Although these customs are changing rapidly, many women and families are attempting to preserve their own valued patterns of experiencing childbirth. For many years, we have understood that nurses and other health professionals must begin to incorporate individuals beliefs and cultural practices into health care in order to reduce some of the cultural conflict and begin to humanize American obstetrics (McClain, 1982).

Pregnancy and Culture

All cultures recognize pregnancy as a special transition period, and many have particular customs and beliefs that dictate activity and behavior during pregnancy. Ford (1964), Mead and Newton (1967), Newton and Newton (1972), and Oakley (1980) have reviewed childbirth from a cross-cultural perspective, surveying literature from traditional non Western societies as well as from Western cultural groups. Recent literature on childbirth customs in the United States has focused on accounts of differing beliefs and practices relative to pregnancy among varying ethnic groups. This section describes some of the biologic and cultural variations that may influence the provision of nursing care during pregnancy.

Biologic Variations

Knowledge of certain biologic variations resulting from genetic and environmental backgrounds is important for nurses caring for childbearing families. For example, pregnant women who have the sickle cell trait and are heterozygous for the sickle cell gene are at increased risk for asymptomatic bacteriuria and urinary tract infections such as pyelonephritis. This places them at greater than normal risk for premature labor as well (Pritchard, MacDonald, & Gant, 1984). It has been established that although heterozygotes are found most commonly among African Americans (8–14 percent), individuals living in the United States who are of Mediterranean ancestry, as well as of Germanic and Native American descent, may occasionally carry the trait (Overfield, 1985; Thompson & Thompson, 1983). If both parents are heterozygous, there is a 1 in 4 chance that the infant will be born with sickle cell disease. Presently, of children born with sickle cell disease, 50 percent live to adulthood (Dickason, Silverman & Kaplan, 1998) Of those surviving the disease, many experience chronic complications throughout their lives.

Another important biologic variation relative to pregnancy is diabetes mellitus. The incidence of both non–insulin-dependent and gestational diabetes is much higher than normal among some Native American groups, a problem that increases maternal and infant morbidity. Illnesses that are common among European Americans may manifest themselves differently in Native American clients. For example, a Native American woman may have a high blood sugar level but be asymptomatic for diabetes mellitus, and the mortality rate in pregnant Native American women with diabetes is higher than whites. Diabetes during pregnancy, particularly with uncontrolled hyperglycemia, is associated with an increased risk of congenital anomalies, stillbirth, macrosomia, birth injury, cesarean section, neonatal hypoglycemia, and other problems. The incidence of gestational diabetes is 10 to 40 times greater among the Pima and Papago Indians of Arizona that in the general U.S. population (Pettit et al., 1980). Early detection and blood glucose screening are mandatory among high risk populations to reduce complications during pregnancy and childbirth.

Other cultural groups whose members may have health conditions that place women or their fetuses at risk are refugees or immigrants from Southeast Asia. Significant numbers of Thais and Cambodians have abnormal hemoglobins (A2 and E), and it is not uncommon to observe a hemoglobinopathic microcytic anemia coexisting with a dietary or folic acid deficiency anemia. Pregnancies in Southeast Asian women who are recent immigrants to the U.S. may be complicated by parasites (45–75 percent), a reactive venereal disease research laboratory (VDRL) test (signifying treponema syphilis or yaws), tuberculosis (62 percent), and symptomatic or asymptomatic hepatitis screen (HbsAg). Obviously, it is important in these cases to rule out active disease or carrier status. Treatment for these conditions may or may not be undertaken during pregnancy as some of the indicated pharmacologic agents may be embryo toxic (Erickson & Hoang, 1980; Nelson & Hewitt, 1983; Pickwell, 1983; Boehme, 1985).

Korea is another area in Southeast Asia where cultural mores may be putting their pregnant women at risk. Research Application 3-1 describes how and why Korea's upper middle class pregnant women may be at an increased risk of HIV transmission to their unborn fetuses.

Research Application 3-1

HIV Knowledge Among Pregnant Korean Women

Chang, S. (1996). HIV/AIDS related knowledge, attitudes, and preventive behavior of pregnant Korean women. *Image: Journal of Nursing Scholarship* 28(4), 321–324.

Findings indicated Korean women were knowledgeable about the diseases HIV and AIDS but were less knowledgeable about transmission. A group singled out in the study as being at particular risk of HIV transmission to their unborn fetuses were Korea's upper middle class pregnant women. Korean women are tolerant of extramarital sex, which is considered a norm within Confucianism. Foreign travel of Korean businessmen along with their higher socioeconomic status makes extramarital sex affordable within and outside of Korea. Contact with prostitutes is increased, with subsequent exposure of the wife to sexually transmitted diseases. Koreans' belief that to go outside the family for help when caring for a family member with the HIV virus will bring shame to the family increases the need for health care providers to be culturally sensitive. In order to prevent rejection and shame the woman may not reveal her diagnosis, which has obvious implications for prenatal care and subsequent care to the mother and baby.

Clinical Application
- Pregnancy is a time when most pregnant women are very aware of the health of their unborn babies. Education focusing on HIV transmission may be especially meaningful to women during this time.

- As the family is the mainstay of the support system in this culture, every effort must be made to include selected members in the care of the pregnant woman and her education.

Cultural Variations That May Impact Childbearing Outcomes

Alternative Lifestyle Choices

Despite recent cultural changes that have made it more acceptable for women to have careers and pursue alternative lifestyles, the dominant cultural expectation for American women remains motherhood within the context of the nuclear family. Changing cultural expectations have influenced many middle class American women and couples to delay childbearing until their late 20s and early 30s and to have small families. Some single women in their 30s are making choices about childbearing that may not involve a marital relationship.

For another group of mothers who choose not to parent, the choices are not as clear. Infant relinquishment is in direct conflict with American ideal cultural values, suggesting that all parents want a child. Nurses must examine their own cultural values when caring for women in this situation, making certain not to negatively stereotype mothers who decide to relinquish their babies for adoption. The decision to relinquish is a difficult one in the majority of circumstances, and is an experience not forgotten by the birth mother. Not all infant relinquishments are due merely to the mother "not wanting the baby." For example, Native Americans living on reservations have been known to relinquish young and older children in the hopes of their child having "a better life off the reservation." Even with such good intentions, the relinquishment is very difficult for all concerned. In a study of the experience of infant relinquishment by Lauderdale and Boyle (1994), the most common reasons given by birthmothers for relinquishment were strictly altruistic, wanting a better life for the baby than birthmothers believed they could offer and wanting the baby to have both a mother and a father. Box 3-1 lists several areas in which nurses can be supportive of women making this difficult decision.

Lesbian couples bearing children are another subculture of pregnant women with special needs. This group of women face psychosocial dilemmas related to their lifestyle and social stigma. The most common fear reported by lesbian mothers is the fear of unsafe and inadequate care from the practitioner once the mother's sexual orientation is revealed (Logan & Dawkins, 1986; Stevens & Hall, 1988; Stevens & Hall, 1991). This situation will require health care providers to examine their own cultural value system. Keep in mind that lesbian parents are dedicated to bringing a new life safely into the world to love and care for to the best of their ability, the same hopes all parents have for their newborns. There are many similarities in lesbian and heterosexual pregnancies, and the parallels should not be overlooked by health care providers. Issues of sexual activity, psychosocial changes related to attaining the maternal tasks of pregnancy (Rubin, 1984) and birth education all need to be addressed with lesbian couples. Special needs of the lesbian couple requiring assessment include social discrimination, family and social support networks, obstacles in becoming pregnant (i.e., coitus versus artificial insemination), lesbian maternal role development, legal issues of adoption by the partner, and coparenting role management (Tash & Kenney, 1993). In order to meet lesbian parents' special needs and provide sensitive and appropriate care, nurses must come to understand the lifestyle of the lesbian couple and work with them in addressing not only their physical but psychosocial concerns as well. Equally important, nurses must understand their own cultural values and norms and be careful not to impose them on their clients.

Box 3-1. *Considerations in the Care of Relinquishing Birth Mothers*

1. During pregnancy, be open to the discussions of single parenting or adoption; be supportive of the woman's decision.
2. Encourage early and appropriate prenatal care.
3. During hospitalization, acknowledge the adoption as a loss; discuss the grief and grieving process with the birth mother.
4. Accept the birth mother as a "real mother," encourage questions, discuss her hospital expectations.
5. Encourage the midwife and/or obstetrician and the pediatrician to provide follow-up care to the birth mother.
6. Include the birth mother in postpartum teaching as appropriate.
7. Assist with the creation of memories in the form of picture taking, locks of hair, footprints, or other acts that have meaning to the birth mother.
8. If desired by the birth mother, allow a formal closure ceremony. Examples of closure could be a quiet "good-bye" between mother and infant or a prayer with family and clergy present. This is important as it facilitates the grief and grieving process.
9. Following relinquishment, it may be helpful for the birth mother to link with other mothers who have successfully coped with a similiar experience. Support groups can be located in association with hospitals, adoption agencies, and other interested community agencies.
10. Encourage postpartum follow-up so that the birth mother's physical and emotional recovery can be monitored.

Nontraditional Support Systems During Pregnancy

A cultural variation that has important implications is a woman's perception of the need for formalized assistance from health care providers during the antepartum period. Western medicine is generally perceived as having a curative rather than a preventive focus. Indeed, many health care providers view pregnancy as a disaster waiting to happen, a physiologic state that at any moment will become pathologic. Because many American subcultural groups perceive pregnancy as a normal physiologic process, not seeing themselves as ill or in need of the curative services of a doctor, pregnant women in these diverse groups often delay seeking or even neglect to seek prenatal care.

Pregnant women and their partners are placing increased emphasis on the quality of pregnancy and childbirth, and many childbearing women rely on nontraditional support systems. For couples who are married, white, middle class, and infrequent users of their extended family for advice and support in childbirth related matters, this may not be crucial. However, for other cultural groups, including African Americans, Hispanics, Filipinos, Asians, and Native Americans, the family and social network (especially the grandmother or other maternal relatives) are of primary importance in advising and supporting the pregnant woman (Rose, 1978; Bryant, 1982; Lantican & Corona, 1992). It is essential for the nurse to do a thorough cultural assessment in order to ascertain to what extent the pregnant woman utilizes nontraditional support systems and/or Western medicine during her pregnancy. Once this assessment is complete and a trusting relationship established, the woman's pregnancy can be managed taking into consideration all the components that both she and the nurse feel are important for a successful outcome. Refer to Chapters 2 and 10 for a review of the components of the cultural assessment.

An example of how women's perceptions for the need of antepartum care may vary is described in a study by Campanella, Korbin, and Acheson (1993). Fifteen Amish women from Ohio described their perinatal beliefs and how they used the available health care system during a total of 76 pregnancies. Prior to the study, local health care providers commonly believed that Amish women underutilized available prenatal and birth care resources. The Amish women utilized perinatal care based on their beliefs about pregnancy and childbirth and in relation to cost, transportation, and child care. The women reported initiating prenatal care earlier for first pregnancies and progressively later with increasing parity and with the increasing knowledge that pregnancy was indeed a "nonproblematic" condition. However, all the women reported seeking immediate medical attention if a serious problem arose, e.g., bleeding. During pregnancy, vitamins and herbal teas were commonly used in preparation for childbirth and usually were recommended by Amish family members/or midwife. Usual daily routines were encouraged to continue throughout pregnancy. A normal pregnancy course for an Amish woman consisted of following recommendations on vitamin and herb use from family and friends, going to a physician for prenatal care, and finally being delivered out of the hospital (either at home or at the Amish birthing center) by a midwife. Hospitals were spoken of positively in terms of "safety" and "getting additional rest." Negative statements about the hospital experience involved "the lack of privacy" and "high cost." Findings also indicated that Amish women are not opposed to the technologic aspects of childbirth but that they selected modern technology to meet their individual and cultural needs. This study emphasized the need to look beyond conformity and homogeneity when providing health care to the culturally different childbearing woman.

In the preceding examples of nontraditional support during pregnancy, it is evident that women utilize a variety of sources including family, friends, and traditional healers. It is the nurse's responsibility to accurately assess each woman's situation, experience and cultural value system so that culturally competent care can be offered.

Cultural Attempts to Control Pregnancy

Cultural variations also involve beliefs about activities during pregnancy. A *belief* is something held to be actual or true on the basis of a specific rationale or explanatory model. *Prescriptive* beliefs, which are phrased positively, describe expectancies of behavior; the more common *restrictive* beliefs, which are phrased negatively, limit choices and behaviors. Many people believe that the activities of the mother, and to a less extent of the father, are influential on newborn outcome. Box 3-2 describes some prescriptive and restrictive beliefs and taboos that provide cultural boundaries for parental activity during pregnancy. These beliefs are attempts to increase a sense of control over the outcome of pregnancy.

Positive or prescriptive beliefs may involve wearing special articles of clothing, such as the *muneco* worn by some traditional Hispanic women to ensure a safe delivery and prevent morning sickness. Other beliefs and practices involve ceremonies and recommendations about physical and sexual activity. One situation in which a pre-

Box 3-2. *Cultural Beliefs About Activity and Pregnancy*

Prescriptive Beliefs

Remain active during pregnancy to aid the baby's circulation (Crow Indian)

Remain happy to bring the baby joy and good fortune (Pueblo and Navajo Indians, Mexican, Japanese).

Sleep flat on your back to protect the baby (Mexican)

Keep active during pregnancy to ensure a small baby and an easy delivery (Mexican)

Continue sexual intercourse to lubricate the birth canal and prevent a dry labor (Haitian, Mexican)

Continue daily baths and frequent shampoos during pregnancy to produce a clean baby (Filipino)

Restrictive Beliefs

Avoid cold air during pregnancy (Mexican, Haitian, Asian)

Do not reach over your head or the cord will wrap around the baby's neck (African American, Hispanic, white, Asian)

Avoid weddings and funerals or you will bring bad fortune to the baby (Vietnamese)

Do not continue sexual intercourse or harm will come to you and baby (Vietnamese, Filipino, Samoan)

Do not tie knots or braid or allow the baby's father to do so because it will cause difficult labor (Navajo Indian)

Do not sew (Pueblo Indian, Asian)

Taboos

Avoid lunar eclipses and moonlight or the baby may be born with a deformity (Mexican)

Do not walk on the streets at noon or 5 o'clock because this may make the spirits angry (Vietnamese)

Do not join in traditional ceremonies like Yei or Squaw dances or spirits will harm the baby (Navajo Indian)

Do not get involved with persons who cast spells or the baby will be eaten in the womb (Haitian)

Do nt say the baby's name before the naming ceremony or harm might come to the baby (Orthodox Jewish)

Do not have your picture taken because it might cause stillbirth (African American)

---

scriptive belief may cause harm occurs when there is a poor neonatal outcome and the mother blames herself. For example, the mother whose fetus has died from a cord accident and who believed that hanging laundry caused the cord to encircle the baby's neck or body, may suffer severe guilt. The nurse who is sensitive to the mother's anguish might say, "Many people say that if you reach over your head during pregnancy, it will cause the cord to wrap around the baby's neck, Have you heard this belief?" Once the woman responds, the nurse can explore her feelings about the practice. Do others in her family or social support network share her belief? The nurse may share her own views by saying, "I have not read in any medical or nursing books that this practice was related to cord problem, although I know many people share your belief." The discussion can then continue, focusing on the feelings and perceptions of the event as it is experienced by the woman and her family.

Negative or restrictive beliefs are widespread and numerous and include activity, work, and sexual, emotional, and environmental prescriptions. *Taboos*, or restrictions with serious supernatural consequences, include the Orthodox Jewish avoidance of baby showers and divulgence of the infant's name before the infant's official naming ceremony (Bash, 1980). A Hispanic taboo involves the traditional belief that an early baby shower will invite bad luck or *mal ojo*, the evil eye (Kay, 1978; Spector, 1996).

Food Taboos and Cravings

Among many subcultural groups, women perceive little personal control over the outcome of pregnancy except through the avoidance of activities and foods that are considered taboo. The evolvement of food taboos in the pregnant Korean woman's diet is thought to stem from the danger and uncertainty associated with pregnancy and childbirth (Bauwens, 1978). Traditional food taboos included chicken, duck, rabbit, goat, crab, sparrow, pork, and blemished fruit. These foods were not eaten in an attempt to guard the child from unwanted physical characteristics; for example, eating chicken may cause bumpy skin or blemished fruit an unpleasant face (Kim & Mo, 1977). A traditional belief in many cultures is that a pregnant woman must be given the food that she smells to eat, otherwise the fetus will move inside of her and a miscarriage will be the result (Spector, 1996).

In a Hindu woman's life pregnancy is considered a hot period. Hot foods (i.e., animal products, chilies, spices, and ginger) and gas-producing foods are avoided because they are believed to cause over excitement, inflammatory reactions, sweating, and fatigue. If eaten too early in pregnancy, hot foods are believed to cause miscarriage and fetal abnormality (Turrell, 1985). Conversely, cold foods (i e., milk products, milk, yogurt, cream, and butter), most vegetables, and foods that are sour in taste are thought to strengthen and calm the pregnant woman. A study in Saudi Arabia found that pregnant Saudi women craved milk, salt and sour foods, sweets and dates. They avoided spicy foods and beverages (al-Kanhal & Bani, 1995).

Some pregnant women experience pica—the craving for and ingestion of nonfood substances, such as clay or laundry starch. Some Hispanic women prefer the solid milk of magnesia that can be purchased in Mexico, whereas other women eat the ice or frost that forms inside refrigerator units. The etiology of pica is poorly understood but there are some cultural implications as women from certain ethnic or cultural groups experience this disorder. It is most common in African American women raised in the rural south and women from lower socioeconomic levels in the U.S. The phenomena of pica has been described in such counties as Kenya, Uganda and Saudi Arabia. Most often, it is seen in women and appears most frequently during pregnancy. It is occasionally seen in children also (Abrahams, 1997; al-Kanhal & Bani, 1995; Greissler, Mwaniki, Thiong'o & Friis, 1997).

Cultural Interpretation of Obstetric Testing

Many women do not understand the emphasis placed on urinalysis, blood pressure readings, and abdominal measurements that occur in Western prenatal care. For traditional women, the vaginal examination may be so intrusive and embarrassing that they may avoid prenatal visits or request a female physician or midwife (Bash, 1980; Meleis & Sorrell, 1981; Nelson & Hewitt, 1983; Lipson et al., 1995). Common discomforts of pregnancy may be managed through folk, herbal, home, or over-the counter remedies on the advice of a relative (generally the maternal grandmother) or friends (Spector, 1996). Recommendations to health care providers include making efforts to meet the needs of women from traditional cultures by explaining health regimens so that they have meaning within the cultural belief system. However, such explanations are only an initial step. Nursing visits can be made to the home, or group prenatal visits may be made based on self-care models instituted by nurses in local community centers. Additionally, nurses can incorporate significant others into the plan of care. Nurses can provide information during prenatal visits on normal fetal growth and development, as well as discuss how the health and behavior of the mother and those around her can influence fetal outcome.

Morgan's (1996) study of African American women explored beliefs, practices and values related to prenatal care. The findings indicated that many of the women in urban areas lacked trust and were apprehensive about their current life circumstances. Establishing a good relationship and providing a safe environment was noted to increase attendance at prenatal clinics. Urban African American women indicated they had less support than their contemporaries in the rural South. Nurses should be encouraged to initiate peer social and educational groups for women who are similar to those in this study. In addition, findings indicated that the use of folk health care beliefs and practices were prevalent among study participants. Nurses must learn more about the practices of their clients and have a nonjudgemental attitude. Acceptance of alternative healers may even be therapeutic and helpful for many clients. Last, barriers to prenatal care were identified such as lack of telephones for communicating with health care providers and lack of transportation to the clinics. Nurses may need to exhibit creativity when solving these problems such as exploring the possibility of city or county governments to provide free transportation to health care sites for citizens who need this kind of assistance.

Cultural Preparation for Childbirth

Preparation for childbirth can be developed through programs that allow for cultural variation, including classes during and after the usual clinic hours in busy urban settings, teen-only classes, single mother classes, group classes combined with prenatal checkups at home, classes on rural reservations, and presentations that incorporate the older, "wise" women of the community. In addition, nurses can organize classes in languages other than English.

Cultural Meaning Attached to Infant Gender

The meaning parents attach to having a son, a daughter, or multiple births varies from culture to culture. Traditionally, the male gender is highly regarded, which places females in a position of "less than favorable." Certain Asian and Islamic cultures feel that a male child is preferable to a female child. Twin births also carry a significance that varies from culture to culture. Twins are viewed as a special blessing by the Yoruba tribe and as a curse by the Ibo tribe in the same West African nation of Nigeria. In these situations the nurse may find the best course of action is simply to point out all the positive attributes of the newborn, regardless of gender.

Nurses must be able to differentiate among beliefs and practices that are harmful, benign, and health promoting. Few cultural customs related to pregnancy are dangerous; although they may cause a woman to limit her activity and her exposure to some aspects of life, they are rarely harmful to her fetus or to her.

Birth and Culture

Beliefs and customs surrounding the experience of labor and delivery are influenced by the fact that the physiologic process is basically the same for all cultures. Factors such as cultural attitudes toward the achievement of birth, methods of dealing with the pain of labor, recommended positions during delivery, the preferred location for the birth, the role of the father and the family, and expectations of the health care practitioner may vary according to degree of acculturation to Western childbirth customs, geographic location, religious beliefs, and individual preference.

The concept of achievement versus atonement in birth refers to the way in which a culture defines the birth process as a praised achievement worthy of celebration or a defilement or state of pollution necessitating ritual purification (Newton & Newton, 1972). In the American culture, birth is often viewed as a achievement, unfortunately, not for the mother but rather for the medical staff. The obstetrician "manages" the labor and "delivers" the infant; for this active role, the doctor is often profusely thanked even before the mother is praised or congratulated. Gifts and celebrations are centered around the newborn rather than the mother. The recent consumer movement in childbirth and the upsurge of feminism have caused some redefinition of the cultural focus and encouraged women and their partners to assume active roles in the management of their own health and birth experiences. Unfortunately, some women who have prepared themselves for a totally "natural" childbirth may feel a sense of personal trauma and failure if they receive analgesic or require a cesarean section delivery (Hott, 1980; Mercer & Stainton, 1984). Nurses must identify how much personal control and involvement are desired by a woman and her family during the birth experience. If expectations and plans made before labor are altered during labor and birth, the nurse should involve the woman and her significant others in all changes and allow the woman to verbalize her feelings following the birth.

Traditional Home Birth

All cultures have an approach to birth rooted in a tradition in which childbirth occurs at home, within the province of women. For generations, traditions among the poor included use of "granny" midwives by rural Appalachian whites and southern African Americans, and "parteras" by Mexican Americans (Frankel, 1977; Kay, 1978; Barry & Boyle 1996). A dependence on self-management, a belief in the normality of labor and birth, and a tradition of delivery at home may influence some women to arrive at the hospital only in advanced labor (Frankel, 1977; Nelson & Hewitt, 1983). The need to travel a long distance to the closest hospital may also be a factor contributing to arrival in late labor or to out-of-hospital delivery from many Native American women living on rural, isolated reservations.

Support During Labor

Despite the traditional emphasis on female support and guidance during labor, the inclusion of spouses and male partners in American labor and birth rooms has been seen as positive by women of many cultures. Women from diverse cultures are reporting a desire to have husbands or partners present for the birth. Unfortunately, many American hospitals still maintain rules that limit the support person to the spouse or prevent a husband from attending the birth unless he has attended a formal childbirth education program with his wife. Another source of conflict is the desire of many women to have their mother or some other female relative or friend present during labor and birth. Because many hospitals have rules limiting the number of persons who may be present, the mother may be forced to make a difficult choice among the people close to her.

Some women and families, particularly those from Orthodox Jewish, Islamic, Chinese, and Asian Indian backgrounds, may follow strict religious and cultural prohibitions against viewing the woman's body by either the husband or any other man, or they may practice separation of the husband and wife once the "bloody show" or cervical dilation has occurred (Bash, 1980, Meleis & Sorrell, 1981; Flint, 1982; Pillsbury, 1982). In cultures in which the husband's presence during labor and delivery is not believed to be appropriate, nurses may mistakenly assume a lack of involvement or interest on his part (Gropper, 1996).

Cultural Expression of Labor Pain

Women from many cultural groups report fear and anxiety about the pain of labor (Affonso, 1978; Kay, 1982; Dempsey & Gesse, 1983). In the past it was commonly

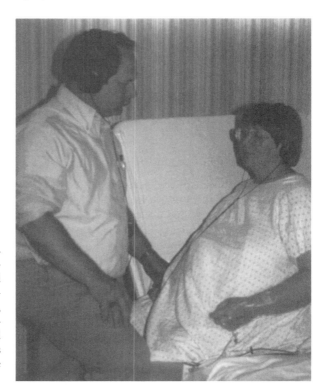

This couple is using music therapy to promote relaxation and to control the pain of labor. Active throughout the pregnancy, labor, and delivery, this husband provides comfort and emotional support and coaches his wife throughout the entire labor and delivery.

believed that women from Asian and Native American cultures were very stoic and did not feel pain in labor (Stanton, 1979); such views are ethnocentric and should be avoided. Many factors interact to influence labor and the perception of pain; these include cultural attitude toward the normalcy and conduct of birth, expectations of how a woman should act in labor, the role of significant others, and the physiologic processes involved. For example, when Filipino women were asked how they would act in labor, many said it was best to lie quietly (Affonso, 1978). By contrast, Middle Eastern women are verbally expressive during labor, sometimes crying and screaming loudly while refusing pain medication (Meleis & Sorrell, 1981). Samoan women may believe that no verbal expressions of pain are permissible, with only "spoiled" Caucasian women needing any analgesia (Clark & Howland, 1979). According to Kay (1978), Hispanic women are traditionally instructed by their *parteras* to endure pain with patience and close the mouth, for opening it to cry out would cause the uterus to rise. Japanese, Chinese, Vietnamese, Laotian, and other women of Asian descent, maintain that screaming or crying out during labor or birth is shameful; birth is believed to be painful but something to be endured (Okamoto, 1978; Rose, 1978; Stringfellow, 1978; Nelson & Hewitt, 1983). Although many of the women from diverse cultures are deemed unprepared by some health professionals because they do not use formal breathing and relaxation techniques, women often employ culturally appropriate ways of preparing for labor and delivery. These culturally approved methods of childbirth preparation may include assisting with or participating in birth from the time of adolescence, listening to birth and baby stories told by respected elderly women, or following special dietary and activity prescriptions in the antepartal period.

Birth Positions

Numerous anecdotal reports in the literature describe "typical" birth positions for women of diverse cultures, from the seated position in a birth chair favored by

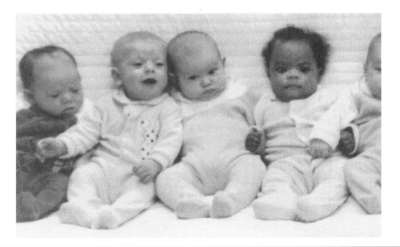

Although historically most deliveries occurred at home, today the majority of infants from all cultural backgrounds are born in hospitals.

> **Box 3-3** *Labor and Delivery Nursing Care for Culturally Diverse Women*
>
> 1. If you are unable to speak the woman's language, talk with an English-speaking relative or arrange for an interpreter.
> 2. If your nursing agency commonly cares for culturally diverse clients, check if other nurses have had experiences with similar clients. Share resources and your expertise with staff members.
> 3. Attempt to gain as much information as possible by completing a cultural assessment.
> 4. Elicit her expectations of her labor and delivery experience.
> 5. Does she want a support person with her? If so, have her identify who that person is.
> 6. Explore with her any cultural rituals she wants incorporated into her plan of care. If requests are manageable, honor them.
> 7. Be patient, draw pictures, gesture. Identify key words from family or the interpreter that you will need to be able to express yourself to her, for example, push, blow, pant, stop.

Mexican American women to the squatting position chosen by Laotian Hmong women. The nurse who cares for laboring women must realize, however, that the choice of positions is influenced by many factors other than culture and that the socialization that takes place on arrival to a labor and delivery unit may prevent women from stating their preference.

Economically disadvantaged women from culturally diverse backgrounds have few birth options; most labor and give birth in large public hospitals. Routinized patterns of care and decreased individualization are common in these institutions. These and other problems, such as language barriers, make the provision of culturally competent care during the birth process an challenge. However, any special provisions or attempts to understand the client from her perspective will be received with cooperation and gratitude. Recommendations for the labor and delivery nursing care of the culturally diverse pregnant woman are presented in Box 3-3.

Culture and the Postpartum Period

Western medicine considers pregnancy and birth the most dangerous and vulnerable time for the childbearing woman. However, other cultures place much more emphasis on the postpartal period. Many cultures have developed practices that balance and cushion this special time of vulnerability for the mother and the infant. Such strategies are thought to serve to mobilize support for the new mother. Interestingly, support that comes from family and friends is usually considered "nontraditional" in approach by Western medicine. These cultural differences, particularly as they relate to restrictive dietary customs, activity levels, and certain taboos and rituals associated with purification and seclusion, may seem unusual to the nurse but have been noted to positively influence the mother's postpartum mental health, thus reducing the incidence of problems such as postpartum depression (Stewart & Jambunathan, 1996). Additional authors (Ross & Mirowsky, 1989; O'Hara, Rehm, & Campbell, 1983) have suggested that lack of social support is one of the highest predictors of both general and postpartum depression. Research Application 3-2 reports on the incidence of postpartum depression among Hmong women.

Research Application 3-2	*Hmong Women and Postpartum Depression*

Stewart, S., & Jumbunathan, J. (1996). Hmong women and postpartum depression. *Health Care for Women International 17*, 319–330.

Postpartum depression in Western culture has been documented in the literature. The literature suggests that one cause of postpartum depression is lack of supportive practices surrounding childbirth. This study explored postpartum depression in Hmong women living in the United States. The results indicated these women perceived themselves to be supported during pregnancy and following delivery. The high levels of support received from spouses and family, combined with the practice of a 30-day rest period, may have made them less vulnerable to depression. The only symptoms of depression reported were related to living in a culture and environment different from their own, and having to use a foreign language.

Clinical Application
- Be sensitive to the fact that Hmong women have difficulty in learning English because of child care responsibilities and possibly lack of a formal education.

- Encourage family involvement in the woman's nursing care plan during and after pregnancy.

- Provide referrals for opportunities to learn English speaking skills and employment skills to facilitate their adjustment to American culture.

Routine nursing care usually includes encouraging a healthy diet, adequate fluid intake, and self-care practices such as good hygiene practices, sitz baths, showering, bathing, ambulation, and exercise. However these practices, common to American obstetric care, may seem strange and even dangerous to women of other cultural groups. Nurses must take time to not only teach, but to listen to their clients, making accommodations and being flexible when possible For many cultures, the concept of postpartum vulnerability is based on one or more beliefs related to imbalance or pollution. *Imbalance* is perceived to be due to disharmony caused by the processes of pregnancy and birth, and *pollution* is seen to be caused by the "unclean" bleeding associated with birth and the postpartum period (Horn, 1981). Restitution of physical balance and purification may occur through many mechanisms, including dietary restrictions, ritual baths, seclusion, restriction of activity, and other ceremonial events.

Hot/Cold Theory

Central to the belief of perceived imbalance in the mother's physical state is adherence to the hot/cold theories of disease causation. Pregnancy is considered a "hot" state. Because a great deal of heat of pregnancy is thought to be lost during the birth process, postpartum practices focus on restoring the balance between the hot/cold beliefs or yin and yang. See Chapter 2 for a more detailed discussion of these concepts. Common components of this theory focus on the avoidance of cold, whether in the form of air or food. An example of a belief concerning immediate harm from cold is the Haitian belief that exposure to cold air may cause a uterine cold; the entrance of air into the vagina is thought to be prevented by use of a sanitary pad (Dempsey & Gesse, 1983).

This real fear of the detrimental effects of cold air and water in the postpartum period can cause cultural conflict when the woman and infant are hospitalized. Nurses must assess the woman's beliefs regarding bathing and other self-care practices in a nonjudgmental manner.

Many women will pretend to follow the activities suggested by nurses, to the point of pretending to shower, while in reality avoiding the nurses' prescriptions. The common use of perineal ice packs and sitz baths to promote healing can be replaced with the use of heat lamps, heat packs, and anesthetic or astringent topical agents for those who prefer to avoid cold influences. The routine distribution of ice water to all postpartum women is another area of care that can be modified to meet culturally diverse women's needs. Offering women a choice of water at room temperature, warm tea or coffee, broth, or other beverage should satisfy most women's needs for warmth, along with the offering of additional bed blankets.

Postpartum Dietary Prescriptions and Activity Levels

Dietary prescriptions are also common in this period. The nurse may note that a woman eats little "hospital" food and relies on family and friends to bring food to her while she is in the hospital. If there are no diet restrictions for health reasons, this practice should be respected. Indeed, the nurse should assess what types of food are being eaten by the woman, documenting as appropriate.

Activity regulation related to the concept of disharmony or imbalance includes the avoidance of air, cold, and evil spirits. Hispanic women are encouraged to stay indoors and avoid strenuous work. Obviously, if pregnancy and birth cause a "hot" state, the woman should avoid "hot" activities such as ironing. Pillsbury (1982) described the Chinese custom of "doing the month," which includes prohibitions against going out into the sunshine, coming into contact with windy drafts, walking about, reading, or crying. Fruits and vegetables may be avoided because they are considered "cold" foods (Matocha, 1998). Many traditional African American women view themselves as "sick" during the postpartal lochial flow. They may avoid heavy work, showering, bathing or washing their hair during this vulnerable time (Carrington, 1978). Cultural prescriptions vary about when women can return to full activity after childbirth, but many traditional cultures suggest that a woman can resume normal activities in as little as 2 weeks, with some taking up to 4 months.

Vulnerability and Seclusion

The period of postpartum vulnerability and seclusion in most nonwestern cultures varies between 7–40 days. Hispanic women, especially primigravidas, may follow a set of dietary and activity rules called *la dieta* (Kay, 1978; Horn, 1981). The Hispanic midwife will stay at the home of the mother for several hours following the delivery, with a follow-up visit the next day.

Philpott's (1979) study of traditional Hispanic postpartum practices described how the midwife disposed of the placenta through burial so that animals would not eat it, as it was believed that if a dog eats the placenta, the mother will be unable to bear subsequent children. Burying the placenta was also believed to prevent the mother from having "afterpains."

In some cultures, women are considered to be in a state of impurity or pollution during the postpartum period. Consequently, ritual seclusion and activity elimination may be practiced to reduce the risk of increasing personal vulnerability to spirit influence or of spreading evil and misfortune. In many cultures this time of seclusion coincides with the period of lochial flow or postpartum bleeding. Common taboos include seclusion and avoidance of contact with others, avoidance of contact with food or objects, and avoidance of sexual relations. A ritual bath may mark the end of the state of pollution; for Navajo women, this may occur on the fourth postpartum day; for Hispanic women, at 2 weeks; and for Orthodox Jewish women, on the seventh day after delivery (Bash, 1980; Kay, 1982).

Pregnancy in Special Populations

Incarceration and Pregnancy

Incarcerated women who are pregnant at the time of their incarceration present health care providers with a unusual set of challenges. This group of women share an unusual and restrictive context that creates a unique subculture. It has been reported that three-fourths of incarcerated women are mothers. Most are young, single, undereducated, unskilled, unemployed, and financially disadvantaged, with 10 percent being pregnant during imprisonment (Osborne, 1995). Normal adaptation to pregnancy is altered by incarceration. According to Hufft (1992), a pregnant woman in prison is vulnerable in four specific areas that include:

1. Increased stress caused from inadequate or poor lifestyle health practices, increased risk of suicide and self-destructive behavior, and if she becomes pregnant while in a federal prison, it is considered an offense punishable at the very least by isolation, which leads to delays in obtaining prenatal care.
2. Women in prison exist in a restricted environment that fosters aggression and violent behavior, leading to ongoing stress. According to Osborne (1995), prisons have ill-defined provisions for prenatal care and/or plans for labor and delivery. The prison environment dictates the inmates' exercise, diet, mandatory workloads and clothing, all of which may need alteration during pregnancy.
3. Social support systems are altered during incarceration. The family and social support that usually helps to guide the woman in decision-making processes during pregnancy are nonexistent, or at least significantly altered. The social support systems in prison are usually anti-authority so that if the health care provider is viewed as part of the "establishment" the in-

mates own support system may encourage responses that result in noncompliance.

4. There is an alteration in maternal role attainment as learning from the usual sources such as observing a "good mother role model" and access to appropriate pregnancy literature is limited.

Rubin (1984) described the maternal role and how it is attained by the pregnant woman. The attainment focuses on the woman's ability to rehearse the anticipated activities after birth. Incarcerated women know they will not care for their infants following birth and understand that they must return to prison upon delivery of their baby to complete their jail time. The incarcerated woman who has an infant during her prison term has two choices: adoption or placing the infant for guardianship. If she relinquishes her infant for adoption, she is faced with yet another loss which must be addressed. Hufft (1992) suggested that development of the maternal role in incarcerated women must be built on the plans that have been made for the placement of the infant after delivery and must include assessment of the new mother's family situation and her cultural beliefs. Prior to the birth, the woman must be counseled and assisted to organize her resources. These assessments should ideally be made by either the woman's health care provider or counselor.

Nurses working in the prison system are in a unique position to assist in the development of prenatal programs designed to provide the care and counseling needed to ensure healthy pregnancy outcomes. An additional benefit of such programs would be that learning new coping skills during pregnancy may help the woman with successful coping skills affecting other areas of the woman's life once out of prison.

Abuse and Pregnancy

There remains a paucity of information regarding women in abusive situations. Important information we do know is that abused women are less likely to seek health care because their abuser limits access to resources (King & Ryan, 1989) or that battering occurs more frequently during pregnancy (Taggert & Mattson, 1996). This has implications for the pregnant woman and places her in double jeopardy, not only for herself but for her baby as well as battering of pregnant women has been associated with adverse pregnancy outcomes (Helton, 1986; Bullock, McFarlane, Bateman & Miller, 1989; Schei, Samuelsen & Bakketeig, 1991). A study by Straus and Gelles (1986) reported that conservative estimates indicated that 20–30 percent of all women in the United States have experienced physical abuse from their partners at least once.

Parker, MacFarlane, Soeken, Torres, and Campbell (1993) estimated that 40–60 percent of abused women incur injuries while pregnant. It is reported that violence often begins or escalates during pregnancy and can result in preterm birth or even fetal demise (Schei, et al., 1991). It has also been confirmed that abused pregnant women have a two to four times greater risk of delivering a low birth weight (LBW) infant (Bullock, et al., 1989). Among the associations between abuse and LBW, is delay in obtaining prenatal care. Research Application 3-3 discusses delays in obtaining prenatal care as a result of battering.

Campbell and Fishwick (1993) suggested that the most appropriate framework for viewing violence in general and specifically wife abuse is the concept of machismo. In Western culture violence can be viewed as a "clandestine masculine ideal" as male

Research
Application 3-3

Prenatal Care Delays Related to Battering

Taggart, L., & Mattson, S. (1996). Delay in prenatal care as a result of battering in pregnancy: Crosscultural implications. *Health Care for Women International 17*, 25–34.

This study evaluated patterns of abuse during the pregnancies of 132 African American, 208 Hispanic, and 162 white American women from low-income clinics in large metropolitan cities in the West. The researchers found that the incidence of abuse did not vary significantly among ethnic groups and that the abused women from these groups sought prenatal care 6.5 weeks later than did the nonabused group. In this study, 1 in 4 women reported they had been physically abused since their current pregnancy began, with African American women suffering the most severe and most frequent abuse.

Clinical Application

* Include questions about abuse in every routine history taken during pregnancy in order to identify abused women. Offer information about abuse and available community resources. Those reporting abuse will need further screening with specific tools.

* Nurses should be aware of subtle signs of abuse. For example, psychosomatic complaints, injuries inconsistent with their explanation, failure to keep clinic appointments, and overprotective partners may be indications of abuse.

* Become familiar with community resources for referrals.

heroes are "Rambo" types and playboys who treat women with disdain. Campbell and Fishwick (1993) suggest that machismo is present to some extent in all men but is more prevalent in lower socioeconomic groups and African Americans. Machismo in African American men resulted from systematic degradation and oppression by white racist society. Machismo is also wide spread in middle class white American society because of the legacy of patriarchy, which is deeply embedded in our culture. Often other factors contribute to violence against women, especially alcohol abuse.

This section will discuss four culturally different groups of women and the experience of abuse during pregnancy. Recommendations for health care providers will follow each discussion and will emphasize the importance of culturally competent care to these high risk clients.

Hispanic Women

Although there are many different Hispanic groups, they do share some important commonalities, e.g., religion, customs, and language. However, as with any cultural group differences do exist among the members. The incidence of wife abuse among pregnant Hispanic women is not clear in the literature. However, Richwald and McClusky (1985) believe that although violence during pregnancy is likely to be the most common form of family violence, it is also the least reported. Campbell and Humphrey (1993) pointed out that it is ironic that prenatal care routinely includes close monitoring for physiologic disorders yet does not routinely include screening for physical abuse from the mother's partner.

Access to health care for pregnant Hispanic women is problematic for many of them. Barriers to prenatal health care include the following: lack of health care insurance, low levels of education that encourages the use of traditional healers and remedies and may foster mistrust of physicians and nurses and lead to noncompliance when pregnant women do use modern medicine, lengthy travel time to clinics followed by long waits, and last, the lack of Spanish speaking health care professionals (Torres,1993). Hispanic women tend to be in low-paying jobs with annual earnings of considerably less than nonHispanic women. They also have less education than whites and large, extended households, often made up of several children and extended family members (Poma, 1987). These many factors place them at a distinct disadvantage when it comes to accessing prenatal care. Furthermore, these same factors would tend to discourage the pregnant Hispanic women from disclosing a situation of abuse and violence. Her choices are the same as those of other women in abusive situations: try to make the relationship work or she can leave her abuser. If you are poor, have no friends or family members nearby and have several little children who depend on you, leaving the family provider will be very difficult.

The Hispanic pregnant woman that chooses to leave her abuser must face the reality of language barriers, a poor economic situation, no insurance and perhaps leaving her traditional family support network. These same factors work to inhibit the seeking of information regarding resources available to abused women. Even when faced with death, it is very difficult for some abused women to expose their private situation to someone outside their cultural circle. Furthermore, certain groups of Hispanic women, such as migrants, are at higher risk because they are separated from family support systems, and other barriers such as poverty and language may be exacerbated (Rodriquez, 1993).

Nurses and other health practitioners in prenatal clinics are in an ideal position to facilitate a trusting relationship with a abused woman. Good assessment skills are crucial, as the first sign of abuse may not be an admission of abuse but physical findings of trauma. It is also helpful that the nurse have strong interpersonal skills and a genuine interest in Hispanic culture. This is a situation where a Spanish-speaking health care provider may be able to form a trusting relationship more quickly, enabling the woman to share information about domestic violence. Recommendations for assistance of abused pregnant Hispanic women include: working with and mobilizing support using the family and kinship structure, educating the abused woman regarding available resources for abused women, encouraging the woman's inner strength, and assisting in the development of skills necessary to mobilize resources (Torres, 1993).

African American Women

Cultural beliefs of African Americans emphasize the larger African American society rather than focusing on individuals, making "all" collectively responsible for one another (McNair, 1992). Therefore, African American women exist in a social context supported by social connectedness versus that of autonomy. There is a paucity of information about domestic violence situations that include African Americans; this makes it very difficult to be specific about an assessment of factors related to domestic violence. However, Roy (1982) has suggested that poor economic conditions may be the major reason violence occurs in African American families. Supporting this view, Carlson (1977) reports that the primary basis for domestic violence is environmental stress related to limited social and economic resources. The risk of wife abuse is thought to be greatest in situations where the woman has a higher educational status than her partner or the situation when the man is unemployed or has trouble keeping a job. This is a familiar social situation in African American male-female relationships.

One of the most difficult barriers confronting African American abused women attempting to get help either from police or from the legal system is the stereotypical view that suggests that violence among African Americans is normal (Hawkins, 1987). This view can lead to an unequal response to African American victims of violence. Another barrier to reporting of wife abuse is that there may be greater than normal consideration by the wife for her abuser. The women are aware of increased male suppression by society at large and thus, may take extra care to protect them (Cazenave & Straus, 1981; Hare, 1979).

The nurse or practitioner in the prenatal setting is again in an ideal position to gather information and initiate a trusting relationship. As has been pointed out, the abused pregnant woman in this culture may not be willing to incriminate her mate as she sees him as already a "victim" of society. The nurse may need to rely heavily on her assessment and history-taking skills, being particularly alert to instances of trauma, problems with past pregnancies. Education must stress that although the women see their men as "victims," women cannot and must not tolerate abuse. Identify shelter facilities in the woman's neighborhood and in other areas. If she feels uncomfortable going outside her neighborhood (many do for fear they will not be understood outside their culture) encourage her to go to extended family, which may be more acceptable within this culture. The important thing is that the woman has a plan of what to do, where to do, who to call for help the next time she is abused and is afraid for her own safety. Last, the nurse must realize that in most instances African American women believe that it is the responsibility of the woman to maintain the family, regardless of other factors. These women have been shown to be more likely to stay in the relationship or work with professionals to modify the abuser's behavior (White, 1985).

Native American Women

Violence within families has not always been part of Native American society. Albers and Medicine (1983) noted that prior to contact with Europeans, Native American society was based on harmony and respect for nature and all living things, sharing, and cooperation. Contributions from both sexes were valued, and many activities were shared, including the roles of warrior and hunter. Traditionally, cruelty to women and children resulted in loss of honor and public humiliation. Cultural disintegration, poverty, isolation, racism, and alcoholism are just a few of the problems that have fostered violence in Native American cultures. Research Application 3-4 discusses Native American women and fetal alcohol syndrome.

Beginning in the 1970s, Native American tribes have made an effort to develop programs to meet the needs of their communities. However, abuse among women has not been addressed adequately due to the male-dominated leadership, other needs of the tribes, and the shame associated with abuse (Bohn, 1993).

Recommendations for health care providers include identification of the abused by direct questioning in a private setting but only after a trusting relationship is established. Assessment of the woman's chart or medical record is critical

Native American Women and Fetal Alcohol Syndrome

Robinson, G., Armstrong, R., Moczuk, B., & Loock, C. (1992). Knowledge of fetal alcohol syndrome among native Indians. *Canadian Journal of Public Health 83*(5), 337–338.

A survey was conducted of 123 native Indians attending a Canadian clinic about their knowledge of how alcohol affects the fetus. The survey revealed limited education about alcohol but substantial knowledge of fetal alcohol syndrome was evident among the respondents. The researchers believe the survey indicated a need for further information about the sequelae of drinking during pregnancy, focusing on families at risk. It was found that education needs to involve the male partner, as they influence the drinking environment of the woman.

Dempster, J. (1996). Continuing education forum. Fetal alcohol syndrome: The nurse practitioner perspective. *Journal of the American Academy of Nurse Practitioners 8*(7), 343–352.

Analysis of the history, incidence, etiology, risk factors, manifestations, diagnosis, and clinical implications of fetal alcohol syndrome in relation to practice issues faced by nurse practitioners as they care for these clients.

Smitherman, C. (1994). The lasting impact of fetal alcohol syndrome and fetal alcohol—effect on children and adolescents. *Journal of Pediatric Health Care 8*(3), 121–126.

Analysis of the impact fetal alcohol syndrome has on children and adolescents. Article describes how fetal alcohol syndrome occurs, how it may be recognized, and the potentially devastating effects it can have on children, adolescents, and their caretakers and how it can be prevented.

Clinical Application

*   Involve the woman's spouse or mate in the education process as the male partner can influence the woman's drinking habits, good and bad.

*   Educate from the perspective of the effect on the developing baby, as women are concerned about the health of their unborn and may be more likely to change their behavior during pregnancy.

*   Educate the "old, wise ones" in the community as they have particular influence over the younger generation. Once educated, incorporate them into the teaching so they are actually the ones who are "teaching" the young.

*   Target families in the education process so that the woman feels support from those persons with whom she has frequent contact.

and may provide an opening for discussion of abuse-related questions. A thorough history may indicate signs of abuse through complaints of prior problems, injuries, depression, suicide attempts, eating disorders, miscarriages and pregnancy complications.

While interviewing Native American women, a sense of humor is most helpful as they view someone with whom they can laugh as easy to talk to. Open-ended questions are preferable. The nurse should also learn to become comfortable with periods of silence following a question. This does not mean that clients are not listening, but rather, just the opposite. They think the question is worthy of thoughtful consideration before answering.

Once abuse has been assessed, the extent of abuse must be ascertained. The nurse/or practitioner must then intervene by providing information, discussing alternatives, and supporting the woman in her decision. Options should focus on Native American resources as they will be culturally sensitive to her needs. If only non Indian sources are available the nurse should determine the experience of Native American women within these agencies (Bohn, 1993). Variables to be considered when discussing options should include her support system, her personal and cultural value system, and her financial status.

Abuse within this culture is traditionally dealt with within the family first. The abused woman may be reluctant to go outside for help as this may cause both families to ostracize her. It is important to note that for a Native American woman, it is considered a virtue to stay with her mate no matter what the circumstance, especially if they were married by a traditional medicine man or woman. Wolk (1982) notes that choosing to stay with her abuser may be done so out of loyalty because he is Indian rather than because he is a man. Essential to understanding is that when a woman is attempting to leave an abusive relationship she must know that her health care provider cares about her. Safety for the woman and her unborn baby is the priority. The woman will need phone numbers of shelters, counselors, legal advisors, and information on job training and educational opportunities. It is important to focus on strengths, her sense of humor, and the skills and resources she has. She must be able to feel hope that both she and her abuser will heal.

An additional factor related to abuse for Native American pregnant women is that of alcohol abuse (Robinson, Armstrong, Moczuk & Loock, 1992). Living with abuse and becoming dependent on alcohol and other drugs are intertwined problems for many women, especially native American women. The use and abuse of alcohol and/or drugs is one way of coping with an abusive relationship, but it is also one that places the woman and her developing fetus at considerable health risk.

Summary

Pregnancy, childbirth and culture have been discussed from many vantage points. Biologic and cultural variations that can impact childbearing outcomes were identified and analyzed. The importance of nontraditional support systems to pregnant women, along with discussions of cultural beliefs and practices as they relate to pregnancy, birth and the postpartum period were presented with suggestions for nursing care.

Special pregnant populations were selected for examination including incarcerated pregnant women, culturally diverse, pregnant, abused women, and women choosing alternative lifestyles. Nursing care recommendations were offered for each. Cultural beliefs and practices are continuously evolving making it necessary for the nurse to acknowledge the various cultures and explore the meaning of childbearing with each family with whom she has contact. It is also important to remember that behavior must be evaluated from within each person's cultural context. Genuine concern, interest and respect is therefore basic as a start toward developing culturally appropriate care for childbearing women and their families.

Review Questions

1. List the biologic variations discussed and the implications for nursing care of the childbearing woman and her family.
2. Identify nursing interventions for women relinquishing infants during the postpartum period. Identify the typical cultural values in American society about women who relinquish their infants.
3. Describe the special needs of lesbian couples choosing to become parents. What are common pejorative values about lesbian mothers?
4. Compare traditional Western medical support for pregnant women with nontraditional support and describe why both may be critical for successful pregnancy outcomes of culturally diverse women.
5. Describe the differences between prescriptive and restrictive beliefs about mothers' behavior during pregnancy.
6. Describe two barriers that face African American women as they attempt to get help in abusive situations.
7. Describe the culturally competent care that must be available to assist pregnant women who experience domestic violence. Why is this care important?

Learning Activities to Promote Critical Thinking

1. Critically analyze the culturally competent nursing interventions for a Hispanic woman following a fetal demise from a cord accident?
2. Develop a prenatal assessment tool that takes account of the cultural context of incarcerated pregnant women. How would you implement use of such a tool? What argument would you use?
3. Analyze the responses the culturally competent postpartum nurse should initiate when an African American woman refuses to get out of bed and shower?
4. Discuss and critically analyze how you would respond to your labor patient's request to allow her lesbian partner to participate in the birth of *their* child? What activities would you include in the plan of care? Why?
5. Describe and analyze how the nurse might offer culturally appropriate support to the husband of a Middle Eastern laboring woman who has followed his cultural traditions and left the labor room once the bloody show occurred?

References

Abrahams, P. W. (1997). Geophagy (soil consumption) and iron supplementation in Uganda. *Tropical Medicine and International Health* 2(7), 624–630.

Affonso, D. D. (1978). The Filipino American. In A. L. Clark (Ed.). *Culture, Childbearing, and Health Professionals.* Philadelphia: F. A. Davis.

Albers, P., & Medicine, B. (1983). *The Hidden Half: Studies of Plains Indian Women.* Lanham, New York: University Press of America.

Al-Kanhal, M. A., & Bani, I. A. (1995). Food habits during pregnancy among Saudi women. *International Journal for Vitamin and Nutrition Research* 65(3), 206–210.

Barry, D., & Boyle, J. S. (1996). An ethnohistory of a granny midwife. *Journal of Transcultural Nursing* 8(1), 13–18.

Bash, D. M. (1980). Jewish religious practices related to childbearing. *Journal of Nurse-Midwifery* 25(5), 39–42.

Bauwens, E. E. (1978). *The Anthropology of Health.* St. Louis. MO: C. V. Mosby.

Berenstein, J. L., & Kidd, Y. A. (1982). Childbearing in Japan. In M. A. Kay (Ed.). *Anthropology of Human Birth*. Philadelphia: F. A. Davis.

Boehme, T. (1985). Hepatitis B: The nurse-midwife's role in management and prevention. *Journal of Nurse-Midwifery* 30(2), 79–87.

Bohn, D. K. (1993). Nursing care of Native American battered women. *AWHONN's Clinical Issues* 4(3), 424–436.

Bryant, C. A. (1982). The impact of kin, friend, and neighbor networks on infant feeding practices. *Social Science & Medicine* 16, 1757–1765.

Bullock, L., McFarlane, J., Bateman, L., & Miller, V. (1989). Characteristics of battered women in a primary care setting. *Nurse Practitioner* 14(6), 47–55.

Campanella, K., Korbin, J., & Acheson, L. (1993). Pregnancy and childbirth among the Amish. *Social Science Medicine* 36(3), 333–342.

Campbell, J., & Fishwick, N. (1993). Abuse of female partners. In J. Campbell, and J. Humphreys (Eds.). *Nursing Care of Survivors of Family Violence* (2nd ed.), pp. 68–104. St. Louis, MO: C. V. Mosby.

Carlson, B. (1977). Battered women and their assailants. *Social Work* 22, 455–471.

Carrington, B. W. (1978). The Afro-American. In A. L. Clark (Ed.). *Culture, Childbearing, and Health Professionals*. Philadelphia: F. A. Davis.

Cazenave, N., & Straus, M. (1979). Race, class and network embeddedness and family violence. *Journal of Comparative Family Studies* 10, 281–300.

Clark, A. L., & Howland, R. I. (1978). The American Samoan. In A. L. Clark (Ed.). *Culture, Childbearing, and Health Professionals*. Philadelphia: F. A. Davis.

Dempsey, P. A., & Gesse, T. (1983). The childbearing Haitian refugee: Cultural applications to clinical nursing. *Public Health Reports* 98(3), 261–267.

Dempster, J. (1996). Continuing education forum. Fetal Alcohol syndrome: the nurse practitioner perspective. *Journal of the American Academy of Nurse Practitioners* 8(7), 343–352.

Dickason, E. J., Silverman, B. L., & Schult, M. O. (1994). *Maternal infant nursing care* (2nd ed.). Philadelphia: Mosby.

Dickason, E. J., Silverman, B. L., & Kaplan, J. A. (1998). *Maternal infant nursing care* (3rd ed.). Philadelphia: Mosby.

Erickson, R. V., & Hoang, G. N. (1980). Health problems among Indochinese refugees. *American Journal of Public Health* 70(9), 1003–1005.

Flint, M. (1982). Lockmi: An Indian midwife. In M. A. Kay (Ed.). *Anthropology of Human Birth*. Philadelphia: F. A. Davis.

Ford, C. S. (1964). *A Comparative Study of Human Reproduction*. New Haven: Human Relations Area Files Press.

Frankel, B. (1977). *Childbirth in the Ghetto: Folk Beliefs of Negro Women in a North Philadelphia Hospital Ward*. San Francisco: R & E Research Associates.

Geissler, P. W., Mwaniki, D. L., Thiong'o, F., & Friis, H. (1997). Geophagy among school children in western Kenya. *Tropical Medicine and International Health* 2(7), 624–630.

Gropper, R. C. (1996). *Culture and the clinical encounter*. Yarmouth, ME: Intercultural Press, Inc.

Hare, N. (1979). The relative psycho-socio-economic suppression of the black male. In W. D. Smith, K. H. Burlew, M. H. Moseley, & W. M. Whitnew (Eds.). *Reflections on Black Psychology*, pp. 359–381. Washington, DC: University Press.

Hawkins, D. F. (1987). Devalued lives and racial stereotypes: Ideological barriers to the prevention of family violence among blacks. In R. H. Hampton (Ed.). *Violence in the Black Family: Correlates and Consequences*, pp. 190–205. Lexington, MA: Lexington Books.

Helton, A. (1986). *Protocol of Care for the Battered Woman*. White Plains, NY: March of Dimes Birth Defects Foundation.

Horn, B. M. (1981). Cultural concepts and postpartal care. *Nursing and Health Care* 2(9), 516–517.

Hott, J. R. (1980). Best laid plans. *Nursing Research* 29, 20–27.

Hufft, A. G. (1992). Psychosocial adaptation to pregnancy in prison. *Journal of Psychosocial Nursing* 30(4), 19–23.

Johnston, M. (1980). Cultural variations in professional and parenting patterns. *JOGYN Nursing* 9(1), 9–13.

Kay, M. A. (1978). The Mexican American. In A. L. Clark (Ed.). *Culture, Childbearing, and Health Professionals*. Philadelphia: F. A. Davis.

Kay, M. A. (1982). Writing an ethnography of birth. In M. A. Kay (Ed.). *Anthropology of Human Birth*. Philadelphia: F. A. Davis.

Kim, K., & Mo, S. (1977). A study of food taboos on the Jeju island: Focused on pregnancy. *Korean Journal of Nutrition* 10, 49–57.

King, M. C., & Ryan, J. (1989). Abused women: Dispelling myths and encouraging intervention. *Nurse Practitioner* 14, 47–58.

Lantican, L. S., & Corona, D. F. (1992). Comparison of the social support networks of Filipino and Mexican-American primigravidas. *Health Care for Women International* 13, 329–338.

Lauderdale, J., & Boyle, J. (1994). Infant relinquishment through adoption. *Image Journal of Nursing Scholarship* 26(3), 213–217.

Lipson, J. G., Hosseini, M. A., Omidian, P. A., & Edmonston, F. (1995). Health issues among Afghan in California. *Health Care for Women International* 16(4), 279–286.

Logan, B. B., & Dawkins, C. E. (1986). *Family Centered Nursing in the Community*. Menlo Park, CA: Addison-Wesley.

Matocha, L. K. (1998). Chinese-Americans. In L. D. Purnell & B. J. Paulanka (Eds.). *Transcultural Nursing: A Culturally Competent Approach*, pp. 163–188. Philadelphia: F. A. Davis.

McClain, C. (1982). Toward a comparative framework for the study of childbirth: A review of the literature. In M. A. Kay (Ed.). *Anthropology of Human Birth*. Philadelphia: F. A. Davis.

McNair, L. D. (1992). African American women in therapy: An Afrocentric and feminist synthesis. *Women and Therapy* 12, 5–19.

Mead, M., & Newton, N. (1967). Cultural patterning of perinatal behavior. In S. A. Richardson & A. F. Guttmacher (Eds.). *Childbearing: Its Social and Psychological Aspects*. Baltimore: Williams & Wilkins.

Meleis, A. I., & Sorrell, L. (1981). Bridging cultures: Arab American women and their birth experiences. *Maternal Child Nursing* 6, 171–176.

Mercer, R. T., & Stainton, M. C. (1984). Perceptions of the birth experience: A cross-cultural comparison. *Health Care for Women International 5*, 29–47.

Milinaire, C. (1974). *Birth*. New York: Crown Publishers.

Morgan, M. (1996). Prenatal care of African American women in selected USA urban and rural cultural contexts. *Journal of Transcultural Nursing 7*(2), 3–9.

Nelson, C. C., & Hewitt, M. A. (1983). An Indochinese refugee population in a nurse-midwifery service. *Journal of Nurse-Midwifery 28*(5), 9–14.

Newton, N., & Newton, M. (1972). Childbirth in crosscultural perspective. In J. G. Howells (Ed.). *Modern Perspectives in Psycho-obstetrics*. New York: Brunner/Mazel.

Oakley, A. (1980). *Women Confined: Towards a Sociology of Childbirth*. New York: Schocken Books.

O'Hara, M., Rehm, L., & Campbell, S. (1983). Postpartum depression: A role for social network and life stress variables. *Journal of Nervous Disorders 171*, 336–341.

Okamoto, N. I. (1978). The Japanese American. In A. L. Clark (Ed.). *Culture, Childbearing, and Health Professionals*. Philadelphia: F. A. Davis.

Osborne, O. (1995). Jailed mothers: Further explorations in public sector nursing. *Journal of Psychosocial Nursing 33*(8), 23–28.

Overfield, T. (1985). *Biologic Variation in Health and Illness*. Menlo Park, CA: Addison-Wesley.

Pettit, D. J., Knowler, W. C., Baird, H. R., & Bennet, P. H. (1980). Gestational diabetes: Infant and maternal complication of pregnancy in relation to third-trimester glucose tolerance in Pima Indians. *Diabetes Care 3*(3), 458–464.

Philpott, L. L. (1979). *A Descriptive Study of Birth Practices and Midwifery in the Lower Rio Grande Valley of Texas*. Ph.D. dissertation, University of Texas Health Science Center, Houston School of Public Health.

Pickwell, S. (1983). Health screening for Indochinese refugees. *Nurse Practitioner 8*(4), 20–21, 25.

Pillsbury, B. (1982). "Doing the month": Confinement and convalescence of Chinese women after childbirth. In M. A. Kay (Ed.). *Anthropology of Human Birth*. Philadelphia: F. A. Davis.

Poma, P. A. (1987). Pregnancy in Hispanic women. *Journal of the National Medical Association 79*, 929–935.

Pritchard, I. A., MacDonald, P. C., & Gant, N. F. (1984). *William's Obstetrics* (17th ed.). Norwalk, CT: Appleton-Century-Crofts.

Raphael, D. (1976). Matrescence, becoming a mother, a new/old rite de passage. In F. X. Grollig & H. B. Haley (Eds.). *Medical Anthropology*. Paris: Mouton Publishers.

Richwald, G. A., & McClusky, T. E. (1985). Family violence during pregnancy. In D. B. Jeliffe & E. F. T. Jeliffe (Eds.). *Advances in International Maternal and Child Health*, pp. 87–96. New York, NY: Oxford University Press.

Robinson, G., Armstrong, R., Moczuk, B., & Loock, C. (1992). Knowledge of fetal alcohol syndrome among native Indians. *Canadian Journal of Public Health 83*(5), 337–338.

Rose, P. A. (1978). The Chinese American. In A. L. Clark (Ed.). *Culture, Childbearing, and Health Professionals*. Philadelphia: F. A. Davis.

Ross, C. E., & Mirowsky, J. (1989). Explaining the social patterns of depression: Control and problem solving—or support and talking? *Journal of Health and Social Behavior 30*, 206–219.

Roy, M. (1982). Four thousand partners in violence: A trend analysis. In M. Roy (Ed.). *The Abusive Partner*, pp. 17–35. New York: Van Nostrand.

Rubin, R. (1984). *Maternal Identity and the Maternal Experience*. New York: Springer Publishing Company.

Schei, B., Samuelsen, S., & Bakketeig, L. (1991). Does spousal physical abuse affect the outcome of pregnancy? *Scandinavian Journal of Social Medicine 19*, 26–31.

Smitherman, C. (1994). The lasting impact of fetal alcohol syndrome and fetal alcohol: Effect on children and adolescents. *Journal of Pediatric Health Care 8*(3), 121–126.

Spector, R. (1996). *Cultural Diversity in Health and Illness* (4th ed.). Norwalk, CN: Appleton & Lange.

Stanton, M. E. (1979). The "myth" of natural childbirth. *Journal of Nurse-Midwifery 24*(2), 25–28.

Stewart, S., & Jambunathan, J. (1996). Hmong women and postpartum depression. *Health Care for Women International 17*, 319–330.

Straus, M. A., & Gelles, R. J. (1986). Societal change and change in family violence from 1975 to 1985 as revealed by two national surveys. *Journal of Marriage and the Family 48*, 465–479.

Stevens, P. E., & Hall, J. M. (1988). Stigma, health beliefs, and experiences with health care in lesbian women. *Image: Journal of Nursing Scholarship 20*(2), 69–73.

Stevens, P. E., & Hall, J. M. (1991). Stigma, health beliefs and experiences with health care in lesbian women. In K. Saucier (Ed.). *Perspectives in Family and Community Health*, pp. 378–385. Hanover, MD: Mosby.

Stringfellow, L. (1978). The Vietnamese. In A. L. Clark (Ed.). *Culture, Childbearing and Health Professionals*. Philadelphia: F. A. Davis.

Taggart, L., & Mattson, S. (1996). Delay in prenatal care as a result of battering in pregnancy: Crosscultural implications. *Health Care for Women International 17*, 25–34.

Tash, D., & Kenney, J. (1993). The lesbian childbearing couple: A case report. *Birth 20*(1), 36–40.

Thompson, J., & Thompson, M. (1983). *Genetics in Medicine* (3rd ed.). Philadelphia: W. B. Saunders.

Torres, S. (1993). Nursing care of low-income battered Hispanic pregnant women. *AWHONN's Clinical Issues 4*(3), 416–425.

Turrell, S. (1985). Asians' expectations: Customs surrounding pregnancy and childbirth. *Nursing Times 81*(18), 44–49.

Wertz, R. W., & Wertz, D. C. (1977). *Lying In: A History of Childbirth in America*. New York: Macmillan.

White, E. (1985). *Chain, Chain, Change*. Seattle: The Leaf Press.

Wolk, L. E. (1982). *Minnesota's American Indian Battered Women: The Cycle of Oppression*. St. Paul: Battered Women's Project, St. Paul American Indian Center.

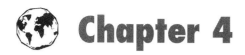

Chapter 4

Transcultural Perspectives in the Nursing Care of Children

Margaret M. Andrews

OBJECTIVES

1. Examine the role of the family in mediating cultural beliefs and practices related to infants, children and adolescents.
2. Explore cultural similarities and differences in normal growth and development.
3. Examine biocultural influences on selected acute and chronic conditions affecting infants, children and adolescents.
4. Apply the concepts of transcultural nursing to the care of infants, children and adolescents from diverse cultures.

ociety depends on its children for its future and provides its offspring with care, nurturance, and socialization. Cultural survival depends on the transmission of values and customs from one generation to the next, a process that relies on children for its success. In this chapter the cultural influences on child growth, development, health and illness will be examined. Figure 4-1 provides a schematic representation of the cultural factors that influence parents' childrearing beliefs and practices. Figure 4-2 provides a visual representation of the interrelationship among culture, communication, and parental decisions and actions related to childrearing. The *clinical relevance* of this information for nurses caring for infants, children and adolescents from diverse cultures will be examined throughout the chapter.

Because the majority of children are cared for by their natural or adoptive parents, the term *parent* is frequently used in the chapter. It should be noted, however, that some children are cared for by grandparents, aunts, uncles, or cousins, or those who are unrelated but function as primary providers of care and/or parent surrogates for varying periods of time. In some cases the primary provider of care looks after the infant, child or adolescent for a brief time, perhaps for an hour or two while the parents are unable to do so. In other cases, this person may function as a long-term or permanent parent substitute even though legal adoption has not occurred. For example, a grandparent might assume responsibility for a child in the event of parental death, illness, disability, or imprisonment. You should be aware that the same factors

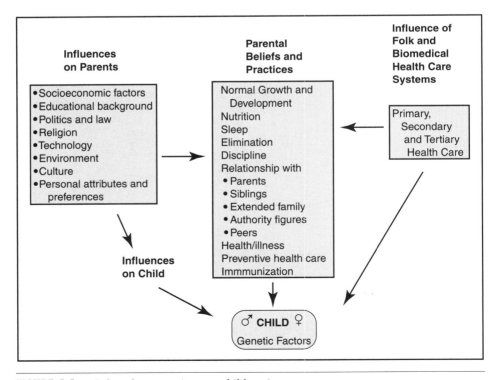

FIGURE 4-1. Cultural perspectives on childrearing.

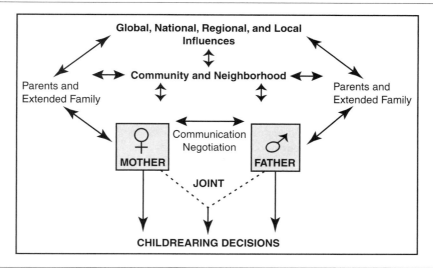

FIGURE 4-2. Culture, communication and parental decisions about childrearing practices.

influencing the parents' cultural perspectives on childrearing also influence others who may care for the child.

Generalizations about children from culturally diverse backgrounds sometimes need to be approached with caution. The observation that children in certain cultural groups are disproportionately poor, unhealthy or otherwise deprived is also of limited usefulness. Statistical data may be ignored or cited selectively to support a particular point of view. For example, although 29 percent of the U.S. poor are African American, 62 percent of the photographs accompanying articles about poverty in *Newsweek, Time* and *US News & World Report* portrayed impoverished African Americans (*Time,* 1997). This sends a subliminal message that exaggerates poverty among African Americans while underrepresenting devastating affects of poverty on people from other cultures. You must be aware of the manner in which subtle and overt racial bias is present in the larger social arena and make efforts to provide culturally competent health care for children from diverse backgrounds.

Family and Culture

Culture, like language, is acquired early in life, and cultural understanding is typically established by age 5. Every interaction, sound, touch, odor, and experience has a cultural component that is absorbed by the child even when it is not directly taught. Lessons learned at such early ages become an integral part of thinking and behavior. Table manners, the proper behavior when interacting with adults, sick role behaviors, and the rules of acceptable emotional response are anchored in culture. There are many beliefs and behaviors learned at an early age that persist into adulthood.

Over time, culture has influenced family functioning in many ways, including marriage forms, choice of mates, postmarital residence, family kinship system, rules governing inheritance, household and family structure, family obligations, family–community dynamics, and alternative family formations. These traditions have given families a sense of stability and support from which members draw comfort, guidance, and a means of coping with the problems of life, including physical and mental illness, handicaps, disability, dying, and death.

Each family modifies the culture of the larger group in ways that are uniquely its own. Some beliefs, practices, and customs are maintained, whereas others are altered or abandoned. Although it is helpful for you to have a basic knowledge of children's cultural backgrounds, it is also necessary to view each family on an individual basis. Assumptions or biased expectations cannot be allowed to replace accurate assessment. It is essential for you to remember that not all members of a cultural group behave in stereotypical fashion. For example, although many Chinese American children behave in the manner congruent with the stereotype, showing respect for authority, polite social behavior, and moderate-to-soft voice, there are some who are disrespectful, impolite, and boisterous. Individual differences, changing norms over time, degree of acculturation, length of time the family has lived in a country, and other factors account for variations from the stereotype.

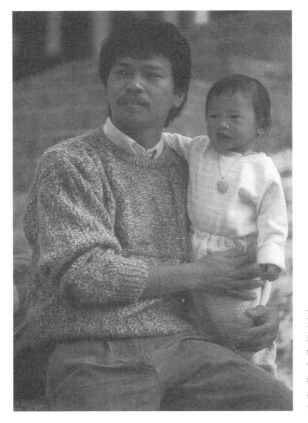

Nurses should avoid gender-related cultural stereotypes about single heads of houshold. Men, as well as women, may find themselves as heads of household, often as a result of spousal death, divorce, or separation.

The behavior of children and adolescents is influenced by childrearing practices, parental beliefs about involvement with children, and type and frequency of disciplinary measures. Although both parents exert an influence on the child's orientation to health, research indicates that a wide cultural variability exists, with the mother being the most influential parent in the majority of cultural groups. Thus, identifying the attitudes, values, and beliefs about health and illness held by the parents and other providers of child care is an important part of the cultural assessment of the family.

According to Richman, Miller, and LeVine (1992), mothers' attitudes toward health and illnesses are related to their educational level. Mothers with little formal education tend to be more fatalistic about illness and less concerned with detecting clinical manifestations of disease in their children than are well-educated mothers. The former also are less likely to follow up on precautionary measures suggested by health care providers. A mother who believes that people have no control over whether they become sick is unlikely to have an approach to health in which there is anticipatory guidance or accident prevention and may not comply with recommended immunization schedules. Nursing interventions with a mother who believes that there is much a person can do to keep from becoming ill will be different with regard to the nature of health education and counseling you provide.

With a knowledge of the belief system(s) of the family, you have data from which to choose approaches and priorities. For a mother who is not oriented to prevention of illness or maintenance of health, focusing energies on teaching might not be very productive; it might be more useful to spend time designing family follow-up or establishing an interpersonal relationship that invites the parent to follow recommended immunization schedules, well-child care, and other aspects of health promotion. You also should be prepared to understand why the mother who is less educated and embraces a fatalistic philosophy may fail to show up for scheduled well-child appointments while arriving for an appointment when she believes her child is sick. You may attempt to improve the attendance at well-child care appointments by offering to send reminders (by mail, phone, computer), encouraging mothers to bring grandparents, cousins, friends or others in a manner that mobilizes the culturally appropriate social support system, and assuring that the waiting period is reasonable and pleasant (e.g., providing magazines and toys that are culturally appropriate).

Extended Family

Early in the nurse–parent relationship, it is necessary to identify members of the extended family who play a significant role in the care of the child. When looking at families worldwide, the nuclear constellation is a rarity. In only 6 percent of the world's societies are families as isolated and nuclear as in the United States and Canada. The extended family is far more universally the norm. Kin residence sharing, for example, has long been acknowledged as characteristic of many African American, Mexican American, Amish, and other groups.

In societies where the extended family is the norm, parents, particularly those who married at a young age, may be considered too inexperienced to make major decisions on behalf of their child. In these groups, key decisions are frequently made in consultation with more mature relatives such as grandparents, uncles, aunts, cousins, or other kin. Sometimes non-kin are considered to be part of the extended family. In many religions, the members of one's church, synagogue, temple, or mosque are viewed as extended family members who may be relied on for various types of support including child care. Not coincidentally, members of some congregations refer to one another as brothers and sisters. The Amish family pattern is referred to as *freindschaft,* the term used for the three-generational family structure. Amish parents know that they can rely on the support of their entire church community. For example, a young Amish couple may turn to that community for assistance with decision making, finances, and emotional and spiritual support when a child is ill.

You should ask the parents if anyone besides themselves will be participating in the decision making that affects their child. Once that information is known, you should include the person(s) identified by the parents in the child's plan of care.

Cultural groups may differ not only in the central role played by families but also in the way they are structured hierarchically. In many parts of the world, distinct lines are drawn between members of society based on family connections, education, and wealth, and all members of the society are keenly aware of where they fit within this hierarchy. For example, in nations such as India, the existence of a caste system has been an integral component of the social order for many centuries. Members of the royal families in many European, Middle Eastern, and African nations enjoy positions of status not afforded to their subjects. Royals, aristocrats and members of the upper class from various nations sometimes seek treatment from U.S. or Canadian specialists for cardiac, renal and other serious or life-threatening diseases. It should be noted that nurses and other health care providers also are assigned a hierarchical position.

The influence of the extended family or of the social support network on the child's development becomes particularly important when considering the number of single-parent households in some culturally diverse groups. According to the U.S. Census Bureau, 55.3 percent of all African American children are born to a single mother, and nearly 60 percent of African American children under the age of 3 are not living with both parents. Among Puerto Ricans living in the United States, 44 percent of families are headed by single women.

The nuclear family is the unit on which most health care programs are designed. Consider the implicit message about the family when noting the number of chairs for visitors typically placed in hospital rooms, physician or nurse practitioner offices, and other health care settings. Although a handful of rural hospitals make special accommodations for the extended and church family of Amish patients to hitch their horses and buggies adjacent to the facility, seldom are the needs of the extended family network accommodated by the majority of health care facilities.

Each family modifies the culture of the larger group in ways that are uniquely its own. Some practices, beliefs, and customs are maintained, whereas others are altered or abandoned. Although it is helpful for you to have a basic knowledge of your clients' cultural backgrounds, it is also necessary for you to view each family they encounter on an individual basis.

Framework for Socialization of Children from Racial and Ethnic Minorities

In socializing their children, parents from racial and ethnic minorities have distinctive beliefs and behaviors that are determined by their cultural and socioeconomic situation. Socialization is often aimed at preparing children for the society they will encounter, a society in which children find out that the color of their skin or parental background determine how others relate to them. How parents socialize their children is influenced by the circumstances in which the parents themselves developed throughout life, experience with prejudice and discrimination, educational opportunities, and historical and political events involving members of their racial or ethnic heritage.

By following culturally influenced values and beliefs, parents try to foster competencies for successful functioning during childhood and in later years. Parents frequently have developed *adaptive strategies* based on their beliefs about what it means to be a member of a racial or ethnic minority group. Adaptive strategies arise from a need to survive and maintain continuity from one generation to the next. These strategies are the observable social behaviors that become linked with cultural patterns. Families formulate *socialization goals* to teach their children the strategies necessary for survival in a multicultural society. These goals are derived essentially from cultural knowledge of the tasks their children will have to face as adults, including ways of dealing with being a member of a racial or ethnic minority in a class- and race-conscious society. Research reveals that some children of African American, Hispanic, Asian, and Native American heritage are socialized to be *bicultural*, i.e., to acquire the skills needed to function in both the minority and majority cultures (Cross, 1987; Zayas & Solari, 1994). By comparison, White parents who are second- or third-generation immigrants tend to embrace a monocultural framework when socializing their children for life in contemporary society. Further study of children from so-called *mixed heritage* needs to be conducted to determine how socialization occurs.

The competencies needed to function in the real world come from socialization goals and are instilled through close interaction between children and older family members, in which more experienced members of the culture guide children to acquire the skills needed to function in the culture. One result of this mentorship and skills development is that the child's *cultural identity* is enhanced. The presence of nurturing, supportive, and disciplined mentors is essential in transmitting the values, beliefs, and behaviors of a culture.

One example of an adaptive strategy and socialization goal occurs when families emphasize solidarity and the individual's sense of obligation to the family. This strategy helps to protect the family's continuity and preserve its culture—or multiple cultures in the case of intermarriage. It should be noted that the extended family members may serve as the primary mentors for transmitting important values of the culture when parents are unavailable or unable to do so, for example, when financial constraints require parents to rely on extended family members for child care while they work outside of the home. The socialization goal that emerges is to have children accept that family is to be the central focus of their lives. A child-rearing practice that incorporates these goals is the insistence on children's conformity to parental and extended-family authority, which often extends to conformity to the authority of other adults as well. In addition to giving esteem to elder members of the culture, this reinforces the importance of family-relatedness and helps in identity development.

Effects of Immigration on Children

According to the U.S. Bureau of the Census, Population Division, Education and Social Stratification Division (1990), more than 2 million U.S. children are foreign-born and millions more are the children of recent immigrants. Many of these children comprise the 6.3 million school-aged children (14 percent of the U.S. population ages 5 to 17) who speak a language other than English at home. Approximately two thirds of these children come from Spanish-speaking homes, and a large percentage of the remainder speak a variety of Asian languages. Some children of immigrants live in *linguistically isolated* households, those in which no member age 14 or older speaks English "very well." Nationwide, 4 percent of children ages 5 to 17 live in such households (U.S. Bureau of the Census, Population Division, Education and Social Stratification Branch, 1990).

Although they may be found throughout the U.S. and Canada, immigrants and their children tend to cluster in certain geographic areas. According to the U.S. Bureau of the Census (1990), California, Texas, and New York are homes for almost two thirds of all foreign-born children. New Mexico, Arizona, New Jersey and Florida also have relatively high numbers of children whose parents recently migrated to the U.S. In Canada, Toronto and Vancouver are home for the majority of children of recent immigrants.

Children are very dependent on their families, and when parents or other adult family members are unfamiliar with the social and health care systems, children are at risk of being underserved. In the current environment, this risk is compounded by the fact that, for some children of immigrants, their parents, siblings, and/or the children themselves may be in the U.S. or Canada illegally. For many undocumented immigrants, frequent contact with public institutions may place them or their continued residence in the U.S. or Canada in jeopardy.

Normal Growth and Development

Although growth and development of infants and children is similar in all cultures, important racial, ethnic, and sex differences can be identified. From the moment of conception, the developmental processes of the human life cycle take place in the context of culture. Throughout life, culture exerts an all-pervasive influence on the developing infant, child, and adolescent. For example, there is similarity cross-culturally in the sequence and timing of developmental milestones in infant development, smiling, separation anxiety, and language acquisition. Developmental researchers who have worked in other cultures have become convinced that human functioning cannot be separated from the cultural and more immediate context in which children develop.

Not all developmental theories formulated on the basis of observations with Western children have cross-cultural generalizability. Investigations of the universality of the stages of development proposed by Piaget, the family role relations emphasized by Freud, and patterns of mother–infant interaction taken to index security of attachment have resulted in modifications as a result of cross-cultural data.

Infant Attachment

In examining infant attachment, cross-cultural differences become apparent in the research that has been conducted on the topic. For example, researchers have discovered that German mothers expect very early autonomy in the child and have few physical interventions as the child plays alone. Among Japanese, there are infrequent mother-child separations and the mother has close physical interaction with the child during play. Japanese mothers tend to stay near a great deal, to do many things for, and have close physical contact with their infants. Similarly, Hispanic mothers of Puerto Rican and Dominican ancestry display close mother–child relationships and more verbal and physical expression of parental affection than European American parents. Anglo American mothers tend to have few physical interventions when the child is playing, and they encourage exploration and independence, behaviors that reflect the cultural values of the mothers. Anglo American mothers tend to give greater emphasis to qualities associated with the mainstream American ideal of individualism such as autonomy, self-control and activity, whereas the Puerto Rican mothers describe children in terms congruent with Puerto Rican cultural emphasis on relatedness, such as affection, dignity, respectfulness, responsiveness to mother and others, and proximity-seeking (Zayas & Solari, 1994). Studies suggest that differences in infant attachment are linked to cultural variation in parenting behavior and life experiences. The parents' socialization, values, beliefs, goals, and behaviors are determined in large measure by what their culture defines as good parenting and preferred child behaviors for each gender.

Crying

Cultural differences exist in mothers' developmental goals for their infants and in the way they perceive, react, and behave in response to their infants' cues, behaviors, and demands. Knowledge of cultural differences in parental responses to crying is relevant for nurses who base their assessment of the severity of an infant's distress according to the parent's interpretation of the crying. You may overestimate or underestimate the seriousness of a problem because of cultural differences in the parent's perception of the infant's distress. You also may misinterpret the degree of concern a parent has for an infant if your cultural beliefs and practices differ from those of the parent or other provider of care.

Cultural Assessment

When assessing infants, children and adolescents, you must understand the relationship between the biologic and cultural aspects of development. In assessing the growth and development of a child, it is important to determine the child's correct age. Stated age may vary according to culture. For example, the Vietnamese consider that infants are 1 year old at birth and that they become another year old at the next *Tet,* or New Year. Furthermore, some Vietnamese who migrated around the time of the Vietnam War learned that it was necessary to give inaccurate information about their children's ages in order to meet legal requirements for entrance into the United States. Thus, an apparently simple question about a child's age is a potential source of miscommunication. Moreover, an apparently straightforward question about a child's age is more complex than you might expect, and it may adversely affect the nurse–parent relationship, particularly if the parent misperceives the reason underlying the question.

Certain *growth patterns* can be identified across cultural boundaries. For example, regardless of culture, there is a pattern of general-to-specific abilities, from the center of the body to the extremities (proximal–distal development) and from the head to the toes (cephalocaudal development). Adult head size is reached by the age of 5 years, whereas the remainder of the body continues to grow through adolescence. Physiologic maturation of organ systems such as the renal, circulatory, and respiratory systems occurs early, whereas maturation of the central nervous system continues beyond childhood.

Other growth patterns seem to be specific to cultural groups. For example, in some cultures, the standard Western developmental pattern of sitting–creeping–crawling–standing–walking–squatting is not followed. The Balinese infant goes from sitting to squatting to standing. Hopi children begin walking about a month and a half later than Anglo American children, which is paradoxical, given the advanced motor development that generally characterizes members of traditional societies. Tooth eruption occurs earlier in Asian and African American infants than in their white counterparts (Overfield, 1995).

Height and Weight

In the U.S., African Americans and whites differ in mean birthweight, with African Americans being 181 to 240 g lighter. This explains, in part, why *prematurity,* defined as birthweight less than 2,500 g (5 lb, 8 oz), is twice as common in African Americans as it is in whites. Chinese, Filipinos, Hawaiians, Japanese, and Puerto Ricans also have lower mean birthweights than whites in the U.S. Significant intertribal variation occurs in the birthweights of Native Americans. For example, the average birthweight among Hopi females is 3097 g whereas Cheyenne females weigh on average 3459. Native Americans from British Columbia and Northwestern Ontario have higher mean birthweights than non-Native Canadians. Overall, Native Americans have a larger number of infants weighing 4000 g or more at birth, a fact that is believed to be associated with the high incidence of diabetes in Native Americans (Overfield, 1995).

Although it is difficult to separate nongenetic from genetic influences, some populations are shorter or taller than others during various periods of growth and in adulthood. African American infants are approximately ¾ inch shorter at birth than whites. In general, African American and white children are tallest followed by Native Americans; Asian children are shortest. Children of higher socioeconomic status are taller in all cultures. Data on African American and white children between 1 and 6 years show that at age 6, African Americans are taller than whites. Around age 9 or 10, white boys begin to catch up in height. White girls catch up with their African

American counterparts around 14 or 15 years of age. Around puberty, African American children begin to slow down in growth, and white children catch up, so that the two races achieve similar heights in adulthood. Their sitting/standing height ratios, however, differ. Mexican American children have sitting/standing height ratios similar to those of white children, indicating similar stature and leg proportions. African American children have longer legs in proportion to height than other groups (Overfield, 1995).

The growth spurt of adolescence involves the skeletal and muscular systems, leading to significant changes in size and strength in both sexes but particularly in males. According to Overfield (1995), North American Caucasian youths aged 12 to 18 years are 22 to 33 lb heavier and 6 in taller than Filipino youths the same age. African American teenagers are somewhat taller and heavier than white teens up to age 15 years. Japanese adolescents born in the United States or Canada are larger and taller than Japanese born and raised in Japan owing to differences in diet, climate, and social milieu. Adolescence also involves changes in the physiologic functioning of body systems, including the reproductive system.

Culture-Universal and Culture-Specific Childrearing

In the following section, some culture-universal and culture-specific childrearing values, attitudes, beliefs, and practices will be examined. In reviewing the literature on cultural perspectives on children and adolescents, you will note similarities and differences in the way parents and other primary providers of care relate during various developmental stages. A discussion of culture-universals in childrearing will be followed by some remarks about culture-specific practices.

Culture-Universal Childrearing Practices

In all cultures, infants and children are valued, treasured, loved and nurtured because they represent the promise that the human race will continue in future generations. From the moment of birth, differentiation between the sexes is recognized. The early differentiation of sex roles is manifest in terms of sex-specific tasks, play, and dress. Throughout infancy, childhood, and adolescence, girls and boys undergo a process of socialization aimed at preparing them to assume adult roles in the larger society into which they have been born or have migrated. Parents and other primary providers of care use various forms of discipline to encourage certain types of behavior and discourage other behaviors in children and adolescents. As children grow and develop, their interaction with others—siblings, extended family members, teachers, religious leaders, peers, and so forth—increases. Children learn communication, language, and other skills needed to interact with people within a cultural context. All parents want to be treated respectfully by their children and want their children to show respect toward selected others in society, the manifestations of which are expressed verbally and non-verbally. When children behave in a manner that is culturally appropriate, they become a source of pride to their parents and bring honor to their family and cultural heritage.

Culture-Specific Childrearing Practices

Although there are many universals, the majority of research has focused on culture-specific childrearing values, attitudes, beliefs and practices. In other words, there has been a greater interest in cultural differences than similarities.

A few caveats will be presented before discussing childrearing practices that are specific to certain groups. First, childrearing practices are interrelated with the social, educational, religious, and cultural backgrounds of the parents or other providers of care. Second, it is important to distinguish between cultural practices and those that reflect the *economic* well-being of the parents and extended family. For example, stereotypes of African Americans suggest that premarital teenage pregnancy is more common and acceptable than it is among counterparts in other cultures. When socio-economic factors are considered, however, the myth is shattered. Although African-American adolescents from the lower socioeconomic class have higher rates of teen pregnancy, this is not the case for middle- and upper-class African Americans. Third, the concept of high context and low context cultures helps to explain some of the similarities and differences observed in childrearing practices.

The following discussion will focus on *clinically significant* childrearing behaviors among families from diverse cultures. Although it may be interesting to know, for example, that children are viewed as a gift from God among various ethnic and religious groups, your primary concern is with knowledge having clinical relevance such as nutrition, sleep, elimination, parent-child relationships, discipline, and related concepts.

Cultural Considerations in Nutrition of Children: Feeding and Eating Behaviors

In many cultures breast-feeding is traditionally practiced for varying lengths of time following the birth of an infant—1 year, 2 years, until the birth of the next child, and so forth. With the growing availability and convenience of bottled formula, manufacturers of these products have launched effective marketing campaigns during the past decade, which has resulted in a decrease in the number of women who breast-feed. Summarized in Research Application 4-1 is a study of the feeding and weaning practices of Cuban and Haitian immigrant mothers.

Research Application 4-1   *Feeding and Weaning Practices of Cuban and Haitian Immigrant Mothers*

Thomas, J. T., & DeSantis, L. (1995). Feeding and weaning practices of Cuban and Haitian immigrant mothers. *Journal of Transcultural Nursing, 6*(2), 34–42.

The reasons for the decline in breast-feeding among immigrant mothers has become the focus of research by transcultural nurses. In a descriptive study of 30 Cuban and 30 Haitian immigrant women residing in Florida, the feeding and weaning practices of mothers were examined using open-ended interviews conducted in Spanish or Haitian Creole. A 110-item questionnaire surveyed sociodemographic characteristics, household structure and function, concepts of child health and illness, and childrearing beliefs and practices related to discipline, expression of emotion, independence, feeding and weaning, and sex role development. Seventy-seven percent (N = 23) of the Cuban mothers considered breast-feeding better than bottle feeding; 10 percent (N = 3) stated that bottle feeding was best; and 10 percent (N = 3) indicated that breast and bottle feeding were equally beneficial. Among the Haitian mothers, 73 percent (N = 22) believed that breast-feeding was best, and 27 percent (N = 8) stated bottle feeding was better. Despite these findings, only 43 percent (N = 13) of Cuban and 60 percent (N = 18) of the Haitian mothers chose to breast-feed one or more of their infants.

Clinical Application

Nurses working with breast-feeding Cuban and Haitian immigrant mothers will find the following data-based recommendations from the study useful in clinical practice.

- Observe for infant obesity due to the combination of early food supplements, prolonged bottle feeding, and the health culture belief that fat children are healthy children.

- When discussing feeding practices with Haitian mothers, ask about adding cereals to bottle feedings because such additives are not regarded as food.

- Observe for dental caries caused by prolonged contact of teeth with carbohydrate-rich fluids used as pacifiers and the sucrose and corn syrup products found in infant formulas.

- Discourage mothers from the cultural practice of sudden breast weaning, most likely to occur among Haitians. Advise the mothers that this practice may result in increasingly frequent temper tantrums and other psychological manifestations of mother–child separation.

- Cognizant of the Haitian practice of purging or using laxatives on children to *clean the blood*, provide parents with information about clinical manifestations of dehydration and provide guidelines to ensure adequate intake of fluids, especially during the neonatal period.

- Recognizing that many Cuban and Haitian mothers give vitamin and mineral supplements, home remedies, or over-the-counter drugs, be sure to assess what the mother is administering before recommending additional medications. It may be necessary to modify either the mother's child-care measures or the routine well-child care recommended by the American Academy of Pediatrics.

You need to be aware that cultural feeding practices may result in threats to the infant's dental health. Studies involving Navajo, African American, Mexican American, and other groups demonstrate that caregivers frequently prop a bottle filled with milk, juice or soda pop when the infant goes to sleep, a practice that is known to cause dental caries. You should teach new mothers about the dangers of propping bottles and encourage them to return to breast-feeding, unless there are contraindications to breast-feeding.

In some cultures, mothers may *pre-masticate* or chew the food for infants and young children with the belief that this will facilitate digestion. The practice has been most frequently reported among African American and Hispanic mothers of lower socioeconomic status. From a nutritional perspective, this practice may remove some of the vitamins and minerals from the food before it reaches the infant and make it more acidic. You should warn the mother to refrain from pre-masticating the food if she has an upper respiratory infection, sore throat or other condition that might be transmitted to the baby.

Health status is, in part, dependent on nutritional intake, thus integrally linking the child's nutritional status and health. Although the United States is the world's greatest food-producing nation, nutritional status has not been a priority for many people in this country. An estimated 1 million U.S. children suffer from malnutrition serious enough to interfere with brain development. Many Southeast Asian refugees, for example, were in a prolonged state of malnutrition before emigrating, and undocumented aliens, migrants, poor African Americans in rural and inner-city areas, Appalachians, and others living at the poverty level may be unable to provide their children with an adequate food intake.

Malnutrition is not found exclusively among children from the lower socioeconomic class. Many middle- and upper-class children, including some obese children, are also malnourished. Obesity frequently begins during infancy, when mothers succumb to pressures to overfeed. For example, among many who identify themselves as Filipino, Vietnamese, and Mexican, to name a few cultures, fat babies generally are considered healthy babies. For the members of most African tribes, fat babies are considered healthy, and mild to moderate obesity is considered a sign of affluence and health later in life.

The popularity of fast-food restaurants and "junk" foods has resulted in a high-calorie, high-fat, high-cholesterol, and high-carbohydrate diet for many children. Parents are frequently involved in numerous activities outside of the house and have

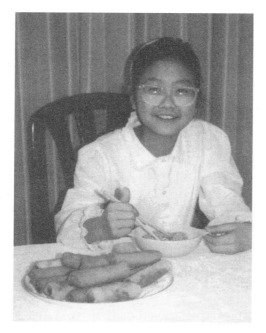

Culture determines the type of foods eaten and the manner in which they are consumed. Many Chinese American children enjoy traditional Chinese cuisine as well as American foods. They are frequently skillful users of both chopsticks and American eating utensils (knife, fork, and spoon).

little time for traditional tasks such as cooking meals. The prevailing attitude among many couples with children is that cooking and housekeeping chores are a choice rather than a necessity. This view toward domestic chores is often held by parents from both affluent and less affluent populations. Because fast foods have intrinsic nutritional value, their benefit needs to be evaluated on the basis of age-specific requirements. For example, the total caloric needs of children of specific ages should be calculated and then compared with total caloric intakes during a typical day.

The extent to which families have retained their cultural practices at mealtime varies widely. Because a hospitalized child's recovery may be enhanced by familiar foods, you need to assess the influence of culture on eating habits. For hospitalized children, you should foster an environment at mealtime that closely simulates the home. Family members can be encouraged to visit during mealtime or to eat with the child, if this is appropriate. For example, the majority of Vietnamese parents believe that children should be fed separately from adults and that they should acquire "good table manners" by age 5 years. Depending on dietary restrictions necessitated by the child's medical condition, parents should be encouraged to prepare familiar foods at home and bring them to the hospital. The child should be encouraged to eat in the manner that is customary at home. For example, the Asian American child who eats with chopsticks at home should be encouraged to do so in the hospital.

Sleep

Although the amount of sleep required at various ages is similar across cultures, differences in sleep patterns and bedtime rituals exist. The sleep practices in a family household reflect some of the deepest moral ideals of a cultural community. Nurses working with families of young children in both community and inpatient settings frequently encounter cultural differences in family sleeping behaviors.

Community health, psychiatric, and pediatric nurses who work with young children and their families often assess the family's sleep and rest patterns. Nurses traditionally have taken a rigid approach on the issue of co-family sleeping that excludes common cultural practices. Although some degree of *cosleeping*, the practice of parents and children sleeping together for all or part of the night, is common in families with young children, there are marked cultural differences in the proportion who cosleep all night regularly (more than 2 to 3 times per week). In a survey of the parents of 3- and 4-year olds from African American, Hispanic, Vietnamese, Russian, Middle Eastern and Eastern European descent, Canuso (1996) found that the majority bring their children into bed with them at some time. Some parents allow the child into their bed only occasionally, as in after a nightmare or if the child is upset, whereas others routinely had children crawl in bed with them. A few parents indicated that they slept with their children all the time.

According to Lozoff, et al. (1996) regular all night cosleeping is most common among African American families (50 percent), intermediate among Hispanic families (21 percent), and lowest among white families (<10 percent). It should be noted that children may also sleep in the same bed with siblings or members of the extended family. Although the socioeconomic status of the family is known to be a factor, with more cosleeping occurring in families of lower socioeconomic status, some middle- and upper-class families practice cosleeping, too. Most white middle-class Americans believe that infants and children should sleep alone. According to Shweder, Jensen and Goldstein (1990), the values that underlie the custom of having children sleep alone—autonomy, privacy, independence, and the primacy of the couple's relationship over the parent–child relationship—are not necessarily shared by parents from diverse cultures who place a higher value on protection of the vulnerable child. As indicated in Research Application 4-2, children who cosleep are more likely to wake at night or have trouble falling asleep alone at bedtime.

To promote rest in the inpatient setting, you need to identify the child's usual pattern by asking the parents about the normal bedtime routine at home. The child

---

Research Application 4-2   *Cultural Perspectives on Cosleeping and Early Childhood Sleep Problems*

Lozoff, B., Askew, G. L., & Wolf, A. W. (1996). **Cosleeping and early childhood sleep problems: Effects of ethnicity and socioeconomic status**. *Developmental and Behavioral Pediatrics, 17*(1), 9–15.

This study examined ethnic differences in the relationship between cosleeping and sleep problems among children, taking socioeconomic status (SES) into consideration. The sample consisted of 186 urban families (N = 90 black and N = 96 white) with a healthy child between the ages of 6 and 48 months who had been seen for well-child care at pediatric health care facilities in a large urban midwestern city. The children were divided into categories based on race and SES, and parents were interviewed about cosleeping and perceived sleep problems. For the purpose of this study cosleeping was defined as parents and children sleeping in body contact with each other for all or part of the night.

The findings reveal that cosleeping was associated with increased night waking and/or bedtime protests among lower SES white children and higher SES black children. Among families who coslept, white parents were more likely than black parents to consider their child's sleep behavior to be a problem, that is, stressful, conflictual, or upsetting as well as regularly occurring. The researchers suggest that one explanation for this is that differing childrearing attitudes and expectations influenced how parents interpreted their children's sleep behavior.

Clinical Application

At the time of each well-child ambulatory visit, home care visit, and pediatric hospital admission, the nurse usually asks how the infant or child has been sleeping. Because difficulties surrounding sleep may indicate the presence of an illness or be the source of concern to parents or other primary providers of care, the nurse must be knowledgeable about cultural beliefs and practices about sleep. Anticipatory guidance aimed at prevention of a problem surrounding the child's sleep is better than rectifying a problem once it has been created. Nurses should examine the cultural context in which cosleeping occurs, assess parental reactions to children's sleep behaviors, and tailor the advice they give about cosleeping and sleep problems. The researchers suggest the following: Ask parents of infants how they feel about cosleeping with a toddler or preschooler or staying with their child at bedtime when he or she is older. If the parents do not like these ideas, suggest that they avoid cosleeping or plan to stop doing so well before the end of the first year of life, when attachment and separation issues become more intense.

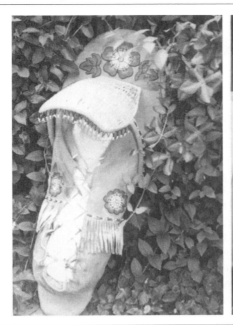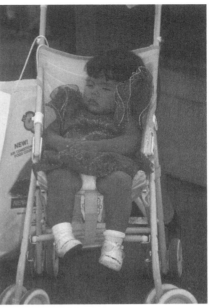

In most cultures, parents and other care providers use devices that enable the child to sleep while being transported from place to place with relative ease. (Left) Use of cradleboards, created many centuries before the infant seat to promote infant mobility and safety, is still prevalent among many Native American tribes. (Right) Mexican American child in a stroller.

may have a favorite toy or story. Depending on the family's religious persuasion, parents may encourage the child to say a prayer at bedtime. You should encourage the child's familiar routine to be continued in the hospital as much as possible.

The type of bed familiar to the child also may vary considerably. In a traditional American Samoan home, infants sleep on a *pandanus mat* covered with a blanket, and sometimes a pillow is used. A *cradleboard* is used by a number of American Indian tribes. Constructed by a family member, a cradleboard is made of cedar, pine, or pinon wood; it may be decorated in various ways, depending on the affluence of the family and on tribal customs. After completion, the cradleboard is blessed in a traditional manner. The cradleboard helps the infant feel secure and can be moved around with ease while the family engages in work, travel, or other activities. Although cradleboards have been blamed for exacerbating hip dysplasias in Native infants, diapering counterbalances this by causing a slight abduction of the hips.

In the United States and Canada, the common developmental milestone of sleeping for 8 uninterrupted hours by age 4 to 5 months is regarded as a sign of neurologic maturity. In many other cultures, however, the infant sleeps with the mother and is allowed to breast-feed on demand with minimal disturbance of adult sleep. In such an arrangement, there is less parental motivation to enforce "sleeping through the night," and infants continue to wake up every 4 hours during the night to feed, which is approximately the frequency of feeding during the day. Thus, it appears that this developmental milestone, in addition to its biologic basis, is a function of the context in which it develops.

Elimination

Elimination refers to ridding the body of wastes, a function that is accomplished by the combined work of the gastrointestinal, genitourinary, respiratory, and integumentary systems. Of primary concern to parents is bowel and bladder control, which is the focus of considerable attention by parents of toddlers and pre-schoolers. Toilet training is a major developmental milestone, perhaps more for the parents than for the child, and is taught through a variety of cultural patterns.

Most children achieve dryness by 2½ to 3 years of age. Bowel training is more easily accomplished than bladder training. Daytime, or diurnal, wetting is less frequent than nighttime, or nocturnal, wetting. Some cultures start toilet training a child before the end of the first year and consider the child a "failure" if dryness is not achieved by 18 months. In other cultures, children are not expected to be dry until 5 years of age. Boys have a more difficult time achieving bladder control than girls.

A child's constipation is a persistent concern among parents who expect a ritualistic daily pattern. In some cultures, infants are given herbs aimed at purging them when they are a few days, weeks, or months of age to remove evil spirits from the body. You should advise the parents against using purgatives in infants because fluid and electrolyte imbalance occurs and dehydration may ensue rapidly.

The role of the nurse is to acknowledge that toilet training can be taught through a variety of cultural patterns but that physical and psychosocial health are promoted by accepting, flexible approaches. A previously toilet-trained child may become incontinent as a result of the stress of hospitalization but will regain control quickly when returned to his or her familiar home environment. You should reassure parents that regression in hospitalized children is normal and expected.

Menstruation

Ethnicity is the strongest determinant of the duration of menstrual bleeding and of the likelihood that heavy bleeding will occur. In a study of 248 12 to 14-year old African American and European American girls, Harlow and Cambell (1996) report that the average duration of bleeding was 5.1 days for African American girls and 5.6 days for European American girls. European American girls were less likely to have an episode of heavy bleeding than were African American girls. These findings reveal that cultural differences exist in menstruation among girls from different groups. The role of diet, exercise, and stress also must be examined because these factors are known to influence menstruation in women of all ages. Further investigation of potential differences in characteristics of bleeding among various cultural groups may help to understand reasons for differences in risk of menstrual and uterine abnormalities.

Attitudes toward menstruation are often culturally based, and the adolescent girl may be taught many folk beliefs at the time of puberty. Among Mexican Americans, menstruation is often considered an unpleasant but natural condition requiring circumspect behavior. For example, in traditional Mexican American families, menstruating females are not permitted to walk barefooted, wash their hair, or take showers or baths. In encouraging hygienic practices, you should respect cultural directives by encouraging sponge bathing, frequent changing of sanitary pads or tampons, and other interventions that promote cleanliness without violating cultural mandates.

Some Mexican Americans believe that sour or iced foods cause menstrual blood to coagulate, and some Puerto Rican teenagers have been taught that drinking lemon or pineapple juice will increase menstrual cramping. You should be aware of these beliefs and should respect personal preferences concerning beverages. The teenager has probably been taught the folk practices by her mother or by another woman in her family, who may be watchful during the girl's menstrual periods. If menstruation coincides with hospitalization, you need to respect the teenager's preferences and may need to reassure the mother or significant other that their cultural practices will be respected.

Some Mexican Americans believe that delayed menses are caused by the stoppage of blood flow, a condition treated by the administration of certain herbs. Among other cultural groups, menstrual cramping may be treated with a wide variety of home remedies. You should ask the adolescent girl whether she takes anything special during menstruation or in the absence of menstrual flow. It may be necessary to verify the amount and type of home remedy and to determine its interactive effect with prescription medicines.

Adolescent girls of Islamic religious persuasion, whose heritage may be Palestinian, Lebanese, Jordanian, Saudi Arabian, and from other Near or Middle Eastern nations or some African nations, have cultural/religious prohibitions and duties during and after menstruation. In Islamic law, blood is considered unclean. The blood of menstruation, as well as blood lost during childbirth, is believed to render the female impure or potentially polluting.

Because one must be in a pure state in order to pray, menstruating girls and women are forbidden to perform certain acts of worship such as touching the *Qur'an* (Koran), entering a mosque, praying, and participating in the feast of Ramadan. During the menstrual period, sexual intercourse is forbidden for both males and females. When the menstrual flow stops, the girl or woman performs a special washing to purify herself (Luna, 1989; Rizvi, 1984).

In Islam, sexual pollution applies equally to males and females. For males, sexual intercourse and the discharge of semen is an act that renders them impure. A *junub* is a man or woman who has become impure because of sexual intercourse. They must perform the ritual washing before being able to perform the prayer (Luna, 1989).

Parent–Child Relationships and Discipline

In some cultures, both parents assume responsibility for the care of children, whereas in other cultures, the relationship with the mother is primary, with the father remaining somewhat distant. With the approach of adolescence, the gender-related aspects of the parent-child relationship may be modified to conform with cultural expectations.

Some cultures encourage children to participate in family decision making and to discuss or even argue points with their parents. Some African American families, for example, encourage children to express opinions verbally and to take an active role in all family activities. Many Asian American parents value respectful, deferential behavior toward adults, who are considered experienced and wise. Many Asian American children are discouraged from making decisions independently. The witty, fast reply that is viewed in some European American cultures as a sign of intelligence and cleverness might be punished in some non-Western circles as a sign of rudeness and disrespect.

Physical punishment of American Indian children is rare. Instead of using loud scoldings and reprimands, Indian parents generally discipline with a quiet voice, telling the child what is expected. During breast-feeding and toilet training Indian children are typically permitted to set their own pace. Parents tend to be permissive and nondemanding.

With the approach of adolescence, parental relationships and discipline generally change. Teens are usually given increasing amounts of freedom and encouraged to try out adult roles but in a supervised way that enables parents to retain considerable control. In many cultures, adolescent boys are permitted more freedom than girls of the same age.

Distinguishing Child Abuse from Folk Healing

Child abuse and neglect have been documented throughout human history and are known across cultures. In the early 1960s, child maltreatment in the United States became prominent as pediatricians documented radiologic evidence and other symptoms of abuse and neglect in well-publicized reports (Kempe et al., 1962). International attention to child maltreatment emerged in the late 1970s, and the International Society for the Prevention of Child Abuse and Neglect (ISPPCAN) has held international congresses and regional meetings to explore physical abuse and neglect, sexual molestation, child prostitution, nutritional deprivation, emotional maltreatment, and institutional abuse from a cross-national perspective (Doek, 1991; Korbin, 1990).

Cross-cultural variability in child-rearing beliefs and practices have created a dilemma that makes establishment of a universal standard for optimal child care, as well as definitions of child abuse and neglect, extremely difficult. The following widely accepted definition of child abuse and neglect in the United States pertains to any person under the age of 18 years: "The injury, sexual abuse, sexual exploitation, or negligent treatment or maltreatment of a child by any person under circumstances which indicate that the child's health, welfare, and safety is harmed thereby. . . . this subsection shall not be construed to authorize interference with child-raising practices, including reasonable parental discipline, which are not proved to be injurious to the child's health, welfare, and safety" (West's Revised Code of Washington Annotated, 1990, p. 121).

Korbin (1991) has identified three levels in formulating culturally appropriate definitions of child maltreatment: (1) cultural differences in child-rearing practices and beliefs, (2) idiosyncratic departure from one's cultural continuum of acceptable behavior, and (3) societal harm to children.

The *first level* encompasses practices that are viewed as acceptable in the culture in which they occur but as abusive or neglectful by outsiders. For example, in Turkey and many Middle Eastern cultures, despite warm temperatures, infants are covered with multiple layers of clothing and may be observed to sweat profusely because parents believe that young children become chilled very easily and die from exposure to the cold. Many African nations continue to practice rites of initiation for boys and girls, usually at the time of puberty. In some cases, ritual circumcision—of both boys and girls—is performed without anesthetic, and the ability to endure the associated pain is considered to be a manifestation of the maturity expected of an adult. In the United States and Canada, the African American family's focus on physical forms of discipline may present controversial and ethical issues for the nurse.

The *second level,* idiosyncratic abuse or neglect, signals a departure from the continuum of culturally acceptable behavior. Some societies (Turkish, Mexican, and others), for example, permit fondling of the genitals of infants and young children to soothe them or encourage sleep. However, such fondling of older children or for the sexual gratification of adults would fall outside of the acceptable cultural continuum (Korbin, 1991).

At the *third level,* societal conditions such as poverty, inadequate housing, poor maternal and child health care, and lack of nutritional resources either contribute powerfully to child maltreatment or are considered maltreatment in and of themselves. African American children are three times as likely as white children to die of child abuse, but considerable disagreement exists about whether race differences exist in the prevalence of child abuse independent of socioeconomic factors such as income and employment status. You need to become knowledgeable about folk beliefs, child-rearing practices, and cultural variability in defining child maltreatment. Summarized in Table 4-1 are four Southeast Asian folk healing practices that produce physical marks on the child's body.

Gender Differences

In all known human societies, adult males differ from adult females in both primary and secondary sex characteristics. On average, males have higher oxygen-carrying capacity in the blood, a higher muscle–fat ratio, more body hair, a larger skeleton, and greater height. Behaviorally, there are also differences between the two sexes, especially in the division of labor.

For children, gender differences can be identified cross-culturally in six classes of behavior: nurturance, responsibility, obedience, self-reliance, achievement, and independence (Barry, Bacon, & Child, 1967). Differences between males and females appear early in life and form the basis for adult roles within a culture. Male neonates are larger and more vigorously active and have more muscle development, a higher basal metabolic rate, and a higher pain threshold. Female neonates react more positively to comforting than do males. By 14 weeks of age, girls may be conditioned through the use of auditory reinforcers, and boys may be conditioned through the use of visual reinforcers but not vice versa. By the age of 4 months, girls focus longer than boys on facelike masks, indicating that girls are more interested in faces or facelike configurations (Overfield, 1995).

Variability in sex-role behavior is a common occurrence. The majority of people in a society adopt most of the behavior defined as appropriate to their biologic sex, but there are many exceptions. Sex roles are themselves highly variable, by age and by social class, among other ways. The stringency of expectations also varies so that females in the United States and Canada can violate sex-role norms with fewer explicit sanctions than can males. Across cultures, even the number of sex roles is subject to variations.

TABLE 4-1
Southeast Asian Folk Healing Practices

Coining (*Cao gio*)

Appearance:	Superficial ecchymotic, nonpainful areas with petechiae usually appearing between the rib bones on the front and back of the body and resembling strap marks. Coining may also be done along the trachea or on either side of the trachea, vertically along the linner aspect of both upper arms, or along both sides of the spine.
Conditions treated:	Pain, colds, heat exhaustion, vomiting, headache
Procedure:	A special menthol oil or ointment is applied to the painful or symptomatic area. Then the edge of a coin is rubbed over the area with firm downward strokes. The procedure is mildly uncomfortable.
Belief:	The "coining" exudes the "bad wind." Appearance of a deep reddish-purple skin color is confirmation that the person indeed had "bad wind" in the body and that coining was the appropriate treatment. If only redness appears, the client must consult a healer or doctor for another treatment.
Age of patient:	Infants a few months old through seniors
Practiced by:	Mien, Vietnamese, Cambodian (rare), Lao (rare), ethnic Chinese
Who applies the treatment:	Any adult

Burning (*Poua*)

Appearance:	Asymmetric, superficial, painful burns ¼ inch diameter appearing either as a single burn in the center of the forehead or as two nearly symmetrical vertical rows down the front or back of the body, often including the neck.
Conditions treated:	Any kind of pain—including pain from a cough or diarrhea—as well as serious conditions such as failure to thrive
Procedure:	A tall, weedlike grass is peeled and allowed to dry. The end is dipped in heated, melted pork lard and the tip is then ignited and applied to the skin in the area requiring treatment (e.g., joints are burned for failure to thrive). The treatment is painful and always the *treatment of last resort.*
Belief:	The burning exudes the noxious element causing the pain or illness.
Age of patient:	Infants a few months old through seniors
Practiced by:	Mien, Cambodian (rare)
Who applies the treatment:	In Mien culture the treatment is performed only by a skilled healer. In Cambodian culture any experienced adult may do it.

Cupping (*Ventouse*)

Appearance:	Circular, nonraised, ecchymotic, painful burn marks 2 in in diameter, usually appearing in symmetric, vertical rows of two to four cups on the left and right sides of the chest, abdomen, and back, or singly as one cup on the forehead. Cupping is rarely practiced in the United States.
Conditions treated:	Pain, bodyache, headache
Procedure:	Though borrowed from the French, the specific procedure in southeast Asia varies among ethnic groups. The principle is to create a vacuum inside a special cup by igniting alcohol-soaked cotton inside the cup. When the flame extinguishes, the cup is immediately applied to the skin of the painful site. Suction is created, and the skin is pulled up inside the mouth of the cup. The cup remains in place 15 to 20 minutes or until the suction can be easily released. The procedure is painful.
Belief:	The suction exudes the noxious element. The greater the "bruise," the greater the seriousness of the illness.
Age of patient:	Adults, occasionally teens
Practiced by:	H'mong, Mien, Lao (rare), Cambodian (rare), Vietnamese, ethnic Chinese

TABLE 4-1 *(Continued)*

Who applies the treatment:	Any adult, except in Vietnamese culture, in which only a skilled nurse or healer may do it.

Pinching (*Bat gio*)

Appearance:	Intensely ecchymotic, isolated, nonsymmetric areas. May be present anywhere on the body, including on the forehead between the eyes, vertically along the trachea, in a "necklace" pattern around the base of the neck, on both sides of the upper chest, on the upper arms (left and right), along the spine, or to either side of the spine.
Conditions treated:	Localized pain and a variety of minor and more serious conditions, including lack of appetite, heat exhaustion, dizziness, fainting, blurred vision, any minor illness, cough, fever. Pinching is a *very common* practice.
Procedure:	Index and middle finger of one hand are flexed and firmly applied to the skin in a quick, pinching motion. Tiger balm, a penetrating, mentholated ointment may be massaged into the area before pinching. The H'mong may pinch first, then prick the area with a sharp needle to draw blood and thus "draw out" the noxious elements.
Belief:	Pinching exudes the bad wind or noxious element.
Age of patient:	Children over 10 years old in most cultures; adults only in H'mong culture
Practiced by:	H'mong, Mien, Laotian, Vietnamese, and Cambodian
Who applies the treatment:	Any adult

From Schreiner, D., Multnomah County Health Services Division. (1981). S.E. Asian folk healing practices/child abuse? Indochinese Health Care Conference, Eugene, Oregon. September 18, 1981, pp. 2–5. Reprinted by permission.

Cultural Perspectives in Affective Development

In an effort to understand how people from various cultures construe their private and social worlds, social scientists have identified various ways to describe the mode that people find comfortable and socially acceptable. For example, there are some cultures in which a predominantly *cognitive* mode prevails, whereas others are characterized by an *emotional* one. For many Anglo Americans, the attributes of cognitive behavior such as their emphasis on logic, rationality, and control are dominant, whereas members of many North American subcultural groups emphasize feeling states, with emotional encounters being of more importance. These different constructions of the world are not accidental cultural developments but rather reflect different philosophical legacies. Also, these constructions occur on a continuum and are not intended to be dichotomous categories.

Among white middle- and upper-class Anglo Americans, for example, children are socialized from a very early age to learn to control their feelings and emotions, especially in public places. On the other hand, they are trained to become independent, self-determining, achievement-oriented, and *work-* and *activity-centered*. In a work- and activity-centered society, relationships are formed on the basis of shared commonalities. One is expected to "work" at a relationship—in a marriage, in a family situation, with colleagues at work, and with friends at a social level.

In a *relationship-oriented* society, feelings and emotions are not repressed, and their expression is generally encouraged. Crying, dependence on others, and high levels of emotionality are socially acceptable. No agenda of shared commonalities is

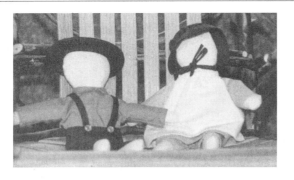

Culture influences the design of children's toys. The Amish belief that prohibits the fashioning of graven images is reflected in these faceless dolls.

necessary for the cultivation of a relationship. Examples of subcultures that are relationship-oriented include Italian, Hispanic, and East Indian.

You need to be sensitive to a wide variety of child-rearing practices when caring for children from different cultural backgrounds. A few examples are presented to illustrate types of child-rearing practices you are likely to encounter. Of course, in addition to being aware of generalized cultural practices, you should observe parent–child interactions and discuss child-rearing practices with the parents.

Health and Health Promotion

The concept of *health* varies widely across cultures. Regardless of culture, most parents desire health for their children and engage in activities that they *believe* to be health-promoting. Because health-related beliefs and practices are such an integral part of culture, parents may persist with culturally based beliefs and practices even when scientific evidence refutes them, or they may modify them to be more congruent with contemporary knowledge of health and illness.

Summarized in Research Application 4-3 are findings of a study on a community-

Research Application 4-3

A Community-Based Health Education Program for Preventive Pediatric Care

DeSantis, L., & Thomas, J. T. (1992). Health education and the immigrant Haitian mother: Cultural insights for community health nurses. *Home Health Nursing* 9(2), 87–96.

In a descriptive survey of 30 Haitian mothers in southeast Florida, informants were interviewed about the value of health education received while seeking preventive health care for infants and preschool children in community health settings, their access to health education, and their perceptions of what community health care providers could do to assist them in improving child health.

Clinical Application
Nurses were considered the best-qualified health care providers to do health teaching. In choosing the appropriate media for reaching Haitian mothers, the research revealed that radio and clinic lectures were preferred to television. Teaching will be valuable if it is *understandable* and *practical, reinforces parenting abilities,* and allows *time for questions.*

based health education program for Haitian mothers in which preventive health care for infants and preschool children was the focus.

Illness

The family is the primary health care provider for infants, children and adolescents. It is the family that determines when a child is ill and decides to seek help in managing an illness. The acceptability of illness and sick-role behaviors for children and adolescents is determined by the family. Societal trends in illness orientation and economic stress both influence the cultural beliefs that are passed from generation to generation. Health, illness, and treatment (cure/healing) are part of every child's cultural heritage. In every society there is an organized response to defined health problems. Certain people are designated as being responsible for deciding who is sick, what kind of sickness the person has, and what kind of treatment is required to restore the person to health.

Research has consistently demonstrated that African American and Hispanic children are less likely to have seen a physician compared with whites, and they have a lower average number of ambulatory visits than their white counterparts. Even when children are hospitalized, minorities receive fewer services compared with whites. Summarized in Research Application 4-4 are findings from a nationwide study of racial and ethnic differences in the use of prescription medications for African American, Hispanic and white children. Unfortunately, the findings reveal that children from federally defined minority groups receive fewer prescription medications than whites, contributing to a disturbing trend in which minority children are deprived of medications that would facilitate their healing, foster recovery from disease, and ameliorate symptoms.

Among many cultural groups, traditional health beliefs coexist with Western medical beliefs. Members of a cultural group choose those components of traditional or folk beliefs that seem appropriate to them. A Mexican American family, for example, may take a child to a physician and either a *curandero* (male) or *curandera* (female), traditional healers. After visiting the physician and the *curandero/a,* the mother may

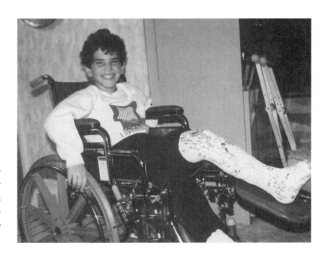

Among the healing rituals associated with fractures in children is having expressions of support and concern written on the cast by family and friends.

Research Application 4-4	*Racial and Ethnic Differences in the Use of Prescription Medications for Children*

Hahn, B. A. (1995). Children's health: Racial and ethnic differences in the use of prescription medications. *Pediatrics* 95(4), 727–732.

This study examines differences in probability and number of prescribed medications for children from African American, Hispanic, and white backgrounds, and whether the differences remain if socioeconomic factors, indicators of need, and number of health care visits are taken into account. Using data from a national survey, multivariate regression analysis was used to examine the probability of receiving a prescription medication for two samples of children, ages 1 to 5 (N = 1347) and ages 6 to 17 (N = 2155).

The findings reveal that when compared with white children, African American and Hispanic children are less likely to receive a prescribed medication and have, on average, fewer medications. These differences persist after adjusting for socioeconomic factors, health conditions, and number of health care visits.

In discussing the findings, the researcher analyzed reasons for the differences in prescribing medications for the groups studied which included five major considerations: (1) better health care access for poor minority children through Medicaid may result in increasing the number of visits and decreasing the number of prescriptions per visit; (2) families without private insurance may increase their use of over-the-counter drugs instead of purchasing prescription medicines; (3) the parents of white, non-Hispanic children are more likely to report repeated ear infections, tonsillitis, pneumonia, and urinary tract infections compared with African American or Hispanic parents, but it is unknown whether these differences are due to socioeconomic, demographic, or biologic characteristics; (4) differences may be due to lack of compliance by African American or Hispanic families compared to whites, which may reflect cultural biases that prohibit prescribed medicines, language differences, and other communication issues; and (5) limitations in the data collection fail to enable the researcher to address all of the unanswered questions without further data collection.

Clinical Application

Pediatric and family nurse practitioners can examine their prescriptive practices for differences when prescribing medicines for children from diverse cultures. If differences are identified, analyze the reasons for them by considering the answer to the following questions. Are differences by race and ethnicity due to factors such as income, insurance, or poor health? If the primary provider of care does not follow the advice given with the prescription, why not?

All nurses, whether they have prescriptive privileges or not, can examine the instructions they provide to the primary provider of care concerning medications. For example, it might be useful to ask, How do I ensure that the instructions have been understood correctly? What resources are available for primary providers of care who do not speak or read English? Is there a pharmacy available to the family that will provide written and verbal instructions in languages other than English? Do I request the primary provider of care to repeat the instructions? Is it clear by what route the medication is to be administered? Is the person who received the instructions the same one who will be responsible for administering the medication at home? Be aware that extended family members or nonrelatives may assist with child care including medication administration.

consult with her own mother and then give her sick child the antibiotics prescribed by the physician and the herbal tea prescribed by the traditional healer. If the problem is viral in origin, the child will recover because of innate immunologic defenses, independent of either treatment. Thus, both the herbal tea of the *curandero/a* and the penicillin prescribed by the physician may be viewed as folk remedies; neither intervention is responsible for the child's recovery.

Belief systems about specific symptoms are culturally unique. In Hispanic culture, *susto* is caused by a frightening experience and is recognized by the symptoms of nervousness, loss of appetite, and loss of sleep. Mexican American babies must be protected from various illnesses. *Pujos* (grunting) is an illness manifested by grunting sounds and protrusion of the umbilicus. It is believed to be caused by contact with a woman who is menstruating or by the infant's own mother if she menstruated before 40 days after delivery.

The evil eye, *mal ojo,* is an affliction feared throughout much of the world. The condition is said to be caused by an individual who voluntarily or involuntarily injures a child by looking at or admiring him or her. The individual has a desire to hold the child, but the wish is frustrated, either by the parent of the infant or by the reserve of the individual. Several hours later, the child may cry and develop symptoms of fever, vomiting, diarrhea, and loss of appetite. The child's eyes may roll back in the head, and he or she will become listless.

Because the most serious threat to the infant with *mal ojo* is dehydration, the nurse encountering this problem in the community health setting needs to assess the severity of the dehydration and initiate a plan for fluid and electrolyte replacement. You should emphasize the potential seriousness of dehydration to the parents and teach them the warning signs that will alert them to impending danger in the future. A simple explanation of the causes and treatment of dehydration is warranted. If the parents adhere strongly to traditional beliefs, you should respect their desire for the

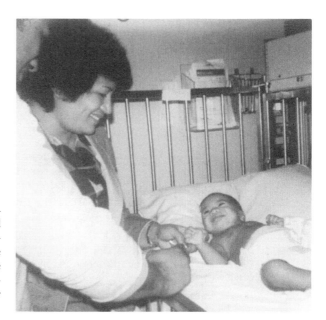

The parents of this hospitalized infant are from the South Pacific island of Tonga. They are visiting their infant and have brought a preschool-aged sibling (not pictured) to see her brother in the hospital.

curandera to participate in the care. Parents or grandparents may wish to place an amulet, talisman, or religious object such as a crucifix or rosary on the child or near the bed.

Caida de la mollera, or fallen fontanel, has a variety of causes for the Mexican American, such as failure of the midwife to press preventively on the palate after delivery. Falling on the head, abrupt removal of the nipple from the infant's mouth, and failure to place a cap on the infant's head also have been identified as causes of *caida de la mollera.* Symptoms of this condition include crying, fever, vomiting, and diarrhea. Given that health care providers frequently note the correspondence of these symptoms with those of dehydration, many parents see *deshidratacion* (dehydration) or *carencia de agua* (lack of water) as synonymous with *caida de la mollera.* Although regional differences exist, treatment usually is directed at raising the fontanel.

Empacho, a digestive condition recognized by Mexicans, is caused by the adherence of undigested food to some part of the gastrointestinal tract. This condition causes an internal fever, which cannot be observed but which betrays its presence by excessive thirst and abdominal swelling caused by drinking water to quench the thirst. Children, who are prone to swallowing chewing gum, are most likely to suffer from *empacho,* but it may affect persons of any age.

Among some Hindus from northern India, there is a strong belief in *ghost illness* and *ghost possession,* culture-bound syndromes or folk illnesses based on the belief that a ghost enters its victim and tries to seize its soul. If successful, the ghost causes death. After conducting extensive field work in India, Freed and Freed (1991) concluded that there is a relationship between infant and childhood illnesses and death caused by ghost illness. Illness and the supernatural world are linked by the concepts of ghosts and fever, a supernatural being in the *Mahabharata* and the *Puranas.*

One of the symptoms of ghost illness is a voice speaking through a delirious victim, a symptom that may be found in children and adults. Other symptoms are convulsions and body movements, indicating pain and discomfort, and choking or difficulty breathing. In the case of an infant, incessant crying is a symptom (Freed and Freed, 1991). The psychological state of the parents is often involved in the diagnosis, and some believe that ghosts may be cultural scapegoats for the illness and death of children. A mother or father may be relieved of psychic tension from feelings of personal guilt when their infant or small child becomes ill and dies by transferring the blame for the death to a ghost.

Biocultural Influences on Childhood Disorders

Children are born with a genetic constitution that has been inherited from their parents, who in turn have inherited their own genetic composition. The child's genetic makeup affects his or her likelihood of both contracting and inheriting specific conditions. Table 4-2 summarizes the distribution of selected genetic traits and disorders by population or ethnic group. The table is intended to be illustrative, not exhaustive.

In both children and adults, genetic composition has been demonstrated to affect the individual's susceptibility to specific diseases and disorders. It is often difficult to separate genetic influences from socioeconomic factors such as poverty, lack of proper nutrition, poor hygiene, and such environmental conditions as lack of ventilation, inadequate sanitary facilities, lack of heating during cold weather, and insufficient clothing to provide protection during winter months. Other factors responsible for

TABLE 4-2
Distribution of Selected Genetic Traits and Disorders by Population or Ethnic Group

Ethnic or Population Group	Genetic or Multifactorial Disorder Present in Relatively High Frequency
Aland Islanders	Ocular albinism (Forsius-Eriksson type)
Amish	Limb girdle muscular dystrophy (IN— Adams, Allen counties)
	Ellis—van Creveld (PA—Lancaster county)
	Pyruvate kinase deficiency (OH—Mifflin county)
	Hemophilia B (PA—Holmes county)
Armenians	Familial Mediterranean fever
	Familial paroxysmal polyserositis
Blacks (African)	Sickle cell disease
	Hemoglobin C disease
	Hereditary persistence of hemoglobin F
	G6PD deficiency African type
	Lactase deficiency, adult
	β-Thalassemia
Burmese	Hemoglobin E disease
Chinese	Alpha thalassemia
	G6PD deficiency, Chinese type
	Lactase deficiency, adult
Costa Ricans	Malignant osteopetrosis
Druze	Alkaptonuria
English	Cystic fibrosis
	Hereditary amyloidosis, type III
Eskimos	Congenital adrenal hyperplasia
	Pseudocholinesterase deficiency
	Methemoglobinemia
French Canadians (Quebec)	Tyrosinemia
	Morquio syndrome
Finns	Congenital nephrosis
	Generalized amyloidosis syndrome, V
	Polycystic liver disease
	Retinoschisis
	Aspartylglycoasaminuria
	Diastrophic dwarfism
Gypsies (Czech)	Congenital glaucoma
Hopi Indians	Tyrosinase-positive albinism
Icelanders	Phenylketonuria
Irish	Phenylketonuria
	Neural tube defects
Japanese	Acatalasemia
	Cleft lip/palate
	Oguchi disease

(*continued*)

TABLE 4-2 *(Continued)*

Ethnic or Population Group	Genetic or Multifactorial Disorder Present in Relatively High Frequency
Jews	
Ashkenazi	Tay-Sachs disease (infantile)
	Niemann-Pick disease (infantile)
	Gaucher disease (adult type)
	Familial dysautonomia (Riley-Day syndrome)
	Bloom syndrome
	Torsion dystonia
	Factor XI (PTA) deficiency
Sephardi	Familial Mediterranean fever
	Ataxia-telangiectasia (Morocco)
	Cystinuria (Libya)
	Glycogen storage disease III (Morocco)
Orientals	Dubin-Johnson syndrome (Iran)
	Ichthyosis vulgaris (Iraq, India)
	Werdnig-Hoffman disease (Karaite Jews)
	G6PD deficiency, Mediterranean type
	Phenylketonuria (Yemen)
	Metachromatic leukodystrophy (Habbanite Jews, Saudi Arabia)
Lapps	Congenital dislocation of hip
Lebanese	Dyggve-Melchoir-Clausen syndrome
Mediterranean people (Italians, Greeks)	G6PD deficiency, Mediterranean type
	β Thalassemia
	Familial Mediterranean fever
Navaho Indians	Ear anomalies
Polynesians	Clubfoot
Poles	Phenylketonuria
Portuguese	Joseph disease
Nova Scotia Acadians	Niemann-Pick disease, type D
Scandinavians (Norwegians, Swedes, Danes)	Cholestasis-lymphedema (Norwegians)
	Sjögren-Larsson syndrome (Swedes)
	Krabbe disease
	Phenylketonuria
Scots	Phenylketonuria
	Cystic fibrosis
	Hereditary amyloidosis, type III
Thai	Lactase deficiency, adult
	Hemoglobin E disease
Zuni Indians	Tyrosinase-positive albinism

From Cohen, F. L. (1984). *Clinical Genetics in Nursing Practice* (pp. 23–24). Philadelphia: J. B. Lippincott. Reprinted by permission.

differing susceptibilities to specific conditions are variations in natural and acquired immunity, intermarriage, geographic/climatic conditions, ethnic background, race, and religious practices. Some studies have attempted to explain differences in susceptibility solely on the basis of the cultural heritage, but they have not succeeded in doing so. This section examines some common conditions in which genetic constitution seems to be a factor and is based on research reported by Overfield (1981, 1985).

IMMUNITY. Perhaps one of the most frequently cited examples of the connection between immunity and race is that of malaria and the sickle cell trait in Africans. Black Africans possessing the sickle cell trait are known to have increased immunity to malaria, a serious endemic disease of the tropics. Thus blacks with the sickle cell trait survived malarial attacks and reproduced offspring who also possessed the sickle cell trait; as dictated by mendelian probability, eventually they developed the disease sickle cell anemia.

INTERMARRIAGE. Intermarriage among certain cultural groups has led to a wide variety of childhood disorders; for example, there is an increased incidence of ventricular septal defects among the Amish and of mental retardation in a number of other groups. In the extreme, intermarriage among groups having few members can lead to total extinction; the number of Samaritans in Israel, for example, has dwindled to a handful of surviving, aging members.

GEOGRAPHY/CLIMATE. Geographic/climatic factors may be illustrated by the classic example of a common communicable disease of childhood, rubeola (measles). Owing either to mutation of the rubeola virus or to increased individual resistance to the virus, measles became a virtually universal benign childhood disease in many parts of the world during the 19th century. Although the majority of children experienced few ill effects from measles, certain populations, such as children in the Hawaiian Islands, were severely or even mortally affected when explorers and missionaries brought the virus to their lands.

ETHNICITY. Although the role of socioeconomic factors in tuberculosis—such as overcrowding and poor nutrition—cannot be disregarded, ethnicity also appears to be a factor in this disease. Groups with a relatively high incidence of tuberculosis are American Indians living in the Southwest, Vietnamese refugees, and Mexican Americans. Ethnicity is also linked to several noncommunicable conditions. For example, Tay-Sachs disease, a neurologic condition affecting Ashkenasic (but not Sephardic) Jews of northeastern European descent, and phenylketonuria (PKU), a metabolic disorder primarily affecting Scandinavians, are congenital abnormalities known to be most prevalent among specific ethnic groups (Overfield, 1981, 1985).

RACE. Race has been linked to the incidence of a variety of disorders of childhood. For example, the endocrine disorder cystic fibrosis primarily affects white children, whereas sickle cell anemia has its primary influence among African Americans and those of Mediterranean descent. African American children are known to be at risk for inherited blood disorders, such as thalassemia, G6PD deficiency, and hemoglobin C disease, and an estimated 70 to 90 percent of African-American children have an enzyme deficiency that results in difficulty with the digestion and metabolism of milk.

HEREDITARY PREDISPOSITION TO DISEASE.   The predisposition to certain diseases also has been linked to cultural influences. For example, the incidences of pneumonia and diabetes are especially high among African Americans, and those of dysentery, alcoholism, and suicide are high among Native American children and adolescents. Mexican American children are known to succumb to pneumonia more frequently than Anglos of similar socioeconomic status.

Chronic Illness and Disability in Children

Chronic illnesses and disabilities have become the dominant health care problem in North America and are the leading causes of morbidity and mortality.

Illness is viewed by many cultures as a form of punishment. The child and/or family with a chronic illness or disability may be perceived to be cursed by a supreme being(s), to have sinned, or to have violated a taboo. In some cultural groups, the affected child is seen as tangible evidence of divine displeasure, and its arrival is accompanied throughout the community by prolonged private and public discussions about what wrongs the family may have committed.

Inherited disorders and illnesses are frequently envisioned as being caused by a family curse that is passed along from one generation to the next through blood. Within such families, the nurse's desire to determine who is the carrier for a particular gene might be interpreted as an attempt to discover who is at fault and may be met with family resistance.

Folk beliefs mingled with eugenics, particularly throughout western and southern Europe, have resulted in the idea that many chronic conditions, particularly mental retardation, are the products of intermarriage among close relatives. The belief that a chronically ill or disabled child may be the product of an incestuous relation may further complicate attempts to encourage parents to seek assistance.

In societies in which belief in reincarnation is strong, such as Indian Southeast Asian groups, a disability is frequently seen as direct evidence of a transgression in a previous life, on the part of either the parents or the child. Those who are disabled are frequently avoided or discounted because of their past lives and are encouraged to lead particularly virtuous lives this time around. Answerable to both the past and the future, too little time and energy are often devoted to improving life in the present.

Among those who believe that chronic illness and disability are caused by an imbalance of hot/cold or yin/yang, the burden of responsibility lies with the affected individual. For many individuals from Latino or Southeast Asian cultures, the cause and potential cure lie within the individual. He or she must try to reestablish equilibrium through regaining balance. Unfortunately for those with permanent disabilities who cannot be fully healed within this conceptual system, society may perceive them as living in a continually impure or diseased state.

Traditional beliefs are tenacious and tend to remain even after genetic inheritance or physiologic patterns of chronic disease progression are explained to the family. Often new information is quickly integrated into the traditional system of folk beliefs, as evidenced by the addition of currently prescribed medications to the hot/cold classification system embraced by many Hispanic families. An explanation of the genetic transmission of disease may be given to a family, but this does not guarantee that the older belief in a curse or bad blood will disappear.

When disability is seen either as a divine punishment, an inherited evil, or the result of a personal state of impurity, the very presence of a child or adult with a disability may be something about which the family is deeply ashamed or with which they are unable to cope. In addition to public disgrace, among some families, especially immigrant groups from eastern Europe and Southeast Asia, parents may fear that disabled children will be taken away and institutionalized against their will.

Finally, it must be emphasized that some cultural explanations of the cause of chronic disease or disability are quite positive. A study of Mexican American parents of chronically ill children found that the informants believed that a certain number of ill and disabled children would always be born into the world (Madiros, 1989). Many Mexican American parents who embrace Roman Catholicism believe that they have been singled out by God for the role because of the past kindnesses to a relative or neighbor who was disabled. They often stated that they welcome the birth of the disabled infant as God's will.

Expectations for Survival

Regardless of cultural heritage, parents of disabled and chronically ill children are concerned with the prognosis for conditions afflicting their loved ones. Although sophisticated technology in North America can now ensure the physical survival of many children with congenital anomalies, the parents may be influenced by cultural attitudes and practices. Such attitudes may compromise attempts to encourage parents to plan realistically for their child's future. Either neglecting or overprotecting an ill or disabled child can have adverse implications for healthy psychological development.

Cultural expectations are not easily categorized or compartmentalized into groups in which long-term survival is expected and groups where it is not. How one is believed to be restored to health is also at times an important issue and has implications for long-term planning. For example, in some African American households, particularly those that are strongly affiliated with Christian churches, hope for even the most critically ill child is frequently encouraged, with families praying for miracles in the face of somber medical prognostications.

Studies of Asian-American children with disabilities indicate that parents tend to be more pessimistic about their child's outcome than peers from other cultural groups whose children have equivalent disabling conditions (Elfert, Anderson, & Lai, 1991; Kelley, 1996). Although infants are treated very indulgently, there are strict demands on school-aged Chinese children to behave and help with household chores; thus, they serve a useful purpose in the family unit. Siblings of disabled and chronically ill children are frequently admonished that it is their obligation to look after the affected child's education and future. Similarly, as an adult member of society, it is expected that one will look after aging parents. The birth of a disabled child may cause Chinese parents to worry about their own future well-being.

For many Chinese-American parents, once the immediate crisis of survival has passed, the child's illness is interpreted in terms of how it will affect the child's future. Parents may be dissatisfied with treatment that they see as only treating the symptoms but not getting at the root of the problem, e.g., asthma, epilepsy. Chinese American parents may not encourage the use of a prosthesis, such as an artificial arm or hearing aid, because they believe it does not really change anything for the child. If the prosthesis is unable to make the child well, why bother with it? Parents may gradually discontinue visits to health care providers when they perceive that "nothing is happening" (i.e., the child is not being restored to "normal"). You should be cautioned against labeling this behavior as noncompliant or neglectful; rather, the cultural context of the parent's behavior needs to be examined carefully.

Culture and Adolescent Development

Adolescence refers to a developmental passage to adulthood marked by major physical, emotional, and social changes. In many ways adolescents from different cultural backgrounds grow and develop in similar ways and experience common physical, emotional, and social changes. It is believed that all adolescents show concerns over changes occurring during puberty such as identity, self-image, increased autonomy, relationships with peers of the opposite sex, and career aspirations. The manner in which adolescents respond to these developmental changes, however, is influenced by cultural forces.

Havighurst (1972) suggests eight subtasks that adolescents must complete before entering adulthood: (1) develop new and more relationships with peers, (2) accept a sex role, (3) accept one's physical appearance, (4) become emotionally independent from parents, (5) prepare for marriage and family life, (6) prepare for economic independence, (7) acquire an ideology and value system, and (8) achieve and accept socially responsible behavior. Each task is believed to be important in accomplishing the central task of adolescence, achieving an identity.

Havighurst indicates that the tasks are both historically and culturally relative and acknowledges that variation exists in the type and timing of the tasks faced by adolescents raised in different cultural or subcultural settings. In a cultural-ecologic model, Ogbu (1981) theorizes that development occurs along multiple pathways and suggests that successful development is defined by the culture's "implicit theory of success." This theory is important because it defines for members of the culture the range of available cultural tasks or social positions, their relative value or importance, the competencies essential for attainment or performance, the strategies for attaining the positions or obtaining the tasks, and the expected penalties and rewards for failure and successes. In order to achieve culturally defined success, individuals must demonstrate competency at the series of tasks that confront them across the life course. Because the demands and opportunities differ in various cultures or subcultures, however, the competencies required for mastery of cultural tasks also may differ.

From a cultural–developmental task perspective, competent development occurs with successful completion of the tasks that confront the individual at different points in the life course and concomitant development of the social and cognitive skills required by the task and permitted by the culture. Adolescents from a wide range of cultural backgrounds are believed to face different tasks at different points in their lives.

As children grow older, they are likely to encounter more people from other cultures, and therefore, become increasingly influenced by factors external to their family. By making comparisons between themselves and members of other cultures, adolescents develop a better awareness of their own culture and may begin to select values, behaviors, or attitudes from cultural groups outside the family. The increased sensitivity to cultural differences experienced by adolescents is largely the result of

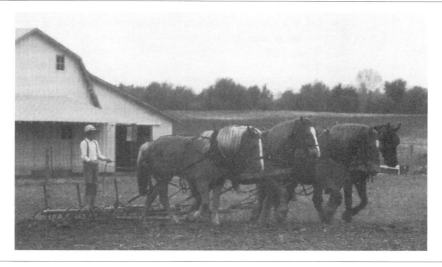

Male and female role differences are taught to children early in life and form the basis for adult roles within a culture. This Amish boy is learning to plough a field, a skill that will later enable him to assume adult responsibilities within a culture whose members reside primarily in rural areas.

three factors: (1) increased mobility and independence, which permits greater exposure to the world outside the home; (2) growing cognitive ability, which permits greater awareness and understanding of cultural issues; and (3) widening social networks in which diversity manifests itself. See Research Application 4-5.

Adolescents who identify with traditionally underrepresented or so-called minority groups are frequently faced with choices about maintaining a separateness or going through the process of assimilation or acculturation to the majority group. In assimilation, the adolescent takes on the values, beliefs, and behaviors of the majority culture and abandons their ethnic traditions. In acculturation, they accept both their own culture and other cultures, adapting elements of each. Acculturated teenagers demonstrate flexibility in adapting their behavior to multiple cultures and are sometimes referred to as having bicultural or multicultural competence.

Research Application 4-5	*Ethnic Identity, Self-Esteem and Assimilation Among Offspring of Immigrants*

Rumbaut, R. G. (1994). The crucible within: Ethnic identity, self-esteem, and segmented assimilation among children of immigrants. *International Migration Review*, 28(4), 748–793.

In a study of ethnic identity formation among 5,000 8th- and 9th-grade offspring of first-generation immigrants from Asia, Latin America, and the Caribbean, Rumbaut (1994) found that instead of a single uniform assimilation path, these adolescents followed multiple or segmented paths to identity formation and resolution. Findings reveal that 27 percent identified by national origin, 40 percent chose a hyphenated-American identity, 11 percent identified as unhyphenated Americans, and 21 percent selected racial or ethnic identity labels. The researcher reports that two thirds of the adolescents ethnically identified with their own or their parents' immigrant origins, with the remaining one third identifying with an American heritage.

The findings indicated that gender is significant in ethnic self-identification. Girls were much more likely to choose additive or hyphenated identities and to choose a Hispanic panethnic label. Boys were more likely to choose an unhyphenated national identity (whether American or national origin), and among those of Mexican descent to identify as Chicano. Gender also was a main determinant of psychological well-being outcomes, with girls being much more likely than boys to report lower self-esteem, higher depression, and a greater level of parent–child conflict.

The researcher found that perceptions of discrimination affect the way the adolescents define their ethnic identities. Those who have experienced being discriminated against and those who believe discrimination will persist regardless of educational level are less likely to identify as American and undercut the prospect that they will assimilate or finish high school. They are also likely to exhibit higher levels of depressive symptoms and greater parent–child conflict.

Youths in inner city schools, where most students are racial or ethnic minorities, are more likely to define themselves in terms of those identities, particularly black and Chicano, and less likely to identify ancestrally by national origin. The opposite effect is seen for those attending upper-middle class private schools. Virtually no Asian-origin youth chose the panethnic labels Asian or Asian American. A black or black American racial identity was chosen by only 10 percent of those from Afro-Caribbean backgrounds. A Hispanic identity was picked by more than 20 percent of those from Spanish-speaking countries.

Clinical Application

In caring for the adolescent offspring of recent immigrants, the nurse should be aware that developing a U.S. or Canadian self-identity takes different forms, has different meanings, and is reached by different paths. The process, however, is one in which all adolescents of immigrants are engaged, in addition to the other developmental tasks appropriate for their age. The process is complex, conflictual, and stressful for parents and teens alike. Based on study findings, the nurse should refrain from using panethnic labels (e.g., black, Hispanic, Asian, or Asian American) when referring to the teen's ethnic identity unless he or she does so. The nurse should be aware that these teens are at higher risk for interpersonal conflict in relationships with parents, teachers, and peers; depression; and suicide. The nurse should provide emotional support for teen offspring of first-generation immigrants struggling with identity issues, observe for clinical manifestations associated with mental disorders, and, when appropriate, refer them to a school guidance counselor, psychiatric nurse, or other mental health professional.

Special Health Care Needs of Adolescents

There are approximately 22 million adolescents in the United States and Canada. Teenagers are in a process of evolving from childhood to adulthood, and they belong not only to the cultural groups that have formed the basis for their values, attitudes, and beliefs but also to the subculture of adolescents. This subculture links the adolescent with other adolescents through a system of socially transmitted behaviors and belongings, such as clothing, music, and status symbols, including motorcycles, automobiles, videocassettes, compact discs, and stereos. The adolescent subculture has its own set of values, beliefs, and practices that may or may not be in harmony with those of the cultural group that previously guided the teenagers' behaviors.

The society of adolescents is a subculture that is vaguely structured, without formal written laws or codes, in which conformity with the peer group is emphasized. One of the most outstanding characteristics of the adolescent subculture is preoccupation with clothing, hairstyles, and grooming. Clothing mirrors the personal feelings of the adolescent and ensures identity with the peer group (Klaczynski, 1990).

In the hospital setting, gowns may stifle the individual's sense of identity, so the adolescent should be permitted to wear familiar clothing whenever the style does not interfere with safety, comfort, or hygiene. There is no harm in allowing a small amount of makeup, jewelry, or other items of apparel that might be important.

Regardless of whether you personally approve of the adolescent's taste in apparel, you should ask the following questions:

Is the preferred clothing or accessory consistent with the teenager's cleanliness and hygiene? You have the right and responsibility to prohibit the wearing of soiled clothing or to request that clothing be laundered before it is worn.

Does the clothing or accessory item permit adequate blood circulation? If clothing is tight or constricting, it may interfere with healing or safety.

In order to gain the cooperation of the adolescent, you should explain the rationale underlying any concerns about clothing. The adolescent's need to conform to peer norms is important. Rejection by members of the peer reference group may be a fate worse than the illness for which the adolescent is hospitalized.

You may notice that some female refugees or recent immigrants prefer to dress in traditional clothing. Some males also may elect to wear traditional clothing, but Western-style attire is likely to be more acceptable for men than for women. It is important for the nurse to determine what the adolescent finds most comfortable to wear during hospitalization.

Because of the relationship between some diseases and socioeconomic status, many low-income adolescents from African American, Puerto Rican, Mexican American, and Native American/Canadian subgroups have a higher than normal incidence of infectious diseases, orthopedic and visual impairments, mental illness, and untreated dental caries. This group of teenagers from low-income, culturally diverse backgrounds is more vulnerable than normal to illness and is more likely to live in an area in which health care is inadequate or absent. Consequently, low-income teenagers have a wide range of diagnosed and undiagnosed diseases. As these adolescents change from dependent children into independent adults, these disorders may interfere with their development of a positive body image, sexual and personal identity, and value system, with their preparation for citizenship, and with their independence from their parents.

Although some adolescent behaviors are believed to be culturally universal—such as the physiologic changes associated with puberty, rebellion, and testing of independence and autonomy—the expression of these changes may vary with the individual and may be related to the individual's cultural heritage; in other words, the cultural expression of the conflicts resulting from the changes of adolescence varies. For example, playing loud music may be an acceptable expression of asserting autonomy for an African-American youth but not for a Southeast Asian teen.

Communicating with Adolescents

Without minimizing the importance of nonverbal communication, this section focuses primarily on verbal communication. For adolescents from many cultural groups, English is a second language. In the case of adolescent members of refugee families, English may not be spoken, written, or understood at all. For example, because of a 1984 agreement between the governments of Vietnam and the United States, many Vietnamese children of American service personnel have emigrated to this country and are now in foster homes throughout the 50 states. Although the majority of Vietnamese teenagers are fluent in English, it is sometimes necessary to use an interpreter, especially during severe illness. It has long been recognized that all people regress under the stress of illness, and this regression may manifest itself as a return of the adolescent to his or her primary language.

The nurse should be aware of gender- and age-related customs before selecting an interpreter. For example, an adolescent girl may be uncomfortable with an older male interpreter, and an older male may find a young interpreter of either sex unacceptable. You must be careful to identify correctly the national origin of the client before seeking an interpreter. Vietnamese, Cambodians, and Laotians, for example, are all Southeast Asians, but there are vast differences in their languages, as well as in their health-related attitudes, values, and beliefs.

Even when English is the client's primary language, you should not take for granted that communication is occurring. People from culturally diverse groups may have their own unique vocabulary that can be misinterpreted by the nurse. For example, the African American adolescent may use the expression "tripping out" to mean intentionally acting silly or foolish. If you erroneously think this refers to substance abuse, the results of the miscommunication may be problematic for both parties. "Black English" is highly functional in some circles of the African American community and is widely spoken and understood.

You should avoid adopting expressions used by teenagers unless you are certain of the meaning of these expressions. A nurse who attempts to use but instead misuses teenage jargon will appear foolish. You may find that teenagers voluntarily abandon jargon when you interact with them. The use of certain vocabulary gives the user a sense of insider status, a feeling of pride and self-worth through group identification. Thus it is frequently more important for you to translate ethnic expressions, slang, black English, or other special language than to use it. It is your responsibility to assess the level of comprehension when providing care for teenagers and to communicate effectively.

Teenagers from non–English-speaking families often have mastered the art of being bicultural (or multicultural). At home they speak, dress, and behave in a manner that will gain them acceptance by their ethnic group, whereas in school or the work world they speak English, dress in keeping with the fashions of the dominant culture, and behave in a manner similar to that of the group from which they seek acceptance.

You should realize that adolescents from different groups may express themselves in different ways. For example, Filipino teenagers often avoid direct expression.

Japanese adolescents may find the open expression of feelings and confrontational behavior to be in direct conflict with cultural values. Some Chinese adolescents are discouraged from showing emotions, especially anger, because this is in conflict with a very deeply rooted belief that harmonious relationships with others are more important than individual feelings.

You must be aware of nonverbal communication when caring for adolescents, especially the significance of touch. Even though many adolescent males exchange hugs with other males as they celebrate athletic victories, some males may perceive this and other types of physical contact as a threat to their masculinity. When touching adolescents, handshakes and gentle taps on the shoulder are usually acceptable. Public expression of any emotion may be prohibited for some Japanese, Chinese, and Filipino Americans. When caring for teenagers from cultural groups in which expression of emotions is encouraged, you may misperceive the intensity of degree of feeling that is being expressed.

For most cultural groups, nudity is unacceptable. The need to undress for a physical examination should be explained, and modesty should be protected. The Hispanic or Latina patient may refuse to be examined by a male physician or nurse. Every effort must be made to have the adolescent and the nurse be of the same gender. If the physician or nurse performing a physical assessment or procedure is of the opposite sex, there should be a health care provider of the same sex present throughout.

Adolescent Health Care

Selected Adolescent Health Problems

A period of growing independence and experimentation, adolescence is a time of changing health hazards. Adolescents are in the process of establishing patterns of behavior that will continue throughout adulthood. Attitudes and behaviors related to diet, physical activity, use of alcohol, tobacco, and other potentially harmful substances, safety, and sexual behavior frequently persist throughout adulthood. Many of the most important risk factors for chronic disease in later years have their roots in youthful behavior. The earlier cigarette smoking begins, for example, the less likely the smoker is to quit. Three-fourths of high school seniors who smoke report that they smoked their first cigarette by grade 9 (USDHHS, 1991).

Irrespective of race or ethnicity, the three leading causes of death during adolescence and young adulthood are *unintentional injuries, homicide,* and *suicide.* Teenagers are also facing health-related problems such as *substance abuse, sexually transmitted diseases,* including AIDS, and *pregnancy.* Summarized in Research Application 4-6 is a study of the perceptions of Mexican American adolescent girls concerning their access to contraceptives.

UNINTENTIONAL INJURIES.   Accidents or unintentional injuries account for approximately one half of all deaths among people aged 15 through 24 years, and three fourths of these deaths involve motor vehicles. More than half of all fatal motor vehicle accidents among people in this age group involve alcohol. Nearly 60 percent of the 10th graders reported not using safety belts on their most recent ride.

Among Native Americans, death from unintentional injuries is 2½ times more common than for the general U.S. population, with motor vehicle accidents accounting for most of these deaths. One study of the Hopi Indians revealed that other accidental causes of death include falls from pickup trucks, mesas, and pueblo roofs, suicide attempts in jails, and assaults (USDHHS, 1991). Efforts to reduce motor vehicle accidents have included raising the minimum drinking age in many states, lowering the speed limit on highways, and requiring safety belt use.

HOMICIDE.   Homicide is the second leading cause of death among all adolescents and young adults, and it is the number one cause of death among African American youths. In recent years, the homicide rate for young African American males has increased by 40 percent to nearly 86 per 100,000, more than 7 times the rate for white males. Since 1914, when U.S. national mortality data were tabulated for the first time by cause of death and race, death rates from homicide among nonwhite males have exceed those for white males by factors as 12 to 1 (USDHHS, 1991).

Homicide rates for nonwhite females have consistently exceeded those for both white males and females. Similarly, data show a consistent annual trend of proportionally decreasing nonwhite victimization. African Americans continue to be greatly overrepresented as homicide victims. Most homicides are committed by persons who are of the same race and ethnicity as their victims. Among African Americans and Native Americans, homicides tend to involve acquaintances more often than family members or strangers and usually involve persons in their 20s. Acquaintance homicides most often occur within a private residence; one-third occur in the street. Among Hispanics, the homicide rate is 22½ times greater than the rate for whites. The risk of a Hispanic male being a homicide victim is 5 to 10 times greater than for a Hispanic female, depending on age (USDHHS, 1991).

Ethnicity and race, however, appear not to be as important a risk factor for violent death as socioeconomic status. Differences in homicide rates among racial and ethnic groups are significantly reduced when socioeconomic factors are taken into account.

As with motor vehicle accidents, about half of all homicides are associated with alcohol use. Nationwide, 10 percent are drug-related, but in many urban areas, the rate is substantially higher. More than half of all homicide victims are relatives or acquaintances of the perpetrators. Most are killed with firearms (USDHHS, 1991).

SUICIDE.   Whereas suicide is the second leading cause of death among young white males aged 15 to 24 years, the rate among African American adolescents and young adults is half that of whites. Both white and African American young women have relatively lower suicide rates (4.7 and 2.3, respectively) than young men. Reviews of suicide patterns among Native American youths reveal wide variations among tribes, variations that are believed to be related to physical environment, the process of imitation, social environment (group integration, cohesion, regulation), poverty, economic change, and rational choice. One study of Crow Indians revealed that as a group, Crow children tended to experience traumatic losses of family members and friends with much greater frequency than children in the population at large, and they responded with characteristic interpersonal distancing/isolation and sadness (loneliness, withdrawal) without anger. There is an almost complete absence of research focusing on depression experienced by Native American adolescents and children, let alone the relationship of depression to suicide in these groups. As is the case with homicides, 60 percent of suicides among adolescents and young adults are committed with firearms (McShane, 1988; USDHHS, 1991).

SUBSTANCE USE AND ABUSE. Conceptualizations of substance abuse and addiction have changed during the past 25 years, with the terms *substance use* and *substance abuse* coming into common usage in the 1970s. Earlier conceptualizations focused on either alcoholism or drug addition as singular addictive disorders. Contemporary trends in theories about the use of substances and associated problems is the identification of core commonalities occurring in a variety of substance use or compulsive behavior syndromes.

The operational definitions of substance use and abuse have been debated widely, along with the substances that various experts believe should be included. Traditionally, alcohol and illicit "street drugs" have been recognized as substance abuse. More recently, however, misuse of prescription medications such as tranquilizers or analgesics and eating disorders such as bulimia and compulsive overeating have been included. As a parenthetical note, I would like to remark that some anthropologists have identified bulimia as a culture-bound syndrome characteristic of the dominant European American white culture as part of its obsession with thinness and youthfulness.

For the purpose of this discussion on selected issues in adolescent health care, abuse of alcohol and illicit drugs will be explored briefly from a transcultural perspective.

ALCOHOLISM. Given that alcohol is associated with 50 percent of deaths caused by motor vehicle accidents, fires, and drownings in U.S. adolescents, the health implications are evident. In a study of American high school seniors by Bachman, Wallace, O'Malley, et al. (1991), alcohol use among white and Native American males was found to be relatively high, whereas use by blacks and Asian Americans was lower, with one-half of the males and one-third of the females reporting use of alcohol during the past month. Heavy drinking is less prevalent among Puerto Rican and other Latin American males, and even lower among black males and Asian American males. The reasons cited for drinking varied cross-culturally. The most common reason given for drinking by white, black, and Hispanic adolescents was to relax; in contrast, Indochinese youth tended to drink to forget.

Most teenagers have their first alcoholic drink between the ages of 12 and 15 years. The median age for the first social drink for white males is 11 years. Alcohol consumption among African American teens sometimes serves as an informal rite of passage from childhood to adulthood, with black males reporting more adverse effects from alcohol than their female counterparts.

Alcohol use and abuse in the adolescent has implications for school performance, suicide, accidents, and many other problems. The nurse should determine the reasons for drinking, the amount consumed and frequency of consumption, and the effects of the drinking on growth and development, particularly on nutritional intake. Positive activities such as sports, social organizations, and other acceptable outlets for adolescent energy are sometimes helpful for adolescents struggling with the early stages of alcohol abuse. For those individuals whom the nurse identifies as alcoholics, professional counseling and assistance from groups such as Alcoholics Anonymous should be encouraged.

DRUG ABUSE. Although adolescents from a variety of cultural backgrounds may be tempted to experiment with drugs, a particularly high degree of addiction among

Puerto Rican youths has been reported. As a result of drug abuse, the Puerto Rican community faces many complex problems. Among the reasons cited for the tendency to abuse drugs are lack of marketable skills, low educational level, and depression, characteristics common among low-income youths of other cultural backgrounds as well.

Hispanic/Latino youths have been identified as indiscriminate users of drugs, with marijuana being the most frequently abused drug. Like many substance abusers, these youths tended to abuse many types of drugs and to combine drug abuse with alcohol abuse. Although the nursing intervention for adolescent drug abuse is beyond the scope of this text, the reader is referred to other references on this topic at the end of this chapter.

TEENAGE PREGNANCY.   One of the major concerns for parents and adolescents during the teen years is pregnancy. Unwed parents are found in all societies. For many years, researchers have studied the problem of teenage pregnancy, which is reportedly at epidemic proportions today. In a study of cultural beliefs of teenagers who became pregnant, Horn (1990) determined that 20 percent of teenagers are sexually active by age 14 years and that 50 percent are active by age 19 years. Thirty-five percent of sexually active female teenagers become pregnant.

In one Midwestern U.S. city, a family service called the Teen Father Program has reported reaching, recruiting, and registering hundreds of young fathers from culturally diverse backgrounds. The young fathers who participated in the program tended to feel alienated from the mainstream of society and faced social and economic problems related to the fulfillment of appropriate masculine roles. In addition, these problems tend to interfere with their fathering role and responsibilities.

No practical means of preventing early sexual activity has been found. Advertising, television, permissive parents, lack of morality, and other factors promote early sexual experimentation. Freeman and associates (1984) found that the more sexual topics were discussed between teenagers and their mothers, the less likely the adolescents would be to have a sexual experience.

In researching the Puerto Rican experience, Cordasco and Bucchioni (1973) found that very little is taught in the household regarding sexuality. This area is considered taboo. Most teenagers are also very shy about discussing this topic in the classroom. This attitude might be due to the adolescents' families' view of the subject or to their ignorance of the subject matter. Hale (1982) reports that sexual competence is generally taught by the peer group. According to Hale, most black males begin sexual exploration between the ages of 10 and 13 years. They tend to be judged by peers on the basis of their success in seduction.

Because most teenagers look to other teenagers for sexual information, the nurse can assist by properly preparing peer counselors, who may effect teen compliance with contraceptive use. These peer counselors might be available on telephone hotlines or in mobile medical vans, since some adolescents may lack money for transportation to reach a clinic. Some experts believe that the optimal setting for the prevention of adolescent pregnancy would be a special teenage clinic that would be open after normal business hours and would allow teenagers to come with a friend. The nurse may have to promote flexible hours to accommodate youngsters. In addition, it is important for the nurse to listen, show interest, and be nonjudgmental when providing information about sex and pregnancy. It is equally important for the nurse to avoid showering the teenager with a lot of advice and information that cannot be absorbed at one time.

In the Native American culture, pregnancy is considered normal; however, the unmarried mother may be ostracized. In a comparison study of attitudes of whites, African Americans, and Native Americans, Horn (1990) found that Caucasian subjects approved of the prevention of pregnancy, whereas Native American teenage girls tended to value pregnancy, believing it validated their feminine role. This value of pregnancy seems to correlate with the findings of Lewis (Staples, 1984), who reported that children are considered sexual beings in African American culture. Interestingly, the African American male child's sexual identity is more easily tied to his definition of himself as a sexual being than to behavior that has been defined arbitrarily as masculine. Staples (1984) observes that traits such as independence and assertiveness do not vary between males and females in African American society. A boy understands that he is a male on the basis of his sexuality, and a girl realizes that she is female on the basis of her sexuality and her ability to bear children. In other words, some African American females think of childbearing as a validation of their femaleness. Consequently, African Americans may have a positive attitude toward childbearing regardless of the circumstances, which may help explain the disproportionate numbers of births among unwed African American teenagers. According to Horn (1990), becoming a mother at a young age, although not highly desirable, has a fairly high level of acceptance among African American teenagers. This orientation to motherhood may account in part for the selection of pregnancy over abortion by most pregnant African American teenagers.

Horn (1990) further reports that beliefs about contraceptives and their availability vary among cultures. For example, African American adolescents tend to believe that contraceptives are appropriate. However, birth control pills and IUDs were not considered acceptable because they are believed to promote illness by altering the menstrual cycle. In addition, some African American adolescents believe that the pill and the IUD dry the mucous membranes, and still others believe that refraining from intercourse for 5 days after menses is an effective method of contraception.

Finally, many Native American teenagers do not believe that contraception should be used until after the first baby is born. The findings of Horn (1990) reveal that pregnancy within Native American culture requires both modern medicine and the medicine man; thus, whenever possible, the nurse should blend folk beliefs with Western biomedicine.

Many adolescents have insufficient knowledge about effective contraceptive use. This illustrates the need for earlier education on contraceptives as well as access to contraceptive services. Summarized in Research Application 4-6 is a study of the perceptions of Mexican American adolescent females concerning their access to contraceptives.

The nurse can help teenagers from culturally diverse backgrounds understand that there are options and provide support for decisions made with respect to those options. Nurses who work with adolescents on a continuing basis are in a good position to counsel adolescents through the chain of sexual decision making.

Research Application 4-6	*Access to Contraception: Perceptions of Mexican American Adolescent Females*

Jackson, E. (1996). Access to contraception: Perceptions of Mexican American adolescent females. *Journal of Multicultural Nursing & Health* 2(4), 19–23.

Mexican American adolescent females are the least likely of all counterparts from diverse cultural backgrounds to become sexually active before marriage. Owing to early marriage and inaccessibility of contraceptives, they are more likely, however, to become adolescent mothers. The purpose of this study was to determine the influence of perceived accessibility to contraceptive methods upon contraceptive use. Using a descriptive survey with multi-staged cluster random sampling design, data were gathered on 250 adolescent Mexican American females. The typical subject was a 16-year-old Catholic Mexican American female residing in a southwestern metropolitan area with her mother, father, and siblings. She had completed the 10th grade within the public school system. Based on the Hollingshead Four Factor Index of Social Status, the social status position was common to unskilled labor and menial service workers.

The findings indicated that 54 percent (N = 136) had never experienced sexual intercourse. Of the 46 percent (N = 114) who had experienced sexual intercourse, 75 percent (N = 85) indicated that they had sex at some time without using any form of contraception. Among those who used contraceptives, the most frequent methods were oral contraceptives (19 percent, N = 22), condom (14 percent, N = 16), withdrawal (12 percent, N = 14), and a combination of withdrawal and condom use (21 percent, N = 34).

The researcher reported that there is a statistically significant relationship between perceived accessibility to contraceptive methods and contraceptive knowledge and between combined influences of perceived accessibility to contraceptive methods and contraceptive knowledge use.

Clinical Application

The researcher concluded that the identification of associations between perceived accessibility to contraceptive methods, contraceptive knowledge, and contraceptive use has implications for nurses who care for adolescent Mexican American female clients in ambulatory care settings such as schools, clinics, and physician or nurse practitioner offices. Tailoring the delivery of health care services to improve Mexican American adolescent females' perceived access to contraception while providing education about contraceptive methods has the potential to increase the likelihood of contraceptive use. Although socioeconomic, religious, and cultural factors will continue to exert a significant influence on the adolescent female's decisions about contraception, the study findings may be useful for nurses when caring for sexually active Mexican American teenage girls who want to avoid becoming pregnant.

Application of Transcultural Nursing Knowledge in the Care of Children and Adolescents: Selected Examples

A few principles of care for specific cultural groups have been provided to illustrate the practical ways in which culturally competent nursing care should be provided. The examples are intended to be illustrative, not exhaustive.

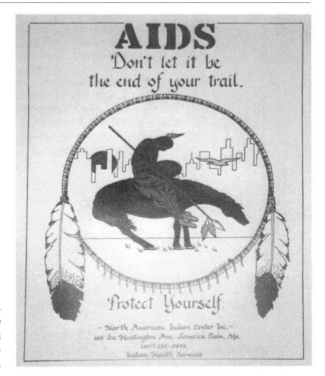

This poster warning about the dangers of AIDS is displayed in many health care facilities serving Native American teenagers.

Hair Care

Despite its importance, hair care is sometimes omitted for African American children because white, Hispanic, Asian, and Native American nurses may be unfamiliar with proper care. The hair of African American children varies widely in texture and is usually fragile. Hair may be long and straight, or it may be short, thick, and kinky. The hair and scalp have a natural tendency to be dry and require daily combing, gentle brushing, and application to the scalp of a light oil, such as Vaseline or mineral oil. For females (and some adolescent males), the hair may be rolled on curlers, braided, or left loose according to personal preference. Bobby pins or combs may be used to keep the hair in place. If an individual has corn-rowed braids, the scalp may be massaged, oiled, and shampooed without unbraiding the hair.

Some African Americans prefer straightened hair, which may be obtained chemically or thermally. Hair that has been straightened with a pressing comb will return to its naturally kinky state when exposed to moisture or humidity or when hair growth occurs. Box 4-1 provides a regimen for shampooing the hair of African American children and adolescents.

Children of Asian descent tend to have straight hair that does not require the same amount of care as the hair of most African Americans or whites. Principles related to personal hygiene apply to children of all racial and ethnic backgrounds, but the specific manner in which care is given may vary widely. When in doubt, you should ask the child's parent or extended family member how hair care is carried out

> ### Box 4-1 *Shampooing the Hair of Black Children and Adolescents*
>
> 1. Select a mild shampoo. Dandruff is best controlled by shampoos containing zinc pyrithione.
> 2. Wet hair and apply shampoo directly to scalp. Lather and rinse with warm water.
> 3. If additional luster and body are desired, add protein conditioner. Allow conditioner to remain in contact with skin for at least 1 full minute, or as directed.
> 4. Rinse with warm water.
> 5. Remove excess water with towel using squeezing motion.
> 6. Apply small amount of light oil to scalp using fingertips. Vaseline or mineral oil may be used unless client has a preference for a commercial formula.*
>
> *Note:* Chemical relaxers should be applied only by licensed beauticians.

at home. Children may feel more secure if a parent or close family member actually provides the care. If you determine that the child would benefit from care by a familiar caregiver from home, the rationale for requesting family intervention should be explained. Comments that the nursing staff is too busy or uninterested in providing hair care should be avoided; rather, the benefit to the child's security and sense of well-being should be emphasized.

Facial Hair Care

Textural variations are found in the facial hair of culturally diverse males during adolescence and adulthood. Many Asian teenage males have light facial hair and require infrequent shaving, whereas African American males tend to have a heavy growth of facial hair requiring regular attention.

Some African American teenage males have tightly curled facial hair, which when shaved curls back on itself and penetrates the skin. This results in a local foreign-body reaction on the face that may lead to the formation of papules, pustules, and multiple small keloids. Some African American males may prefer to grow beards rather than shave, particularly when they are ill.

Before shaving a client, you should determine the client's usual method of facial grooming and should attempt to shave or apply depilatories (agents that remove hair) in a similar manner. When using depilatories, you should protect the skin from irritation by keeping the chemical from contacting the client's nose, mouth, eyes, and ears. Straight and safety razors are contraindicated when depilatories are used because they may cause local irritation to the skin.

Skin Care

When bathing a client, you should remember that some parts of the outermost skin layer are removed by the washcloth. Such sloughed skin, which will be evident on the washcloth and in the bathwater, will vary in color depending on the ethnic group of the person being bathed. The sloughed skin of an African American child, for example, will be a brownish black color. This does not mean that the child was dirty; the normal sloughing of skin is simply more evident in African Americans than other lightly pigmented groups . The more melanin present, the darker the skin color will be. Because dryness is more evident on darkly pigmented skin, Vaseline, baby oil, lanolin cream, and lotions can be applied after the bath to give the skin a shiny, healthy appearance.

Evaluation of the Nursing Care Plan

To evaluate the effectiveness of the nursing care plan in providing culturally competent care, you should first ask a few probing questions to determine whether the plan was successful in achieving the desired *outcomes*, including the mutual goals established with the child's parents. Second, if the goals were not met, you should ask a few probing questions to determine the reasons for failure. Were the child's parents included in the planning and implementation of the nursing care? Were extended family members included in the plan? Did the true decision maker in the family participate in the care plan? For example, it may be that the grandmother, grandfather, uncle, aunt, or other extended family member—not the biologic mother or father— may be the family decision maker. Third, if the goals were met, the reasons for their success should be evaluated and communicated to other nurses for future reference. Other members of the health care team should be involved in the evaluation, including traditional healers or folk practitioners.

Application of Cultural Concepts to Nursing Care

The following case study is presented to demonstrate the application of transcultural nursing concepts, theories and research findings to clinical nursing practice.

CASE STUDY 4.1

Maria Gonzalez, an enthusiastic new graduate, argues heatedly with her nursing supervisor, certain that her persuasive, rational approach will win her case, if not the pure "rightness" of her cause. Located approximately 50 miles from a sophisticated urban university medical center is a rural Amish community. With frequent intermarriage has come some serious, but surgically correctable, cardiac defects among the offspring of the Amish. Members of the Amish community have become a familiar nursing "problem" for the staff of this large children's hospital. Arriving in "unreasonably large groups," several adults, adolescent girls, and younger children often come to visit Jeremiah, a 6-month-old with ventricular septal defect. The problem of overnight accommodation for the extended family, which includes members of the biologic family as well as of the extended Amish community, has become a topic of lively debate among the nursing staff. Sensitive to the cultural practices and beliefs of the Amish child and his family, the new graduate begins her argument on behalf of the family's right to adhere to Amish cultural practices.

The supervisor listens impatiently as Maria argues her case for cultural sensitivity and quickly interrupts with her decision. "These people are such a nuisance. They don't even know how to flush the toilets when they visit the hospital. This isn't a hotel. They can just go back to their horses and buggies, outhouses, and old-fashioned ways. The answer is *No!* The natural, biologic mother or father may spend the night. Everyone else is to go home. And that's final."

The use of the Amish in this case is illustrative of many cultural groups characterized by an extended family network and by cultural beliefs and practices that differ from those of the health care providers of the dominant health care delivery system. The case example warrants attention for the many issues it raises. The cultural concepts relevant to nursing practice in this situation are illustrated in Box 4-2. As shown, the nature of the nursing problem is complex and multifaceted. The interconnectedness of the various components of the child's situation with the larger system is often minimized or disregarded. The values and beliefs of both the nurses within the health care delivery system and the Amish extended social network must be considered. For the purpose of analysis, some fundamental conflicts in values and beliefs have been identified. Similarities and differences also have been indicated in the nursing plan of care (Box 4-2).

Box 4-2 *Nursing Plan of Care: Hospitalization of an Amish Child*

Goal: Child's recovery and ultimate discharge from the hospital (return to parents) in an optimal state of health.

This is a mutual goal of the Amish child's parents and of the health care providers within the health care system.

In order to plan care for this child, the nurse needs to examine the underlying attitudes, values, and beliefs of the two groups that are in conflict. Points on which there is agreement must be identified as well.

Amish	**Health Care Providers**
Family	
Large families; agricultural lifestyle; extended sociocultural-religious network of Amish community members who can be counted on to assist the natural parents.	Small family units; urban lifestyle; nuclear family
Cooperation and support among extended family, especially in stressful "crisis" times such as hospitalization of a child	Individual responsibility by nuclear family; mother and father primarily responsible
Amish community members show interest and concern by visiting.	Visiting by grandparents and siblings accepted only under specified conditions (i.e., at times and places convenient for the nurses)
Concept of family includes nonblood relatives.	Concept of family includes only biologically related persons.
Parental Obligations	
Children are a part of a larger cultural group; adult members of the larger community have various relationships and obligations to the children and parents even though they are not biologically related.	Mother and father are responsible for children; *one* adult may stay with patient overnight, preferably natural mother or father. Hospital facilities do not allow for a larger number of visitors, who clutter rooms, violate fire safety rules, and hinder work. A request for information from every visitor is time-consuming and perceived as an interruption to the nurse's work.

Box 4-2. *(Continued)*

Economic Considerations

Communal sharing of resources; hospital bill is paid from a common fund; entire bill is paid in cash upon discharge.

Health insurance; bureaucratic, moderately "slow" in processing claims after discharge. Sense of anonymity and impersonal. Large amounts of cash are available for claims; decreasing with diagnostic related groups (DRGs) and government regulation of health care but still viewed as large, rich, source of money

Traditional and Religious Values

Religious values permeate all aspects of daily living; time set aside daily for prayer and reading of scripture.

Religion is important, in some families often in proportion to the degree of illness; usually worship is limited to a single day of the week, such as Saturday or Sunday.

Illness afflicts both the just and the less righteous and is to be endured with patience and faith.

Illness is part of a cause-effect relationship; science and technology will one day conquer illness.

Protestant work ethic (in an agricultural, rural sense)

Protestant work ethic (in an urban sense)

Dress is according to 19th-century traditions; specific colors and styles indicate marital status.

Fashions occur in trends; wide range of "acceptable" dress

Married men wear beards; single men are clean-shaven.

Whether a man shaves is a matter of personal preference.

Simple, rural lifestyle; family-oriented living. For religious reasons, avoid "modern" conveniences such as electricity; use candle/kerosene lights, outdoor sanitary facilities.

Use electricity/nuclear energy; indoor plumbing is the norm; view flush toilets as "ordinary."

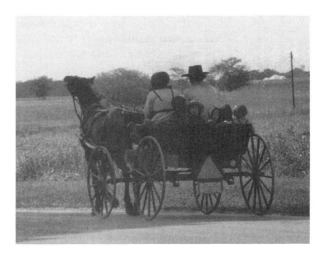

The use of horse and buggy exemplifies the traditional values of the Amish.

Having conducted a cultural assessment, identified mutual goals, and compared underlying attitudes, values, and beliefs among the Amish parents and the health care providers, you are ready to engage in activities that will promote health or identify nursing care problems (sometimes referred to as nursing diagnoses). Having done this, you examine potential nursing interventions from a transcultural perspective. When making nursing care decisions or actions, Leininger's cultural care preservation/maintenance, cultural care accommodation/negotiation, and cultural care repatterning/restructuring will be useful in providing culture-congruent care. Finally, the nurse, in collaboration with the parents and significant others who may be members of the extended family, should evaluate the effectiveness of the nursing care from a transcultural nursing perspective.

The key to successful nursing care is conducting a comprehensive cultural assessment during which appropriate and relevant cultural information is gathered. In addition, you need to compare these data with what you know about the health care system within your institution or agency. How does change occur? What parts of the system need to be manipulated to bring about the desired change? Who are key persons to involve in effecting change? In the case involving the Amish child, the nurse is clearly pushing for a policy change, for which she has no support from her immediate nursing supervisor. Is a compromise possible? How legitimate are the arguments against having the extended family room in with the child? Are there legal implications? What ramifications does the proposed change have for the welfare of other patients? Can fire safety regulations be met without necessitating expensive changes in the hospital building? What are the adverse effects on the child if the extended family cannot spend the night? Are the natural parents able to understand the rules of the hospital and to adapt to the situation?

There are no definitive solutions or answers to these questions. The purpose of this case study has been to demonstrate the complexity of the problem and to emphasize the necessity for thoughtful analysis of various facets of the problem. The ability to apply knowledge from the liberal arts—psychology, anthropology, religion/theology, history, economics, sociology, and others—to the nursing care of children from culturally diverse backgrounds is invaluable.

If nurses want to provide excellent transcultural nursing care, cultural assessment is the foundation upon which it is based. With practice and repeated experiences assessing children and adolescents from various cultural backgrounds, you will gain the knowledge and skill needed to conduct comprehensive, meaningful cultural assessments. In reflecting on the practical aspects of conducting cultural assessments, some nurses comment on the busy and rapid pace of a typical pediatric unit and argue that there is insufficient time to conduct cultural assessments on their patients. The few minutes needed to take a cursory admission history may be the only time a professional nurse spends assessing those aspects of the child and family which have cultural significance. Cultural assessment should be an integral part of the admission routine for all children and adolescents, not an additional data category that is perceived to be optional. Cultural information that the nurse fails to obtain during the cultural assessment is frequently overlooked by other members of the health team as well. The missing cultural data may result in an unnecessarily prolonged period of recovery or in care that is culturally inappropriate.

Summary

Culture exerts an all-pervasive influence on infants, children and adolescents and determines the nursing care appropriate for the individual child, parents, and extended family members. Knowledge of the cultural background of the child and family is necessary for the provision of excellent transcultural nursing care. Your cross-cultural communication must convey genuine interest and allow for expression of expectations, concerns, and questions.

Culture influences the child's physical and psychosocial growth and development. Basic physiologic needs such as nutrition, sleep, and elimination have aspects that are culturally determined. Parent–child relationships vary significantly among families of different cultural and individual differences among those with the same background add to the complexity. Cultural beliefs and values related to health and illness influence health-seeking behaviors by parents and determine the nature of caring and curing expected.

There is a dearth of information specifically about adolescents from different cultures. Therefore, health professionals need to learn about, study, and document findings about teenagers. Regardless of the cultural background of an adolescent, the transition has to be made from childhood to adulthood. This may be complicated when the adolescent's values, beliefs, and practices conflict with traditional cultural values or with those of the dominant U.S. or Canadian culture in which the teenager lives. The blending of an old and a new culture by an adolescent presents problems for the family as well as for the individual.

Review Questions

1. Analyze the cultural factors that influence parents' childrearing beliefs and practices. From a transcultural perspective, explore the ways in which parental beliefs influence their children's growth and development.

2. Critically examine the framework for socialization of children from racial and ethnic minorities presented in this chapter. Identify the strengths and limitations of the framework. What challenges do adolescents who are the offspring of mixed marriages face in the process of cultural identification?

3. Compare and contrast the childrearing practices of at least three cultural groups. Explore the role of extended family members in raising children for each of the three groups. How does the nurse identify key decision makers in the child's family? Critically examine the ways in which extended family members can assist parents during a child's illness.

4. Critically examine the culturally perceived causes of chronic illness and disability in children from diverse cultures. How are the parents' philosophical and religious beliefs interconnected with their explanations for the cause of chronic illness and disability?

5. Compare and contrast the following Hispanic culture-bound syndromes affecting children:

   a. *pujos* (grunting)   c. *caida de la mollera* (fallen fontanel)

   b. *mal ojo* (evil eye)   d. the digestive disorder known as *empacho*

6. Critically explore the cultural influences on teen pregnancy. Compare and contrast cultural beliefs about contraceptives for adolescents from different cultures.

7. Analyze the major three causes of death during adolescence and young adulthood—unintentional injuries, homicide, and suicide. Critically examine the risk factors for teens from diverse cultural backgrounds that contribute to their early deaths.

Learning Activities to Promote Critical Thinking

1. Arrange for an observational experience in a classroom at a school known to have children from various cultures. Compare and contrast the behaviors observed. Does the student–teacher interaction vary according to cultural background? What culturally based attitudes, values, and beliefs are reflected in the children's behaviors? If possible, ask the students how they believe they should relate to teachers, nurses, and other adults. Ask the teacher(s) to discuss cultural similarities and differences in the classroom.

2. When caring for a child from a cultural background different from your own, spend time talking with the child's parents or primary provider of care about child-rearing beliefs and practices (e.g., discipline, toilet training, diet, and related topics). Who is primary provider of care? Compare and contrast the parental responses with your own beliefs and practices.

3. When assigned to the Pediatric Unit, observe the number and relationship of visitors for children from various cultures. Who visits the child? If non-related visitors come, what is their relationship to the child? How do various visitors interact with the child? With the parent(s)?

4. When caring for a child from a cultural background different from your own, ask the parent(s) or primary provider(s) of care to tell you what they believe causes the child to be healthy and unhealthy. To what cause(s) do they attribute the current illness/hospitalization? What interventions do they believe will help the child to recover? Are there any healers outside of the professional health care system (e.g., folk, indigenous, or traditional healers) whom they believe could help the child return to health?

5. If your hospital has a play room, observe the types of toys and books available. For which group(s) are the majority of these items intended? Do books and toys represent various cultures? What is the role of nurses in determining culturally appropriate books and toys? Are there any items you believe should be added to (or removed from) the play room to better meet the cultural needs of hospitalized children?

References

Bachman, J. G., Wallace, J. M., O'Malley, P. M., et al. (1991). Racial/ethnic differences in smoking, drinking, and illicit drug use among American high school seniors, 1976–1989. *American Journal of Public Health 81*(3), 372–377.

Barry, H., Bacon, M. K., & Child, I. L. (1967). Definitions, ratings, and bibliographic sources of child-training prac-

tices of 110 cultures. In C. S. Ford (Ed.). *Cross-Cultural Approaches* (pp. 293–331). New Haven: HRAF Press.

Brindis, C. (1992). Adolescent pregnancy prevention for Hispanic youth: The role of schools. *Journal of School Health 62*(7), 345–351.

Campinha-Bacote, J., & Ferguson, S. (1991). Cultural considerations in child-rearing practices: A transcultural perspective. *Journal of the National Black Nurses Association* 5(1), 11–16.

Canuso, R. (1996). Co-family sleeping: Strange bedfellows or culturally acceptable behavior? *Journal of Cultural Diversity* 3(4), 109–111.

Cordasco, F., & Bucchioni, E. (1973). *The Puerto Rican Experience.* New York: Littlefield, Adam & Co.

Cross, W. E. (1987). A two-factor theory of black identity: Implications for the study of identity development in minority children. In J. S. Phinney and J. M. Rotherman (Eds.). *Children's Ethnic Socialzation: Pluralism and Development* (pp. 117–133). Newbury Park, CA: Sage.

DeSantis, L., and Thomas, J. (1994). Childhood independence: Views of Cuban and Haitian immigrant mothers. *Journal of Pediatric Nursing* 9(4), 258–267.

Doek, J. E. (1991). Management of child abuse and neglect at the international level: Trends and perspectives. *Child Abuse and Neglect* 15(Suppl. 1), 51–56.

Elfert, H., Anderson, J. M., & Lai, M. (1991). Parents' perceptions of children with chronic illness: A study of immigrant Chinese families. *Journal of Pediatric Nursing* 6(2), 114–120.

Erikson, E. H. (1969). *Identity, youth and crisis.* New York: Norton.

Freed, R. S., & Freed, S. A. (1991). Ghost illness of children in North India. *Medical Anthropology* 12, 401–417.

Freeman, E. W. et al. (1984). Urban Black adolescents who obtain contraceptive services before and after their first pregnancy. *Journal of Adolescent Health Care* 5(3), 183–190.

Hale, J. E. (1982). *Black Children: Their Roots, Culture and Learning Styles.* Provo, UT: Brigham Young University Press.

Horn, B. M. (1990). Cultural concepts and postpartal care. *Journal of Transcultural Nursing* 2(1), 48–51.

Kelley, B. R. (1996). Cultural considerations in Cambodian childrearing. *Journal of Pediatric Health Care* 10(1), 2–9.

Kempe, C. H., Silverman, F. N., Steele, B. F., et al. (1962). Child abuse. *Journal of the American Medical Association* 181, 17–24.

Klaczynski, P. A. (1990). Cultural–developmental tasks and adolescent development: Theoretical and methodological considerations. *Adolescence* 25(100), 811–823.

Korbin, J. E. (1991). Cross-cultural perspectives and research directions for the 21st century. *Child Abuse and Neglect* 15 (Suppl. 1), 67–77.

Leininger, M. M. (1990). Issues, questions, and concerns related to the nursing diagnosis cultural movement from a transcultural nursing perspective. *Journal of Transcultural Nursing* 2(1), 23–32.

Lozoff, B., Askew, G. L., and Wolf, A. W. (1996). Cosleeping and early childhood sleep problems: Effects of ethnicity and socioeconomic status. *Developmental and Behavioral Pediatrics* 17(1), 9–15.

Luna, L. J. (1989). *Care and Cultural Context of Lebanese Muslims in an Urban U.S. Community: An Ethnographic and Ethnonursing Study Conceptualized Within Leininger's Theory.* Doctoral dissertation, Wayne State University, Detroit, MI.

McShane, D. (1988). An analysis of mental health research with American Indian youth. *Journal of Adolescence* 11, 87–116.

Mead, M. (1928). *Coming of Age in Samoa.* New York: William Morrow.

Ogbu, J. (1981). Origins of human competence: A cultural–ecological perspective. *Child Development* 52, 413–429.

Oneha, M. F., & Magyary, D. L. (1992). Transcultural nursing considerations of child abuse/maltreatment in American Samoa and the Federated States of Micronesia. *Journal of Transcultural Nursing* 4(2), 11–17.

Overfield, T. (1981). Biological variation: Concepts from physical anthropology. In G. Henderson and M. Primeaux (Eds.). *Transcultural Health Care.* Menlo Park, CA: Addison-Wesley.

Overfield, T. (1985). *Biologic Variation in Health and Illness: Race, Age and Sex Differences.* Menlo Park, CA: Addison-Wesley.

Overfield, T. (1995). *Biologic Variation in Health and Illness: Race, Age and Sex Differences.* New York: CRC.

Richman, A. L., Miller, P. M., & LeVine, R. A. (1992). Cultural and educational variations in maternal responsiveness. *Developmental Psychology* 28, 614–621.

Rivzi, S. (1984). *Taharat and Najasat: The Book of Cleanliness.* Toronto, Ontario: Sexsmith.

Rogoff, B., & Morelli, G. (1989). Perspectives on children's development from cultural psychology. *American Psychologist* 44(2), 343–348.

Rumbaut, R. G. (1994). The crucible within: Ethnic identity, self-esteem, and segmented assimilation among children of immigrants. *The International Migration Review* 28(4), 748–793.

Staples, R. (1984). The mother-son relationship in the black family. *Ebony* 84(October), 74–78.

Time (September 1, 1997). Numbers. p. 25.

U.S. Bureau of the Census (1990). A comparison of child-rearing practices among Chinese, immigrant Chinese, and Caucasian American parents. *Child Development* 61, 429–433.

U.S. Bureau of the Census, Population Division, Education and Social Stratification Branch (1990). *Language Use and English Ability, Persons 5 to 17 Years, by State, 1990 Census.* Washington, DC: U.S. Government Printing Office.

U.S. Department of Health and Human Services, Public Health Service (1991). *Healthy People 2000: National Health Promotion and Disease Prevention Objectives.* Washington, DC: U.S. Government Printing Office, DHHS Publication No. (PHS) 91–50212.

Zayas, L. H., and Solari, F. (1994). Early childhood socialization in Hispanic families: Context, culture, and practice implications. *Professional Psychology: Research and Practice* 25(3), 2100–2206.

Chapter 5

Transcultural Perspectives in the Nursing Care of Middle-Aged Adults

Joyceen S. Boyle

OBJECTIVES

1. Understand how culture influences adult development.
2. Explore how health-related situational crises might influence adult development.
3. Analyze how culture influences caregiving in the African American culture.
4. Analyze how culture influences early adult development in a Haitian refugee family.
5. Evaluate cultural responses in adulthood that assist individuals and families to manage during health-related situational crises.
6. Assess ways that gender and culture influence adult development.

This chapter discusses transcultural aspects of health and nursing care associated with developmental events in middle age and the adult years. The first section presents an overview of cultural influences on adulthood, followed by a discussion of the stages of psychosocial development and cultural variations. The second section gives examples of problems faced by middle-aged adults of different cultures who are experiencing health problems and developmental transitions. How culture influences

161

individual and family responses to health problems and developmental transitions will be described.

Until recently, little interest, attention, or research has been directed toward developmental processes and health concerns in adulthood. In the last two or three decades, there has been an interest in women's health and numerous studies have focused on middle-aged women undergoing menopause. In the United States, many concerns related to menopause and our responses to them are shaped by a cultural emphasis on health care technology and pharmaceutical interventions. In addition, some nursing textbooks now include a chapter on men's health problems, many of which develop in middle age. However, developmental differences among adults have not been examined cross-culturally and most existing theoretical and conceptual models of adult health do not provide insight into cultural differences. The lack of specific descriptive terms for such a significant portion of the life span is in itself an interesting cultural phenomenon.

Cultural Influences on Adulthood

Development in adulthood has been termed "the empty middle" by Bronfenbrenner (1977), another indication of Western culture's lack of interest in the adult years. Traditionally, these years have been viewed as one long plateau that separates childhood from old age. It was assumed that decisions affecting marriage and career were made in the late teens and drastic changes seldom occurred afterward. However, over the past two or three decades, the pattern of a stable adulthood in American society has changed dramatically. Sociocultural factors have precipitated tremendous changes, producing crises and other unpredictable events in adult lives. Divorce, career change, increased mobility, the sexual revolution, and the women's movement have had a profound impact on the adult years. Middle age can be a time of reassessment, turmoil and change. Society acknowledges this with common terms such as "mid-life crises" or "empty nest syndrome" along with others that imply stress, dissatisfaction, and unrest.

Myerhoff (1978) noted that although there are no universal criteria for any of the identified life stages and associated milestones, and attributed experiences may differ considerably, all known societies have an age known as "adulthood." Neugarten (1968) observed that each culture has quite specific chronologic standards for appropriate adult behavior; these cultural standards prescribe the ideal ages at which to leave the protection of one's parents, to choose a vocation, to marry, to have children, and so on. Neugarten (1968) argued that the events themselves do not necessarily precipitate crises or change. What is more important is the timing of these events. As a result of each culture's sense of social time, individuals tend to measure their accomplishments and adjust their behavior according to a kind of social clock. Awareness of the social timetable is frequently reinforced by the judgments and urging of friends and family, who say, "It's time for you to . . ." or "You are getting too old to . . ." or "Act your age." Problems often arise when social timetables change for unpredictable reasons. An example is the recent trend of adult children, frequently divorced or unemployed, or both, returning to live with their parents, often bringing along their own children. Being widowed in young adulthood or fired close to retirement are other examples that are more likely to cause trauma and conflict when they occur outside of our notions of social order.

Culture exerts important influences on human development in that it provides a means for recognizing stages in the continuum of individual development throughout the life span. It is culture that defines "social age," or what is judged appropriate behavior for each stage of development during the phases of the life cycle. In some societies, adult role expectations are placed on young people when they reach a certain age. A number of cultures have defined rites of passage that mark the line between youth and adulthood. In modern American society, however, there are no definitive boundaries, although legal sanctions confer some rights and responsibilities at ages 18 and 21 years. Examples are the age requirements for a driver's license and for purchasing alcohol and tobacco. In our culture, there is no single criterion for the determination of when young adulthood begins, since individuals experience and cope with growth and development differently and at different chronologic ages. Even though there are broad norms, social time varies even by subculture in the United States.

Adulthood as such is usually divided into young adulthood and middle adulthood. Generally, young adults in their late teens and early twenties struggle with issues related to intimacy and relationships outside their family of origin while pursuing their education and establishing a career. In middle age, considered to include the years between ages 35 to 65 years, adults concentrate on making a contribution to society through work and/or family (Behler, Tippett, & Mandle, 1994). Exactly how individuals pursue these developmental tasks and how they cope with and manage the challenges of adulthood are influenced by their cultural values, traditions, and background.

Many personality theorists, such as Freud, Erikson, and Fromm, cite maturity as the major criterion of adulthood. Jung recognized young adulthood as a time of coping with the demands of emotional involvements in family, work, and community (Hill & Humphrey, 1982). According to Erikson (1963), the developmental task at middle adulthood is the attainment of generativity versus stagnation. Generativity is accomplished through parenting, working in one's career, participating in community activities, or working cooperatively with peers, spouse, family members, and others to reach mutually determined goals. Hill and Humphrey (1982) suggested that the mature adult has a well-developed philosophy of life that serves as a basis for leadership, stability, and objectivity. Individuals in adulthood assume numerous social roles, such as spouse, parent, child of aging parent, worker, friend, organization member, and citizen. Each of these social roles involves expected behaviors established by the values and norms of society. Through the process of socialization, the individual is expected to learn the behaviors appropriate to the new role. See Research Application 5-1.

In the United States, young adults are usually able to establish goals that are relatively specific and definitive; however, life experiences obviously play a major part in determining whether an individual can establish and maintain these goals. In many ways, Erikson's and other theorists' views of what occurs in adulthood are the biases of middle-class "Anglo" values and experiences. This constellation of characteristics has been attributed to predominantly white, Anglo-Saxon, Protestant (WASP) views and behaviors. For many cultural groups in this country, mastery of "mainstream" developmental tasks is not easily managed, and in some cases, it may even be undesirable. For some groups, developmental tasks may be accomplished through culturally defined patterns that are different from or outside the norm of what is expected in the dominant culture. Furthermore, there are now some authors who suggest that developmental stages and the associated developmental tasks of adulthood have been derived primarily from studies of men, and thus women may experience adult development somewhat differently (Gilligan, 1982a, 1982b; Belenky, Clinchy, Goldberger, & Tarule, 1986). Women's traditional location of responsibility was in the home, nurturing children and husband, as well as parents. This view is changing, prompted by societal changes and informed by scholars who are addressing women's psychosocial development in new ways. Some of these differences are described in the next section.

Research Application 5-1

Grey Glasses: Sadness in Young Women

Gramling, L. F., and McCain, N. L. (1997). Grey glasses: Sadness in young women. *Journal of Advanced Nursing, 26,* 312–319.

This study suggests that young women may experience sadness as a developmental phenomenon. Sadness occurs before the age-30 transition and appears to be a particularly decisive time of evaluation when the individual woman decides to extend current life pathways or seek new ones. Sadness was conceptualized as a pervasive feeling of disillusionment and unhappiness that influences the meaning of life events and decision making. Sadness can be likened to failed expectations, a disillusionment about life. For most women in the study, sadness was self-limited as most women in the sample successfully integrated the dream of adult life which they held in childhood and adolescence with the realities of adulthood. Yet some women were unable to resolve sadness and became depressed. The transitional relationship of sadness to depression has important implications for women's mental health.

Clinical Application

- Recognizing sadness in young women is important. Nurses can help by assisting clients to realistically appraise their lives and how they relate to their world.

- Young clients can be helped to identify a personal network of support people, including both men and women, that can help them understand what is attainable in life and how to set realistic goals.

- Nurses can carefully assess sadness in young women as an antecedent to potential depression. Early intervention based on a developmental perspective could reduce the risk of depression in young women.

- Recognize that studying adult development is important to clinical practice. Previous theories of adult development were from a male perspective. They may or may not be appropriate for women.

- From a clinical perspective, nurses must learn to recognize variety among men and women across all of society as well as acknowledge the positive quality of diversity in gender attributes.

Psychosocial Development During Adulthood

Throughout life, each individual is confronted with developmental tasks—responses to life situations encountered by all persons experiencing physiologic, psychological, spiritual and sociologic changes. Although the developmental tasks of childhood are widely known and have long been studied, the critical experiences of adulthood are less familiar to most nurses. Havighurst (1974) identified seven developmental tasks or stages of middle adulthood. While the applicability of his work to diverse cultural groups within the United States and Canada can certainly be called into question, his work does reflect traditional thinking about adulthood and the norms that are associated with that particular stage of life.

Havighurst's first task is reaching and maintaining satisfactory performance in one's career. Success in a career seems based on behaviors and attitudes that arise in a traditional white, middle-class value system that emphasizes the male working role. A successful career is enhanced for a middle-aged male if his wife has assumed primary responsibility for management of the household and supervision of their children. For men and women without "spouses" (or an equivalent person to manage domestic tasks and child rearing), success in a career may seem less important or may be more difficult because of division of time and energy. It could also be argued that economic goals may be more quickly attained if both husband and wife are employed outside of the home.

Lipson (1991) and Lipson, Hosseini, Kabir, Omidian, et al. (1995), in studies of Afghan refugees, have found that while family life is the core of Afghan culture, role conflict and stress occur within the family as gender roles begin to change during contact with American culture. For example, sometimes the male head of household is unable to find employment; if he was a professional in Afghanistan, he may be reluctant to accept the menial jobs that are traditionally filled by immigrants or refugees when they first come to this country. Frequently, low status jobs are more available to immigrant women. When the Afghan woman seeks employment (e.g., as a hotel maid), this threatens her husband's traditional patriarchal role and alters the power structure between them as well as changing her role as wife and mother. The lack of adequate social supports such as affordable day care, adequate compensation for work, and the additional physical and emotional stress results in an unacknowledged toll on refugee women and their families, including their husbands. See Box 5-1.

At the present time in the United States, to expect members of certain groups, such as ethnic minorities, newly arrived immigrants or refugees, or the homeless or unemployed to achieve satisfaction from jobs that interest them or from status derived from succeeding in a career is unrealistic and indicates a lack of sensitivity to the problems faced by these groups. In addition, plant closings, "downscaling" in workplaces, decreased production, and high unemployment have posed problems for many workers, including health care professionals. Thus, although the work role is valued in American society, the attainment of a successful career may not be realistic for some minority groups or even certain individuals within the majority culture, many of whom are returning to school, hoping to prepare for a "second career."

Havighurst (1974) defines the second major task of adulthood as achieving social and civic responsibility. Social and civic responsibilities are in part culturally defined.

Box 5-1. *Some Characteristics of Immigrant and Refugee Families*

1. Traditional family values are evident; for example, roles of men and women are differentiated. Women's role is in the home, with the family. Men are heads of household and family providers.
2. Families tend to be extended; if members are not actually living in the same household, there is frequent visiting and contact.
3. Many immigrants come to this country because they already have family members here.
4. Most immigrants and refugees are poor and struggle to earn an adequate income. Often men in refugee communities have been professionals in their home country but are unable to be employed in the same capacity in this country.
5. Refugees may be fleeing war and political persecution. Many may experience symptoms of post traumatic stress syndrome.
6. Traditional health and illness beliefs may influence behavior. Immigrant and refugee families may combine traditional health practices with U.S. health care. Use of traditional practices is fairly common in some groups.
7. Language is a significant barrier for the first few years immigrants and refugees live in the United States. Children tend to learn English more quickly and acculturate faster than their parents.

Whereas members of the dominant American culture may value achieving an elected office in the local PTA or Rotary Club, other cultures may emphasize different goals. For example, in some groups, religious obligations may be given priority over civic responsibilities. Becoming an elder or a lay pastor may be highly valued by some African Americans. Among religious groups such as the Latter-Day Saints (Mormons) or the Amish, being appointed a lay bishop may be more valued than career success. Usually, traditional religious groups have not encouraged the emergence of women in leadership roles within the church structure or the wider society.

For women to seek roles outside of the traditional family often results in censure or criticism as broadly defined developmental tasks that include recognition and acknowledgment outside the family group may conflict with the traditionally defined role for women. Some religious and ethnic or cultural groups believe that a woman's place is in the home, and women who attempt to succeed in a career or in activities outside the home or group are frowned on by other members of the group. Civic responsibilities that relate to children or domestic matters may be viewed as appropriate for women to assume, whereas others may be viewed as more within the province of men. Middle Eastern and Southeast Asian cultures emphasize responsibilities and contributions to the extended family or clan rather than to the wider society. Family ties are of great importance to many traditional cultural groups residing in the United States.

The third developmental task of adulthood is to accept and adjust to the physiologic changes of middle age. Age-related physical changes begin in middle adulthood and ultimately necessitate adjustments in activities of daily living, lifestyle, and attitude. The rapid acceptance of hair coloring, contact lenses versus eyeglasses, cosmetic surgery and the interest in procedures such as suction lipectomies tell much about the way some members of American culture resist or attempt to delay the physiologic changes associated with late adulthood. On the other hand, the effects of aging may be more easily accepted by members of cultural groups such as Native Americans or Asian Americans, whose traditional values include respect for and deference to the elderly.

The fourth developmental task of middle-aged adults is to help teenage children become responsible adults. The age at which young persons marry and become independent varies by custom or cultural norm as well as by socioeconomic status. Generally speaking, adults of lower socioeconomic status leave school, begin work, marry, and become parents and grandparents at earlier ages than middle- or upper class adults. It is relatively common in American society for an 18-year-old, for example, to marry and move away from home or to leave home to pursue higher education or to find employment. Indeed, early independence, or "leaving home," is encouraged by many American families, although this trend has decreased as the American economy has declined. Other cultural groups, such as those from the Middle East and Latin America, place more emphasis on the extended family; even after marriage, a son and his new wife may choose to live very close to both families and to visit relatives several times each day. Families from some cultural groups such as Hispanics may be reluctant to allow their young daughters to leave home until they marry.

Many couples who have delayed childbearing, perhaps because of the woman's career or other reasons, or couples who have chosen to have children in a second marriage are having children in later childbearing years. These parents confront many unique issues. They may have less in common with parents of their children's playmates or even their own peers whose children are grown. Parental energy, agility and emotional flexibility may be lacking as parents nearing 50 years of age attempt to keep up with their young children. Young children born to older parents may not know their grandparents who have played an important role in extended family relationships in the past.

Havighurst's fifth developmental task of adulthood involves a change in the roles and relationships of individuals with their parents. This stage in life has been described as the "sandwich" generation. Caring for and launching their own children as well as caring for their own parents places some middle-age adults between the demands of caregiving from parents and from children. Primarily, caregivers have been women and the excessive stress resulting from caregiving demands place them at increased risk to health problems. Cultures that value and maintain extended family networks can share the responsibilities of caring for both children and older parents.

Adjusting to aging parents and responsibilities toward them, as well as finding appropriate solutions to problems created by aging parents, are challenges faced by many adult Americans as they approach middle age. Placing an aged mother or father in a nursing home may be a decision made with reluctance and only when all other alternatives have been exhausted. Such actions may be totally unacceptable to some members of other cultural groups, in which family and community structures would facilitate the complex care required by an aged ill person and would exert a great deal of social pressure on an adult son or especially a daughter who failed in this obligation.

The sixth and seventh developmental tasks defined by Havighurst place emphasis on the role of wife or husband and establishment of strong friendships along with increasing enjoyment of leisure activities. The relationship of wife and husband is often enhanced in middle adulthood, although divorce at this time is becoming a more frequent occurrence in the United States. The frequent need for both spouses to work may conflict with traditional roles and cause feelings of guilt and shame on the part of the husband. Some women continue to assume all responsibility for domestic chores while working outside the home, and experience considerable stress and fatigue as a result of multiple role demands. If either or both spouses are working in low-paying jobs and still struggling to make ends meet, the enjoyment of leisure activities may be sharply curtailed.

In addition, an emphasis on an emotionally close interpersonal relationship between a husband and wife may be a culturally defined value. Studies have suggested that in some groups, such as Hispanic cultures, women develop more intense relationships or affective bonds with their children or relatives than with their husbands. Latin men, in turn, may form close bonds with siblings or friends, ties that meet the needs for companionship, emotional support, and caring that might otherwise be expected from their wives (O'Kelly, 1980). Gender roles and how men and women go about establishing personal ties with either sex are heavily influenced by culture. New paradigms that examine women's development suggest that female identity is formed, not by individuation, but within relationship contexts (Lewis & Bernstein, 1996). In North American society, women are more likely to have intimate, self-disclosing friendships with other women than men have with other men. A man's male friends are likely to be working, drinking, or playing "buddies." In southern Europe and the Middle East, men are allowed to express their friendship with each other with words and embraces. Such expressions of affection between men are uncommon in American culture and might be attributed to homosexuality.

Thus, affiliation and friendship needs in adulthood and the satisfaction of these needs are facilitated or hindered by cultural expectations. How individuals are approached and greeted as well as the kind and type of relationship established may be closely tied to culture expectations and norms. Health professionals should inquire about the appropriate manner to use in approaching clients and their family members. Table 5-1 provides some suggestions and guidelines to use in approaching clients and using their names in interpersonal relationships. Social support, family ties, and friendship needs can be met through the extended family and kinship system or through other culturally prescribed groups such as churches, singles bars, work, and civic associations. An individual's health may be affected by such ties, since persons who have a reliable set of close friends and an extensive network of acquaintances are usually healthier—both emotionally and physically—than those without friends. Lifestyle, a powerful influence on health status, involves the practice of health habits and a guiding philosophy of life to promote a positive outlook. Individual and family lifestyles vary according to resources and cultural values and traditions. Changing North American lifestyles are creating realignment of the division of labor, roles, and values of the family. In turn, adult growth and development in middle age are undergoing profound changes.

TABLE 5-1

Guidelines for Names

Arab	Both males and females are given a first name. The father's first name is used as the middle name; the last name is the family name. Usually, a person is called formally by the first name as Mr. Mohammed or Dr. Anwar.
Chinese	The family name is stated or written first and then the given name, just opposite of European American tradition. Only very close friends use the given name. Politeness and formality are stressed; always use the whole name or family name. Use only the family name to address men, e.g., if the family name is Chin and the man's given name is Wei-jing, address the man as Chin. Many Asians take an English name that they use in this country. Use the title Mr. or Mrs. preceding their English name as the use of just the first name is considered rude. Some Asians switch the order of their names to be like Western names and this can be very confusing to outsiders.
	Women in China do not use their husband's name after marriage. If the woman has lived in Hong Kong, Taiwan, or a Western country for a long time, her name may be the same as her husband's name.
Latin American	The use of surnames may differ by country. Many Latin Americans use two surnames representing the mother's and father's sides of the family. Maria Cordoba Lopez indicates her father's name is Cordoba and her mother's surname is Lopez. When Maria marries, she will retain her father's name and add the last name of her husband. Thus, Maria becomes Maria Cordoba de Recinos.
	Many Latin Americans drop their mother's surname after they immigrate to the United States. In approaching clients of traditional Latin cultures, it would be appropriate to use the Spanish terms *Señor* or *Señora* followed by the primary surname (the husband's) assuming the nurse is comfortable with those terms.
Native American	Native American names differ by tribal affiliation. Many tend to follow the dominant cultural norms. In the Navajo culture, a health care provider may call an older Navajo client "grandfather" or "grandmother" as a sign of respect. In the past, some tribes have tended to convert traditional names into English surnames. Thus there are names like Joe Calf, Phyllis Greywolf, etc.

The above-mentioned examples are very general; if in doubt, always ask, as it can be embarrassing for the nurse and the client if the nurse uses a name in an inappropriate manner. Members of cultures that adhere to traditional values might be confused by our current practice of using Ms. as a designation for women. Generally speaking, it is *always best and most appropriate* to be formal and use the surname with the appropriate title of Mr. or Mrs. preceding the name. Adapted from Purnell, L. D., & Paulanka, B. J. (1998). *Transcultural Health Care: A Culturally Competent Approach.* Philadelphia: F. A. Davis.

Health-Related Situational Crises

The preceding section described cultural influences, developmental tasks, and selected cultural variations in adulthood. This section contains two case studies of adults from different cultural groups who experienced health problems compounded by social and cultural factors as well as by situational or developmental crises. In addition to the developmental or maturational changes discussed in the preceding section, situational crises resulting from a serious illness may impinge on individuals in middle age. For example, the leading causes of death in middle adulthood are heart diseases, lung cancer, cerebrovascular disease, breast cancer, colorectal cancer, and obstructive lung disease (U.S. Department of Health and Human Services, 1990). These conditions affect individuals but they also occur within a family system and affect children, spouse, aging parents, or other close relatives. Since middle-aged adults may be responsible for aging parents or ill adult children, the illness of any one individual must be evaluated very carefully for the myriad ways that it impacts on all members of the family.

Danielson, Hamel-Bissell and Winstead-Fry (1993) indicated that health professionals need a better understanding of how families influence the health-related behavior of their members because definitions of health and illness and reactions to them form during childhood within the family context. Health promotion, disease prevention and the treatment of illness are influenced by cultural beliefs and values. When the illness has cultural connotations, the issues become more complex; medical treatment and nursing care must take into account the cultural history, values, beliefs, and practices that influence the client and family's ability to cope with the illness as well as assessing whether the interventions are congruent with their culture.

Caregiving and African American Women

African American women, like all women, receive and provide health care in the context of the families in which they perform multiple caregiving roles—as wives, mothers, daughters, widows, single childless women, and so on. Caregiving roles of women often predispose them to interrupted employment, and limited access to health care insurance and pension and retirement plans. Leigh (1995) observed that these general problems and characteristics of caregivers are compounded for African American women by the special circumstances of their lives and the lives of the men about whom they care. In the case of African American caregivers, "prejudice, discrimination, and poverty all interact to generate the daily diet of stresses that bear on their health" (pp. 112–113).

Caregiving implies the provision of long-term help to an impaired family member or close friend (Wright, Clipp, & George, 1993). Caregiving usually is labor intensive, timeconsuming, and stressful, although the exact effects on the physical and emotional health of caregivers is still being documented. The most commonly studied caregiving situation has been that of an elderly individual, usually a woman, caring for a spouse with Alzheimer's disease. When caregiving activities for other family members are necessary in middle adulthood, the roles and challenges obviously are different although this factor has not been extensively documented. In addition, culture and ethnicity influence beliefs, attitudes, and perceptions of what is normal and what is sickness. Culture and ethnicity also influence how often individuals engage in self-care versus seeking formal health services, how many medications they take, how often they rest and exercise and what type of foods they consume (Wykle & Haug, 1993). Wright (1997) observed that "caregiver research is based predominantly on white subjects, and ethnic differences are rarely analyzed. Further, very few studies focus specifically on minority caregivers" (p. 277).

The few studies that have been conducted on African American caregivers have found that they tend to use religious beliefs to help them cope with the stress of caregiving. Picot (1995) for example, reported that African American caregivers indicated that God and their religious beliefs were most helpful to them even in such aspects of caregiving as physical care. Boyle, Ferrell, Hodnicki and Muller (1996) found that African American caregivers' belief in a personal God and their intense, daily relationship with Him provided them with support during the illness of a family member and helped them cope with death and loss. Data on caregiver depression show that African Americans are less depressed than whites (Haley, et al., 1995) and Hispanic caregivers (Cox & Monk, 1990). There is also some indication that African American caregivers may solve the problems of caregiving differently and that these differences may be due to social and cultural factors. For example, African American mothers who care for adult children with HIV disease may not always exhibit a proactive, problem-solving approach in regard to their adult child's HIV disease (Boyle, Ferrell, Hodnicki & Muller, 1998). This is not because African American caregivers are not interested in their adult child's health or cannot understand the complexity of medical regimens. Such behavior may be related more to the racial discrimination and racism that have remained significant factors in the health care of African Americans over time. In addition, there may be cultural influences that shape human behavior in such a way that problems arising from illness and caregiving are solved by different approaches.

HIV/AIDS and the African American Community

Quam (1994) argued that the epidemic of HIV/AIDS must be viewed in the larger context of developments in the political economy of the United States. This context includes a close examination of the distribution of wealth and changes in control over production that have eroded the living standards of most American citizens and undermined the ability of the federal and state governments to meet the health needs of the American people. Other groups, both governmental and private, also have insisted that the AIDS epidemic cannot be understood apart from the context of racism, homophobia, poverty and unemployment (National Commission on Acquired Immune Deficiency Syndrome, 1991). Although there is often a fine line between what is "cultural," what is "political," and what is "economic," it is important for health professionals to become advocates for new policies that provide services needed for the health and wellbeing of everyone, especially for those whose lives have been blighted by social and economic deprivation. From a public health standpoint, education has been stymied by an unwillingness to talk frankly about sexual and drug use behaviors and this has been a substantial barrier in effective HIV preventive programs. In essence, the AIDS epidemic has forced society to examine and attempt to alter cultural behaviors and values that were largely ignored in the past.

Over the past few years in the United States, the practice of high risk HIV behaviors has changed from selected populations of white homosexual men with no history of drug use to heterosexuals having multiple sex partners and using drugs (Siegal, Carlson, & Falck, 1993). HIV disease disproportionately affects selected groups, especially African Americans and Hispanics and risk patterns are different for males and females (Centers for Disease Control, 1993). Of equal concern, HIV infection rates are "giving way" to rural areas from large epicenters (Kalichman, 1995) and minority women seem at particular risk. It is generally agreed by most researchers and public health officials that preventive efforts and other interventions should match the social, cultural, linguistic, psychological, developmental, and behavioral characteristics of the risk group of interest (Sumartojo, Carey, Doll, & Gayle, 1997). However, implementing such interventions has proven extremely difficult.

Caregiving in the African American Culture: Mothers Who Care for Adult Children with HIV Disease

Much of the caregiving literature has focused on predominantly European American caregivers who provided care to elderly spouses or parents. In the last decade or so, the nature of caregiving has changed with the impact of the AIDS epidemic as AIDS affects a much younger population. At first, caregivers to persons with AIDS often were men; however, mothers and other family members have become more involved as the incidence of HIV disease has changed from white homosexual men to the heterosexual population. Many African Americans living in the rural South first learned about HIV/AIDS from television programs, and many thought of AIDS as a disease that was common in large cities; few thought it was something that could happen in small southern towns or to a member of their own family. Like many other Americans, most African Americans thought AIDS was a disease of white, homosexual men, so it was somewhat of a shock when rural African American families learned that one of their own family members had HIV disease. Many African Americans, especially younger adults or teenagers, now commonly refer to HIV/AIDS as "the virus."

CASE STUDY 5.1

Mrs. Ernestine Pollard, a 52-year-old African American woman, lives in a small town in rural South Carolina. Mrs. Pollard has always cared for an older sister, who is now 65 years old. Mrs. Pollard explains that her sister "can't talk and her mind's not good." Her mentally retarded sister has always lived with her, but recently the sister's health has been deteriorating because of a series of "little strokes." Then, just a few months ago, Mrs. Pollard's 26-year-old son, Steve, returned home to live with her. Steve was living and working in Florida, where he became very ill. He was taken by friends to the emergency room and then admitted to the hospital. It was during this hospitalization that he tested positive for HIV disease. After discharge from the hospital, he returned to his home town to live with his mother.

Mrs. Pollard explains that sometimes with the stress of caregiving and worry about Steve, her "pressure goes sky high." She has had "high blood" for a number of years. Her physician prescribed medication for her blood pressure, and she tries to take it on a regular basis. Lately, as Steve has become more ill, Mrs. Pollard is not sleeping well and is very worried about Steve's condition. She told her doctor that she has "bad nerves" and explained that she was unable to sleep at night. The physician prescribed sleeping pills for her, but Mrs. Pollard is unwilling to take them because she fears that she will not hear Steve during the night if he needs her. In addition to her worry about Steve, she is concerned about her sister's health also. Mrs. Pollard has two daughters who are older than Steve and they try to help their mother with her caregiving activities.

....

Health Promotion Strategies and Nursing Interventions

Priorities of nursing management for Mrs. Pollard would be support of her caregiving role and health promotion strategies to control her blood pressure and reduce the stress she is currently experiencing. In terms of blood pressure management, a nurse might advise Mrs. Pollard to lose weight and incorporate changes in eating habits and regular exercise into her lifestyle. However, these health goals may be compromised by social and cultural factors as well as the caregiving situation. Nurses can become more culturally sensitive to cultural norms and values of clients such as Mrs. Pollard by listening carefully, being empathetic, recognizing the client's self-interest and needs of her family members, being flexible, having a sense of timing, using the client's and family's resources, and giving relevant information at the appropriate time.

While Mrs. Pollard does have a private physician and tries to seek care when appropriate, she considers Steve's needs before her own. Steve is the only member of the Pollard family who is receiving regular health care. He attends an Infectious Disease clinic at Health Science Center located about 50 miles away from where his mother lives. His medications are provided through Ryan White legislation, a state and federal cooperative agreement to provide care for persons with AIDS. As his illness progresses, a home health care nurse visits several times each week. Even though the nurse's focus is on Steve's illness, he or she will want to support and help Mrs. Pollard care for her son as she is directly responsible for most of his care and is with him much of the time. Of considerable importance, Mrs. Pollard knows his health history and probably understands him better than anyone else.

Like many other adults, Mrs. Pollard has fairly definite preferences about food and the way it is prepared and served. She believes that the proper kinds of food will promote and enhance good health. The Pollard family frequently eats foods that are high in fat; for example they enjoy servings of fatback or "fat meat" for breakfast several times each week. They prefer their vegetables cooked with bacon for flavoring. Mrs. Pollard is primarily concerned about Steve's appetite and his ability to eat on a regular basis. One morning, Steve told his mother that he thought he would like a steak. Mrs. Pollard hurried to the grocery store to buy a steak and cook for him, and he obviously enjoyed eating it. Symbolism is attached to food in every culture and Mrs. Pollard believes that Steve will gain some of his strength back by eating healthy foods like meat. In her concern for Steve, she neglects her own diet or eats whatever is available and needs to be gently reminded by the nurse that it is important that she pay some attention to her own nutrition also.

Clark (1996) suggested that "food can function as a focus of emotional association [and as] a channel for interpersonal relationships, or as a means of communicating love, disapproval, or discrimination" (p. 303). Being able to prepare food that her son will eat and enjoy is a source of relief for Mrs. Pollard and a reinforcement of her successful caregiving. Her focus is now on Steve and his worsening health problems. Encouraging Mrs. Pollard to take her medication regularly, to rest as often as she can and to avoid or eat only a small amount of foods that are high in fat and/or sodium may be realistic goals for Mrs. Pollard during Steve's illness.

Nurses providing care to clients such as Mrs. Pollard will need to consider other cultural factors that ultimately influence the nursing goals. Rural African Americans often have cultural ways to view health and illness. Cultural bound syndromes were discussed in Chapter 2 and several can be identified in the assessment data provided by Mrs. Pollard. "High blood" is an illness condition that is associated with African Americans in the rural south. Many health professionals make the wrong assumption that high blood is the same as high blood pressure, and while there are similarities, the cultural explanation for high blood is different than the biomedical explanation for high blood pressure. High blood is conceptualized in terms of blood volume, thickness, or even elevations of the blood in the body (e.g., "blood rushes to your head").

Causation is due primarily to factors that "run blood up," such as salt, fat, meats, and sweets. This condition results in an increased "pressure" or high blood pressure. Sometimes high blood leads to a feeling of faintness that might cause the afflicted person "to fall out" or faint. Other causal factors that result in high blood are emotional upsets or prolonged stress. Sometimes the cause is thought to be a falling out with God, or eternal forces, such as enemies putting a "hex" on someone. Many older African American clients believe that eating slightly acidic foods, such as greens with vinegar or dill pickles, will lower high blood. Thus, while there are similarities between high blood and high blood pressure, the explanations and treatments are not always the same in the cultural prescriptions as in the biomedical model. Mrs. Pollard tries to be conscientious about taking her blood pressure medication, but she does forget when she becomes distracted with caring for Steve and her sister. The nurse should acknowledge Mrs. Pollard's concern and active involvement in her own health promotion and encourage her to take her blood pressure medication as prescribed.

"Nerves" or even "bad nerves," while not unique to the rural south, are commonly described by many southerners. Bad nerves are often equated with anxiety and worry but may refer to something as serious as a "mental breakdown" or severe emotional disorder. Mrs. Pollard uses the term to refer to her worry, concern, and anxiety about Steve's deteriorating health status and anticipation of loss. Sometimes she has "crying spells" that she describes as "just crying and crying, and not being able to stop." She gets up several times at night to answer Steve's call or to check on him and make certain that he is all right. Lack of sleep and continued worry and anxiety accelerate her psychological distress. Again, recognition from the nurse that she is providing excellent care to her son is reassuring for her. She should be encouraged to rest and assured that crying and feeling sad are normal reactions to her son's illness and impending death.

African American midlife women are more likely to be subjected to a number of stressful life events due to a lack of economic resources, such as job and marital instability, lack of male companions as head of households, erratic income, and frequent changes and relocations (Jackson, 1985; Lewis & Bernstein, 1996). Even before Steve's illness, Mrs. Pollard experienced many life stresses that were related to the lack of economic resources. In the beginning of Steve's course of illness with HIV disease, Mrs. Pollard continued working in the housekeeping department of a local technical college. However, as Steve's illness progressed and he became increasingly unable to care for himself, Mrs. Pollard quit her job to stay home and take care of him. She faces numerous situational crises; Steve's illness and impending death, the aging of her older sister, as well as economic hardship because she is the family provider.

Stress and anxiety are normal reactions in the lives of middle-aged adults like Mrs. Pollard. However, limited resources, lack of access to quality health care and discrimination during a severe illness of a family member compound the stress and complicate a situational crises. Mrs. Pollard's physician prescribed sleeping medication for her, assuming that would take care of her inability to sleep. Unfortunately this reaction is fairly common as physicians sometimes tend to prescribe medications for the symptoms reported by clients rather than probing more deeply into the situation. The nurse can reinforce Mrs. Pollard's decision not to take this medication and explore with her how to set aside time during the day when she might be able to take a nap. In addition, Mrs. Pollard's anxiety and inability to sleep well are directly related to the stress of caregiving. This can be dealt with in a more culturally acceptable manner than the routine prescription of sleeping medication. Some ways to support and help Mrs. Pollard deal with stress and anxiety may be family support and participation in religious activities.

Close family and spiritual ties within the African American family and community support the caregiving role. Extended and nuclear family members willingly care for sick persons and assume these roles without hesitation. Mrs. Pollard's two daughters try to help their mother and Steve as much as possible. They visit daily and bring their children with them. Steve enjoys being with his nieces and nephews and Steve enjoys reading to the younger ones. The teenagers can help him with small tasks such as folding his clothes when they have helped with the laundry. Even Mrs. Pollard's sister tries to help out as best she can by sweeping the floor and wiping the dishes. After a family discussion that involved Steve, Mrs. Pollard, and his two older sisters, it was decided to disclose Steve's HIV diagnosis to his older teenage nieces and nephews.

Many individuals with HIV disease and their close family members are reluctant to disclose the diagnosis to others outside of the family as the stigma of disclosure in a small community can affect all members of the family. Mrs. Pollard's minister is aware of Steve's conditions, as are a few members of Mrs. Pollard's "church family." The primary stressor of women during the midlife years is the loss of relationships and friendship networks, often because of competing demands on time (Lewis & Bernstein, 1996). It is extremely important for Mrs. Pollard's health and coping abilities that she continue to participate in church activities and to maintain those friendships and networks.

Spiritual beliefs form a foundation for Mrs. Pollard's daily life. Like other African Americans who live in the same rural community, Mrs. Pollard attends a small Protestant church whose membership is exclusively African American. Many, but not all, African Americans strongly believe in the use of prayer for all situations they may encounter. They use prayer as a means of dealing with everyday problems and concerns. Mrs. Pollard relies a great deal on prayer and her religious beliefs and practices provide her with support and strength in her caregiving role.

Mrs. Pollard has a lifetime experience with her church; she attended church services as a child and has continued this pattern in her adult years. The role of the church in the black community has always been important as it was the center of activities for African Americans for decades (Dressler, 1991). Mrs. Pollard's religious beliefs are integrated in her daily life as a caregiver and her belief in God enhances her ability to care for Steve. She, like many other African Americans, has a personal relationship with God and is able to share her worries and concerns through prayer. Her religious beliefs provide the foundation for an active approach to coping with problems.

Psychosocial Development and Nursing Interventions

The first priority of nursing care for Steve and his family is to help them understand and adjust to the impact of HIV disease. The diagnosis of HIV/AIDS precipitated a situational crisis for the Pollard family. Such a situation can best be resolved by the provision of culturally relevant health-promotion and risk-reduction strategies. The health teaching and nursing interventions provided to the Pollard family should focus on wellness and health promotion. The nurse can continue this emphasis by helping Mrs. Pollard successfully manage the situational crises as well as the developmental tasks common to adulthood.

Mrs. Pollard may face problems in the completion of the developmental tasks discussed earlier. Havighurst suggests that an important developmental task for middle-aged adults is career success. Mrs. Pollard has worked outside of the home most of her adult life; yet rural African American culture does not place the kind of emphasis on work and career that the wider American society does. Mrs. Pollard's ties of affection to Steve and her maternal role are reinforced by African American cultural values. Families ties and the lifelong attachments, as well as the extension of the maternal role to an adult child, are valued in the African American culture. These values are emphasized over woman's careers outside of the home. Many African American women of Mrs. Pollard's generation obtain meaning in their lives by caring for family members. Their feelings, behavior, and attitudes go beyond a simple sentiment of affection or of family ties. In explaining why she cares for her older retarded sister, Mrs. Pollard says " We were little girls together. I always knew that I was going to take care of her." In many societies, women disproportionally provide caregiving services and social policies, and programs are organized around the assumption of women's availability and willingness to provide care (Guberman, Maheu, & Maille, 1992). At the same time, it is important to understand that Mrs. Pollard values the traditional caregiving role and she needs support and assistance in providing the care she believes that her family members need.

Family caregivers should be recognized for their unique knowledge of the care receiver's preferences, values, needs and life history (Rutman, 1996). What is important for the nurse to assess and acknowledge is that Mrs. Pollard is valued, recognized, and respected for her competence and expertise as a caregiver. The nurse could begin by including Mrs. Pollard, Steve, and his sisters in developing mutual goals for his care. Mrs. Pollard should be encouraged in her role of providing help and care to family members and in promoting the health of her son and others. It is also important that her attention be directed toward her own needs on occasion, as she tends to focus on meeting the needs of Steve and her sister before her own. Of particular concern is the timing of Steve's serious illness. Having a young, previously healthy adult child with a terminal condition will cause unique trauma and conflict as society's expectations are that older parents will die before their adult children.

The second task of adulthood defined by Havighurst involves relationships with others and the community. Social and civic responsibilities among rural, older African Americans in the South are met almost entirely at the level of the extended family and the African American church. These ties and associations are very strong, are often complex, and are not readily understood by outsiders. African American pastors are key players in the lives of their congregation and in their communities. Mrs. Pollard should be encouraged to attend church services and to seek the help and support available to her through this important cultural resource. Mrs. Pollard sings in the church choir and tries to attend choir practice every Wednesday evening. Perhaps, the nurse could help set up a blood pressure clinic for church members. Several women who are active in the church are also nurses and they could be included in the planning and implementation of the clinic.

The third developmental task of adulthood proposed by Havighurst is acceptance and adjustment to the physiologic changes of middle age. Because hypertension is common in African Americans, it is sometimes seen as a normal occurrence in middle age. The health-promotion strategies and nursing interventions described earlier will help Mrs. Pollard adjust to other health-related changes. Havighurst's fourth developmental task is that of helping teenagers become responsible adults. In Mrs. Pollard's situation, two of her daughters and her son Steve have attained adulthood. However, this developmental task is complicated by Steve's illness and his returning home for care during a terminal illness. Although he has lived independently for a number of years, he is now dependent on his mother for support and care. Different stressors, however, may have different effects on caregivers because personality factors and experience influence each person's perception of and reaction to a stressful situation. Coping strategies such as prayer and resources such as family and church support mediate Mrs. Pollard's reaction to this stressful situation.

Havighurst's other developmental tasks pertinent to this case study involve relationships with spouse and friends. Mrs. Pollard's life revolves around her family and church. The nurse must understand the importance of cultural ties with kin and others so as to also understand that support is crucial when an illness develops and is a necessary factor for successful health promotion and maintenance in caregiving activities.

The last task suggested by Havighurst involves increased enjoyment of leisure activities. Mrs. Pollard can be encouraged to continue with leisure activities that are congruent with cultural practices. It is important for her to attend church services and activities as her social life is derived from her participation in the activities of her church. Arranging for one of Steve's sisters to stay with him while Mrs. Pollard attends church services would be appropriate. It will be the church family who will be instrumental in providing emotional support and help when Steve's condition worsens. After his death, the church will offer spiritual support as well as the opportunity for Mrs. Pollard to find meaning and to cope with her loss and grief.

The Refugee Experience: Haitian American Culture

During the last 25 years, the United States and Canada have experienced the influx of considerable numbers of individuals (both legally and illegally) from such diverse areas of the world as Southeast Asia, Central America, Eastern Europe, the Balkans, the Middle East, Cuba, and Haiti. For some refugees and immigrants, traumatic life events have been followed by the stress of coping with a new culture and a different environment. These experiences may predispose individuals to problems in adult development, as well as to certain health problems. The following case study illustrates how a situational crisis created by the refugee experience has hindered the psychosocial development of one individual (the mother of the family) by disrupting developmental tasks related to family and work patterns. Nursing interventions that are based on cultural implications and a development framework are discussed.

Haitian Refugees: Background and Context

To provide appropriate care to Haitian Americans, nurses must have some knowledge about the social and political events that have occurred in Haiti and must understand the issues that have influenced Haitian migration to the United States. Haiti has experienced a very troubled social and political history that has produced crippling poverty, economic insecurity, revolutions, and political turmoil. Many Haitians, seeing little opportunity for improvement in miserable living conditions and the overall economic situation, have fled their country.

Although Haitians have been migrating to the United States for many years, most of them who came before 1980 were upper class individuals who were able to obtain permanent residence and citizenship with little difficulty and usually assimilated rather quickly into the dominant culture. This changed in 1980 as a result of a change in U.S. immigration policies. From April to October of 1980, the Mariel boat lift from Cuba took place. In order not to be discriminatory, the State Department created a special status called "Cuban Haitian entrant, status pending." The "entrant" category described a temporary status and was used rather than political asylum. However, the "entrant" status created its own problems, since Haitian immigrants were placed in a bureaucratic limbo because they could not apply for resident status or citizenship (U.S. Committee for Refugees, 1986). In October of 1980, the immigration policies were changed again to prevent further migration of Haitian refugees, and a maritime interdiction program was later initiated to turn back Haitian refugees at sea. However, during the years 1980 to 1982, over 36,000 Haitians arrived in southeast Florida, some of them through legal channels, but the majority of them entered this country illegally (Frankenhoff, 1985).

At the present time, many adult Haitian women leave their children with relatives in Haiti and come to the United States by themselves. Leaving children behind is not unusual as Haitian mothers fear interdiction and detention in the United States and do not want their children placed with strangers. Their intent is to send for their children once they get settled in the United States; however, to date, immigration policies of the U.S. government have not permitted this. As a result, many Haitian women have entered new consensual unions and have had additional children after settling in this country (DeSantis, 1986). Restrictive as well as changing immigration policies have created many difficulties for Haitian refugees. Haitians who have managed to make it to the United States face a very real risk of being arrested, detained, and deported by immigration officials.

In addition to these fears, the federal government's refusal to grant political asylum or allow them to apply for residency or citizenship status has deprived the refugees of benefits. DeSantis (1990) noted that Haitian refugees placed additional demands on community resources already under pressure from the needs of the area. Local taxpayers have often resented the additional demands when the federal government was reluctant or refused to reimburse local and state governments for monies expended on the care and resettlement of Haitian refugees. These policies helped create and reinforce hostility and resentment toward the newly arrived Haitians. In addition, Haitians have been subjected to prejudice and discrimination because they are black; they are also very poor and lack the educational skills necessary to do well in U.S. society. Furthermore, they have been stigmatized by their early classification as an at-risk group for AIDS/HIV disease (Nachman & Dreyfuss, 1986; Cosgray, 1991).

All entrants who applied for residency in the United States were required to be tested for AIDS, and this requirement has had a negative impact in the Haitian community. DeSantis (1990) reported that health care professionals experienced considerable frustration and difficulty in meeting the health care needs of Haitian refugees in part because the large numbers of Haitians overwhelmed the health care system. Furthermore, most health professionals did not understand their language, culture, or health beliefs and practices.

CASE STUDY 5.2

Monique St. Clair is the 35-year-old mother of two young girls, ages 2 and 4 years. The family lives with relatives in a large apartment complex in Miami, Florida. Mrs. St. Clair was born in Haiti and grew up in a poor family who lived on the outskirts of Port Au Prince, the capital city. Mrs. St. Clair left her oldest child, a boy now 17 years old, in the care of family members and came to the United States with a maternal aunt and a cousin. Together the three of them have comprised an extended family that has grown by the addition of the cousin's spouse, their children, and Mrs. St. Clair's conjugal mate and their two children.

The term *conjugal mate* is used by DeSantis (1990) to refer to unmarried adult males who live in a conjugal relationship with women in the household. Such a common-law marriage is common in Haitian families living in the United States and Haiti and is predominant among the poor (Cosgray, 1991). This kind of arrangement imposes much of the responsibility for caring for and meeting the needs of the family on the mother. Child rearing is shared by older children and extended family members, but by and large, it is the mother who bears much of the burden and responsibility for the children. Often in the United States and Canada, we tend to use the designation "Ms." rather than "Mrs." when addressing female clients, especially if there is no "official" husband in the home. Other cultures, such those from Latin American and the Caribbean, are not as sensitive as North Americans about the manner in which married versus unmarried women are addressed. In fact, some Latin women might be offended by a "neutral" salutation that does not acknowledge their marital status. It is always appropriate for the nurse to ask clients how they prefer to be addressed. See Table 5-1 for some general guidelines.

Like other poor Haitian women, Mrs. St. Clair and her aunt are employed as maids in a motel in a poor section of the city. These are low-paying, low-status jobs with no benefits such as sick leave or health insurance. Studies of Haitian families in southeast Florida determined that the median household income was only $8500 yearly despite the fact that two or more persons from the household were employed (DeSantis, 1990). Obviously, this limited income is way below the poverty level set by the U.S. government for families of similar size. Few licensed day-care centers are available in the Miami Haitian community. When her cousin is not employed, she will babysit Mrs. St. Clair's two little girls, but when her cousin is working, Mrs. St. Clair pays one of her neighbors to watch the children. Family resources for child care that might have been available in Haiti are unavailable to mothers in the United States, so Mrs. St. Clair feels fortunate that she has female kin that are intermittently available to help her with the children.

Traditional Haitian Health Beliefs

Many of the illnesses affecting the HaitianAmerican community are potentially preventable or controllable through self-care measures. DeSantis and Halberstein (1992) and DeSantis (1985, 1988) have described many of the health problems in the Haitian population. They include a high prevalence of general malnutrition, hypertension, pediatric and adult HIV/AIDS, infant diarrhea and nursing bottle caries, measles and other childhood communicable diseases, suicide, and depression, as well as tuberculosis. Like other cultural groups, many Haitian Americans rely on traditional health beliefs and practices, and this has major implications for nursing practice not only for illness care but also for health promotion and wellness.

The practice of voodoo, an African-Haitian religious belief system, is not uncommon. Cosgray (1991) described voodoo as a religious system practice that dates back to the preslavery days of Africa; it was brought by slaves to Haiti in the 17th and 18th centuries. Voodoo practitioners are *houngans* (male) or *mambos* (female) and are further divided into other classifications that are not as well defined. The voodoo practitioners of Haiti are powerful figures with magical powers; they claim to be able to change themselves into animals, to pass through locked doors, and to perform other supernatural acts. Because of its association with black magic, voodoo is perceived as superstition by health care providers, and many Haitian Americans will not readily admit that they practice voodoo for fear of ridicule. The importance of voodoo in daily life and as a therapeutic system is pervasive and cannot be overemphasized. Over a period of several visits, the nurse must assess if Mrs. St. Clair uses voodoo practices and to what degree these practices might influence health practices within the family.

Generally speaking, Haitian folk diseases or traditional illnesses can be divided into illnesses that result from natural causes and those which result from supernatural causes. Since the causes are attributed to different sources, treatment is sought from different caregivers. Probably the most frequently used traditional practitioner is the herbalist who prescribes various herbs and home remedies to treat natural illnesses. Diseases of supernatural origin are believed to have been brought about because the individual had a breach with his or her "spirit protector." Haitians brought the belief from Africa that an individual is surrounded or enveloped by a variety of powerful, dominate spirits (Cosgray, 1991). When this protection is disturbed, the individual or a close family member becomes ill. Magical powers may be employed for the purposes of destroying one's enemies or healing the sick. Haitian Americans frequently hold a holistic conceptualization of humanity's relationship to God and to the external environment. In traditional Haitian belief systems, supernatural entities are a part of the external world.

Thus reliance on God and prayer to affect everyday life—i.e., money, a job, health, sickness—is a central element in the Haitian world view. DeSantis (1993) noted that Haitians in her study stressed the social, behavioral, and feeling dimensions of health. A core theme in the Haitian health belief system is the status of one's blood as an indicator of illness (Laguerre, 1981; Farmer, 1988; DeSantis, 1993). DeSantis (1993) stated that

> the amount [of blood] (too much or too little), color viscosity (thick or thin), turbulence (quiet or rushing) of flow, degree of impurities (good/bad or clean/dirty), and rise and fall of blood in the body are diagnostic of health and illness in traditional Haitian ethnomedicine. (p. 15)

These beliefs about blood and body fluids extend to menstruation, whereby the monthly menstrual flow is believed to cleanse the body of impurities and restore a woman to a healthy "clean" state. DeSantis and Tappen (1990) stated that Haitian women believe that they need to be extra careful during menstruation because they are more vulnerable to illness at this time. Likewise, the diagnosis of HIV/AIDS is frequently termed "bad blood" (DeSantis, 1993).

Many Haitian Americans believe in the hot and cold theory of disease that is prevalent in Latin American countries. This theory classifies food, medications, illness, and other body conditions as either "hot" or "cold." The assignment to hot or cold categories has nothing to do with the temperature of the object but rather its essence or essential qualities. The basic idea is an attempt to achieve balance between the hot and cold forces. For example, if a person had a "hot" disease, it would be appropriate to treat it with a "cold" medication or food. The postpartum period is considered one of the hottest states possible, and the patient is restricted from eating hot foods, which would make the condition unhealthy (Kirkpatrick & Cobb, 1990). Examples of "cold" foods that would be encouraged by those who believe in traditional health practices during the postpartum period would include avocado, cashew nuts, mango, pineapple, banana, and grapefruit and orange juice (Wiese, 1976).

In a study of infant feeding practices among Haitian mothers, DeSantis (1986) described another belief related to breast milk that has implications for the health and nutrition of breast-fed babies. It is believed that mothers may suffer from a condition that causes their milk to "spoil," and when this happens, it is believed that the breast milk turns into a poisonous substance, making the baby very ill. The obvious cure is to wean the baby from the breast immediately.

These traditional beliefs influence Mrs. St. Clair's child-rearing practices, and she is careful that her children do not become too hot or too cold and that they take care to avoid drafts of cold air. When they were babies, Mrs. St. Clair kept them heavily clothed to prevent cold air from entering the body through the umbilical cord while it was healing or through the sutures of the fontanel line. She also used numerous magicoreligious measures such as a multicolored bead necklace to ward off harm or spells of bad luck as well as curses from evil people. In addition, Mrs. St. Clair frequently prayed to God to protect her children, to grant them good health, and to prevent evil or harm from befalling them.

Mrs. St. Clair uses the professional health care system on occasion, usually only for the children rather than for herself. The cost of an office visit to a physician has been a tremendous barrier, so she has tended to use public health facilities. She has taken the children to the health department for their immunizations, but this has been sporadic because of her work schedule. As a result, the children's immunizations are not complete, and they have lacked continuous well-child care. When they are ill, Mrs. St. Clair treats them with home remedies such as poultices, herbal baths, and home-brewed teas. She is extra cautious during their illnesses about the effects of hot and cold foods and other factors on their health status. Sometimes when she can afford them, she will purchase over-the-counter medications such as cough syrup or laxatives. Purgatives or laxatives are often administered on a routine basis because periodic purging is central to Haitian health culture and is seen as a method of ridding the blood and body of impurities (DeSantis, 1988, 1990).

Developmental Assessment and Nursing Interventions

The following discussion focuses on Mrs. St. Clair's role and psychosocial development in relation to the social and cultural expectations that are placed on Haitian mothers. It is very important that the nurse be open and sensitive to Mrs. St. Clair's needs and concerns about her family. Mrs. St. Clair must be included in mutual goal setting in order to set realistic goals that are culturally relevant and appropriate. The preceding example of a mother caring for an adult child with AIDS used Havighurst's list of developmental tasks to assess the psychosocial adult needs of an African American woman; the next discussion uses Erikson's (1963, 1980) view of middle adult development.

According to Erikson, the developmental task of middle adulthood is the attainment of generativity rather than stagnation. *Generativity,* in Erikson's terms, is a concern for oneself, as well as for the growth and development of one's children, peers, the community, and society. According to Berger (1983), all of Erikson's stages share one general characteristic: They are centered on each person's relationship to the social environment. Generativity is accomplished through parenting, success in one's career, participation in community activities, and working cooperatively with peers, spouse, family members, and others to reach mutually determined goals.

Haitian American women often are the major providers for their families in terms of financial contributions as well as emotional and social support. The strength of the family structure develops from a sense of obligation of its members to the family unit. This sense of obligation can be easily identified in Haitian mothers, but Haitian fathers, even though they may be absent from the family a great deal, also feel deep pride and a sense of obligation to their families. As described earlier, the social, political, and economic situation of Haitian refugees is such that women often have what could be described as two families. The first family consists of the children left behind in Haiti with relatives, and the second family consists of children born in the United States in consensual unions. Often the children's father is unable to assume economic responsibility for his family, primarily because of the migratory nature of his work or the lack of steady employment. Many HaitianAmerican mothers and fathers, however, try to send a small amount of money back to Haiti each month to help their family's meager financial resources or to support children left behind with family, friends, or distant kin.

Because of the refugee experience, Mrs. St. Clair is stressed in multiple ways and is unable to successfully complete adult development tasks. However, nurses must realize that notions about adult development and what adults should do are influenced by our own cultural views of what is proper or normal for men, women, and families. Our traditional values suggest that men are the providers, support their families, and are heads of households. Women should marry, bear and raise children, manage the household, depend on men for economic support, and accept a subordinate position in the home. While traditional values are changing, particularly the roles of women, there is still a strong cultural norm in middle class America that stipulates women should not have children or a family outside of marriage.

Although poverty, racism, and discriminatory immigration policies have kept Haitian women from complying with the traditional American family ethic, they are nevertheless judged by its terms. The nurse might wonder why Mrs. St. Clair does not insist on marriage or why she continues to allow her conjugal mate to live with her family when he appears to contribute little financial assistance. For that matter, how could a "good" mother ever leave her child behind in Haiti for relatives to care for? In addition, our values in the United States are oriented toward individualism—an emphasis on individual worth, individual attainment, and individual growth and development.

Other cultures, such as Haitian culture, emphasize families and kinship more than individuals, and the Haitian is taught to be subordinate to family, church, and government authorities. They are more comfortable when cooperating with others rather than taking the initiative in any activity. An individual's self-worth as such is directly related to his or her position within the family unit. One way for the nurse to promote Mrs. St. Clair's growth and development is to emphasize her success as a parent and her positive relationship with her mate, her immediate family members, and neighbors. In addition, Mrs. St. Clair is fulfilling her obligations to her family in Haiti. Haitian parents never really abandon their children emotionally or financially.

New Ways of Coping

Laguerre, 1981 and DeSantis, 1990, 1993 have pointed out that Haitian Americans lost the emotional and social support of extended kin when they left Haiti. They have endured poverty in the United States and have experienced discrimination here because they are black and have been stigmatized because of their early association with AIDS and/or HIV disease. With such high-risk and culturally diverse groups, nursing interventions to support growth and development and promote health must be directed at both individuals and families as well as at the community level. The refugee experience has mandated that Mrs. St. Clair learn to manage on her own in a new culture.

In some ways, the refugee experience has empowered Haitian women like Mrs. St. Clair. They have learned new ways of coping and have developed new skills that have enabled them to manage in a new environment. On the other hand, the refugee experience has not been as beneficial for the Haitian men. Some of them may resent the growing financial, social, and independent role of women and the changing concepts of gender roles. Traditionally, Haitian men were heads of households, made decisions about their families, and handled the family finances. This situation changed with the refugee experience, and often men now find themselves peripheral to family life. Although many Haitian men do help with child care and household chores, these are new roles for them. It is especially important not to condemn the Haitian refugee woman for allowing the male to remain in the household and to make many decisions about the family. These new kind of relationships are often fragile, and frequently there is a potential for domestic violence, a phenomenon of concern in the Haitian community.

There are a number of things that Mrs. St. Clair can do to enhance her coping skills and thus enable her to better provide for herself and her family. DeSantis (1990) has pointed out that much of the stress affecting the Haitian community, such as poverty and an undefined residency status, are external to and beyond the direct control of health care professionals. However, these are the very factors that contribute to illness and raise significant barriers to preventive care. Nurturing cultural networks that exist in the Haitian community and the sense of interdependence that exists will strengthen the community and the individuals who live there. Helping the community mobilize its efforts to develop day-care facilities and other needed resources is an important nursing intervention. Members of the Haitian community share a common bond arising from the refugee experience, and they want to help themselves as a community. Health care professionals who wish to effect change for the Haitian community must work in the sociopolitical arena to bring about those needed changes.

Helping Mrs. St. Clair find health care for her children, including well-child care, that is available and affordable is important, but it is equally important that Mrs. St. Clair be encouraged to take actions that will promote her own health. Often a way for the nurse to win a Haitian mother's trust is to show interest and concern about her children. Once a trusting relationship is established, then Mrs. St. Clair will be able to focus on her own needs and concerns. Enhancing her coping skills will decrease psychological and emotional stress, but Mrs. St. Clair needs to be concerned with her physical health also. A sensitive nurse can help Mrs. St. Clair understand that rest, exercise, and an adequate diet will help her manage her family and work more expeditiously. Teaching her how to do breast self-examination and encouraging an annual pap smear are appropriate interventions that should be followed by helping Mrs. St. Clair find appropriate care that is low in cost and convenient. Numerous factors contribute to the decision as to whether or not to use family planning methods, and a holistic, culturally sensitive approach that considers her traditional health beliefs is needed to assist Mrs. St. Clair in choosing a method that she believes will be safe and comfortable. It is important to take into account that traditional Haitian beliefs suggest that the number of children a family has depends on God, not on the use of contraceptive practices. Since Mrs. St. Clair may become pregnant again, given her age, the importance of seeking early prenatal care to ensure both maternal and infant health must be incorporated in health teaching.

In addition to increasing resources and services, Jones and Meleis (1993) have suggested that something more is needed. They stated, "If individuals are not active participants in creating and using these resources, gaps between the resources and the individual's health will continue to grow" (p. 7). Thus, empowerment of individuals may be that necessary link. Empowerment includes helping Mrs. St. Clair develop a critical awareness of her situation and enables her to master her environment to achieve and maintain health for herself and her family. The most culturally appropriate way to empower Mrs. St. Clair is to help her make certain that her children are healthy and can take advantage of the resources available in the community for them. Enhancing generativity for Mrs. St. Clair means recognizing, promoting, and enhancing her abilities to meet her own and her family's needs, solve their own problems, and mobilize necessary resources to take control of their own lives.

Summary

The challenge to create new paradigms of adult development reflecting a more holistic picture of adult life seems evident in the examples just described. It may well be that existing models of adult development are androcentric, meaning they are based on men's life experiences and situations. Using these models to understand and interpret women's lives may obscure women's life structures and developmental pathways. Bryant (1989) suggested that we need to examine more closely those persons, "both men and women, who are out of sync with their time, the forerunners of new criteria for normal adult development—the women who could not be patently subservient to men, the men who could not be independent of emotions, the oldsters in physical and sexual vigor . . ." (pp. 3–4).

All individuals are confronted with developmental tasks, those culturally defined ways of responding to life situations. The example of a middle-aged African American woman who was providing care to her retarded sister and to her 26-year-old son with AIDS was presented. Culturally appropriate ways that the nurse might implement nursing care were suggested. Use of traditional family and religious systems were encouraged, since these ties are of particular significance in rural African American culture.

The second transcultural case study concerned a Haitian-American family living in the United States. The major nursing role with this family was promoting successful completion of adult developmental tasks by enhancing the mother's ability to cope with her many responsibilities and tasks. Although these developmentally specific interventions will not solve all the problems facing this family, such nursing guidance will help family members plan ahead, realistically anticipate outcomes, and cope with them in a manner that decreases stress and pressure, particularly on the mother. In this example, the mother was experiencing difficulties related to the adult stage of development, such as rearing children and adequately providing for the financial support of her family. These difficulties were embodied in the multiple crises confronted by the family in the last few years as well as the diminished support system outside of the immediate kin group.

Review Questions

1. List and describe the developmental tasks proposed by Havighurst (1974) and outlined in this chapter.
2. How are these developmental tasks of adulthood influenced by culture? For example, explain how a woman from a traditional culture such as those in the Middle East might experience adulthood differently.

3. Discuss how gender might influence adult development in white "mainstream" American culture.

4. Describe how social factors such as mobility, increased education, and changes in the economy have influenced adult development in U.S. culture.

5. How might caregiving for a family member influence development in middle aged adults? Would this differ for cultural groups such as Chinese American or Mexican American? How?

6. Describe how culture influences the role of the caregiver in some African American cultures.

7. Identify ways that the refugee experience might influence adult development in the Haitian culture.

8. How might family constellation differ among Haitian refugees? How might this influence adult development?

9. Define the terms *immigrant, refugee,* and *entrant.* What are the similarities and differences in these terms?

Learning Activities to Promote Critical Thinking

1. Interview a middle-aged colleague, a client, or a person from another cultural group. Ask about family adult roles and how they are depicted. How are these role descriptions typical of traditional roles that are described in the literature? If not, how are they different? What are some of the reasons why they have changed?

2. Interview a middle-aged client from another cultural group. Ask about the client's experiences within the health care system? What were the differences the client noted in health beliefs and practices? Ask the client about his or her health needs during middle age.

3. Using the cultural assessment guidelines provided in Chapter 2, conduct a cultural assessment of a middle-aged client of another cultural group. Critically analyze how the client's culture affect the client's role within the family and the timing of developmental tasks. How might the assessment data differ if the client were older? Or younger?

4. Review the literature on Mexican-American culture. Describe the traditional Mexican-American family. What are the cultural characteristics of Mexican Americans to consider in assessing developmental tasks of adulthood in this group?

5. Christina Calderon Salazar is a refugee from El Salvador who now lives in California and has residency status in the U.S. Several weeks ago she underwent a mastectomy. Señora Calderon has recently experienced menopause. She lives with her husband in a small suburb of Los Angeles, fairly near her two grown sons and their families. Critically analyze the cultural factors that are important to consider in providing nursing care to Señora Calderon. For example, how does Latin American culture view breast surgery? Menopause? How might you assist her in meeting her developmental tasks? What will be some problems that Señora Salazar might encounter in the U.S. Health care system?

References

Behler, D., Tippett, T., & Mandle, C. L. (1994). Middle adult. In Edelman, C. L. & Mandle, C. L. (Eds.), *Health Promotion Through the Lifespan*, (3rd ed., pp. 607–631). St. Louis, MO: C. V. Mosby.

Belenky, M. F., Clinchy, B. M., Goldberger, N. R., & Tarule, J. M. (1986). *Women's Ways of Knowing*. New York: Basic Books.

Berger, K. S. (1983). *The Developing Person Through the Life Span*. New York: Worth.

Boyle, J. S., Ferrell, J. A., Hodnicki, D. R., & Muller, R. B. (1997), Going home: African-American caregiving for adult children with human immunodeficiency virus disease. *Holistic Nursing Practice, 11*(2), 27–35.

Boyle, J. S., Ferrell, J. A., Hodnicki, D. R., & Muller, R. B. (1998). *Connections of Care: African American Mothers and Adult Children with HIV Disease*. Manuscript submitted for publication.

Bronfenbrenner, U. (1977). Toward an experimental econology of human development. *American Psychologist, 32*, 513–531.

Bryant, J. (1989). Normal adult development: But what about the rest of us? Unpublished paper, Norfolk, VA: Virginia Commonwealth University.

Centers for Disease Control (CDC) (1993, October). *HIV/AIDS Surveillance Report*. Atlanta: Department of Health and Human Services, Public Health Service.

Clark, M. J. (1996). Cultural influences on community health. In Clark, M. J. (Ed.), *Nursing in the Community* (pp. 273–333). East Norwalk, CN: Appleton & Lange.

Cosgray, R. E. (1991). Haitian Americans. In J. N. Giger and R. E. Davidhizer (Eds.), *Transcultural Nursing: Assessment and Intervention*. St. Louis: C. V. Mosby.

Cox, C., & Monk, A. (1990). Minority caregivers of dementia victims: A comparison of black and hispanic families. *Journal of Applied Gerontology, 9*(3), 340–354.

Danielson, C. B., Hamel-Bissell, S., & Winstead-Fry, P. (1993). *Families, Health and Illness: Perspectives on Coping and Intervention*. St. Louis: C. V. Mosby.

DeSantis, L. (1985). Childrearing beliefs and practices of Cuban and Haitian parents: Implications for nurses. In M. A. Carter (Ed.). *Proceedings of the Tenth Annual Transcultural Nursing Conference*, (pp. 54–79). Salt Lake City, UT: The Transcultural Nursing Society.

DeSantis, L. (1986). Infant feeding practices of Haitian mothers in South Florida: Cultural beliefs and acculturation. *Maternal-Child Nursing Journal, 15*, 77–89.

DeSantis, L. (1988). Cultural factors affecting newborn and infant diarrhea. *Journal of Pediatric Nursing, 3*(6), 391–398.

DeSantis, L. (1990). The immigrant Haitian mother: Transcultural nursing perspectives on preventive health care for children. *Journal of Transcultural Nursing, 2*(1): 2–15.

DeSantis, L. (1993). Haitian immigrant concepts of health. *Health Values, 17*(6), 3–16.

DeSantis, L., & Halberstein, R. (1992). The effects of immigration on the health care system of South Florida. *Human Organization, 51* (3), 223–234.

DeSantis, L., & Tappen, R. M. (1990) . Preventive health practices of Haitian immigrants. In J. F. Wang, P. S. Simoni, and C. L. Nath (Eds), *Proceedings of the West Virginia Nurses Association Research Symposium. Vision of Excellence: The Decade of the Nineties* (pp. 7–15) .

Charleston, WV: West Virginia Nurses' Association Research Conference Group.

Dressler, W. W. (1991). *Stress and Adaptation in the Context of Culture*. Albany, NY: State University of New York Press.

Erikson, E. (1963). *Childhood and Society,* 2nd Ed. New York: Norton.

Erikson, E. H. (1980). *Identity and the Life Cycle*. New York: Norton.

Farmer, P. (1988). Bad blood, spoiled milk: Bodily fluids as moral barometers in rural Haiti. *American Ethnologist, 15*(1), 62–83.

Frankenhoff, C. A. (1985). Cuban, Haitian refugees in Miami: Public policy needs for growth from welfare to mainstream. *Migration Today, 13*(3), 7–13.

Gilligan, C. (1982a). Adult development and women's development: Arrangement for a marriage. In J. Z. Giele (Ed.), *Women in the Middle Years* (pp. 89–114). New York: John Wiley & Sons.

Gilligan, C. (1982b). *In a Different Voice: Psychological Theory and Women's Development*. Cambridge, MA: Harvard University Press.

Gramling, L. F., & McCain, N. L. (1997). Grey glasses: Sadness in young women. *Journal of Advanced Nursing, 26*, 312–319.

Guberman, N., Maheu, P., & Maille, C. (1992). Women as family caregivers: Why do they care? *The Gerontologist, 32*(5), 607–617.

Haley, W. E., West, C. A. C., Wadley, V. G., Ford, G. R., White, E. A., Barrett, J. J., Harrell, L. E., & Roth, D. L. (1995). Psychological, social, and health impact of caregiving: A comparison of black and white dementia family caregivers and noncaregivers. *Psychology and Aging, 10*, 540–552.

Havighurst, R. J. (1974). *Developmental Tasks and Education*. New York: David McKay.

Hill, P. M., & Humphrey, P. (1982). *Human Growth and Development Throughout Life: A Nursing Perspective*. New York: John Wiley & Sons.

Jackson, B. (1985). Role of social resource variables upon life satisfaction in black climacteric hysterectomized women. *Nursing Papers, 17*(1), 4–22.

Jones, P. S., & Meleis, A. I. (1993). Health is empowerment. *Advances in Nursing Science, 15*(3), 1–14.

Kalichman, S. C. (1995). *Understanding AIDS: A guide for mental health professionals*. Washington, DC: American Psychological Association.

Kirkpatrick, S., & Cobb, A. (1990). Health beliefs related to diarrhea in Haitian children: Building transcultural nursing knowledge. *Journal of Transcultural Nursing, 1*(2), 2–12.

Laguerre, M. S. (1981). Haitian Americans. In A. Harwood, (Ed.), *Ethnicity and Medical Care* (pp. 172–210). Cambridge, MA: Harvard University Press.

Leigh, W. A. (1995). The health of African American Women. In Adams, D. L. (Ed.), *Health Issues for Women of Color*, (pp. 112–132). Thousand Oaks, CA: Sage.

Lewis, J. A., & Bernstein, J. (1996). *Women's Health: A Relational Perspective Across the Life cycle*. Sudbury, MA: Jones and Bartlett Publishers.

Lipson, J. G. (1991). Afghan refugee health: Some findings and suggestions. *Qualitative Health Research 1*(3), 349–369.

Lipson, J. G. Hosseini, M. A., Kabir, S., Omidian, P. A., & Edmonston, F. (1995). Health issues among Afghan women in California. *Health Care for Women International 16*(4), 279–286.

Myerhoff, B. (1978). Aging and the aged in other cultures: An anthropological perspective. In E. Bauwen (Ed.), *The Anthropology of Health.* (pp. 151–166). St. Louis: C. V. Mosby.

Nachman, S. R., & Dreyfuss, G. (1986). Haitians and AIDS in South Florida. *Medical Anthropology Quarterly, 17*(2), 32–33.

National Commission on Acquired Immune Deficiency Syndrome. 1991. *America Living with AIDS: Report of the National Commission.* Washington, DC: U.S. Government Print Office.

Neugarten, B. (1968). *Middle Age and Aging: A Reader in Social Psychology.* Chicago: University of Chicago Press.

O'Kelly, C. G. (1980). *Women and Men in Society.* New York: Van Nostrand.

Picot, S. J. (1995). Rewards, costs, and coping of African American caregivers. *Nursing Research, 44,* 147–152.

Purnell, L. D., & Paulanka, B. J. (1998). *Transcultural Health Care: A Culturally Competent Approach.* Philadelphia, PA: F. A. Davis.

Quam, M. D. (1994). AIDS policy and the United States political economy. In Feldman, D. A. (Ed.). *Global AIDS Policy.* Westport, CN: Bergin & Garvey.

Rutman, D. (1996). Caregiving as women's work: Women's experiences of powerfulness and powerlessness as caregivers. *Qualitative Health Research, 6,* 90–111.

Siegal, H. A., Carlson, R. G., & Falck, R. S. (1993). HIV infection/Serostatus outside epicenters. Human immunodeficiency virus (HIV-1) infection: A comparison among injection drug users in high and low seroprevalence areas. In B. S. Brown & G. M. Beschner, (Eds.), *Handbook on Risk of AIDS: Injection Drug Users and Sexual Partners,* (pp. 38–71). Westport, CT; Greenwood Press.

Sumartojo, E., Carey, J. W., Doll, L. S., & Gayle, H. (1997). Targeted and general population interventions for HIV prevention: Towards a comprehensive approach. *AIDS, 11,* 1201–1209.

U.S. Committee for Refugees (December, 1986). *Despite a Generous Spirit: Denying Asylum in the United States.* Washington, DC: American Council for Nationalities Service.

U. S. Department of Health and Human Services. (1990). *Healthy People 2000: National Health Promotion and Disease Prevention Objectives,* DHHS Pub. No. (PHS) 91-50212.

Wiese, J. (1976). Maternal nutrition and traditional food behavior in Haiti. *Human Organization, 35*(2), 193–200.

Wright, L. K. (1997). Health behavior of caregivers. In Gochman, D. S. (Ed.), *Handbook of Health Behavior Research III: Demography, Development, and Diversity,* (pp. 267–283). New York, NY: Plenum Press.

Wright, L. K., Clipp, E. C., & George, L. K. (1993). Health consequences of caregiver stress. *Medicine, Exercise, Nutrition, and Health, 2,* 181–195.

Wykle, M., & Haug, M. R. (1993). Multicultural and social-class aspects of self-care. *Generations* (Fall), 25–28.

Chapter 6

Caring for the Older Adult Client: Nursing Challenges in a Changing Context

Margaret A. McKenna

KEY TERMS

Formal Support Networks	Illness Behavior	Popular Health Care
Functional Age	Informal Social Support	Traditional Medicine or Practices
Hispanic	Older Adult	

OBJECTIVES

1. Demonstrate knowledge of factors at a societal level and at a community level that influence the experiences of older adult clients in the health care system.
2. Apply concepts of social support and cultural variation in planning and implementing nursing care for the older adult client.
3. Integrate concepts of cultural variation, life experiences, and available resources into planning appropriate nursing care of the older adult in community and institutional settings.
4. Develop nursing interventions with older adult clients that will be perceived as culturally appropriate and acceptable.

C are of the older adult client is becoming an increasingly important focus in the education and clinical training of nurses in response to the expected demands that the older sector of the population will place on the health care system. Nurses have traditionally cared for the older adult client in acute care hospitals and in long-term care facilities, but currently nurses are expanding their roles in the care of individuals and groups of older adults in community-based settings. Nurses may expand their roles as resource persons, case managers, direct care providers, discharge planners, or nursing consultants as care of the older client in different community settings, including residential centers, housing projects, and board and care facilities, will become more commonplace. Older adults are a heterogeneous sector of our population and as such will have a range of strengths as well as various needs that require different levels of care, assistance, and support.

The premise of this chapter is that culture shapes the way individuals view aging and explains the variability between groups of older clients in their adjustments to aging and in their health- and illness-related behavior and practices. Culture is not the sole determinant of behavior but is a critical dimension in understanding the interactions of older clients in their families and in an encompassing societal context. Nurses will implement care that is more individualized to the strengths and needs of each client, and care will be most appropriate to each individual's circumstances when attention is given to the client's cultural background.

In the current environment of human services, nurses are caring for older adult clients in a greater variety of settings including different residential options in communities. The framework for this chapter is that to appropriately plan and implement care in challenging settings, nurses should assess the social, cultural, and family contexts in which the older adult exists. By examining the variations that occur in the interactions of the older adult client in encompassing family contexts and in the broad community and society contexts nurses can determine the relative impact of these variables on the status of the individual. Nurses should develop an increased understanding that the older client is a participant in the culturally influenced patterns of care within a family. The available resources in the community as well as institutions and interventions at a societal level will affect the older clients' options for care and will affect the individual's movement on a continuum of care.

This chapter is organized in three sections that emphasize the dimensions that nurses will find relevant in planning appropriate and acceptable care for older adults: (1) the social and economic factors that influence the illness response and help-seeking behavior of the older client, (2) how the resources including informal and formal sources of help that are available to older clients will vary in their community contexts and will determine the older clients' immediate and long-term plans for care, and (3) how individuals who are impacted by society and local community–level factors are also members of families and are individuals whose responses to health and illness and whose actions to seek help will be influenced by their cultural beliefs, values, and practices.

Within the broadest societal context, nurses must assess cultural variations that should be included in planning and implementing nursing care of older adults. The older clients' cultural traditions and their values that are underlying their actions will influence their preferences for their residence, their lifestyles, and their expectations for who will be their caregivers. The cultural traditions and related practices among older adults are, of course, varied. The influence that social, economic, and other factors, including acculturation, have on the retention of these traditional cultural values and practices will be considered in this chapter. In assessing the needs of older adults, nurses must consider individuals in a broad societal context, in the context of their cultural upbringing, and as members of families who have varying strengths, resources, and capacities for care of aging family members. Several implications are drawn for how nurses can assess and plan nursing care for individuals in community and institutional care settings.

As a starting point in a framework for developing culturally appropriate care for older clients, the broadest context is society. The help-seeking behavior of the older adult population has been influenced by social and economic factors that include government interventions that were intended to improve the situations of older adults. Some of these factors are briefly reviewed as they influence the experiences of older adults in the health care system. See Box 6-1 for highlights of multiple factors that interact and shape the context for older adult clients who seek care or use health care services.

Box 6-1 *Factors that Influence Older Adults' Responses in Seeking Health Care*

At a broad societal level:

- Social and economic factors and changes that have occurred over time impact the experiences of older adults in the health care system:
  - Interventions to control Medicare expenditures force shorter hospital stays.
  - Gaps in health care services put greater burden on older patients for home and community-based care.

Cultural variation within a societal context:

- Different cultural traditions have values that influence patterns in caring for older adult family members as they require more assistance.
- Younger family members become acculturated and change traditional behaviors that may differ from older adults' expectations.

At the individual level:

- Female family members who were considered primary caregivers for older family members are entering the work force.
- Families' economic situations, proximity to the older adult, and sources of formal support in the community will determine options for residence and care needs of the older adult.

The Older Adult in Contemporary Society: Multiple Factors Impact the Experiences of Older Adults in the Health Care System

This section addresses selected factors that form the encompassing context that surrounds and influences older adult clients: demographic factors of the aging population, variables that increase the proportion of older adults to be served in the human services system, and psychosocial theories of aging that shape how older adults in Western society perceive growing older.

Several factors including improved living conditions and improvements in public health are contributing to an increase in the proportion of older adults in the population of the United States and Canada, as well as in other developed countries. Life expectancies are increasing, and in many nations, including the United States, the fertility rates are declining, which further adds to what may be called an aging of the population. At the beginning of the 20th century, a newborn could expect to live until age 47. As we approach the end of the 20th century, a white infant born in the United States has a life expectancy of 75.8 years.

By the year 2025, nearly 21 percent of Canadians will be 65 years of age and older. In 2025, projections are that 19 percent of the United States population will be 65 years and older (U.S. Bureau of the Census, 1992, 1993). The Hispanic older adult population is also increasing at a high rate. In both the United States and Canada, the percent of citizens over the age of 85 years is a fast-growing segment of the population (U.S. Bureau of the Census, 1992, 1993). The aging phenomenon is not limited to North American nations. In Japan, which is the nation with the longest life expectancy at birth, more than 25 percent of the population will be aged 65 or older by the year 2025 (Angel & Angel, 1997). In the Northern European nations, Iceland, Finland, Norway, Sweden and Denmark, a projected 20.5 percent of the population will be over the age of 65 years in 2025 (Giarchi, 1996).

To serve the growing proportion of older clients, nurses should consider that social and economic factors, cultural variation, and available support will interact and will impact the illness behavior and related help-seeking responses of older clients. As nurses prepare to care for older clients, they must assess the heterogeneity of the population as ethnicity, cultural traditions, social and economic situations, living arrangements, employment status, and migration history of older adults are as varied as for younger adults. These background factors contribute to varied responses among older adults to illnesses that require care and management in the health care system.

The aging sector of our population also poses special concerns that focus primarily on the care and management of chronic conditions. Disability associated with chronic conditions is not an inevitable result of growing older. Actually, the majority of older adults in North American settings do not suffer from disabling conditions. This finding is true cross-culturally as well. In the United Kingdom, approximately 80 percent of the population 75 years and older are not disabled, which compares with 70 percent of the older adult population in Belgium and France that are similarly able (Giarchi, 1996)

However, for approximately 20 to 25 percent of the older adult population, the care and management of chronic conditions becomes more problematic and costly with advancing age. The health care systems in the United States, Canada, and other developed countries must face expanded demands made by some older clients that includes care for multiple chronic conditions. There are three explanations that account for increasing life expectancy and rates of disability among sectors of the older population (Rice & Laplant, 1988). These explanations are (1) costly medical interventions have successfully resuscitated and prolonged life for individuals who would otherwise have died; (2) chronic illnesses that previously were fatal have been treated successfully, which has led to some older people living longer with a chronic disease; (3) lifestyle changes, including healthier diet, exercise regimens, and smoking cessation, have diminished the risks for acquiring some diseases (Verbrugge, 1989).

There is no simple correlation between the need for care and increased age because the need for care and health status are affected by many dimensions in an older person's life, including social class and ethnicity factors. Elderly African Americans often have suffered functional declines at earlier ages than have white Americans. African American older women have a much higher proportion of disabling conditions than African American older men (Chatters, 1993) and white older adults (Edmonds 1990). African American older women in the Southern United States are at higher risk for functional impairments than are African American women living in other regions (Gibson & Jackson, 1987; Martin & Panicucci 1996). The demands that the older population will place on the health care field are complex but a sub group of the population of older adults will experience some aspects of physical decline or functional disability that requires use of hospital, community, or home-based personal health services.

Economic Factors

The cost of long-term care for older adults in the United States, has contributed to growing Medicare expenditures. Medicare was intended to provide health care insurance for individuals aged 65 years and older. The percent of the federal budget spent on Medicare expenditures more than doubled from 1970 (3.5 percent) to 1990 (8.6 percent) (Moon, 1993). Given that the numbers of older adults who may require long-term community-based or institutional care is very likely to rise, this can only mean increasing financial burdens at national, state, and local systems to finance health care.

The provision of the health care services including an appropriate intensity of services to older clients in community settings will be a challenge. The need for health care services and support services was a focus of the White House Conference on Aging convened in 1995. The representatives to this conference addressed means to be developed that will (1) ensure comprehensive health care, (2) promote economic security, (3) maximize support service options, and (4) identify develop options for quality of life for older Americans. Nurses working with older clients are developing more roles in the provision of comprehensive services (first point in the White House Conference on Aging) in acute or community settings, and in short-term and long-term care settings.

Nurses who work with older clients in their homes often find that ethnic elderly clients cannot afford personal health care costs. There is a pattern that fewer older Hispanics have Medicare coverage than do their non-Hispanic peers. Only 21 percent of older Hispanics purchased supplemental Medicare insurance compared with 65 percent of all elders (Commonwealth Fund Commission, 1989).

Some examples from the caseload of a nurse who provides preventive care and assessments in a housing complex for older adults will illustrate that individuals have different experiences regarding health care and Medicare that is intended to provide for older adults. An 85-year-old man visits the nurse and requests to have his blood pressure checked. He complains about pain in his hip and shoulders and recollects many memories of his life's work. He was 17 years old when the stock market crashed and went to work to support his family. He worked as a laborer loading and unloading boxes and later became a roofer. He is sure that his pains now are due to arthritis from many years of hauling wood and supplies, and he accepts the discomfort as a natural sign of aging. He is quite proud that he was a union worker and receives a pension. He has not been in a hospital, and while he has Part A Medicare coverage, he has not had to rely on that coverage for health care needs.

Another resident in the housing project has different experiences related to economic factors and government funded health care insurance. A 70-year-old woman who worked as a housekeeper did not seek health care until she had a stroke related to untreated hypertension 4 years ago. She had limited contributions to Social Security owing to an episodic work history and her illness depleted any savings. She received Medicare funded services and continues to receive home health care through Medicaid, which is state-funded health care coverage for individuals with low income. These two residents are representative of the situations faced by many older adults who are affected by the societal interventions, namely Medicare, that aim to provide health care for older clients. These residents are like many other older clients for whom affordable health care and available health care services are a necessity. These brief examples illustrate that nurses must consider the effects of lower socioeconomic status on maintenance of health and management of chronic illnesses.

Impact of Changing Regulations on the Settings for Delivery of Health Care

There are interesting debates about the economic social burden of paying for health care for the older population, but rather than focusing on financial issues, the focus in this chapter is on the impact these changes in regulation have on nursing care for older adults. The Diagnostic Related Groups (DRGs) is one system for classifying diagnoses for use in determining money to be reimbursed to hospitals by a government payer. The DRG system was an intervention to contain elderly health care costs, but it has exerted a significant influence on the continuity of care for older adults. A primary impact has been shorter hospital stays for older adult patients. Older adults must then be cared for at home or in subacute units, or nursing facilities and patients are faced with many challenges to piece services together. Nurses may be providing short-term care for older adults in nursing facilities who have very recently had surgery and may then be involved in planning the post-facility discharge care for this patient. As a home health nurse, you may assess that older patients on your caseload would benefit from nursing assessments and medication monitoring, but you are informed that the patient's insurance and Medicare will not cover such services. Medicare pays only a small portion of home health care services, and the patient must be medically eligible to quality. Older adults who have other insurance may have some additional home health services covered.

The care that older adults may receive will be influenced and determined by economic necessity as well as environmental situations such as resources for nursing services, homemaker resources, as well as rural and urban locations that will affect resource availability. The needs that older adults have for care, their requests for assistance, and the sources of caregivers are also dimensions that are culturally influenced. Within the United States, nurses and health care professionals would see numerous variations in the types of caregiving support resources, both formal and informal, that are provided for older adults. Culturally influenced variations in care giving patterns for older clients are discussed in the next section. Before moving to the commuinty level, it is worthwhile to consider that at this encompassing societal level, there are psychosocial concepts that shape the experiences of older adults. This is to say that in addition to the demographic and economic factors that influence the older population, there are other dimensions to the experience of growing older.

Western Theories of Aging

The older adult clients' requests for services and the reactions of others to older adults are shaped in part by the prevailing psychosocial theories of aging in Western society. There are three theories that have been developed in Western culture that have some relevance in planning nursing care for older adults: activity theory, continuity theory, and disengagement theory. The theories provide a framework for assessing the older clients' responses to growing older and to making decisions about living arrangements and anticipated care needs that will be influenced by their cultural values. In American society, the values of independence, self-reliance, and productivity contribute to the attitude that the aged, who no longer contribute to society as workers, have less esteem and may be ignored. According to this view, older adults who continue to volunteer or produce services are valued. Often the contributions of older family members to intergenerational interactions and as bearers of wisdom are overlooked. Whereas some Americans reflect these values, there are of course variations, for many people value family roles and do not place such a strong emphasis on productivity. The theoretical frameworks are highlighted in Box 6-2.

Box 6-2 *Western Psychosocial Theories that Explain Older Adults' Reactions to Aging*

Disengagement Theory:

- A pattern of withdrawal that is usually considered desirable by the older person (Havighurst, 1968).
- Time allocated for reflection and leisure activities.

Activity Theory:

- Substitute activities for the tasks, including employment, that are regulated and withdrawn from the worker.
- Maintain activity levels and resist changes that would mean withdrawal.

Continuity Theory:

- Continue the relationships from earlier years and maintain lifelong activities that contribute to their self-perceptions (Atchley, 1989).
- Find meaning in adapting behaviors from younger adulthood.
- Personality make-up does not change, and behavior becomes more predictable.

These theories were developed years ago, and support among nursing researchers as to the applicability of these theories with different cultural groups has been mixed. On a positive side, the conclusions of a study of older Japanese showed that the most satisfied and healthy persons were the most active, which is consistent with the concepts of activity theory (Palmore & Maeda, 1985). A study of Puerto Rican elderly women living in Boston indicates that the women maintained family relationships and roles as they aged, which is a finding that supports the dimensions of the continuity theory (Sanchez-Ayandez, 1989). The Gray Panthers support the activity theory and advocate for creative, productive older adult lifestyles that are aimed at counteracting the losses of roles and status suffered by many older clients. The findings of a recent study of 213 women who were followed for over 30 years were that women with more roles had higher self-esteem and more optimal health as they grew older, which lends support to the activity theory (Moen, Dempster-McClain, & Williams 1995; Cutillo-Schmitter, 1996). In mainstream American culture, many older individuals experience their occupations and status withdrawing from them and the older person is disengaging from society through a reduction in social interaction due to retirement.

The theoretical frameworks may be most useful in working with older adults in North American contexts who have been raised with Western values. An example from Saudi older clients illustrates that theories are based on culturally influenced expectations of behavior that are not common in all groups. Whereas the continuity theory posits that the individual's personality does not change significantly as one ages, the Saudi subjects saw their personalities changing as they aged (Mansour & Laing, 1994). There were differences among older subjects in their employment and educational status. The lower educational group who were unable to read or write did not feel they were more reflective as they aged (Mansour & Laing, 1994). The finding that the continuity theory of aging was not supported among a sample of Saudi patients confirms that nurses should treat each client as an individual and assess the influence of the individual's culture on behavior, but it is imperative not to impose Western aging theories on members of other cultural groups.

Accommodating to Cultural Diversity at the Community Level: Older Adults in Different Ethnic and Cultural Contexts

Nurses will be increasingly challenged to plan and implement culturally appropriate care for the acute and long-term care needs of older adults who represent different cultural and ethnic groups as well as varied socioeconomic lifestyles. Nurses and health care professionals will also identify that older adults in our society represent diverse traditions. The life experiences of older adults will shape their responses in seeking health care and these experiences may include living through the depression; seeing the invention of television, computers, and video teleconferences; migrating to find employment; and fighting in an international conflict. European Americans in their 70s may have been adolescents fleeing Poland or Czechoslovakia before World War II. Many Southeast Asians who left Cambodia fled as conflict and political unrest enclosed around them. The stressful life experiences that some older adults have endured may make them reluctant to seek services and to lack trust in the care provided by health care professionals who are very different than themselves. Political refugees who have lived through civil wars and political revolution could well have depleted their coping mechanisms and experienced adjustment problems that may warrant care in the health care system, but at the same time, the clients distrust the system.

Culture influences the ways individuals view aging and affects how persons manage interpersonal crises and the alterations in health that often accompany aging.

Culture will influence the expectations the older person has of what constitutes illness and will also influence if the older adult maintains the use of traditional sources of health care in place of or in addition to the use of biomedical sources of care. Some older clients will prefer the use of traditional medicine from their native country or practices that they recall from their childhood traditions. The use of traditional sources of health care concurrently with or in place of the biomedical health care system is not limited to members of recently migrated cultural groups but is common to nearly all individuals. The lingering chronic conditions that often accompany age increase the likelihood that older adults will use traditional sources to treat their symptoms. The older adult may resort to an over-the-counter medication and may use other popular remedies before, during, or after the use of prescribed sources of care. Nurses can show an interest in the client and can ask clients about any actions they take to treat their conditions, in order to assess the older client's concurrent use of traditional practices, folk medicine, or popular medicine. See Research Application 6-1.

Older adult clients may also make use of traditional medicine that they recall from their cultural upbringing as a means to prevent illness. Preventive measures may combine a magical or religious element, such as burning a candle, offering cornmeal to the spirits, wearing an amulet or reciting a prayer. The nurse may reinforce these preventive actions that the older client views as promoting health with other actions to prevent illness and maintain health. To assess cultural beliefs and practices, the nurse can demonstrate a nonjudgmental attitude and ask questions that are similar in intent to the following:

Have you eaten any foods that made your problem better?
Have you used some herbs to make you feel better?
Have you bought or used pills or medicine to help your problem?
Did you talk to someone else and follow his or her advice about your problem? What do you expect your treatment to be?
What would you like us to do to make you comfortable?

A brief example in Case Study 6.1 illustrates that assessing the client's use of alternative sources of treatment is useful in developing a care plan that the client will find to be acceptable.

CASE STUDY 6.1
Use of Alternative Sources of Care

 Mr. S.L. was a 78-year-old man who was a retired machinist and had degenerative joint disease that caused recurring pain in his elbows and knees. He referred to his condition as "arthritis" and attributed his pain to the wear and tear of his long career around machinery, hauling parts, handling equipment, and standing for long intervals. He was raised in West Virginia, and recalled that his mother used rubbing liniment and kerosene to relieve aching joints. Mr. S.L. lived outside of a major Northwest city when he was interviewed by a nurse researcher about his use of alternative sources of treatment for his joint pain. He said that beside over-the-counter pain medication, he regularly rubbed kerosene and sheep liniment on his affected joints. He explained that his joints were not well lubricated and that they felt like gears that were clashing. An oil-based rubbing compound penetrated the joints and relieved his discomfort.

CLINICAL APPLICATION

The nurse assessed that the use of the rubbing compound did not interfere with the prescribed medications. His belief that the rubbing compound improved his condition and decreased his pain allowed him to participate in a prescribed exercise program. The nurse would continue to assess the treatment if the use of an alternative source of treatment interfered with the prescribed care plan.

....

Older clients who select to use alternative sources of care and who decide not to follow prescribed treatment plans may do so based on their beliefs about the causes of their illness and their expectations for treatment. Older clients may blend some biomedical beliefs about the cause of illness with some traditional and popular notions about illness, so it follows that clients may adhere to some traditional practices and to some biomedical treatments. For example, the findings of a study of rural African American older clients found that study participants had ideas about high blood pressure that were fairly congruent with biomedical concepts. Even though the clients acknowledged their traditional practices surrounding "high blood," they preferred prescribed medications. This study is described in Research Application 6-1 and indicates how important it is for nurses to assess each client's beliefs and practices as there are intra-group variations.

Research Application 6-1

Health Beliefs of African American Rural Elders

Schoenberg, N. E. (1997). A convergence of health beliefs: An "ethnography of adherence" of African-American rural elders with hypertension. *Human Organization, 56*(2), 174–181.

A sample of African American elders living in a rural area in Florida maintained selected traditional beliefs along with biomedical explanations about what caused high blood pressure. Most study participants believed that high intake of certain foods and a genetic predisposition could cause hypertension. They also believed that they would always have high blood pressure, and although they knew of the "old way remedies to reduce high blood," the participants tended to prefer to use prescribed medications. This finding, although limited in its generalizability, is useful as it describes the beliefs and practices of one group of African Americans and therefore highlights the heterogeneity of this population. The research findings remind nurses to (1) assess rather than to assume knowledge of older clients' beliefs about the cause of an illness and treatment expectation; (2) avoid the stereotypical views from prior research that clients are homogeneous and adhere to traditional ways; and (3) recognize that culture is dynamic so older clients' views of illness will change as they blend some biomedical explanations with traditional concepts.

Clinical Application
* The views and advice that nurses offered were highly regarded and were well received by study participants, which reminds nurses to take appropriate responsibility to work with the older clients toward mutually agreed-upon goals for care.

- Nurses who are culturally competent will recognize that prescribed diets such as low-sodium diets may not be region-specific, or might not include foods common in rural older clients' diets, so nurses would do well to help clients with adjustments.

- Nurses should also assess how older clients prepare their foods, as "greens" may be prepared with pork and may be high in sodium.

- Nurses are in a good position to reinforce the older clients' beliefs (that may be based in religion) that they should live life in moderation and modify their dietary intake as these behaviors will support a prescribed regimen that is intended to improve the clients' well-being.

Culture will also determine the older adult's expectations for family caregiving. Culture is not the only determinant of behavior, but it significantly influences the interaction of the older client in encompassing society, including access to and use of the health care system, as well as the relationships that the older clients has with family members and friends in a support network.

Several recent studies have described the implications for appropriate health care of older adult clients from different cultural backgrounds. While the situations of the groups are unique, there are some similarities across cultural groups that are relevant in planning nursing care. Older clients from different backgrounds may share in experiences of migration, changing social and family structures, structural forces that include discrimination, and historical events that include political conflict.

The hardships that the older clients have endured may increase their striving for autonomy in later years. The desire to remain autonomous may diminish the readiness of the older client to accept health restorative care from the nurse and may push the client toward self-reliance. The older client may prefer autonomy and needs time to reflect on decisions. A study of older Appalachian adults supported this finding as these clients tended to regard health care very cautiously. The harsh life led the clients to be fatalistic about many losses in life, and they weighed any options about health care in relation to their fatalistic views and in relation to their roles and interactions in their families (Lewis, Messner, & McDowell, 1985).

The findings of multi-cultural studies indicated that older clients retained their traditional beliefs while they modified aspects of their behavior to adapt to new surroundings. Older adult clients may vary from total acceptance of their traditional practices to some blending of traditional and biomedical care to total acceptance of biomedical care. The finding that the older clients preserved their traditional values indicated that a connection to their origins gave meaning to their lives. These studies are highlighted in Table 6-1.

Nurses can provide culturally appropriate care after assessing if the older client retains traditional values or blends traditional values and practices with biomedical beliefs and practices. Many older clients, now in their 80s, could have grown up with limited preventive care and associate health care only with emergent conditions, so nurses should assess the older client's previous experiences in the health care system.

Situations of Older Adults Who Migrate

Some older adults have been lifelong residents of this country and have resided in the same city or state for all of their adult life. Other older adults have migrated to

TABLE 6-1
Highlights of Selected Transcultural Studies of Older Adult Clients, 1990–1997

Study (Author, Date) and Group Studied	Cultural Values Relevant in Care of Older Adult Client	Implications for Nursing Care
Brod & Heurtin-Roberts (1992) Russian Jewish emigres in San Francisco seen in a medical clinic	Older emigres might have immigrated to be with children, and their status is compromised by immigration. May believe illness due to social causes, loss, food shortage, poor housing.	Assess the extent that clients may be accustomed to demanding care, to not seek counseling services but prefer attention from physician. Assess client's life experiences and immigration circumstances to assess for psychosocial needs.
Mansour & Laing (1994) Saudi patients on medical and surgical units, 25 percent of the sample over 60 years	Women in Saudi Arabia more involved with children, had less time for introspection. Men had different lifestyles, agreed that ego energy and style decreased with age.	Saudi subjects perceived aging differently from the Western subjects referred to in the continuity theory of aging. Nurses need to assess individuals for their beliefs, perceptions about aging.
Martin & Panicucci (1996) 40 black women, over 65 years old, members of a Southern, urban Baptist church	Sample had a high adherence to 20 recommended health behaviors that included abstinence from alcohol and smoking that may have been related to participants' religious doctrines.	Assess each client's interest in preventive behavior and make preventive practices relevant for client's lifestyle. Identify whether cost is a factor that explains lack of preventive care. Tailor approaches for individuals, not a global approach.
O'Hara & Zhan (1994) Pharmacologic considerations in care of Chinese elders	Traditional medicine includes herbal treatments, diet therapy, acupuncture, usually used only when symptoms occur.	Assess length of time that client has been in the country; assess retention of traditional beliefs and use of traditional therapies, folk medicine. Assess for interaction of these treatments with biomedicine.
Rosenbaum (1990) Greek Canadian widows, 12 subjects studied intensively and 30 additional informants	Family and religion were important. Church provides community care and prayer also important for well-being.	Reciprocation, love, companionship, hospitality, helping are culturally learned and are care constructs. Spiritual care is important.
Shiaveneto (1997) Hispanic elders, distinguishes cultural heritage among Mexican, Spanish, Central American, South American, Cuban, Spanish	Traditional gender roles, value respect, courtesy, features of Hispanic culture positively affect an individual's health status. "Hispanic" masks cultural identities, traditions of diverse groups.	Assess for increased severity of the illness that may be related to delay in seeking treatment. Communication barriers may lead to distrust. Assess use of traditional medicine that may be incorporated in plan of care.
Wilson & Billones (1994) New elder Filipino immigrant (NEFI)	Belief in destiny beyond one's control, conflict avoided, high value on privacy, esteem of the family system is highly valued, expect filial responsibility.	Older migrant changes status upon relocation, younger and older family members accommodate, elder has diminished social network. Consider the elder's role, assess home environment.

different regions of the country or have made a significant transition and relocation in their late adult years to be close to younger family members. Older clients may have the common experience of relocating or migrating, but the length of time that they have resided in one area may vary. There are other sectors of the older adult population who are recent immigrants and refugees. Whereas the notions of a melting pot formerly brought images of immigrants from northern and western European countries, currently there are increasing numbers of older adults who migrate from nations all over the world to relocate with other immigrating family members in the United States and Canada. Nurses and health care professionals may find that recent immigrants have a stronger family orientation and expectation of caregiving by adult children to their parents.

Older immigrants may have lost their social positions and may be clinging to family roles in light of the stress of acculturation that reduces their status. The psychological stress related to cultural change is more intense for older refugees (Moon & Pearl, 1991). In a study of 258 elderly Indochinese refugees, including ethnic Vietnamese, Chinese Vietnamese, and Laotians, those refugees who resided with immediate family members had a higher sense of social adjustment (Tran, 1991). However, older refugees who shared a living space with many extended family members and non-kin had a lower sense of social adjustment. The older refugee has sometimes left behind a career and a status associated with that career. The older refugee has a greater loss of status and status inconsistency that supports an inverse relationship between age and social adjustment (Tran, 1991). In Case Study 6.2, an older immigrant parent assumes a new role and acquires a new source of status in the family.

CASE STUDY 6.2

Immigration and Loss of Status in Family

 Mrs. D.R. is a 79-year-old native of the Philippines. She moved to an urban area in California to be near her four children who lived in the same state. She had lived in the same town in the Philippines for her adult life and had stayed there to care for her husband and later her sister who had both required care for chronic conditions. She is representative of the Filipino who migrates at a later age to join family members in North America. Whereas she was a much needed and highly esteemed member of her household in the Philippines, she like many other migrants, suffered role reversal as the elder lost the once dominant position within the family and became financially dependent on adult children during relocation (Wilson & Billones, 1994). Mrs. D.R. was also like other older Filipino adults who had a more active social network before relocation. She, like many older Filipinos, spoke a dialect and did not speak Tagalog, which many younger residents of the Philippines speak. After her relocation to the United States, her communication and interaction became restricted to her extended family due to language differences as she did not feel confident in using her limited English and she did not find other speakers of her dialect. Mrs. D.R. found increasing comfort through prayer and attendance at the Catholic Church to buffer the disequilibrium she felt due to her migration.

The older Filipino adult's status changes if the older migrant assumes child care or other duties within an adult child's home, which maintains the older member's respect within the family. This reciprocal relationship may lead to the perception of filial obligation between the generations of family members. Mrs. D.R. assumed the care of her two daughters' children, which increased Mrs. D.R.'s self-esteem, personal dignity, and pride in her family. The nurse who took care of Mrs. D.R. in the emergency department owing to a fractured wrist that she received in a fall assessed that Mrs.D.R.'s injury would actually place a stress to the family as they would temporarily be without their child care provider. The nurse was able to involve the family members in the discharge plan for Mrs. D.R. so her recovery could be assured, she would not lose respect, and she would not feel responsible to assume her usual duties until she felt better.

CLINICAL APPLICATION

The nurse caring for Mrs. D.R. did very well to assess the following areas, which are relevant concerns for any older adult client:

Dynamics of the family system
Interaction of the older client within the family
Environment that the older client will return to
Adherence of the client and the family to traditional values

All of the above-mentioned factors may vary among older Filipino migrants, and nurses must assess the extent to which individuals retain their traditional practices and the related underlying values.

Under the current immigration policies, some recent immigrants do have a financial responsibility to their older family members. The older adult usually does not have an option to work, nor is public assistance an option, so the family must provide for the older adult members. Older family members may reciprocate services for younger family members. A national sample of older Hispanics reported that 30 percent of the respondents provided child care to younger family members and 50 percent reported assisting in family decisions (Westat, 1989). As part of a nursing assessment, the nurse notes if older adults are primary care providers for grandchildren or other family members and if an illness episode in the older adult disrupts the family.

Many immigrants, who have migrated after the age of 50 years, experience more depression associated in part with their increased dependence. One study of Mexican American elderly found that the rate of depression among those immigrants who came to the United States after they were 50 years old was nearly 35 percent. In this study, the immigrants who were between the ages of 40 and 49 had the lowest rates of depression, but that was still significant at 23 percent. The rate of depression among those Mexican Americans born in the United States was 22.8 percent (Markides, 1992).

For many Mexican American older adults, there are socioeconomic factors that would indicate they would be at risk for higher morbidity and mortality than whites. However, their rates of heart disease and cancer are actually somewhat lower than those of non-Hispanic whites. This is suggestive of protective aspects of traditional Mexican American culture that may include their integration into the extended family and their care at home that contributes to a slightly better than expected health status (Scribner, 1996; Schiavenato, 1997). The protective aspects of Mexican American culture may diminish over time among families as they become more acculturated. As the length of residence and extent of acculturation increases for the families with older adult members, the families may face the economic necessities of the adults working outside of the house that will lessen their availability for family care of the older adult. The family may come to rely on community and institutional sources of care.

Membership in a cultural group or the shared experience of immigrating from the same country does not imply that older adults are similar. The life experiences of the individuals, including their occupations and education, and their acculturation will affect what are their needs and what are their expectations for care in their advancing years. Thus, there are tremendous differences among individuals within a cultural group as well as between cultural groups.

Consistency of Behavior With Underlying Values

In a homogeneous society, where three values— respect for the aging, inter-generational duty, and family loyalty—are widely accepted, the majority of individuals would expect and find that care for older adult family members is assumed by younger family members. Traditional Japanese culture offers us an example of the shared culturally influenced expectation that daughters and daughters-in-law would care for older family members as they face declines in personal health. Some families who are Japanese American may continue to uphold traditional values.

While the traditional values may be desirable, other factors, including increasing education and career opportunities for women as well as economic necessity to enter the labor force, may influence the behavior of female family members to work outside the home and not to be full-time caregivers. There are other patterns that include the suburbanization of Japanese Americans and more varied geographic locations that reduce the relevance of traditional values in the lives of the Nisei (second-generation) Japanese Americans, which may impact lowered status and reduced authority for the Issei (first-generation) Japanese American elderly (Osako, 1979). Nurses may need to assess what could be disparities in what the older client expects for care and what the younger family members can realistically provide.

Family Responsibility for Older Adults

The importance of involving the family in the care of the older adult member is considered central to the discussion of cultural variation. Family members are participants in informal social support networks that often nurture and maintain older adults in their preferred community residences. It is also vital to consider the preferences of the older person and his or her family members, as well as the capacities of the older adult for self-care, and the willingness and capabilities of the families to offer support and assistance with care. The type and duration of support than can be provided by family members must be considered in relation to sources of formal support that could be used to sustain the family care. This includes the skilled assessment, care, and evaluation of care that are provided by nurses and other health care professionals in different settings.

The nature of what constitutes formal support and the contexts for formal support and health care for the older adult have been evolving rather steadily over the last two decades. The old image of care for older adults in skilled nursing facilities has given way to a continuum of services for older adults that includes self-care, supported self-care, assisted care, and skilled care. The roles that family members take in each of these levels of care certainly vary according to cultural, socioeconomic, and demographic characteristics, which are discussed later in this chapter. Family members are learning more about the care of older family members from books that have been written by and for adults caring for aging parents. We hear of adults who are sandwiched between the layers of care of their own children and in the care of aging parents. All families have culturally influenced patterns of responsibility to meet the care needs of older family members. Culture definitely influences the role that the family members will take in the care of older family members. Nurses and health care professionals must be increasingly aware of the social and economic factors that alter families' retention of traditional values that affect caring for older family members. The economic necessity that two adults in many households must work to provide adequate household income has contributed to a decline in the former take-for-granted availability of adult female children as caregivers to parents, grandparents.

The participation of women in the work place and the decline in the numbers of adult children in many families have contributed to families who are not available to provide personal care to the older adult family members. Adult children and other family members may be available to provide episodic assistance, emotional support through short visits, or some financial assistance to purchase in-home services. It is not possible to talk about older adults or their families as if they were a homogeneous group, in similar life situations. Rather it is necessary to consider that cultural diversity and lifestyle choices may actually influence and determine many different options for care of the older adult. Nurses working in acute, community, and long-term care settings will be asked to support family members who are involved and contributing to the care of older family members in different ways: tangible support, emotional support, financial assistance, personal caregivers, and relief caregivers.

The majority of older adults experience some forms of disabilities in their functional status. Culture can influence the extent that functional disabilities will be perceived as disabling or merely annoying, and will influence the extent that individuals seek help for their disabilities. Families have often developed culturally influenced patterns of caregiving and social support.

Dimensions of Social Support

The concept of social support has been studied by different disciplines for more than two decades, resulting in well-supported findings that individuals with adequate support systems may maintain their health and avoid institutionalization (Kaplan, Cassel & Gore, 1977; Crawford,1987; Ryan & Austin, 1989; Sutherland & Murphy, 1995). Social support assumes special relevance for the older client, as many older clients sustain social deprivation from several sources:

Separation from immediate family members due to geographic mobility
Age-related segregation due to increased nuclear families in neighborhoods
Loss of spouse due to death or illness
Loss of leisure pursuits or entertainment due to illness or loss of income

It is especially important for many older adults to have social, emotional, and physical sources of support to assist them to remain as independent as possible. Social support for an older client in a continuum of care may mean that the individual remains in a community-based setting indefinitely or for a longer period of time before institutional care becomes necessary. Understanding the patterns of support that older adults might need and assessing the cultural variations in these patterns of support is good preparation for nurses who may be working in acute, extended-care, or community settings. Norbeck (1981) initially described three types of social support in young adults, but they are applicable for the older client:

Affective support: expressions of respect, love
Affirmational support: receiving endorsement of one's behavior, perceptions
Tangible support: receiving some kind of aid, physical assistance such as accompanying a person to an appointment

One implication is to identify the importance that the older client places on these types of social support. In a study of older clients in two community settings, the clients indicated that the need for affective support (love and respect) was highest followed by tangible support (Sutherland & Murphy, 1995). Another implication for nursing care is to assess what the older client identifies as his or her sources of affective, affirmational, and tangible support. One nursing study of older adult participants in a community center group and in a geriatric day treatment center group identified the members of their respective groups as important sources of social support (Sutherland & Murphy, 1995). The community center group identified that family, friends, and clergy were sources of social support.

Nurses and other health care professionals can gain insight into understanding the older adult's social support network by learning from cross-cultural work in nursing and in anthropology. Anthropologists that studied the structure and functions of support networks described the intricacies and multiple relations that individuals have within a support network. Nursing researchers have identified that kinds, amounts, and sources of social support vary in health and illness situations and are situation specific (Sutherland & Murphy, 1995). Several dimensions of support networks are adapted into a matrix of support networks that are common among many older adults who are in community settings including living in their own residence. This matrix is discussed in Table 6-2 and is useful for nurses to assess strengths of older clients as well as to anticipate the type of support that older clients might need.

To understand that culture may influence the types of social support that family members offer to older clients, nurses may assess the concept that the structure of families affects how informal support is provided. Some families, including the Yankee Americans, German Americans, and families of English extraction often have a linear structure. The expectation is that adult children will assume care responsibilities for aging parents, and grandchildren will assume caregiving for aging parents and grandparents when needed. Another family structure is collateral when the perceived bonds are more diffuse and include parents, aunts, uncles, grandparents and family friends may be part of the collateral bonds of families. Among families with a collateral structure are those of Irish, Polish, and African American families, who expect to receive and to provide informal support among all collateral contacts. The expectation for care among many Irish families is that relatives must assist each other when needed. Many Irish and Irish American families would agree with two assumptions that describe mutual support within kinship relations: (1) a person must act like a relative in order to be thought of as one, and (2) their relatives are obliged to enter into generalized reciprocity (Giarchi, 1996).

TABLE 6-2

Dimensions of Social Support Networks Common to Older Clients in Community Settings

Network	Participants in the Network	Characteristics of the Network
Integrated support network with local support	Family members living nearby, friends, neighbors	Based on long-term local residence of the older adult, frequent contact with available kin, usually a large network; older client remains involved in community. Friends may offer tangible assistance, affirmational support. Family offers affective support.
Community-based support network	Family members do not live in proximity, friends may be available, neighbors more accessible	Family members accessible by phone for affective support, friends may not be in good health to help, younger neighbors who are available help as they can for tangible support
Family-dependent network	Adult children, other relatives, minimal or no contact with friends, contact with neighbors for emergencies or occasional relief support	Adult children and other relatives provide most sources of support. Network may depend on a primary caregiver with planned relief. Would benefit from some formal source of support: homemaker, aide.
Restricted support network	Spouse or adult children of the older client are primary caregivers. Friends do not maintain contact or are not available owing to their own illness or distance.	Older client may be out of touch with peers. Older client may live in adult child's home. Usually frailer older adult. Network may fall apart if the one primary caregiver becomes ill or unable to provide support. Usually needs formal source of support to be maintained.

One implication for the nursing care of older African American adults, for example, is that more caregiving tasks may be assumed by more individuals in the older adult's collateral bonds (White-Means & Thornton, 1990). Research among African American families has indicated that church members may provide assistance that supports family members' support (Walls & Zarit, 1991). Non-kin, that is individuals who are friends but are not related, may be very significant helpers in the informal network for older African Americans (Johnson & Barer, 1990). Two researchers (White-Means & Thornton,1990) found that persons of German and English heritage were less involved as caregivers than were African Americans in similar situations when the time constraints and work restrictions were taken into account.

In addition to cultural variation in patterns of giving help and support, it is not surprising that socioeconomic status will influence the amount and level of assistance that family members provide to older adult family members. It is important to identify the relative influence of two types of factors on patterns of family members providing support to their older members. These are (1) demographic factors such as family size, migration patterns, rural/urban residence, and (2) the second category is socioeconomic factors including income and educational level. Both of these sets of factors may determine the availability of family members to offer assistance and may influence the type of support that is offered. Thus, nurses must assess the relative influence of these factors on the older adult's social support network and identify that demographic factors and socioeconomic factors may be blended with culturally influenced patterns of behavior.

Generally, more older adults in rural areas tend to live with their family members than does a comparative group of urban older adults. The older adults in rural areas are also more likely to see their adult children every day than are urban older adults (Angel, De Long,Cornwell, & Wilmoth, 1995).

Socioeconomic Levels

Researchers who have studied the elderly in our society found that working class families were more inclined to provide assistance with activities of daily living and with household chores. Families in higher socioeconomic levels were more inclined to purchase goods or gifts for older family members (Cantor & Little, 1985).

Influence of Family Size

It is more likely that an older Mexican American or Chinese American in a traditional or immigrant family will live with an adult child and receive help from an adult child than a white older individual (Lubben & Becerra, 1987). This is not a definitive finding that can be attributed to specific factors, but it is suggestive that economic necessity or the presence of larger families may lead to the observed pattern of residence and assistance for some families. Nurses and other health care professionals must also be very cautious to identify the variations within groups and not just between groups. We should not assume that all Hispanic families are familistic, nor should assume this is a characteristic among only Hispanic families. We would find that other groups are just as familistic in their attention to older adults and that some Hispanic families are not demonstrating that characteristic to any greater extent than other families.

Intragroup Variations

Nurses and health care professionals can certainly move beyond generalizations toward appreciating the cultural differences among groups of older adults who are in the general term "Hispanic." One implication for nurses is to understand differences among the groups classified as Hispanic, in patterns of their older adults to have daily contacts, church attendance, and socialization with friends (Angel & Angel, 1992). Older Cuban Americans are more likely than Mexican Americans and older Puerto Ricans to get together often with friends. Older Mexican Americans are more likely than either Cuban Americans or Puerto Ricans to attend church and to have daily contact with their children (Angel & Angel, 1997).

The Individual Level: Integrating Social and Cultural Factors in the Care of Older Adults

The purpose of this section is to identify that the variables that are present at a societal level and the concepts of cultural variation that have been discussed in the previous sections impact older clients as individuals. More specifically, social and cultural factors influence most older clients' progress in meeting the developmental tasks of aging. The developmental tasks that older adults achieve include the satisfaction of basic needs, such as safety, security and dignity, and the fulfillment of integrity and self-actualization. For the majority of older adults, these needs are intertwined with the lifestyle and the residence of the older adult. For that reason, this section focuses on the options that older adults have for community or institutional care as these options provide older clients with safety, security, and an opportunity to possess dignity and autonomy. The older adult also usually exerts some control over planning where he or she will live and exercises self-determination and self-esteem. Usually in conjunction with the community or institutional residence of the older client, the individual may find an outlet for individual or group activity, volunteer efforts, artistic activity, or socialization that are sources of self-esteem, give meaning to one's life, and contribute to positive fulfillment of the developmental tasks of aging.

Nurses are especially well prepared to work with older clients as they demonstrate a professional understanding that aging is a positive developmental experience for individuals who are in a stage of reflecting on life experiences and finding meaning in their lives. Older adults may have many transitions that are chosen or are inevitable with growing older. These include retirement, grandchildren, changed living arrangements, family mobility, declining health, deaths of family members including spouse, siblings, or children. Older adults may assume new roles, and nurses can do much to normalize the changing roles and reframe the challenges as opportunities for positive growth (Cutillo-Schmitter, 1996). Nurses often view the strengths and residual abilities that older clients possess rather than dwelling on the losses, and in doing so, the nurse promotes optimal functioning when the older adult may be experiencing unavoidable dependency.

Cultural factors, including the cultural group history, and life experiences, including immigration, will interact and will determine the older client's efforts to achieve security, autonomy, and integrity. In achieving integrity, the older client has a need to bring closure to life and acceptance of an eventual death. A nurse may assess this need in a patient's family and be a sensitive listener when the client works through the steps of achieving integrity. Older clients need time for a purposeful life review. The older adult may relinquish some aspects such as paying bills to an adult child, so the older person is free to reflect on life successes and failures.

All older clients require culturally appropriate communication and intervention that is specific to their background. Additionally, the older population will require three types of care that can be summarized as (1) intensive personal health service, depending on the presence of acute and chronic conditions; (2) health maintenance and restorative care, depending on the presence of chronic conditions; and (3) coordinated nursing, social services, and ancillary services that may be provided on an episodic basis for older clients in the community.

Decisions on a Continuum of Care

Depending on the level of disability that an older person suffers, he or she may be faced with a decision to continue to live in one's home with assistance, with family members, in an assisted living residence, or in a skilled nursing facility. Nurses will observe that older clients express different attitudes that range from resignation to acceptance when they must change residences. The nurse can assess that the older client's attitudes about community or facility residence have been influenced by social and peer groups, and the nurse can be sensitive to the older client's reactions.

Researchers who have studied the elderly in America have found that for nearly two decades, the most consistent factor in determining the placement of the older person into a skilled nursing facility is the lack of an adequate informal network (Shanas, 1979). Nurses who provide care to older clients and families from different cultural backgrounds will notice that functional abilities required for family participation vary by cultural context. For example, members of some cultural groups will provide care that maintains the older family member at home.

The nurse may assess the following: Does the family modify the environment and assist in home care so that the older adult remains at home? Do children and grandchildren share tasks, provide meals, and run errands so the grandparents can live alone? Some differences have been noted in the patterns of living arrangements according to ethnic background. Even when single older African Americans lost functional abilities, they were less likely than whites with similar losses to enter skilled nursing facilities (Angel, Angel, & Himes, 1992).

That finding indicates that some older Black Americans may be able to reside in the community with family assistance, and informal and formal social support for a longer duration than white clients. In one study of Puerto Ricans in skilled nursing facilities in New York City, the residents had higher levels of disability than did a comparison group of other facility residents. That finding suggested that Puerto Rican family members may have been more inclined to care for family members with declining health status and for a period of time longer than non-Puerto Rican families (Espino, Neufeld, Mulvihill, & Libow, 1988). Nurses must also asses that the values of independence and self-reliance may be very strong for some older clients, and they may refuse any assistance from family members, so the nurse should evaluate clients' behaviors relative to underlying values.

According to 1990 census data, while 6 percent of whites over the age of 65 years may reside in a nursing home on a typical day, the percent of Hispanics older than 65 residing in a nursing home is half that, or 3 percent. The census category subsumes many different cultural groups under a very broad category of Asian Americans, and only 2 percent of those older than the age of 65 years would reside in a nursing facility on a representative day (Angel, Angel, & Himes, 1992). White elderly clients aged 85 years old and older comprise 23 percent of the nursing home residents in the United States (Wray, 1992). Hispanic and Asian/Pacific Islander older adult clients comprise 10 percent of the nursing home population aged 85 years or older (Wray, 1992).

Among different ethnic and cultural groups, cultural traditions may influence the perceived responsibility of adult children to care for their parents at home. Historically, a higher proportion of older adults from diverse cultures have been cared for in home environments than have elders who are white (Wray, 1992). The interaction of other factors including the availability, acceptability, and affordability of a skilled nursing facility that is in proximity to the ethnic populations also definitely impacts the overall residence patterns by members of cultural and ethnic groups.

Older adults who for the majority, if not all, of their lifetime have spoken their native language and surrounded themselves with friends who also shared their customs could find it enormously difficult to enter a skilled nursing facility that would appear quite foreign in its practices. Much of the professionals' actions and behavior that occurs in health care facilities is the result of acculturation in the biomedical culture. Nurses and other health care professionals are not always aware that their behavior such as an insistence on schedules, order, and cleanliness would not be valued equally by older adults from different cultural groups. Thus, ethnic elders may feel especially uncomfortable if they do not understand why they are awakened at a certain time, required to be dressed, and asked to participate in group socialization. The ethnic elder may find the skilled nursing facility to be hostile and unfriendly.

Some older adults who have immigrated to North America from other nations may have negative perceptions of skilled nursing facilities based on their experiences in their native countries. The situation in a Russian nursing home, while it may not be typical, does illustrate that a Russian immigrant might have a negative perception of anticipated nursing care in a facility. In a Moscow residential home, there were 300 bedridden older adults, and 200 residents had dementia. The facility was to be staffed by 7 doctors, 44 nurses and 96 auxiliary personnel, but 45 percent of the positions were vacant at the time of a visit in 1990 (Giarchi, 1996). If the prospective nursing home resident had this type of negative perception, it would clearly contribute to the reluctance or refusal of the older adult to be admitted to a facility.

Nurses can do much to ease the entry of ethnic elders into skilled nursing facilities when they assess each resident's cultural background, food preferences, choices for daily care and personal schedule, and interaction with family members. The individual's life experiences and personality will certainly shape the reaction to being in a skilled care facility. In order to better understand the older client's perspective, nurses could adapt some aspects of an ethnographic research approach and ask open-ended questions of the older client as part of a holistic nursing assessment. These questions could focus on topics that were meaningful to the older client, for example, what was most important for them to maintain in their daily routines, and what would they like to do so they were as independent as possible. For more information about applying aspects of an ethnographic approach in nursing practice see Research Application 6-2.

Research Application 6-2

Applying Ethnography to Care of Older Adults

Brandriet, L. M. (1994). Gerontological nursing: Application of ethnography and grounded theory. *Journal of Gerontological Nursing 20*(7), 33–40.

Ethnography is a qualitative research approach that uses a holistic, inductive method, participant observation, and in-depth interviews in a naturalistic setting to collect data. Ethnography would be especially useful in understanding older clients in relation to their cultures of origin and to the culture of technological, impersonal health care settings. Nurses may adapt aspects of this approach to collect and analyze client information to better understand the older client's perspective, reactions, and culturally influenced decisions. An ethnographic approach would lead to the discovery of the inside reality or "emic" view that an older client has of his or her daily experience, for example, chronic illness and self-care, technological treatment, long-term care placement, and decisions pertaining to care.

Clinical Application

- Nurses could use participant observation to observe and record the interaction of staff and older clients in nursing facilities or in assisted living centers.

- Nurses may ask older clients about a domain of interest: what concerns them about their daily experiences, what gives them hope each day, what makes them feel independent, or what aspects of care they wish to control.

- Studying technology from the older client's perspective might give the nurse insight into its impact as an intrusion into the older person's life.

- Using an ethnographic approach could inform the nurse about the client's cultural beliefs about illness causation and expectation for treatment that the nurse could compare with a biomedical explanation.

- Nurses who become familiar with an ethnographic approach could practice viewing biomedical care as outsiders to appreciate how the older clients view the realm of in-home treatment, medication monitoring, and health assessments that are provided by nurses.

Community-Based Services for Older Adults

The skilled nursing facility represents only one option for extended care of the older adult. The current nursing facility resident is regarded by experts in the field as an individual that has generally exhausted the opportunities for care in the community. This individual usually only enters a facility after home care, and levels of assisted living have been implemented. Long-term care nursing consultants and nurses working in ambulatory care settings often are asked to assess older clients to help determine the best care option for an aging individuals with declining functional abilities. Criteria that the nurse often considers to recommend the level of care or residential placement that would be most appropriate for an older client include mental orientation, physical mobility restrictions (use of assistive devices and ability to walk unaided), degree of assistance needed to complete activities of daily living (ADLs), frequency of incontinence, and level of risk for accident or injury if living independently.

Assessing the Older Adult's Needs

Nurses can assess the factors that determine the care needs of older adults, the resources to meet those needs and the locations for residence and care that are most appropriate. Nurses must assess the physiologic status of the older adult and consider the safety of the client in a residential setting. The nurse must also consider medication management of the older client, and there are physiologic changes in aging that must be considered for every client. Those changes that indicate to medication management include decrease in lean mass, possible decline in renal function, and overall sensitivities that may increase with age (Katzung, 1992). Additionally, approaches that will reduce misunderstandings due to language differences should be integrated in a care plan for any older client. The nurse should assess for the older clients' understanding of medication directions as the client's eyesight may be failing and the directions such as "Take with meals" may be open to multiple interpretations. There are other factors to assess that include

Cultural values that affect the expectation of the older adult and the family members

Available resources including informal sources of support: children, grandchildren able to provide personal care, assistance with ADLs, financial support.

Nurses and health care professionals who are aware of the older adult client's preferences for in-home care or for residence in skilled nursing facilities are realizing that the client's economic resources may affect preferred care options. The reality is that many ethnic elderly of color have accumulated fewer financial assets, that is, they have a lower household income, fewer dividends, and less income from private pensions than do elderly whites (Angel & Angel, 1997; Even, 1994). One of five ethnic elderly of color rely on Supplemental Security Income (SSI) as the primary source of income after age 65, while a much smaller number of elderly white clients (1 out of 20) relies on this source for their retirement income (Angel & Angel, 1997). One of the major problems that many ethnic older adults and their families face is limited tangible assets and lower equity in their homes that may limit possible care options as families cannot afford costly long-term care or community-based care of the older adult family member.

For the poor elderly person, purchasing part-time personal health care services or attendant care that would enable one to remain at home may not be an option, so the older adult manages in less than desirable or potentially unsafe living situations. Nurses who are working with individual clients and those who are assigned a caseload of groups of older adults in community settings, such as apartment complexes and assisted living centers, will assess the client's needs, available sources of support from the family, and formal sources of support that are affordable to the client in a total plan of care for the client. Local programs through the Division of Aging or Aging Services or comparable agency may leverage available state or federal funds in innovative programs to reduce rental costs to assist elderly clients so they can remain in the community.

Local or church affiliated agencies that recruit and train volunteer visitors and caregivers to the elderly may be utilized in conjunction with the aging agency programs to enable the fragile older adult to function at home with formal sources of support. These organized sources of support that may include a weekly visitor or a person to do chores for the elderly client may supplement the care and support that family members may provide. Nearly all older adults indicate their preferences for remaining in the community and in their homes rather than institutional care (Kendig & Yan, 1993). The desire to be independent is a cultural value that is highly regarded by many older adults who proudly proclaim how they have supported and cared for themselves for years. For the majority of older American adults, the long-held value to be independent is so strong that the person would rather live alone even in poor health than be a burden to one's family.

Options for Community Residence

Older individuals who are independent or self-sufficient in the above-mentioned areas are most likely candidates for what are termed Continuing Care Retirement

Communities. These are common residential locations that offer the older adult a comfortable apartment, a range of levels of assistance with ADLs, meals, social activities, and supervised exercise programs. Some residential communities have the capacity to ease the transition of the older client to a higher level of care that may include the administration of medications or treatments by a licensed nurse. There are some residential communities that have an attached facility or an arrangement with a facility in close proximity for the skilled nursing care of the older client. Many of these communities have provisions to move the older client through the levels of care with accommodation to move the client to higher and lower levels of care based on the older client's needs, which may change over time. Factors that could cause changes in the older client's condition that would warrant transfers from one level of care to another would include acute exacerbations of chronic illness, new illness episodes, surgical care, declines in functional abilities associated with falls or accidents.

These continuing care retirement communities offer many older adults the security of responsible adults to summon health care assistance if needed, the opportunity to interact with peers, and the option to remain in a community setting with an increased likelihood of participating in community resources, including cultural events, shopping trips, or entertainment provided by younger adults or school children. But, some older adults would feel stigmatized by residence in such a facility and would prefer to live in an independent location in the community. Other perspective residents might prefer the stimulation of intergenerational contact outside of an age-related residence and would prefer living on their own with other means of informal and formal support.

The challenge that the majority of older individuals will face is the high cost of paying for levels of care in residential communities or in skilled nursing facilities. Many older clients and their families assume that Medicare will be the means for paying for such care. However, Medicare is limited to reimbursement for post-hospital acute nursing facility stays and does not cover what is termed custodial or maintenance care of the older client. Older individuals and their families may exhaust their personal resources to cover extended care needs and custodial care. Nurses working in ambulatory care are finding many new work experiences in caring for older adult clients for short term post-hospital care or for assessment of clients who need extended care.

Options for Formal Support for Community-Based Care

One study estimated that millions of hours are provided weekly to older family members by children and other relatives (Liu, Manton, & Liu, 1985). In the last decade, there has been an increase in the development of day programs in communities that provide nursing assessment, physical or occupational therapy, group socialization, and nutrition to older adults. These programs may supplement the affective support and tangible assistance that families give, and the programs provide settings that affirm the older clients' dignity. The range of these services provided at each site varies according to the support of the local community including volunteers and professional staff. Some sites provide group socialization and nutrition for a lunch time meal. The older adults may be transported to the sites by public or private transportation. Older adults attending that type of nutrition program are usually independently ambulatory and are oriented.

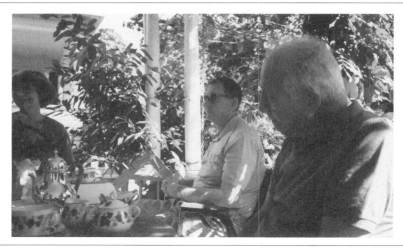

Opportunities to recall and share life experiences affirm the older client's identity and self-esteem. (Elderwise, Seattle, Washington.)

Other locales may offer more comprehensive programs. One of the longestrunning and most established type of programs is the On Lok adult day care program that pioneered in Chinatown in San Francisco. It is very unique in providing a multi-disciplinary team to provide comprehensive services to the very frail elderly who would be at risk of nursing home placement. The participants who are transported from their homes to centers may receive occupational and physical therapy as part of coordinated services in a treatment plan that is monitored and evaluated for participant progress. Other programs have adapted dimensions of the On Lok service delivery model for different locations. The On Lok program has been successful in that it operates under a Medicaid waiver and receives a higher per capita Medicaid payment for serving high-risk clients.

The options are expanding for the older client to continue to reside in the community and to participate in an adult day program. One such program is Elderwise, which offers older adults the opportunities to share experiences, to talk, and to be heard by others in a nurturing environment. Activities at Elderwise include artwork in watercolors and clay, exercise, lunch, and discussion topics. Discussion of current events, history, and psychological issues stimulate the older participants to reflect and to learn with each other. As older adults review events in their personal histories, they are validated as the authorities on their lives, their needs, and their abilities. Program participants receive affirmational support from their peers that reinforces their self-esteem and dignity.

Elderwise is a local program in Seattle, Washington, and is an example of a senior enrichment program. Nurses may want to assess the availability of a program similar to Elderwise in local settings and encourage attendance at such a program for older adult clients. Some colleges provide programs for older adult residents to audit courses or to attend short-term courses during the summer. Many community centers provide pottery classes, art classes, exercise groups, water exercise classes, or dance classes for the older adults. These center-based programs and similar church-affiliated older adult programs often include day trips or special holiday-focused celebrations.

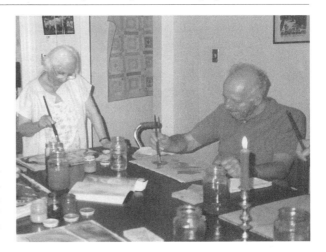

Creative expression through painting stimulates discussion among participants in an older adult enrichment program. (Elderwise, Seattle, Washington.)

Other programs are intergenerational and support older adults becoming involved within the community and the educational system. These types of program include the Older American Volunteer Program, the Retired Senior Volunteer Program, and the Foster Grandparents Program. The first intergenerational child care center began in 1976. These programs demonstrate that older volunteers are resources in the community, and the younger generation of children in child care settings and schools will benefit. The older participants also benefit. The evaluations that were conducted of multigenerational programs found that the older volunteers had a high level of life satisfaction including psychosocial adjustment and self-esteem. Rather than concluding that a high level of life satisfaction could be attributed to program participation, research showed that the volunteers may have previously had a high level of life satisfaction, which suggests that older volunteers are a self-selected group. They are activists who demonstrate the activity theory of aging and not the disengagement theory. Selected resources for multi-generational programs and for resources that might be of interest to practitioners working with older adult clients are included in Box 6-3.

Some nurses working in community settings will have more opportunities to be population based practitioners. In such a position with a local health department, the nurse may need to address and evaluate the cost effectiveness of day care programs, such as the On Lok program, that are options to the long-term care placement of the frail older client. An evaluation of the On Lok program indicated that day care services were between 5 and 40 percent lower than the cost of caring for the person with similar needs in a skilled nursing facility (Menagh, 1993). The results of cost-effectiveness studies of providing nursing care and support services at home for elderly clients who would otherwise be at risk for nursing facility placement indicate that community-based care is not necessarily less expensive than facility placement (Weissert & Hedrick, 1994). Advocates for community-based care, which often includes nurses, will argue that life satisfaction may be higher for clients and their family members.

The state of Washington implemented a demonstration project more than a decade ago to check the effectiveness of community-based services that would extend the residence of older adults in the community before skilled nursing facility placement

> **Box 6-3** *Resources for Multigenerational Programs and Other Resources of Interest for Nurses Working with Older Adult Clients*
>
> A Guide to Intergenerational Programs
> The National Association of State Units on Aging
> 600 Maryland Ave., S.W.
> West Wing, Suite 208
> Washington, DC 20024
> 202–898-2578
>
> The National Council on the Aging, Inc.
> 600 Maryland Ave., S.W.
> Washington, DC 20024
> 202–479-1200
>
> Web Sites
> **Senior Net (www.seniornet.org).** Book clubs and a forum on successful aging.
> **National Senior Citizens Law Center (www.nsclc.org).** Legal issues that affect the security and welfare of older persons of limited income.
> **SeniorLaw Home Page (www.seniorlaw.com).** Elder law, Medicare, Medicaid, rights of the elderly.

became necessary. Several individual successes occurred, and clients benefited from chore services and skilled nursing care that offered them more independence while remaining at home, but proving cost-effectiveness remained a challenge. Other states and regions have developed similar programs, and nurses will continue to be involved as caregivers and will also develop their roles in evaluating the effectiveness of these types of community-based programs. The importance of volunteers to provide meals, transportation, and social support to complement the provision of professional services is expected to continue. Nurses may function in the role as manager for home-based services that integrate volunteer services with professional assessment, intervention, and evaluation.

Evaluating Services to Improve Delivery of Care

The nurse manager who evaluates the use of services by older clients can assess the cultural appropriateness and acceptability of services. Clients may be reluctant to use services for various reasons that include internal barriers, contextual barriers, and service barriers. These barriers are summarized in Box 6-4.

To overcome the barriers that are perceived by older clients, nurses can assume several approaches to interact effectively with older adults from diverse groups. These approaches include

Be sensitive to the life experiences and the previous health care experiences of the older clients.

Listen attentively to the older client's experiences, complaints, and recollections.

Listen to related conversations to assess for underlying depression.

Box 6-4 *Barriers that Impede Service Delivery to the Older Adult Client*

Internal barriers

Lack of knowledge of perceived need for service
Lack of knowledge of existing services
Lack of knowledge needed to enroll in a service
Perception that one is not entitled to services
Desire to remain self-sufficient
Perception that providers are rude, address older clients in overly familiar terms, and interrupt the elderly

Contextual barriers

Space: lack of private space for most interactions that occur in clinical settings
Position: embarrassing position of the client in relation to the health care provider
Technology overload: presence of signs, contact with many personnel
Sensory overload: printed instructions, verbal messages, visual cues, video-tapes

Service barriers

Lack of access
Affordability of care
Availability of services

Elicit information about the older client's preferences for care, including diet and use of self-care remedies and include them when appropriate.
Identify available sources of informal sources of support and confirm availability.

Summary

A cultural approach to the older client recognizes that individuals are the products of, as well as the participants in, an encompassing societal framework. Within the societal framework, the cultural backgrounds of the older clients will influence their variations in their perceptions, behavior, and practices. Culture serves as a guide to the older client to determine what choices and actions are appropriate and acceptable. Within cultural groups contexts, individual variation is quite evident in response to the physiologic signs and the psychosocial demands of increasing age. The examples of older immigrant clients demonstrate that the clients views and perceptions may differ from those of family members and from the views of the nurse. The different attitudes, practices, and behaviors among older clients are the result of their heritage, experiences, education acculturation, and socioeconomic status. Nursing care is not acceptable if it is based on assumptions that members of cultural groups are all the same. Instead, nursing care must be based on the assessment of individual differences in the variables that influence responses to illness and help-seeking behavior. Nurses who are providing care in acute care settings or in the community often ask several questions as part of the nursing assessment:

1. Is the older adult isolated from culturally relevant supportive people, or is the older client enmeshed in a caring network of relatives and friends?
2. Has a culturally appropriate network replaced family members in performing some tasks for the older adult client?
3. Does the older adult expect family members to provide care, including nurturance and emotional support, that the family members are unable to provide?
4. Does language create a barrier in the older client's receipt of services from formal resources?

Older adult clients have often developed their own systems including informal supports for coping with illness and with changes associated with age. Nurses who are working with older clients in a variety of settings will want to assess who provides affirmation, affective, or tangible support that maintains the older client in an optimal level of functioning. Formal resources may be used to sustain the informal support systems to promote the lifestyle preferred by the older client. It is increasingly important for nurses to recognize the expanded roles that the older client may have in their family as a caretaker of young grandchildren or another family member. Nurses caring for older adult clients should give attention to the client's family and social roles and develop care plans that maintain and restore the individual to his or her usual roles and patterns of activity. In the future, nurses will assess and work with more older clients as they progress along a continuum of services and through more than one type of residence in the community. By assessing the client's cultural background and available support resources, nurses will plan appropriate care that will help older clients to optimize their self-esteem and dignity based on the client's functional abilities, affective support, and affirmational support.

Review Questions

1. What constraints and factors should be assessed and considered by the nurse who has been assigned to develop a care plan for a recently discharged 80-year-old chronically ill man who is living in a downtown hotel?
2. As the nurse who does health assessments for frail older adults who attend a community comprehensive day program, what are the types of information used to assess to determine the cultural appropriateness of the elderly Filipino and Chinese-American clients' care plans?
3. The short-term subacute unit where you are the nurse manager serves a multi-national group of older clients who are admitted for orthopedic surgery, what cultural assessments do you teach the staff to use in identifying the needs of clients and their families?

Learning Activities to Promote Critical Thinking

1. Many local communities offer exercise classes or an occupational health/physical activity session for community-based older adults. Many programs are day programs for older adults with some degree of impaired mobility

or chronic health care problems. Request permission and plan to attend an activity as an observer and attentive listener. Through observation and if possible, conversation with a participant, try to assess the levels of self-care that session participants possess and identify the types of assistance that these clients require to remain in the community.

2. As a case manager for a managed care organization, you receive many requests for authorization for in-home nursing services for older adults who have been discharged home following hospitalization for acute illnesses or surgical treatment. List the factors that you will consider and the types of data that you would want to make an informed decision about the nursing and health-related services and the duration of services that the older client should receive while at home.

3. Continuity of care is a challenge for nurses for the older client who may move from home to hospital to extended care facility and return to home. As a community nurse who is assigned to the population of older adults in a low-income housing complex, your clients are often in different stages of these transitions. You are asked by the housing agency and your health agency employer to develop plans to maintain the optimal levels of self-sufficiency for your clients. Consider their needs for safety, their preferences for independence, and any sources of community support that are available.

4. Some health care sites and skilled nursing facilities have developed intergenerational care centers that provide extended care for the older client and daily child care for a limited number of children. Identify if your community offers such a program, and request permission to observe the interaction for a portion of a day. What can you infer from this observation about the needs of the older client for love and belongingness, self-actualization?

5. Critical thinking: With your awareness that cultural traditions and life experiences influence many older adults to prefer independent living, what arguments would you develop as a home health care nurse to support extended government funding of home health services for older adults?

References

Angel, J. L., & Angel, R. J. (1992). Age at migration, social connections, and well-being among elderly Hispanics. *Journal of Aging and Health, 4,* 480–99.

Angel, J. L., DeLong, G. F., Cornwell, G. T., & Wilmoth, J. M. (1995). Diminished health and living arrangement of rural elderly Americans. *National Journal of Sociology, 9*(1), 31–57.

Angel, R. J., & Angel, J. L. (1997). *Who will Care for Us? Aging and Long-Term Care in Multicultural America.* New York: University Press.

Atchley, R. C. (1989). A continuity theory of normal aging. *The Gerontologist, 29,* 183–189.

Bould, S., Sanborn, B., & Reif, L. (1989). *Eighty-five Plus: The Oldest Old.* Belmont, CA: Wadsworth.

Brandriet, L. M. (1994). Gerontological nursing: Application of ethnography and grounded theory. *Journal of Gerontological Nursing, 20*(7), 33–40.

Brod, M. & Heurtin-Roberts, S. (1992). Older Russian emigres and medical care. *Western Journal of Medicine, 157*(3), 333–337.

Chatters, L. M. (1993). Health disability and its consequences for subjective stress. In J. S. Jackson, L. M. Taylor, & R. J. Taylor (Eds.). *Aging in Black America* (pp. 51–77). Newbury Park, CA: Sage Publications.

Crawford, G. (1987). Support Networks and health related changes in the elderly: Theory based nursing strategies. *Family & Community Health, 10*(2), 30–48.

Cutillo-Schmitter, T. A. (1996). Aging: Broadening our view for improved nursing care. *Journal of Gerontological Nursing, 22*(7), 31–42.

Day, J. C. (1993). *Population Projections of the United States, by Age, Sex, Race and Hispanic Origin: 1993–2050.* U.S. Bureau of the Census Population Reports, p. 25–1104. Washington, D.C. U.S. Government Printing Office.

Giarchi, G. C. (1996). *Caring for Older Europeans: Comparative Studies in 29 Countries.* Honts, England: Ashgate Publishing Limited.

Gibson, R. C., & Jackson, J. S. (1987). The health, physical functioning, and informal supports of the Black elderly. *The Milbank Quarterly, 65*(2), 421–454.

Havighurst, R. (1968). Disengagement and patterns of aging. In B. Neugarten (Ed.) *Middle Age and Aging. Chicago*: University of Chicago Press.

Johnson, C. L., & Barer, B. M. (1990). Families and networks among older inner-city Blacks. *Gerontologist, 30,* 726–733.

Kaplan, B. H., Cassel, J. C., & Gore, S. (1977). Social support and health. *Medical Care, 15*(5), 47–57.

Katzung, B. (1992). *Basic and clinical pharmacology.* Norwalk, CT: Appleton & Lange.

Lewis, S., Messner, R., & McDowell, W. A. (1985). An unchanging culture. *Journal of Gerontological Nursing, 11*(8), 21–26.

Mansour, A., & Laing, G. (1994). Research Concerns Aging as Perceived by Saudi Elders. *Journal of Gerontological Nursing, 20*(6), 11–16.

Markides, K. S. (1992). *A Longitudinal Study of Mexican American Elderly Health.* Washington, D.C. National Institute on Aging.

Martin, J. C., & Panicucci, C. L. (1996). Health Related Practices and Priorities: The Health Behaviors and Beliefs of Community-Living Black Older Women. *Journal of Gerontological Nursing, 22*(4), 41–48.

Menagh, M. (1993). Heroes of Health Care. *Omni, 15,* 34–41.

Moen, P. Dempster-McClain, D., & Williams, R. (1995). Pathways to women's well being in later adulthood. A life course perspective. Unpublished manuscript. Available from Cornell University. In Cutillo-Schmitter, T. A. (1996). Aging: Broadening Our View for Improved Nursing Care. *Journal of Gerontological Nursing, 22*(7), 31–42.

Moon, M. (1993). *Medicare Now and in the Future.* Washington, D.C. Urban Institute.

O'Hara, E. M., & Zhan, L. (1994). Cultural and pharmacologic considerations when caring for Chinese elders. *Journal of Gerontological Nursing, 20*(10), 11–16.

Osako, M. (1979). Aging and family among japanese americans: The role of ethnic tradition in the adjustment to old age. *The Gerontologist, 19*(5), 448–455.

Rice, D. P., & LaPlante, M. P. (1988). Chronic illness, disability, and increasing longevity. In S. Sullivan and M. E. Lewin (Eds.). *The Economics of Long Tern Care and Disability* (pp. 9–55). Washington: American Enterprise Institute for Public Policy Research.

Ringsven, M. K., & Bond, D. (1997). *Gerontology and Leadership Skills for Nurses* (2nd Ed.) Albany: Delmar Publishers.

Rosenbaum, J. (1990). Cultural care of older greek canadian widows within Leininger's theory of culture care. *Journal of Transcultural Nursing, 2*(1), 37–47.

Ryan, M. C., & Austin, A. G. (1989). Social support and social networks in the aged. *Image Journal of Nursing Scholarship, 21,* 176–180.

Schiavenato, M. (1997). The Hispanic elderly: Implications for nursing care, *Journal of Gerontological Nursing, 23* (6), 10–15.

Schoenberg, N. E. (1997). A convergence of health beliefs: An "ethnography of adherence" of African-American rural elders with hypertension. *Human Organization, 56*(2), 174–181.

Scribner, R. (1996). Editorial: Paradox as paradigm—The health outcomes of Mexican Americans. *American Journal of Public Health, 86*(3), 303–305.

Sutherland, D., & Murphy, E. (1995). Social support among elderly in two community programs. *Journal of Gerontological Nursing, 21*(2), 31–38.

Tran, T. V. (1991). Family living arrangement and social adjustment among three ethnic groups of elderly Indochinese refugees. *International Journal of Aging and Human Development, 32*(2), 91–102.

Verbrugge, L. M. (1989). Recent, present, and future health of American adults. In J. E. Breslow and J. E. Fielding (Eds.). In *Annual Review of Public Health* (pp. 333–362.). Palo Alto, California: Annual Review.

Walls, C. T., & Zarit, S. H. (1991). Informal support from black churches and the well-being of elderly blacks. *Gerontologist, 31,* 490–95.

Weissert, W. G., & Hedrick, S. C. (1994). Lessons learned from research on effects of community based long term care," *Journal of the American Geriatrics Society, 42,* 348–53.

White-Means, S. I., & Thornton, M. C. (1990). Ethnic Differences in the production of informal health care. *Gerontologist, 30,* 758–768.

Wilson, S., & Billones, H. (1994). The Filipino elder: Implications for nursing practice. *Journal of Gerontological Nursing, 20*(8), 31–36.

Wray, L. A. (1992). Health policy and ethnic diversity in older Americans. Dissonance or harmony? *Western Journal of Medicine,* Special Edition, 157, 357–361.

Three

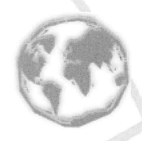

Applications of Transcultural Concepts in Nursing Care Delivery

Chapter 7

Transcultural Perspectives in Mental Health

Kathryn Hopkins Kavanagh

KEY TERMS

Acculturation	Diversity	"Isms"
Affiliation Group	Diversity Management	Language of Distress
Cultural Competence	Explanatory Models	Somatization
Culture-Bound Syndromes	Illness versus Disease	Stereotypes

OBJECTIVES

1. Provide a sense of mental health and mental illness as varying with culture, time, and place.
2. Relate issues related to mental health and mental illness as fully integrated into other aspects of living, health, and health care.
3. Realize the wide variability in expression of symptoms, interpretations, explanations, and expectations associated with phenomena related to mental health and mental illness.
4. Emphasize the potential that interactive processes and communication have for facilitating effective transcultural mental health care.
5. Suggest and use strategies to facilitate effective transcultural mental health care.

There was a time when mental illness did not exist in western society. People had problems and some were psychotic, but whether tolerated, pitied, shunned, or punished, and whether they lived out their years or died, the "mad" were more likely to be viewed as fools, or possessed, than ill. With the social conscience of the 18th century, the mentally ill were given refuge in asylums, where, isolated and in large part gratefully forgotten by society, they received little more than shelter (Conrad & Schneider, 1992).

Today's mentally ill are, for the most part, in the community, which encourages an emphasis on primary and preventive care (Matteson, 1995; Oakley & Potter, 1997), as well as on crisis intervention and care management that is specific to client needs. Most mentally ill individuals are not psychotic, although of course some are. Overall, however, other problems are far more numerous in today's society, such as severe stress, violence, anxiety, anger, mood disturbances (for example, depression, suicidal thoughts, or intense and prolonged grieving), confusion (related to aging, drug use, or other issues), and substance abuse. People often have problems relating to others, sex, food, pain, chronic illness, and physical health problems. Spiritual distress also comes under the rubric of mental health.

Given the interrelatedness of mental health phenomena in everyday life and with physical illness, it is not surprising that most mentally distressed and ill people are encountered in health care settings, both in-patient and out-patient, that are not labeled "psychiatry" or "mental health" (Gorman, Sultan, & Raines, 1996). Wherever they occur, today nearly all services that support mental health are short term (Marmor, 1994). Meanwhile, the mentally ill often confront severe social and economic strains, while mental health needs and care resources are in flux (Billings, 1993; Marmor, 1994; Gorman, Sultan, & Raines, 1996; Oakley & Potter, 1997).

The U.S. population also continuously changes. The "browning of America" refers to projections that by the middle of the 21st century the average resident (as defined by Census Bureau statistics) will trace his or her ancestry to Africa, Asia, the Pacific Islands, or the Hispanic or Arab worlds, rather than to European roots (Henry, 1990). By 2050, one out of every five Americans will be Hispanic (U.S. Census Bureau as cited by United States Department of Health and Human Services, 1991). Each person learns from those around him one or more languages; ethical, religious or other guidelines for living; and other meaningful and systematic ways of relating to the world that compose their cultural orientation. Culture is, therefore, learned, transmitted, shared, integrated, both ideal and real, and constantly changing (Campinha-Bacote, 1997). Often ethnicity is the basis of such an orientation. However, human diversity is not limited to culture or ethnicity. It exists everywhere that there are differences, which includes age, sex, experience, socioeconomic status, social view, gender preference, race and so on. It is important to keep in mind that transcultural nursing is limited to neither health care nor culture in the sense of ethnicity; it involves all human diversity.

While the U.S. may be the most diverse society that has ever existed and continues to include large refugee and immigrant populations (Lipson, 1996), the nation is moving away from stereotyped "one-size-fits-all" expectations of medical treatment and nursing care. New themes related to diversity in mental health care are developing, such as advocacy and empowerment (Rose & Black, 1985; Dunst, Trivette, & Deal, 1988), participatory decision making, diversity (Kavanagh & Kennedy, 1992), pluralism, multi-culturalism (Locke, 1992; Wali, 1992), and mind/body holism (Anderson, 1996). Both providers and clients are increasingly committed to recognition of rights of affiliative groups (that is, the groups with which people identify or to which they reference themselves), as well as involved in health care. This means that care is expected to meet the standards of the groups with which people are affiliated. Culturally competent nurses learn to use effectively cultural sensitivity, knowledge, and skills in cultural encounters (Campinha-Bacote, 1997).

This chapter discusses transcultural nursing as it relates specifically to psychiatric and mental health nursing. It presents a practical and flexible framework based on a balance of sensitivity, knowledge, and skills (Pedersen, 1988; Kavanagh & Kennedy, 1992). The approach used is premised on the value of respectful, open, mutual

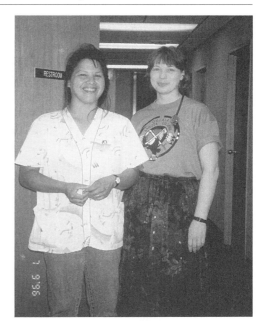

Transcultural nurses bring together sensitivity, knowledge, and skill to promote health and care for the ill in culturally congruent ways. Pictured are Evie Weston and Lucia Schliessmann, nurses working together at Porcupine Clinic on the Pine Ridge Reservation, South Dakota.

communication and collaborative relationships between nurses and clients. The medium for both collaborative treatment and diversity management is mutual communication. This approach portrays the client as someone more expert about his or her or their situation than the health care provider is, and from whom the nurse can learn to understand the situation as the client does. The culturally competent transcultural nurse has the ability to manage diversity effectively, when management of diversity is defined as helping each person to reach his or her full potential (Thomas, 1991).

A balance of cultural sensitivity, knowledge, and skills allows nurses to link awareness and sensitivity with knowledge of typical, expectable group patterns. Sensitivity and knowledge, in combination with cultural assessment, communication, and other mental health nursing skills, can produce respectful, culturally acceptable and effective nursing interventions for diverse peoples in specific, individual situations.

However, limiting attention to sensitivity leaves the sensitive nurse powerless, as he or she still lacks the knowledge and skills required to act knowingly on the issue. Knowledge of expectable cultural patterns provides starting places against which the reality of a given situation can be tested. Such knowledge differs from stereotypes, which lock out real evidence through acknowledgment of only that which was expected. Lack of sensitivity, knowledge, and skill may be involved when people are labeled "noncompliant," "problem patients," or too resistant or defensive to benefit from treatment or to recognize the value of the care being offered. Might it be that the client's ideas (and their expression) about care and caring simply differ from those of the nurse?

Mental Illness and Mental Disease

In many ways, health and illness are more central to transcultural psychiatric/mental health nursing than are mental diseases. Much of the counseling, therapy, and other care given by mental health professionals focuses on illness prevention and making everyday life better. The distinction between illness and disease is important. Illness emphasizes subjective behavioral, psychological, sociocultural, and experiential dimensions of disorders. Disease, in contrast, pertains to chemical, physiologic, and other organic and objective phenomena related to sickness (Helman, 1990; Tseng, 1997). Biologic disorders of memory, perception and feeling surely exist, as do compensatory processes of rationalization and action that are strongly influenced by social and cultural factors (Kiev, 1972; Tseng & Streltzer, 1997). Rates of mental illness and of mental diseases do not seem to vary much among groups when social and economic factors are controlled. There is no conclusive evidence that mental illness rates vary with race or other intrinsic human characteristics, although they are clearly associated with low socioeconomic status, low educational level, separation, and loss.

Four-fifths of the global population lives in non-Western countries, while most psychiatric resources are in western societies. The schizophrenias, manic-depressive disorders, major depressions, and anxiety disorders are thought to occur throughout the world. Depression anxieties and somatiform disorders (that is, the expressions of problems in physical rather than psychologic signs and symptoms) are probably more prevalent in the non-Western world than are infectious diseases (Kleinman, 1991). However, despite international epidemiological and research efforts, there are at present no international centers focused on mental health treatment programs comparable to, for example, the World Health Organization. The global emphasis has been on physical health (Kleinman, 1991), although somatic disorders are interwoven with both culture and mental illness (Chaplin, 1997).

Every society has systems of beliefs and practices related to health care, and specific persons trained as healers. There are many places where biomedicine is not widely available and most people depend on traditional healers, although they also exist (and are depended on) in modern westernized societies. Whereas shamans and traditional healers are often not very effective in treating chronic mental disorders, the outcome for some conditions tends to be more positive in those societies where clients are not negatively stigmatized and are not alone with their problems. Where persons with mental illness are devalued, they are more likely to be demoralized and isolated, to feel dehumanized, and to curtail the development of potential support systems (Beiser, Waxler-Morrison, Iacono, Lin, Fleming, & Husted, 1987; Lipson & Steiger, 1996). American individualism and self-reliance further reinforce a tendency toward social isolation and alienation. Additionally, many individuals cross cultures, which requires special psychosocial resilience and adaptation (Kim & Gudykunst, 1988; McCubbin & McCubbin, 1988; Ory, Simons, Verhulst, Leenders, and Wolters, 1991; Tseng & Streltzer, 1997).

There is probably more variation among etiological beliefs of mental health care professionals than is commonly acknowledged, but belief in relatively impersonal, environmental, and natural causation generally prevails. For a variety of reasons or simply by chance, parts, systems, families, or individuals take on characteristics that are assessed as dysfunctional. In contrast, members of many cultural groups believe illness is caused by a supernatural being (a deity or god), a nonhuman being (such as an ancestor, a ghost, or an evil spirit), or another human being (a witch or sorcerer) (Foster & Anderson, 1978). The sick person in such a case is viewed as a victim who is not responsible for his or her condition or its resolution. Some peoples have no concept of accident or spontaneous internal disease processes, so every phenomenon is accounted for as the result of intent by an outside force.

Diagnosis: Problems with Normality and Abnormality

The division of illnesses into physical and mental categories is Western, although every society labels some behaviors as abnormal. The cultural assumption that mind and body are somehow separate, which is now increasingly challenged in terms of relationships between healing and the mind (Moyers, 1993; Goleman & Gurin, 1993), has for several centuries strongly swayed Western ideas about normality and abnormality. What is considered "normal" and what is "abnormal" is always based on cultural perspective. Culture influences (that is, it shapes but does not determine) expression, presentation, recognition, labeling, explanations for, and distributions of mental illnesses. See Research Application 7-1.

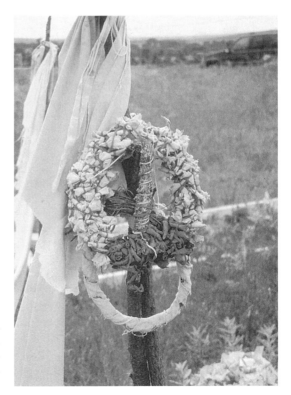

Cultural groups honor life stages in diverse ways. Here tobacco ties and sage, circular in form to reflect unity, mark a traditional Lakota grave.

Interpretations of health and of even overt signs of physical disease vary widely. Mental health and mental illnesses are more difficult than physical disorders to delineate because of the lack of readily observable, discrete, and organic phenomena. The symptoms of mental illness, dependent as they are on behavioral expression, vary because they depend on social definitions rather than physical measures. Assessment is based on the appropriateness of behaviors (for example, dress, posture, smell, gestures, speech, and facial expression) that lack fixed standards and depend upon context and social relationships to differentiate what is considered normal from what is viewed as abnormal. Although psychiatry is part of western biomedicine, it deals with ambiguous areas such as self and symbolic behavior, deviance and marginality, power and control (Fabrega, 1989).

Diagnoses involve social competence, which, to be sensitively evaluated, must be assessed against culture-specific criteria. Many cultures do not dichotomize normality and abnormality as rigidly as western societies often tend to, or even distinguish health from illness. These may be viewed as multidimensional, continual, and perhaps overlapping (Helman, 1990), with ideas about mental health and mental illness mixed with those about health and medicine in general. To members of such societies, concepts such as mental health have little meaning. The distinction between illness and health may be based on ability to perform one's normal roles in society. A physician's diagnosis, prognosis and treatment, based on imprecise and unobservable phenomena, may seem ludicrous.

| Research Application 7-1 | *Mental Health Issues Among Vietnam Amerasians* |

Nuguyen, M. N., & Organista, K. C. (1997). **Vietnam Amerasians: Assimilation and adjustment problems in the United States.** *Journal of Multicultural Social Work* 6 (1/2), 77–91.

Although the Vietnam War ended in 1975, its legacy remains a factor in the lives of the offspring of American fathers and Vietnamese mothers. Currently, more than 21,000 Vietnam Amerasians and 50,000 of their accompanying family members reside in the United States. Research indicates that Amerasians from Vietnam tend to experience more psychological distress and mental health risk factors during resettlement than members of other refugee and immigrant groups. Although a variety of experiences both before and after migration strongly affect their current mental health, one of the most important predictors of adjustment is the fit between premigration expectations of life in the United States and the post-migration reality. A discrepancy between those often leads to higher rates of anxiety and depression.

Clinical Application

- Be sensitive and attuned to symptoms of psychological distress and mental health risk when providing care to Vietnam Amerasians who are resettling in the United States.

- Explore family and community support systems available to Vietnam Amerasians who seek health care services. Be cognizant of community resources and services for referral purposes.

- Gently ask the Vietnam Amerasian refugee to describe his or her premigration expectations of life in the United States and to contrast that view with the reality they encountered when they migrated to this country. Based on the discrepancies described, the nurse will be able to understand how well the person has adjusted to life in the United States.

- Identify resources such as Vietnamese-speaking mental health professionals in your community or state. If these resources are not available locally in your community, are they available via telehealth/telemedicine sites?

- Be knowledgeable about how symptoms are expressed and how they are perceived and treated by others in this cultural group.

- Somatization likely occurs in this cultural group. Headaches, backaches, and stomach aches may reflect depression rather than an underlying physiologic cause. Although physiologic symptoms warrant careful examination, they may be a sign that the client needs a careful mental and emotional health evaluation.

- Support family relationships, and encourage clients to engage in cultural practices that provide a connection to their Vietnamese cultural traditions.

The pattern used by a client to express concern or disorder is referred to as a language of distress (Helman, 1990). Close examination of how people express themselves and interact is essential in understanding relationships between psychiatric and social factors. The same phenomena (for example, visions and dream states, trance states, hallucinations, delusions, belief in spirits, speaking in "tongues," drug or alcohol intoxication, or suicide) may be judged normal or abnormal according to the settings and circumstances in which they occur (Conrad & Schneider, 1992). At times cultural groups encourage altered states of consciousness that may be viewed as mental disturbances to others. However, because addictive substances (such as alcohol, tobacco, and opiates) in most societies were traditionally reserved for use during special times or rituals, widespread related health problems seldom occurred. Today, on the other hand, Western redefinition of deviant alcohol and drug use as disease (rather than as a social, moral, or legal issue [Conrad & Schneider, 1992]) has made this a primary mental health concern.

How symptoms are expressed and how they are perceived and treated by others varies widely. Although psychotic disorders occur in every society and the primary symptoms (that is, social and emotional withdrawal, auditory hallucinations, general delusions, flat affect, mood changes, and insomnia) occur across cultures, the secondary features of these disorders are highly influenced by culture (Tripp-Reimer, 1984; Tseng & Streltzer, 1997). For example, in some groups, guilt and suicidal ideation do not accompany depression; in others they frequently do (Harrison, 1997). In some societies, suicide is an acceptable escape from problems ranging from marital dissension, illness, sorcery, loneliness, and hopelessness to criticism from others.

Analogously, in some groups, somatic (physical) rather than psychological symptoms are prominent among depressed individuals; in others, such as middle class European Americans, psychological "blues" prevail. Somatization pertains to a preoccupation with physical symptoms that are thought to have a psychological rather than physical cause (Chaplin, 1997). Somatic symptoms that express psychological distress occur at high rates, for example, among clients who are Hispanic (Escobar, 1987) or Chinese (Kleinman, 1988). It is not unusual for nurses to encounter clients who deny being depressed but complain of headaches, backaches, stomach aches and other physical phenomena prompted by (and sometimes consciously associated with) sorrow and suffering.

The content of delusions and hallucinations also reflects cultural patterns. For instance, the content may be primarily psychological, religious or spiritual, moral or social, naturalistic or supernatural, or physical or medical. In Western Ireland, psychiatric patients tend to have delusions of a religious nature (Scheper-Hughes, 1978), while American schizophrenics more often have persecution delusions involving electromagnetic or other secular phenomena (Oltmanns & Maher, 1988; Helman, 1990), believing perhaps that their toasters talk to them or current from electrical outlets is altering their thinking. Likewise, some groups may associate sex with guilt, while others do not (Sanday & Goodenough, 1990; Bohannan, 1992). For example, middle class European American criticism of sex and pregnancy outside of marriage among African Americans does not take into account the social history that made many black women vulnerable to unwanted sexual activity and that, over time, helped many to redefine extramarital sex and pregnancy as events apart from moral apprehension.

Some conditions, such as post-traumatic stress disorder, can occur in various forms anywhere. Others, known as culture bound syndromes, exist within specific cultural groups. Some conditions may represent labeling differences, as in China where the term neurasthenia is widely used for symptoms produced by social stressors and may correspond to what Western medicine refers to as depression. Some conditions fall into categories of folk illnesses that defy western psychiatric identification, although they are very real to the persons experiencing them. Examples of folk illnesses include fright or soul loss (susto), which is often associated by Hispanics with a sudden start or sneeze (Foster & Anderson, 1978). Various conditions thought to result from the evil eye (mal ojo) are believed to occur unintentionally when, for instance, a nurse fails to touch a child he or she has noticed or examined. Herbal remedies, rubbing, massage, and other physical manipulations by curanderos (curanderas, if they are women) are typical treatments. These might be used with home remedies (such as teas) or prayers and trips to religious shrines or charismatic folk healers to alleviate distress. See Research Application 7-2.

Research Application 7-2

Race and the History of Race Continue to Influence Relationships Today

Vontress, C. E., & Epp, L. R. (1997). Historical hostility in the African American client: Implications for counseling. *Journal of Multicultural Counseling and Development, 25*, 170–184.

Centuries of slavery, discrimination, and fear of unequal treatment by members of the dominant culture result in a collective psychology that requires special sensitivity, knowledge, and skills. Known as "historical hostility," this phenomenon may be expressed as hostility, hopelessness, and a paranoid perception of discrimination in cross-racial encounters with health care providers. Members of African American and other groups may manifest such a response pattern, particularly if they are from cultures that were formerly oppressed by colonization.

Managing historical hostility starts with recognition that a client is both a unique individual and a member of a historically oppressed group. Although everyone deserves equal opportunities for culturally congruent care, care must also be specific to patterns of reaction and outlooks on reality. In psychiatry, as in the rest of health care, "One size does *not* fit all!" It is important to remember that there is a wide variation within any group. The effective transcultural psychiatric nurse realizes that the defensiveness known as historical hostility may or may not be manifest by clients. If it is anticipated, it can be recognized and managed. However, if it is expected, the nurse may project defensiveness that generates client resistance.

Clinical Application

• Accept and work with the fact that some African American clients will be hostile toward white, middle-class health care professionals.

• Recognize that although the client is a unique person with special attributes, he or she may also have patterns of reaction and outlooks that reflect a historical oppression. If hostility is recognized, it can be recognized and managed in the milieu of the therapeutic relationship.

• Mental health professionals must be accepting and sensitive to cultural variations in their clients, and willing to explore clients' perceptions of "white" culture.

• Cultural influences on stress and coping constitute important information for dealing with mental health problems, and these cultural influences should be understood by the culturally competent nurse.

The U.S. has numerous folk illnesses, such as "nervous breakdown," that occur throughout the society. There are also culture-bound syndromes. Anorexia nervosa, for example, occurs only where food is abundant, although in various forms. Other culture-bound syndromes are seen more often in traditional, nonindustrialized societies and in immigrants from those. Despite the exotic nature of many of the classic culture-bound syndromes, it is useful to know of the existence of these ethnic or "reactive psychoses" (Yap, 1977). Several culture bound syndromes are described in Box 7-1.

Misdiagnosis (for example, with overdiagnosis of antisocial disorders and psychoses and underdiagnosis of depressions [Brown, 1990]) is a major problem among members of groups that differ from the European American, middle class, Christian, and male orientation that dominates American culture (Pinderhughes, 1982; Collins, Sorel, Brent, & Mathura, 1990; Secundy, 1992). An example of a commonly misdiagnosed folk illness is falling out, a stress-relieving pattern of shaking and falling that typically occurs when sympathetic others are present; it is seen among African Americans, Haitians, whites, and other southern ethnic groups (Weidman, 1979; Gaines, 1992). Adding to the complexity of psychiatric diagnosis is the fact that, despite the influence of culture in patterned psychological and physical conditions, there are also individual or idiosyncratic explanations and expressions of behavior.

There is a new cultural and cross-cultural psychiatry (Kleinman, 1988; Tseng & Streltzer, 1997) that extends the thinking of many psychiatrists to allow for culturally based explanations of client behavior. However, at the same time, the widely used series of *Diagnostic and Statistical Manuals of Mental Disorders* (American Psychiatric Association, 1994), the "DSM- IV" and its previous versions, requires surrender of many cultural insights (Conrad & Schneider, 1992; Eisenbruch, 1992). Works such as the DSM-IV organize symbolic and instrumental evidence of those forms of deviance that are considered medical concerns (Conrad & Schneider, 1992) and provide the medical community with administratively useful classifications for diagnosis and record keeping.

However, despite varying cultural expressions of psychiatric problems, in less affluent countries than the U.S. where library funds are particularly limited, the *Diagnostic and Statistical Manuals of Mental Disorders* standards tend to be used as the ultimate text on psychiatric diagnoses and categories (Littlewood, 1991; Eisenbruch,

Box 7-1. *Culture-Bound Syndromes and Variants*

Amok: an acute reaction resulting from hostility (Yap, 1977) and dissociative amnesia (Castillo, 1997). Our term "running amok" comes from the frenzied lashing out associated with this syndrome.

Anorexia nervosa: an eating disorder associated in Western societies, but not in Eastern cultures, with fear of obesity (Gorman, Sultan, & Raines, 1996; Tseng & Streltzer, 1997).

Homophobia: an anxiety-related syndrome based on fear of homosexuals (Ficarrotto, 1990; Bernstein, 1997).

Malignant anxiety: acute anxiety states with panic and varying degrees of ego disorganization (Yap, 1977) that have been associated with criminality and loss of stable culture due to colonialism or other extreme societal disruption.

Pibloktoq: "arctic hysteria" among Polar Eskimos. Accounts are of bizarre, dramatized behavior, such as running naked through the snow (Parker, 1977).

Susto: a traumatic, anxiety-depressive state with psychophysiologic changes; "fright sickness" that results from such stimuli as a fall, a thunderclap, meeting some threat, or other frightening experiences. Susto causes anxiety, insomnia, listlessness, loss of appetite, and social withdrawal. This folk illness occurs throughout Latin America (Rubel, 1977; Uzzell, 1977).

Trance dissociation: possession syndromes occurring in various parts of the world with varying degrees of social sanction (Yap, 1977). This differs from primary schizophrenic reactions and is believed to be caused by disease, the loss of one's soul, or the invasion of a benign or evil spirit. In some circumstances it is viewed as a mystical state. Some American Indian vision quests resulted in altered states of consciousness similar to this.

Voodoo death: "magical" or sociocultural death that has been explained as a result of "flight or fight" response, belief in the power of threat and suggestion, and the acceptance of hopelessness (Lex, 1977).

1992). This seems contradictory to the evidence that, although medical involvement in madness has been recorded for at least 2000 years, those aspects of treatment and care that foster transcultural understanding emerge more as humanitarian reform than biomedical accomplishment (Conrad & Schneider, 1992).

Mental Health Needs, Beliefs, and Practices

Realizing that perspectives are shaped by specific values and beliefs rooted in specific cultures and subcultures allows objective assessment of diverse practices that people employ to promote health and cope with illness. Whether or not they are understood, people have reasons for their behavior. They may, for example, refuse to have blood drawn owing to a belief that it could be used for sorcery or, as was traditionally believed in Asian societies, that blood contains the personality. It does not make sense to risk personality loss with blood (or other organ) donation or confusion with some else's. On the other hand, it does make sense for clients to alter their medication dosages when they believe that the "large" American physicians who prescribe medicines are likely to order too large a dose for someone of smaller stature (Goode, 1993). Appreciating that what is to one individual a "superstition" may be to someone else a firmly held explanation or belief allows the culturally competent nurse to objectively consider the behavior associated with that belief for its own merit, neutrality, or harm. Automatic discrediting of ideas or practices because they are unfamiliar, "old fashioned," or not scientific risks alienation of clients, as well as loss of potentially useful resources. See Research Application 7-3.

Mental health care is not the same for everyone. Parenting is only one of myriad areas of concern to transcultural nurses, but it provides a useful example of the diversity inherent in fulfilling a universal need. Understanding parenting patterns requires discerning parents' ideas and expectations about their children, child rearing traditions, and knowledge and beliefs about human development (Steinhausen, Offer, Ostrov, & Howard, 1988), as well as assessment of the child and actual situation. Not everyone parents the same way; some, for example, may view "good parenting" as keeping a child safe, fed, and clean, but not including activities that stimulate cognitive, affective, and physical development. Parents, particularly those who are single, are more alone with childrearing responsibilities in industrialized societies than is the case in societies in which extended families are more common and socialization responsibilities are shared with other adults. Growth and development are additionally influenced by cultural patterns that encourage protecting children from some facts of life while exposing them very early to others. In the U.S. for example, children typically learn little about economically productive roles when they are young. However, although they may not observe their parents working, they are likely to be exposed at a tender age to adult sexual roles and to violence via the media.

Research Application 7-3	*There Are Many Views of the History of Psychiatric and Mental Health Care*

Russell, D. (1997). An oral history project in mental health nursing. *Journal of Advanced Nursing 26*, 489–495.

Oral histories have been collected as data for several books on the history of psychiatric and mental health nursing. Interviews of staff or former staff reveal opinions, attitudes, feelings, and practices of care. One wonders why the recollections of former patients are not collected as well as those of the staff. However, it is race and ethnicity that the author addresses, noting that "Differences of ethnic origin, surprisingly, do not seem to have been much discussed, in spite of the many different nationalities of nurses working at various times in the hospital" (p. 493). Russell speculates that the notable racial mix among both nurses and physicians may have facilitated tolerance and acceptance within the setting. Although that may be the case, other research has suggested that race, ethnicity, and gender issues may actually be avoided in psychiatric settings (Kavanagh, 1991). Culturally competent nurses realize that diversity-related issues can play important parts in communication, relationships, mental health, and mental illness. It is questionable, therefore, whether a care setting can truly be therapeutic if such issues are not openly and comfortably discussed.

Clinical Application

- Issues related to diversity, such as race, ethnicity, and gender must be identified, and health care professionals must make an effort to move beyond such issues. They can best do this by openly identifying the issues and discussing them with colleagues. Such a discussion calls for openness and sensitivity with other health care providers as well as clients.

Social and environmental conditions often lead to mental health problems. Substantial proportions of children and adolescents live in poverty, with severe mental health effects (Scheper-Hughes, 1987). Children and adolescents or every social class and ethnic background are vulnerable to sexual and physical abuse (Levinson, 1989). High rates of depression are associated with problems in areas of family and personal relationships, finances, and general living conditions. Crime, drug use, and suicide are prevalent problems that may be associated with limited perceived hope (Jackson, 1990; Poussaint, 1990; Harrison, 1997). Although disorganized and dysfunctional families are not specific to the poor, the poor often have higher mortality and morbidity rates (Levinson, 1989) and relatively few treatment resources. Painful separation, torture, loss, bereavement, uncertainty, and violence have made post-traumatic stress syndrome a popular diagnosis for persons of any age and any traumatic background (Eisenbruch, 1992; Schultz-Ross, 1997).

Demographic shifts have implications for mental health. Lower levels of fertility mean that future elders will have fewer adult children and kin as potential caregivers. Increased geographical mobility and separate living styles result in loose social networks and increased social alienation. Immigration can lead to conflict between traditional and modern roles (Takeshita, 1997). Similarly, increased divorce rates often disrupt the flow of personal support. Today many members of groups that were traditionally cohesive find themselves isolated from culturally relevant support persons (Bond & Harvey, 1991; Lipson & Steiger, 1996). Rapid increases in the populations of older adults have led to ethnogerontology, the study of relationships between culture and age and their impact on physical and mental well-being as contexts, roles, prestige, and social interaction patterns change (Myerhoff & Simic, 1978; Sokolovsky, 1985, 1990; Fry, 1990; Dewit, Wister, & Burch, 1988; Ahmed, 1997; Oakley & Potter, 1997).

The Challenge of Categories

Understanding social interactive processes that facilitate culturally competent communication and care, as well as those that perpetuate social distance and inequality, is important since those patterns strongly influence people's experiences. Everyone handles huge amounts of information every day. Categories must be used to organize related items so that information does not become totally overwhelming. The problem with these groupings is that they may be based on, or become, stereotypes.

Stereotypes are simple links in memory between a person and a particular trait (Brislin, 1993). They create broad categories that often capture characteristics that are real and common in the group (Rothenberg, 1988; Seelye, 1993). However, stereotypes may also be out of date and dangerously limited. People tend to see what they expect to see, and stereotypes narrow vision by ignoring variations that occur naturally within groups. If one stereotypes all psychiatric patients as dangerous, for example, the generalization does not accurately represent the high percentage of patients who are not. When seen through stereotypic lenses, various realities are oversimplified. Aspects of individuality get left out that may be important to understanding and to providing care.

There is an important difference between stereotypes and generalizations. Stereotypes are like images frozen in time and cause one to see what one expects to see, even when reality differs from that. Descriptive generalizations, in contrast, serve only as changeable starting places. There are group patterns that are valuable to know. Nurses must be flexible enough to know those general patterns **and** to recognize variations when they occur. For instance, being aware that in many traditional societies women are expected (and expect) to follow the lead of the men in their families (whether father, husband, brother, or son) is helpful when caring for a female patient who defers to her male relatives for answers to questions even about herself. The same behavior among members of Westernized, modern societies may have different implications. One would have to explore the situation further to avoid risking intervening on the basis of stereotypes that may not fit the individuals involved.

The ways that these interactive processes relate to each other is condensed in the following display.

Box 7-2. *Interactive Processes That Facilitate Cultural Communication or Barriers*

OBSERVATIONS AND INFORMATION PROCESSING
↓

NATURAL BIAS
Some things are noticed but not others.
↓

GENERALIZATIONS
Changeable starting places for comparing typical behavioral patterns with what is actually observed (the facts).
↓

OPEN, MUTUAL RELATIONSHIPS; UNDERSTANDING CLIENTS' VIEWS; AND PROVIDING CULTURALLY APPROPRIATE CARE

NEGATIVE BIAS
Some views and strengths get left out.
↓

STEREOTYPES
Seeing what is expected and missing what is not expected. When stereotypes are negative, they lead to prejudice.
↓

PREJUDICIAL ATTITUDES
Negative expectations about a group that are applied to individual situations.
↓

DISCRIMINATORY BEHAVIORS
Treating people unfairly; the "isms"

Stereotypes are particularly dangerous when they involve negative beliefs about a group. These lead to "prejudgment" (or prejudice) that ignores actual evidence. Prejudice involves negative feelings about groups different from one's own, regardless of how they are different. These attitudes are based on limited knowledge, limited contact, and emotional responses rather than on careful observation and thought. They are beliefs, opinions, or points of view that are formed before the facts are known. Facts that contradict a prejudice may be left unexplored or be ignored (Kluegel & Smith, 1986). For example, a student nurse expected a Chinese patient to like rice, drink tea, and use chopsticks to eat. When he grabbed a fork off someone else's tray, it was interpreted as aggressive behavior due to a combination of the student's fixed cultural expectations and negative stereotypes about both psychiatric patients and people who are ethnically and racially different than she is. Actually, the frustrated patient was angry about being expected to "act Chinese."

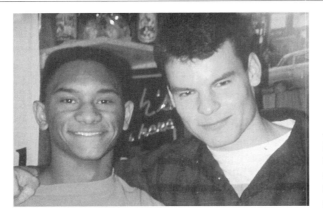

Developing lasting meaningful relationships across potential social barriers such as race contributes to improved social communication.

Stereotypes can be favorable as well as unfavorable, although both types disregard real facts for preconceived notions. Take, for example, a situation in which an individual of Asian or Asian American background is expected to excel in school due to stereotypes that associate Asians with scholarly accomplishments. Since every group has some individuals who do well in school and in math, and others who do not, Asian individuals who struggle academically must contend with a sense of group as well as individual failure. The same process is seen in many forms: a child may be expected to do well because his or her older siblings did, people with glasses to read a lot of books, or all blacks to be great dancers or athletes. These are not negative stereotypes, but they are potentially harmful because they impose expectations that are unrealistic, just as negative stereotypes do.

There are several types of prejudice that are commonly observed in health care and can lead to discriminatory behavior there. Discrimination is prejudice that is expressed behaviorally.

The time when African Americans and other Blacks, Asians, and Native Americans were overtly discriminated against and prevented from entering the social and economic mainstream of the U.S. is officially over. However, the stereotypes and prejudices associated with racial status may have mellowed, but they remain despite formal integration. For instance, negative stereotypes associating African Americans with poverty, drugs, and violence do not do justice to the fact that most African Americans are not poor and do not engage in drug-related or violent behavior. Assuming that a patient is on welfare because he or she is black, or that addiction is an issue or physical aggression a likelihood, may lead to treatment that is different than that given clients who are not African American. Similarly, other negative stereotypes and prejudices result in unequal treatment.

These discriminatory interaction patterns have acquired the label "Isms" because of their common word endings. Each "ism" involves a tendency to judge others according to similarity with or dissimilarity from a standard considered ideal or normal. Whatever the issue or level (personal or group), an "ism" is centered on one's own or a group's judgment (Brislin, 1993). Centered on oneself, for example, one is egocentric. When an entire society puts forth one way of doing or thinking as best, it is sociocentric, as in "Eurocentric" or "Afrocentric" education. Ethnic groups are groups that share historical and sociocultural backgrounds while existing within a larger society (Essed, 1991). We frequently run into "ethnocentric" views; nearly every group sees itself as "best" or most deserving. However, in a society composed of multiple groups, care must be taken to counteract such biases, or discrimination and social injustices occur. See Box 7-3.

Box 7-3. *The "Isms"*

Egocentrism: the assumption that oneself is superior to others. An example of this involves someone who has never been diagnosed as mentally ill (a staff member, for instance) who thinks he or she is better than those who are diagnosed as mentally ill.

Ethnocentrism: the assumption that one's own cultural or ethnic group is superior to that of others. Ethnicity refers to cultural differences and should not be confused with race. Ethnocentrism occurs, for example, when everyone is expected to speak English and to know the rules (many of which are implicit) for living in this society.

Racism: the assumption that members of one race are superior to those of another. (Race refers to biologic differences that are presumed to be significant.)

Sexism: the assumption that members of one sex are superior to those of the other. For example, women have historically been viewed as less rational and more emotional and subject to mental illness than men.

Heterosexism: the assumption that everyone is or should be heterosexual and that heterosexuality is superior and expectable. It is relatively recently that homosexuality was redefined as a lifestyle rather than a disease.

Ageism: the assumption that members of one age group are superior to those of others. Young patients and staff may not be taken as seriously as those who are older.

Adultism: the assumption that adults are superior to youths and can or should control, direct, reprimand, reward, or deprive them of respect. Children in American society are, for example, often interrupted or ignored by adults. They may not be given choices that allow them to learn how to cope with specific situations.

Sizism: The assumption that people of one body size are superior to or better than those of other shapes and sizes. Positions involving interaction with the public, for example, may be denied individuals who are very heavy or who otherwise fail to meet the standards of ideal appearance.

Classism/elitism: the assumption that certain people are superior because of their social and economic status or position in a group or organization. This often assumes that those with more money or education are superior. A poorly dressed high school drop-out, for example, may not be given the same treatment options offered to a well-dressed college graduate.

"Ableism": the assumption that the ablebodied and sound of mind are physically or developmentally superior to those who are disabled, retarded, or otherwise different. An example of "ableism" is not offering a chronically ill patient choices owing to the assumption that he or she does not want to or cannot make decisions.

Ethnicity

In the early part of this century, the goal was to Americanize the many peoples who came from all over the world to make their homes in the U.S. They had to learn English and become as much a part of the dominant culture as they could, which often meant compromising or even giving up their original cultures. Times have changed. As the century closes, people from diverse ethnic and other backgrounds expect, demand, and are viewed as deserving opportunities to preserve their various lifestyles, beliefs, and practices. Some people find the trend toward increased diversity (particularly recognition of ethnic, racial, and gender-oriented groups) threatening. Others view it as an opportunity to make America live up to its democratic ideals (Wali, 1992). In any event, this transition is occurring. And nurses must be prepared to care for this diverse population.

Many differences in mental health care needs are attributable to ethnic variation (Ho, 1987; Comas-Diaz & Griffith, 1988), although it must be remembered that there is significant diversity within each group, as well as between groups, and that many people cross groups, identifying with and belonging to several. Another important factor is that some peoples are very traditional in their views, while others are more acculturated and modern, although again there can be great variation within groups and even families. Despite the limitations imposed because ethnic categories are not mutually exclusive in a diverse society such as that of the U.S. it is useful for transcultural nurses to be aware of the generalized patterns associated with those aggregates who represent increasingly large proportions of the total population.

African Americans

Distinguished from others who come to the U.S. from the Caribbean Islands or from Africa, African Americans today are very diverse. Centuries of discrimination in a predominately "white" culture has perpetuated a focus on differences and leaves "blacks" and "whites" artificially divided. The mental health movement has drawn attention to African American resilience and strengths, and away from association of difference with psychopathology (Ruiz, 1990). Contemporary African Americans often remain enthusiastic about religion and spirituality, are characterized as adaptable and bicultural (that is, able to function in two worlds, one black and one white, which requires considerable effort and energy), and typically value work and education despite a history of limited opportunity to acquire or utilize those institutions. Strong networks tend to extend beyond households to multiple collateral relationships. Expectations for culturally congruent care among African Americans generally includes general concern for one another (the "brothers and sisters") (Leininger, 1984). In a society in which dark skin rendered people socially invisible for centuries, genuine respect, and acknowledgment are essential to acceptable care.

African American folk medicine, traditionally not separated into mental and physical components, contains elements of various origins (Snow, 1993). In the early 19th century, Haitian slaves rebelling against French masters brought with them a form of voodoo (a blend of European Catholicism and African tribal religions with modified aspects of humoral pathology). This spread through the Protestant American south and assimilated practices from 17th- and 18th-century European occultism, probably due to the insistence on using English rather than African languages (Foster & Anderson, 1978). Reflecting its multiple origins, black folk medicine today provides widely varied terms and methods, including, for example, "root" medicine, "rootwork," "mojo," "conjuring," "voodoo," and "hoodoo." There remains a tendency to bring to the health care situation a mixture of somatic, psychological, and spiritual problems (Capers, 1985; Snow, 1993).

In African American folk systems, diseases may be from natural causes or spiritual in nature (e.g., punishment for sins or violation of sacred beliefs) (Wood, 1989). Etiologies may be viewed as natural (such as failure to protect the body against inclement weather) or unnatural (for instance, divine punishment for sin) and tend to represent a perspective that holds the world to be a dangerous and hostile place. The individual is traditionally viewed as vulnerable to outside attack and as dependent upon outside help (Snow, 1977, 1993). This perspective was reinforced by nearly three centuries of slavery and then one of struggle for full rights.

American Indians

There are more than 500 different Native American and Alaskan Native tribes and nations. Also referred to as American Indians, First Nations, or Indigenous Americans, some groups are recognized by the federal government and others at only the state or local level. Most Native populations shared a traditional orientation to being in the present (rather than to doing and to the future, which is more typical of European Americans), to cooperation rather than competition, to giving rather than keeping, and to respect for age rather than youth (Attneave, 1982). Traditionally, the life cycle emphasizes rhythmic, natural phenomena aimed at a balance between living and working toward achieving Indian goals; self development is never completed. Noninterference is valued, and behaviors that imply manipulation or control may be offen-

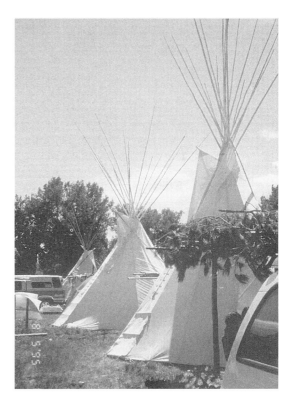

Traditional peoples bring cultures together in contemporary life in many ways. Ideally, individuals with more than one cultural affiliation can bring parts of each culture together without conflict. Tipis at a Lakota Nation Powwow, Pine Ridge, South Dakota.

sive. The astute clinician makes sure that the Indian client is aware of the consequences of behavior but then leaves it to the individual to decide how to proceed. Silence and a conservative show of interest (including, for example, minimizing eye contact) are respectful, caring behaviors.

The potential for personal confusion is obvious in a situation where mainstream society devalues most of the concepts integral to traditional Native American philosophies and ideologies. American Indian ideas about health and illness place less emphasis on dysfunction of the body than is typical of biomedicine, and more on relationships within society. For many American Indians, health typically denotes a special, balanced relationship between humankind and its physical, relational, and supernatural environment; illness implies having fallen out of balance with the world.

Traditional self-care prevention measures may include religious or magical elements (for example, burning candles, wearing amulets, reciting prayers, or making offerings) (McKenna, 1989). Although the prevalence of alcohol and drug use varies by tribe and by age within tribes, Native Americans tend to have higher rates of alcoholism than those presented by other groups. Associated phenomena include high suicide rates among the young, domestic (spouse and child abuse) violence (Baker, 1988; Myers, 1990), and homicide (Bell, 1990). However, many tribes today pride themselves in rates of sobriety that are higher than in the past. Stress-producing socioeconomic situations accompanied by psychological, cultural, and spiritual stressors lead to perceptions of loss and depression. Those who are least acculturated to white society and who have strong tribal identity tend to have the fewest problems. Group therapies with an emphasis on society have been found especially useful for treatment (Giago, 1984). Often those are family-network therapy and traditional Indian group talking and purification therapies (Vogel, 1970; Manson, Walker, & Kivlahan, 1987; Lewis, 1990; DuBray, 1992).

Hispanic Americans

Generally, the terms Latino and Hispanic refer to Spanish ethnicity, language skills, and ancestry, but also imply significant cultural variation. Some common themes among Hispanic Americans include Catholicism (although increasing numbers of Hispanics are turning to Protestant religions and Pentecostal sects), orientation toward extended family systems (which may include godparents [compadres] and other non-biologic kin), distinctly different roles for men and women, a high value of respect for self and others, the priority of spiritual and humanistic over commercial values, clear hierarchy and patriarchy, and fairly common reliance on folk systems of medicine. Since Hispanic Americans tend to value being listened to and having time spent with them, task-oriented hurrying about is viewed as noncaring. Involvement, loving, and empathy are valued caring behaviors (Leininger, 1984). There is wide variability in levels of acculturation (that is, integration into the mainstream American system). While the average Mexican American was born in the U.S. and many members of other Hispanic groups are American by birth, numerous others are immigrants.

Spanish American folk medicine, despite some variation with place and group, clearly reflects its humoral antecedents, as well as Catholic ritual and beliefs about supernatural influences. Many illnesses are "hot" or "cold," so sufferers are treated with medicines and foods of opposite characteristics. These qualities do not refer to temperature but to symbolic properties. Care and treatment regimens can be negotiated with patients within that framework.

Asian Americans

Americans of Asian ancestry represent diverse cultures from Japan, China, Korea, India, the Philippines and other Pacific islands, and southeast Asia. Education and hard work have paid off for many Asian immigrants, although the "Asian success story" fails to take into account that there are many poor Asian Americans (despite relatively low rates of dependence on public assistance and welfare) and a notable discrepancy between education level and income persists.

Strong Asian values generally involve harmonious interpersonal relationships, webs of obligation, and fear of shame (which is a social concept, in contrast to the Westernized notion of guilt, which is more individualized) (Shon & Ja, 1982). The family is of great importance, and family sharing is a major construct in care. Respect, especially for family, elders, and those in authority, is seen as vital. Respect is expressed through recognition of family members and in listening to and valuing their input (Leininger, 1984). Reciprocity and generosity are highly valued. Disruptive and conflict situations are viewed as noncaring (Leininger, 1984).

Traditional Asian health care practices include such varied preventative strategies as worshipping gods and ancestors and striving for balance in all aspects of life (Burnside, 1988). The goal of balance also permeates all culturally congruent treatments. Asian societies share a tradition of Chinese medicine (which is more general than western medicine because it has a single unifying theoretical basis), as well as of shamanism. There is a strong reliance on Chinese medicine for specific problems and for prevention. Traditional healers draw on biologic, psychological, social, and ecological evidence to diagnosis conditions arising from disruptions in the client's life; his brain and body may be out of balance, for example, and his relationships with past lives, ancestors, and destiny disturbed in some way (Kuo & Kavanagh, 1994). Inappropriate behavior may leave the patient vulnerable to brain collapse, ancestral vengeance, and interference from evil spirits and people. Communication is viewed as fundamental to the healer–patient relationship.

The Chinese have characteristic ways of dealing with mental illness in the family, starting with a protracted period of intrafamilial coping with even serious psychiatric illness, followed by recourse to friends, elders, and neighbors in the community; consultation with traditional specialists, religious healers or general physicians, and finally treatment from western specialists. Although it may conflict with western practices of multiple dosage in tablet or capsule form, many Asians prefer to use over the counter drugs that come in liquid form, as well as in single-doses, as was typical of liquid preparations in Chinese folk practices (Rempusheski, 1989). Others believe that only injections will be effective.

For many Asian Americans, the forces of tradition are entangled with those of modernization. Traditionally providing most care within families despite the shame associated with mental illness, the strains and changes of recent urbanization and industrialization have led to increasingly diverse lifestyles and a need to discard stereotypes of well-satisfied, well-cared for and respected ill and elders (Hirayama, 1985–86; Lee, 1985–86; Moon & Pearl, 1991). See Research Application 7-4.

| Research Application 7-4 | *Mental Health Care for Asian and Pacific Islander Americans* |

Sandhu, D. S. (1997). Psychocultural profiles of Asian and Pacific Islander Americans: Implications for counseling and psychotherapy. *Journal of Multicultural Counseling and Development, 25*, 7–22.

Demographically, the category "Asian and Pacific Islander Americans" includes more than 40 different cultural groups. What they share in common is either ancient or recent roots in Asia. Asians are so often described as "model" or "successful minorities" that actual problems experienced by individuals, families, and subgroups may be overlooked or minimized. Levels of acculturation vary widely. The families of some Asian Americans have been in the United States for four or more generations; others may be new immigrants. Generally, more acculturated peoples tend to higher levels of mental health–seeking behaviors. Ancestral values and language patterns also differ greatly. Training to increase cultural competence is important for non-Asian mental health practitioners.

Clinical Application

- Explore with the client just how he or she views himself or herself culturally. For example, how does the individual client "name" his or her culture?

- Ask the client to describe his or her culture for you and explain cultural characteristics for your benefit.

- Understand that by the act of seeking mental health, your client is probably more acculturated than others of the same cultural group.

- Organize a training session at your worksite and invite members of the Asian and Pacific Islander community to come and talk with you about themselves and their culture.

Middle Eastern Cultural Groups

In recent decades, the U.S. has experienced an influx of peoples from Middle Eastern and Northern African cultures. This has increased the traditionally Judeo-Christian American awareness of the complex cultural beliefs, values, and lifeways of members of predominately Islamic societies. Despite considerable cultural diversity among Middle Eastern peoples (Meleis, Lipson, & Paul, 1992), generally shared value orientations include Moslem (Muslim or Islamic) submission and obedience to God and prescribed rituals of prayer and washing. Strict concepts of what is allowed and forbidden (that is, clean and unclean, good and bad) impose important dietary and other rules that should be verified and accommodated as much as possible in health care situations. Class, status, education, modesty, and emotional expression are generally valued. Patriarchy and the centrality of religion typify Middle Eastern social and familial organizations. Elders are honored, gain in status, and interestingly, tend not to experience the senility common to more youth-oriented cultures (Luna, 1989).

Oriented traditionally to the present, making plans may not be valued by some Middle Easterners because the future is seen as neither uncertain nor preordained but as something that one accepts with fatalistic grace (Jalali, 1982). Nursing research indicates that Egyptian, Yemeni, Iranian, Armenian, and Arab immigrants to the U.S. who are more traditional in social integration, cultural attitudes, and family orientation tend to have less positive morale that those who are more acculturated (Meleis, Lipson, & Paul, 1992).

The Appeal of Alternative Systems

Folk and popular systems of health care continue to serve, to a greater extent than is often recognized by mental health personnel, to smooth harsh cultural gaps between traditional societies and the predominant American system. They are available in every American city, do not require going to unfamiliar places or being seen by people who are strangers, and are readily understandable to someone socialized to the group. Folk systems are also simply organized, relative to scientific systems, and relatively devoid of intimidating testing, technology, lengthy history taking (which often seems irrelevant to patients and families), and invasive diagnostic procedures. Interpersonal, social, and kinship relationships are emphasized, rather than the isolated individual. Traditionally, a focus on groups minimized the discomfort associated with unaccustomed attention to individuals outside of the context of the family.

Experienced as more humanistic than scientific, traditional systems of knowing and healing are usually less mechanized, less urbanized, and less intellectualized than biomedicine, which is often focused on fixing dysfunctional parts or systems, limited in access, and dependent upon rationality to the extent that emotional needs may be overlooked. Use of psychiatric resources may be discouraged by professionals' intolerance for magical and religious orientations and practices, which is common when science and systems of symbolic beliefs and faith compete. Interest in traditional healing beliefs and practices is in no way limited to immigrant or indigenous groups. Today, Americans of every ethnic heritage are expressing increasing interest in alternative or complementary health care and healing traditions.

Communication

The crux of transcultural psychiatric/mental health nursing is communication, the style of which varies greatly with culture. Some of these differences are quickly evident, as when mental health practitioners expect a degree of openness, verbosity, self-disclosure, emotional expression and insight that reflect the dominant American culture (Tripp-Reimer, 1984; Young, 1988) rather than the client's orientation. Groups also vary widely in their ideas about appropriate stance, gestures, language, listening styles, and eye contact. Traditional Asian Americans, African Americans, Native Americans (Wood, 1989), and Appalachians (Tripp-Reimer, 1984) typically consider direct eye contact inappropriate and disrespectful.

Language differences can cause treatment to take much longer than treatment for English-speaking patients (Sherer, 1993) and it is often tempting to use the most available person to facilitate this process. However, dependence on family members to translate may complicate the situation. Particularly when the patient and translator are not of the same sex, new problems may be fabricated to avoid stating the real ones in front of the individual who was solicited to translate. Although linguistic assistance is vital, some translators may actually interpret rather than translate what the client says. The nurse unfamiliar with the language may not realize whose views are being expressed. See Box 7-4.

Box 7-4. *Information Box*

AT&T's Language Line Services offers translations in nearly 150 languages. Call (800) 752-6096 to learn more about this service. You might want to share the information you learn with the local mental health facility.

As complex as they may be, crossing communication barriers and mutual identification of the problem or offending agent are only parts of the process. Transcultural care requires cultural negotiation and compromise. This may involve understanding how the client views and explains the problem, and may extend, for example, to advocating use of folk healers and herbal remedies along with prescribed treatments and medications, or helping clients arrange traditional ceremonies associated with grieving and loss. In addition to accepting that communication is possible but that mistakes will at times occur, effective intervention requires sensitivity to the communication process, knowledge of expectable client-specific patterns of communication and care, and a set of practiced skills (Pedersen, 1985, 1988).

There are four primary transcultural communication skill areas (Pedersen, 1985, 1988; Kavanagh & Kennedy, 1992). The first is the ability to understand and state an issue or problem as it is perceived from the client's perspective. Nursing's advocacy role frequently involves articulation of problems or issues from clients' points of view to decrease risk of misunderstanding and imposition of values and norms that are not those of the client. Knowing a client's explanation for his or her problems allows the nurse to work with the client to resolve them (Pedersen, 1988; Kavanagh & Kennedy, 1992). Otherwise, the ideas that the client has about those problems may not articulate with the priorities, goals, and interventions posed by the nurse, who may become frustrated with the client's lack of "compliance."

The second and third skill areas involve recognizing and reducing resistance and defensiveness, which directly impede development of productive relationships between nurses and clients and further contribute to the basis for negative attitudes and labels such as "noncompliance." Accusations made by clients about practitioners' incompetence often stem directly from clients' perceptions that those providers are pursuing their own goals and do not acknowledge the clients' as important. Providers may be defensive about this; after all, they are doing what they have been instructed to do, just as clients expect to have their needs met and not the providers'.

Developing skills to decrease resistance or defensiveness includes learning to recognize specific ways in which such interactive processes are displayed. Sensitivity to only generalized forms of these phenomena does not facilitate effective intervention. Consider the difference between "He is always so nasty to me!" and "I feel defensive when he tells me I am too young to help him." The specific behavioral information contained in the latter version allows work to begin on problem resolution.

The fourth transcultural communication skill area involves recognition that everyone makes interactive mistakes from time to time. Although taking the risk of making an error is preferable to playing it so safe that communication is inhibited, venturing into unknown territory may go against the way some nurses were socialized to behave. Communication recovery skills involving, for example, apology, humor and redirection (Pedersen, 1988) are reclamation techniques to use after a blunder. They reinforce confidence as well as competence because, when it is known that there is something to fall back on, one is less likely to avoid interactions that may prove difficult. Being able to admit that one does not know everything is a powerful skill. Why should nurses expect themselves to know everything? There are more than 3000 cultures and untold numbers of cultural variations and interpretations. Using a learning stance, that is, letting clients know that they are experts about their cultures and that we wish to learn from them, allows space for real learning, as well as respectful communication and recover from honest mistakes. See Research Application 7-5.

Humor can help bridge communicative gaps in transcultural settings even when direct communication is viewed as impertinent or otherwise offensive (Durant & Miller, 1988). For example, chiding the self for one's own silly ineptness can humanize situations that are otherwise intimidating and distancing. Nurses who can chide themselves with a chuckle when realizing that they just wished a Jewish client a "Merry Christmas" are unlikely to be considered insensitive. However, it must be remembered that respect is the essential ingredient to mutual communication. Awareness of the meaning of any experience from others' points of view is crucial. Humor related to some topics (for instance, race, sex or ethnicity) is often considered socially unacceptable.

Research Application 7-5	## "*Lunatics*" *and the Moon: Nature and Madness, or Just a Phase?*

Mason, T. (1997). **Seclusion and the lunar cycles.** *Journal of Psychosocial Nursing, 35* (6), 14–18.

For centuries (at least since Hippocrates posited the relationship some 2500 years ago) people have associated increases in violence and aggression in psychiatric patients with the full moon. Over time, this came to be known as the Transylvanian effect. Research examined the use of seclusion in various phases of the moon as a way of investigating the relationship (if any) between the moon and madness. Seclusion, in various forms, is used universally for disturbed patients, and in psychiatric settings for control and management of violence and aggression. If the Transylvanian effect actually occurs, there should be a demonstrable relationship between lunar cycles and the use of seclusion. Although staff members may use seclusion when they fear they or others may be in danger and thus may be hypervigilent during the full moon (whether or not the moon has any effect on patients' behavior), no such correlation was found between the full moon and use of seclusion for the mentally ill.

Clinical Application

- Seclusion may be used appropriately when mental health professionals believe they are in danger from a client's violent and aggressive behavior.

- Violent behavior in clients is triggered by such factors as noncompliance with medication or perhaps stress or other events in the clients' environment rather than the full moon.

- Seclusion, in various forms, is used universally for violent clients and has been used with some success for centuries.

Communicating across cultures requires testing stereotypes against reality. When cognition and affect are impaired by mental illness, communication can be especially time consuming and complex, although it is no less important. Assumptions must be avoided. Unusual language use may, for example, represent cultural differences rather than thinking or hearing impairments, although those explanations might also be valid. The skilled communicator learns how to identify and bridge differences.

Transcultural nurses elicit clients' explanatory models through open-ended questions in lay terms (Kleinman, 1982). Explanatory models consist of clients' ideas about the cause of the illness; the reason for its onset at a given time; its pathophysiology, expected course, and prognosis; their ideas about such concepts as stress, coping, ethnicity and spirituality; past experiences with health care workers and treatment modalities, illness behavior, and patterns of help seeking; and the treatment that they believe should be administered. A patient who believes, for example, that his illness is the result of having broken the rules (perhaps by committing a sin or breaking a taboo) may not believe that medication is going to resolve the problem. Some cathartic or purification ritual may be needed. Often such a remedy works best in conjunction with the biomedical approach.

Learning clients' perspectives reduces risk of conflict between and imposition of nurses' and other care providers' values and enables assessment of cultural orientation and related needs. Clinicians must express genuine interest in clients' views before most will share their ideas about their circumstances and beliefs, yet once they are established, many cultural and psychosocial themes in clients' lives can be effectively explored with even moderately disturbed individuals. Understanding specific explanatory models also allows access to conflicts, support and communication patterns that may be key elements in the client's situation (Kleinman, 1982).

In mental health care, the goal of mutual communication as effective and appropriate intervention implies that it must be acceptable to the client as well as to health care professionals. It takes skill to examine communication patterns and their potential for creating either communicative barriers or mutually respectful interactions. Although traditionally nurse-client communication was often oneway, participatory health care requires that setup to change.

Sometimes clients are expected to follow different interactive rules than those used by non-clients, which prohibits mutual communication. A double set of standards is especially noticeable when clients who are seriously ill, mentally ill, or of different national origin or social class than the provider are not expected to respect basic rules of common decency (Kavanagh, 1988, 1991). Differences in social status, hierarchy, and the fact that mental health personnel who are members of majority groups may never have experienced or critically examined the meaning of clients' minority status (which may involve any combination of gender, race, ethnicity, economic and social status, diagnosis, or health status) all have tremendous impact on relationships, perceptions of problems, and perceptions of alternative interventions. Although members of ethnic and racial minority groups compose 22 percent of the U.S. population, only 8 percent of practicing physicians and 14.2 percent of people who enroll in RN programs come from those minority backgrounds (Sabatino, 1993). It is important that sincere (not patronizing) interest be taken in the client's views and experiences, and that they be taken seriously.

In short, mutual communication involves awareness and knowledge of social process, and sensitivity to and recognition of barriers to acceptance and sharing, as well as skill in communication techniques. Most important is the ability to empathize, that is, to understand others' beliefs, assumptions, perspectives, and feelings (Pedersen, 1985, 1988). The effective communicator learns to acquire and to understand, to the greatest extent possible, multiple perspectives. Tolerance and acceptance of others' attitudes, beliefs and behaviors, and the willingness to expose oneself as interested but still learning sensitivity, knowledge and skills are important strategies.

Nurse, Know Thyself

Culture is learned and shared. It is learned both formally, as in class or religious instruction, and informally by observation and experience. Culture is constantly changing yet not easily changed. It strongly influences, but does not determine, ideas and behavior. Cultural values and social norms may be stressors as well as media for expression. Culture does not involve biologic or personal characteristics but only those values, beliefs, and ideals that people share. We all have culture, not only others who are "different." Culture is not always neat and orderly; various cultures and subcultures overlap. Values, attitudes, ideas, and patterns of behavior are shared in this time of instant and visual communication when many people are exposed to multiple cultures. We give little thought to eating Chinese food one day and Mexican food the next.

Caring behaviors exist in every culture, so nursing is sometimes misconstrued as essentially culture-free. However, specific nursing behaviors, as well as nurses themselves, reflect the cultural contexts in which they occur (Leininger, 1988). The dominant values of the U.S. shape its professional orientations. For example, Americans emphasize individualism and self-reliance, and these are reflected in the goals generally set forth for mental health clients. However, independence is not valued universally, and dependence in non-industrial societies has different meanings. Where households are not so differentiated, there is a more obvious norm of generalized reciprocity, and life is more cohesive and collective. In much of the world, interdependence is valued and independence viewed with ambivalence or as pathologic.

Learning to understand the cultures of clients requires learning about your own cultural orientation and about yourself. "The one who would change others must himself be changed" (Milio, 1970, p. xi). The culture of the nurse interacts with those of clients. It is important to realize that culture includes the values and norms learned in the process of becoming a nurse (or a member of any other group) as well as those associated with ethnicity, age, class, or gender background. Understanding who we are requires close examination of one's own orientation to recognize where one's own sense of personal and social identity comes from and how it was formed. Ask yourself what kind of person you were socialized to be and how your social identity has changed and is it changing. They are never static.

Such self-knowledge is critical to realizing which cultures or groups one tends to favor or avoid, and which groups one negatively or unrealistically positively stereotypes. Such blind spots (that is, biases) can keep one from considering, for example, that a "nice, middle-class grandmother" might also be a much conflicted lesbian woman who is addicted to cocaine. Each of us has attitudinal limitations that obscure facts from our consideration and vision. With whom do you feel strange and uncomfortable, and why? How do your concerns and biases affect who gets care and what type of care you give? It is well known than there are cultural preferences among mental health providers for clients who are young, attractive, verbal, intelligent, and successful (also known as YAVIS) (Wilson & Kneisl, 1983), while those who are considered quiet, unattractive, old, indigent, different, and stupid (that is, the QUOIDS) often get less attention.

Commitment to transcultural nursing assumes the recognition and value of human dignity, cultural relativism (that is, the idea that all perspectives have worth) as an acceptable and preferred philosophy, willingness to alter personal behavior in response to the cross-cultural interactive process, and willingness to monitor personal resistance and defensiveness. Consider how you feel about those criteria.

People may avoid professional mental health care because of incompatible values and beliefs, poverty, social stresses that occur among special populations but are not well understood by professionals, language barriers, lack of education, social isolation, stigma, bureaucratic barriers, and the unequal distribution of services. It is crucial that the nursing process be examined from the cultural perspectives of health care providers **and** consumers to maximize appropriate utilization and quality care. Care can then be provided by informed practitioners in ways that are perceived as both acceptable and appropriate. See Research Application 7-6.

Culture and Psychiatric/Mental Health Nursing

Transcultural nurses utilize multiple ways of understanding to move beyond the rigidity of trying to fit diverse experiences, interpretations, and expectations into a few ready-made (but culture bound) categories. All cultural groups share time-honored systems of health beliefs and practices; it is often nurses who can interpret expectations between groups. Sensitive cultural interviews are required to know who clients are. Nursing, to provide culturally congruent care, attends to relationships between the self and others; between mental illness and such phenomena as poverty, suffering, violence, chronic illness, and aging; between the cultures of nursing and psychiatry and those of our clientele; and between nursing ethics and the provision of appropriate care. When nurses and clients come from different cultural backgrounds, accurate diagnosis, treatment, and care depends on time-consuming special knowledge and skills (Westermeyer, 1987; Benner, Tanner, & Chesla, 1996; Lipson & Steiger, 1996).

Research Application 7-6	*Urban/Rural Differences Are Important too*

Hauenstein, E. J. (1997). **A nursing practice paradigm for depressed rural women: The women's affective illness treatment program.** *Archives of Psychiatric Nursing, 1,* 37–45.

When major depressive disorders occur in rural areas where few professional mental health treatment resources exist and clients may be hard to access and treat, effective psychosocial interventions must be adapted for specific populations. A primary care setting providing screening, diagnostic care, brief treatment, and follow-up can produce significant symptom reduction, improved functional ability of clients, and programs of relapse prevention. This was done in the rural Piedmont area of the South by training generalist nurses with psychoeducational skills to work with a culturally competent advanced practice psychiatric nurse and by designing a program for specific care needs. Field testing and evaluation of the program for rural women in the area studied indicated that a combination of self-care skills (including self-assessment, stress reduction, and health behavior modification) and minimum psychiatric resources can create a promising and powerful partnership.

Clinical Application

- Rural clients can be treated effectively in primary care settings in their own communities. These services should include screening and diagnostic and brief treatment services. Follow-up services can be provided as needed. This model has been shown to improve functional ability of clients and reduce their symptoms.

- Nurses can be trained to provide culturally competent psychiatric services in rural areas.

- Self-care skills that can be taught to rural women include self-assessment, stress reduction, and health behavior modification. These practices can decrease symptoms in clients who live in hard-to-access rural areas.

Transcultural nursing may involve collecting information about specific cultures; acquiring a culturally acceptable ally or advocate for the client and/or a cultural consultant for the nurse; work with a translator; learning clients' behavioral, attitudinal and cognitive norms; or ensuring that only culturally fair psychometric tests are used (Geller, 1988). Standardized tests are appropriate only when they are properly modified to fit cultural heritage and experiences. Some transcultural nurses view culture brokering as part of their roles, bridging, linking or mediating between groups that differ in background or orientation (LaFargue, 1985; Jezewski, 1990, 1993). Ideally this is done with information from the client's perspective, for which the nurse serves merely to facilitate the opportunity to be heard. Other transcultural nurses define their responsibility more in terms of expediting situations in which clients can do their own negotiating.

Since psychopathology occurs at roughly the same rate in every society (World Health Organization, 1973; Hughes, 1990; Tseng & Streltzer, 1997), it stands to reason that a transcultural perspective is essential to appropriate mental health and psychiatric nursing care. The value of psychiatry is questionable if it is limited to middle class Europeans and European Americans (Kleinman, 1988). In its current thinking, ethnopsychiatry, which involves culture-specific constructions of psychiatric systems (Devereux, 1980), attempts to move beyond the assumption that Western ways of understanding and treating are universally applicable. Mental health and mental illness are instead understood within the cultural contexts in which they develop (Gaines, 1992; Tseng & Streltzer, 1997). The same challenge faces nursing; ethnonursing methods foster understanding of care-related phenomena from the perspectives of those people who experience the phenomena (Leininger, 1991).

It is essential for clients to feel accepted if they are to share with providers what they believe and practice outside of the biomedical system. This will not happen if clients are left to assume that their beliefs and activities are not of interest to health care providers, or will be rejected by them. It may be important, however, to know what the patient or client believes and does to minimize the possibility of harm from treatments or medicines that interact disadvantageously with those of the alternative systems. Although it is dangerous to assume that all indigenous approaches are innocuous, most practices are harmless, whether or not they are effective cures. Often such treatments provide valuable psychological support and, due to that contribution, should not be discouraged.

Assumptions that coping patterns of clients and patients are or should be similar to those of nurses (and others socialized to the health care system) simplify care. Differences may be overlooked in efforts to avoid time-consuming complications. The risk involved in such behavior is that clients and providers may work with different strategies or toward dissimilar goals. The nurse, for example, may hurry to include all items relevant to health promotion for high-risk clients, when it is the presence and time spent with them that the clients value, not the information.

The two largest consumer groups of mental health care today are the chronically, seriously mentally ill and the aged. New care management and case management strategies are making significant inroads with both populations. The field of geropsychiatric nursing will require more and more skilled psychiatric nurses in the future, for work both with the elderly and with their caregivers. Nurses are increasingly involved in rehabilitative training, resocialization programs, partial hospitalization centers, and support groups, in addition to one-to-one relationships. Hospital admissions have become increasingly brief, despite increased acuity and the management problems that presents. Most clients diagnosed with chronic schizophrenia and other major psychiatric illnesses can be maintained on psychotropic drugs in community and ambulatory settings (Franks & Faux, 1990). Psychiatric/mental health nurses are liaisons among clients, health care facilities, and families (Baldwin, 1993). As such, they can facilitate effective integration of multiple belief systems, or they can impose preset expectations that lead to interventions oriented toward the practitioner's and health care system's values and goals rather than the client's.

Nurses sometimes question how they can learn all of the relevant characteristics of the clients they care for (they cannot and should not try) and why they should know about group patterns when it is individuals with whom they work. The important thing is to ascertain a client's cultural orientation and what it means to him or her (or them, since many nurses work with families or other groups). It is not a matter of matching clients to their reference groups, but of learning about and understanding the relationships involved. For example, is it more useful and accurate to ask "How is this client Norwegian or Lutheran?" than it is to ask "How Norwegian or Lutheran is this client?"

The former question allows comparison of the answer against the expectable patterns (that is, generalizations about Norwegians and Lutherans), whereas the latter question seeks a match between the client and stereotypic standards for his or her reference groups. Always, easy stereotypes should be avoided: Chinese do this and Latinos do that. Stereotypes simply do not work effectively. While every group has discernable patterns that help distinguish it from other groups, most individuals also express beliefs or traits that do not match the group norm. One may be very traditional in one aspect and quite modern in others. Sometimes when people are ill they become more traditional in their expectations and thinking. There is also significant variation within as well as between groups. Knowledge of the group is valuable in as much as it provides a set of realistic expectations. However, only by learning about the individual or family at hand can the clinician understand in what ways the group patterns are meaningful.

Before 1950, psychiatric services in the U.S. were provided primarily at state hospitals (Mollica, 1983). Today, 60 percent of patients hospitalized in the U.S. with a primary psychiatric diagnosis are treated in general hospitals, and many of those occupy beds scattered throughout various areas rather than on designated psychiatric units (Summergrad, 1991; Gorman, Sultan, & Raines, 1996). This means that many nurses who do not identify with care of the mentally ill are exposed to that population. Another reason that it is important for nurses to be culturally sensitive, knowledgeable, and skillful is that they are instrumental in the export of mental health concepts to other societies (e.g., Stanley, 1993). Nurses educated in the U.S. work throughout the world, as well as with people who come to North America from elsewhere. We must be aware of our potential as communicators of more than we intend.

Culture-Specific Care

It may be tempting to avoid close examination of basic values and beliefs because they seem amorphous, complex, or too intimate. However, a grasp of the concepts of normality, abnormality, ethnocentrism, relativism, pluralism, stereotyping, prejudice, and discrimination provides a basis for understanding how society handles differences in attitude and behavior. Social ranking (that is, social stratification) and its consequence, social inequality, affect human experience, opportunities, and availability, acceptability, and utilization of mental health care resources.

It is a myth that treating people differently because of racial, religious, ethnic, cultural, gender, or other characteristics implies prejudice and discrimination. That is an overused excuse to avoid dealing with issues that are part of social process. The problem with not acknowledging diversity is that it denies meaningful variations in real life experience. It is not necessarily irrational for the individual who has been discriminated against because of his or her dark skin, or the woman who has been raped, to be paranoid. On the other hand, having one's experience discredited or made to seem unimportant is painful, and situations do not go away simply because they are ignored or avoided. Aspects of them may eventually surface.

In trying to satisfy the basic needs of his or her client, the transcultural nurse asks: "What do you expect (or want) the nurse to do for you?" (McKenna, 1989). In other words, "How do you want to be cared for?" Culturally congruent nursing care decisions and actions have the potential to intervene in three ways: cultural care preservation, accommodation, or repatterning (Leininger, 1988).

The need for cultural maintenance or preservation was demonstrated, for example, when a student from New Zealand came to a university mental health clinic with complaints of chronic headaches, sleeplessness, and inability to focus on his school work. He explained that the onset of these symptoms coincided with his father's death, about which he did not learn until it was too late to return for the burial rites. Owing to his failure to be there when his mother especially needed his support, a relative "pointed a bone" at him and that action, he believed, resulted in his present problems. A thorough assessment failed to produce additional reasons for the young man's somatic complaints, decreased academic achievement, and social discomfort.

Fortunately, a clinician was located who previously worked in New Zealand and made herself available to work with both the clinic staff and the disturbed student. Together they delineated the problem, worked to understand what it would take to alleviate it, and participated in an adapted ceremony that allowed the client to believe that the effect of the bone-pointing had been neutralized. The student was at peace with the knowledge that it was through no fault of his that he had missed his father's funeral. He knew that further amends for the social transgression could wait until after successful completion of his studies. This would allow him to serve his reference group more effectively than would his premature return as an academic failure.

The second mode of nursing intervention involves assisting clients to negotiate or adapt new cultural ways (Leininger, 1988). As nurses become sensitive to the complex factors that influence clients' responses to care, they learn to negotiate. This mode of intervention is illustrated by the example of a 15-year-old Mexican American girl who was referred to the mental health clinic after a suicide attempt. Her school attendance was sporadic, her grades were poor, and she was depressed. Both parents worked outside the home, and her older brothers had moved out, leaving her as primary caretaker for several young siblings. Although she had been dating a boy for several months, her parents planned to send her to Mexico to marry a man they knew there. After she argued with them about her household chores and her future, her boy-friend ended their relationship, and the school threatened to suspend her for nonattendance, she cut her wrists. Maria verbalized anger, identity and role confusion, her guilt over rejection of her family, and her resentment of her parents' expectations and of her limited choices.

Individual and family therapy with mental health clinical nurse specialists helped negotiate a realistic and acceptable plan that would keep Maria in school (thus increasing her life choices later) while helping her bridge the gap between traditional and more modern ways. In a group with other young women, Maria was empowered by sharing and learning that there were aspects of her culture and her circumstances that she could accept, reject, ignore, and change.

A third approach to intervention involves culturally acceptable and appropriate care that enables change to new or different behavioral patterns that are meaningful, satisfying, and beneficial (Leininger, 1988). Changing the view that a person has of events requires altering the meaning of the situation (Pesut, 1991). However, the need for such restructuring is less common than that for cultural preservation and negotiation, and involves only partial behavioral repatterning. Those cultural attributes that are useful are preserved, as was observed in an urban program designed to strengthen family processes. Families were encouraged to spend social time in its community center. When parents were confronted in writing (as well as with reprimand) with the program's expectation that there would be no hitting on the premises, several families stopped coming. It was not until the staff realized the parents' need to learn alternative ways to set limits for children that those families began to feel comfortable at the center.

For many program participants, physical recourse was the only mode of discipline with which they were familiar; the no-hitting policy had been interpreted as meaning no discipline. Parents had to learn alternative ways of dealing with disciplinary issues and with stress, and children eventually learned that their parents would be consistent in their non-physical limit setting, that punishments would correlate with the transgression, and that the expression of caring was not limited to physical evidence. With repatterning over time, meaningful verbal and other non-physical ways of disciplining were modeled, learned, and implemented.

Ideological Conflict in Psychiatric/Mental Health Nursing

A growing awareness of the changing and complex nature of illness, the influence of social context, and the importance of holistic perspectives leave nurses in a quandary when the dominant model in psychiatry focuses on organic and genetic factors as underlying causes of mental disease (Lutzen, 1990). For some, "the decade of the brain," with its high-tech brain scans and powerful new drugs, threatens to forget the patient as a person (Goode, 1988). This may lead nurses who are surrounded by others who think differently to question their ability and worth (Arena & Page, 1992) or to resent psychiatry's role in social control (Brown, 1989; Morrison, 1990).

Ideological conflict is not new in psychiatric/mental health care and continues to shadow nurse–physician and nurse–client relationships (Kavanagh, 1988, 1991). Continued frustration with a plethora of phenomena, many of them (such as poverty and discrimination) beyond the usual scope of medical treatment, confront public psychiatric/mental health systems. Despite the medicalization of mental health, nurses often feel they must balance structural requirements (which may conflict) with operationalizing knowledge of care and therapy (which may be ambiguous), all the while communicating with persons who may communicate abnormally (Bunch, 1983). All of this occurs in a society that is ambivalent toward individuals who exhibit unpopular differences. Nurses must continue to explore diverse models of caring and attend closely to the practices they actually employ.

Being an applied profession with a humanistic ethic, nursing grapples with tension between the outsider (etic) values of the nursing and medical subcultures (which reflect the dominant society) and an insider (emic) view reflecting the values of individuals, families, communities, and other affiliation and cultural groups for whom nurses advocate. Transcultural nursing helps bring emic perspectives together with the etic.

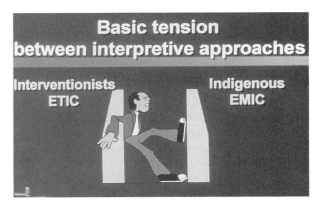

Implications for Transcultural Mental Health/Psychiatric Nursing Practice

As a practical science of caring (Bottorff, 1991), nursing strives to use strategies that lead to positive outcomes. How does the nurse incorporate cultural beliefs and practices into daily practice? Key points for the transcultural mental health nurse are summarized here using Diekelmann's (1991, 1994, 1995) framework of "concernful practices."

Welcoming, gathering, and *accepting* involve creating effective relationships and establishing open communication. The nurse's role is to suggest illness prevention and health maintenance practices, as well as treatment strategies that fit with and reinforce clients' cultural beliefs and practices. Understand clients' desire to please and their motivations to comply or not to comply. Often "noncompliance" occurs because clients are trying to preserve their own priorities (Morrison, 1990; "Culture clash," 1996). Understand relationships between clients and authority, health care institutions, and bureaucracies. Whenever possible and appropriate, involve significant others and leaders of relevant local groups. Confidentiality is important, but ethnic and other leaders know the problems and often can suggest acceptable interventions. Try to make the setting comfortable. Consider colors, sound, atmosphere, scheduling expectations, seating arrangements, pace, tone, and other environmental variables. Be prepared for the fact that children go everywhere with members of some cultural groups, as well as with families who do not have options due to economic limitations; include them.

Knowing, connecting, and *staying* involve finding meaningful ways that clients, families, and others can contribute their own cultural input and goals, while both patterns and variations are recognized. As nurses become more mindful of managing their own diversity, questions initiated by "Why don't they . . .?" are gradually balanced with "Why do we . . .?," often prompting on-going discussion of various approaches and perspectives. Becoming more aware of the potency of cultural expectations as well as personal choices, all participants in cross-cultural relationships find themselves consciously setting priorities and considering options regarding what to accept, reject, ignore, or try to change.

Prescencing, attending, and *staying open* are confounded with time, which harangues modern health care and nursing. Routinization and efficiency are valued by the dominant culture, while caring, connecting, and learning take time. Visiting, sharing stories, and many other simple encounters are useful strategies for learning what care and caring mean to the client and family. Understand what members of the cultural or subcultural group consider "caring," both attitudinally and behaviorally. Ask what they would like and expect to have happen. Acquire basic knowledge about cultural values, health beliefs, and traditional health-related practices common to the group you are working with. Learn about expectations for personal hygiene, ideas about health and illness, and eating (Rempusheski, 1989). Language and food are important symbols; respect and use them. Also know the folk illnesses and remedies common to the cultural group with which you are working. Inquire about over-the-counter and folk remedies being used; research indicates that up to 80 percent of treatments used by clients are not reported because professionals do not ask about them (Wood, 1989). Build on cultural practices, reinforcing those that are positive;

do not discredit any beliefs or practices unless you know for sure that specific practices are harmful.

Creating a place and *keeping open possibilities* entail working to establish caring relationships and increasing sensitivity to our own implicit understandings and expectations. Present yourself with confidence. Shake hands if it is appropriate. Ask how clients prefer to be addressed. Allow them to choose seating for comfortable personal space and culturally appropriate eye contact. Avoid assumptions about where people come from; let them tell you. Most people are pleased when others show sincere interest in them. Strive to gain the other's trust, but do not resent it if you do not get it. Avoid body language that may be offensive or misunderstood. Determine the patient's level of fluency in English and arrange for an interpreter if needed. Speak directly to the client, even if an interpreter is present. Choose a speech rate and style that promotes understanding and demonstrates respect for the client. Avoid jargon, slang, and complex sentences. Do not expect clients to share your medical orientation. Use open-ended questions or questions phrased in several ways to obtain information, but be aware that some groups do not consider direct questions to be polite. Invite individuals to tell you stories about their problems and themselves. Determine the patient's English reading ability before using any written materials.

Safeguarding, preserving, advocating, and *protecting* guide awareness that people tend to see what they expect to see, and that stereotypes narrow vision by ignoring variations that occur naturally. Learning about diversity and caring involves recognizing and replacing stereotypes with informed, expectable patterns that serve merely as starting points for inquiry and comparison. Advocacy roles require cultural sensitivity, knowledge, and skill—including a willingness to examine personal values and those of the subcultures of nursing and biomedicine, as well as those of other individuals and cultural groups. Negotiate goals that are explicit and realistic. Check for client understanding and acceptance of recommendations. Be patient; do not expect rapid change. Be sensitive when describing or writing about groups. Present a generally comprehensive perspective that emphasizes the positive over the negative. Relate social organization, structure and process to each group's unique history. Acknowledge the diversity that occurs within as well as between and among groups. Beware of literature that uses deviant models rather than unbiased and fair information about groups. There is much of value to be found in both classic and modern literature, but it must be used critically owing to the propensity for bias.

The need for *engendering mutuality* and *community* reflects ways that health care providers and clients come together, get to know and value differences as well as commonalities, and form flexible, open, and creative relationships and caring communities. Avoid stereotypes by sex, age, race, ethnicity, socioeconomic status, and other characteristics. Remember that cultural generalizations may not differ much from stereotypes and may lead to prejudice if they are not open to being revised, that some people do not like having ethnic labels attached to them and wish to "be treated like everyone else," that culture is not restricted to people of color, that differences within groups may be greater than differences between groups, and that our own attitudes and blind spots may be more important than those of clients in terms of outcome. Understand your own cultural values and biases. Emphasize positive points and strengths of health beliefs and practices. Be respectful of values, beliefs, rights, and practices. Express interest in and understanding of other cultures without being judgmental. Some ideas may conflict with your own or with your determination to make changes, but every group and individual wants respect above all else. Show respect, especially for males, even if it is females or children you are particularly interested in. Males are often decision makers about health care.

Transcultural mental health nursing also necessitates an additional genre of practices that comprise *letting be* and *letting go* to expedite openness to learning. Learn to appreciate the richness of diversity as an asset rather than viewing it as a hindrance to communication and effective intervention. Honor the uniqueness of clients and their dignity and worth. Attempt to establish caring relationships that can overcome any cultural misstep, and strive to help clients obtain their self-determined goals, to learn clients' explanatory models, and to get to know yourself as an effective transcultural nurse.

Review Questions

1. How has the interpretation of mental health and mental illness changed with time?
2. Describe three ways in which diversity influences mental health and mental illness.
3. How are culture and mental health integrated into other aspects of living?
4. Describe how interactive processes and communication facilitate effective transcultural mental health care. How might interactive processes and communication erect barriers to effective transcultural mental health care?
5. Describe seven strategies that nurses can use to facilitate effective transcultural mental health care.

Learning Activities to Promote Critical Thinking

1. Write a story or a narrative about a personal experience that you have had or observed in which a cultural misunderstanding occurred. Critically evaluate and discuss how you felt as an observer and how you suppose the others involved in the situation felt? Discuss how the situation might have been more effectively managed?
2. Students often describe situations in which they work very diligently and then get ill when their work is finished or it is the weekend or vacation time. With two or three friends, share personal stories related to this or related phenomena. Reflect on how you and others explain these situations? Where did each of you learn the explanations that you provided? Now critically discuss how you have divided illnesses into physical and mental categories.
3. Having a family member with a severe mental illness often poses a strain on the entire family. Ask someone who has a family member with a psychiatric diagnosis to share his or her story. Critically analyze what the situation has that been like for the family? An excellent model or example for this is *Imagining Robert (My brother, madness, and survival): A memoir* by J. Neugeboren.

4. An excellent exercise to help pull together cultural sensitivity, knowledge, and skills for effective transcultural mental health nursing involves interviewing someone from a culture significantly different from your own. Practice your communication skills to ask about ideas and practices related to mental health and illness. Then delve into the literature about that person's affiliation or cultural group(s). Whether your interviewee is from Tibet, gay, or a century old, discuss how what you have read fails to represent (or successfully represents) the individual that you interviewed.

5. Compile a list of the groups that you affiliate with and in which you feel you are an "insider." Then list several groups with which you are not affiliated and where you would feel and "outsider." As honestly and comprehensively as you can, critically analyze why you are comfortable with some groups and not with others. If possible, get an insider's perspective of the group(s) to which you do not belong. Critically analyze the traits and attributes with which you might be comfortable (or uncomfortable). Evaluate the strengths and vulnerabilities of each group.

6. Rafael Campo includes the following poem in his 1996 book, *What the body was told*. Write down your interpretations of the poem from various perspectives, for instance, the culture of the elderly, an ethnic viewpoint, a holistic and humanistic nursing perspective, and others.

    Ten Patients, And Another
    I. Mrs. G.
    The patient is a sixty-odd-year-old
    White female, who presents with fever, cough
    And shaking chills. No further history
    Could be elicited; she doesn't speak.
    The patient's social history was non-
    Contributory: Someone left her here.
    The intern on the case heard crackles in
    Both lungs. An EKG was done, which showed
    A heart was beating in the normal sinus
    Rhythm, except for an occasional Dropped beat. An intravenous line was placed.
    The intern found a bruise behind her ear.
    She then became quite agitated, and
    Began to sob without producing tears.
    We think she's dry. She's resting quietly
    On Haldol, waiting for a bed upstairs.
    (Campo, 1996, p. 61)

7. Psychiatric symptoms typically reflect the cultural orientation of the mentally ill individual. How would you manage the following situation? You realize that your next door neighbor, a retired European American electrical engineer, has lined the interior walls of his house with aluminum foil to protect himself against the "beams" of the neighbors on the other side of him who are immigrants from another country and speak little English. What assessment strategies would you employ to distinguish the mental health issues from confounding cultural issues?

8. Role play is an effective strategy for developing cultural competence. With three colleagues, simulate a cultural encounter in which each of you takes

a different role: one is the client, one is the nurse who does not know what the client's cultural background is, one is a backup for the client and can say the things that the client is thinking but might hesitate to articulate, and one is the backup person for the nurse and provides ideas for questions or approaches when the nurse is stumped. Each person can see and hear each of the others as they role play encounters that are as realistic as possible. (Adapted from Pedersen, 1985, 1988; Kavanagh & Kennedy, 1992).

9. Effective communication involves listening attentively to people, accepting and acting upon what they say, ensuring that all communication can be understood by everyone, being trustful and sincere, acting in socially and culturally appropriate ways, and regularly advising others about what is happening (Stringer, 1996, p. 38). Discuss with someone you consider culturally competent how each of these criteria contributes to understanding in mental health settings.

References

Ahmed, I. (1997). Geriatric psychopathology. In W-S. Tseng & J. Streltzer (Eds.) *Culture and Psychopathology* (pp. 223–240). New York: Brunner/Mazel.

American Psychiatric Association. (1994). *Diagnostic and Statistical Manual—Fourth Edition.* (DSM-IV). Washington, DC: American Psychiatric Association.

Anderson, R. (1996). *Magic, Science, and Health: The Aims and Achievements of Medical Anthropology.* Fort Worth, TX: Harcourt Brace.

Arena, D. M., & Page, N. E. (1992). The imposter phenomenon in the clinical nurse specialist role. *Image,* 24(2), 121–125.

Attneave, C. (1982). American Indians and Alaskan Native families: Emigrants in their own homeland. In M. McGoldrick, J. K. Pearce, & J. Giordano (Eds.), *Ethnicity and Family Therapy* (pp. 55–83). New York: Guilford Press.

Baker, F. M. (1988). Afro-Americans. In L. Comas-Diaz & E. E. H. Griffith (Eds.), *Clinical Guidelines in Cross-Cultural Mental Health* (pp. 151–181). New York: John Wiley and Sons.

Baldwin, A. (1993, February). Psychiatric liaison nursing: A ready help in organizational change. *American Nurse,* p. 14.

Beiser, M., Waxler-Morrison, N., Iacono, W. G., Lin, T-Y., Fleming, J. A. E., & Husted, J. (1987). A measure of the 'sick' label in psychiatric disorder and physical illness. *Social Science and Medicine,* 25(3), 251–261.

Bell, C. C. (1990). Black-black homicide: The implications for black community mental health. In D. S. Ruiz (Ed.), *Handbook of Mental Health and Mental Disorder among Black Americans* (pp. 192–207). New York: Greenwood Press.

Benner, P., Tanner, C. A., & Chesla, C. A. (1996). *Expertise in Nursing Practice: Caring, Clinical Judgment, and Ethics.* New York: Springer.

Bernstein, D. M. (1997). Anxiety disorders. In W-S. Tseng & J. Streltzer (Eds.). *Culture and Psychopathology* (pp. 46–66). New York: Brunner/Mazel.

Billings, C. (1993, February). The "possible" dream of mental health reform. *American Nurse,* pp. 5, 9.

Bohannan, P. (1992). *We, the Alien: An Introduction to Cultural Anthropology.* Prospect Heights, IL: Waveland.

Bond, J. B., & Harvey, C. D. H. (1991). Ethnicity and intergenerational perceptions of family solidarity. *International Journal of Aging and Human Development,* 33(1), 33–44.

Bottorff, J. L. (1991). Nursing: A practical science of caring. *Advances in Nursing Science,* 14(1), 26–39.

Brislin, R. (1993). *Understanding Culture's Influence on Behavior.* Fort Worth: Harcourt Brace.

Brown, D. R. (1990). Depression among Blacks: An epidemiologic perspective. In D. S. Ruiz (Ed.), *Handbook of Mental Health and Mental Disorders among Black Americans* (pp. 71–93). New York: Greenwood Press.

Brown, P. (1989). Psychiatric dirty work revisited: Conflicts in servicing nonpsychiatric agencies. *Journal of Contemporary Ethnography,* 18(2), 182–201.

Bunch, E. H. (1983). *Everyday Reality and the Psychiatric Nurses: A Study of Communication Patterns Between the Schizophrenic and the Psychiatric Nurse.* Oslo, Norway: Gyldendal Norsk Forlag.

Burnside, I. M. (1988). *Nursing and the Aged.* New York: McGraw Hill.

Campinha-Bacote, J. (1997). Understanding the influence of culture. In J. Haber, B. Krainovich-Miller, A. L. McMahon, & P. Price-Hoskins (Eds.). *Comprehensive Psychiatric Nursing,* (5th Ed., pp. 75–90). St. Louis: Mosby.

Campo, R. (1996). *What the Body Told.* Durham, NC: Duke University Press.

Capers, C. F. (1985). Nursing and the Afro-American client. *Topics in Clinical Nursing,* 7(3), 11–17.

Chaplin, S. L. (1997). Somatization. In W-S. Tseng & J. Streltzer (Eds.). *Culture and Psychopathology* (pp. 67–86). New York: Brunner/Mazel.

Collins, J. L., Sorel, E., Brent, J., & Mathura, C. B. (1990). Ethnic and cultural factors in psychiatric diagnosis and treatment. In D. S. Ruiz (Ed.), *Handbook of Mental Health* and *Mental Disorder among Black Americans* (pp. 151–165). New York: Greenwood Press.

Comas-Diaz, L., & Griffith, E. E. H. (Eds.). (1988). *Clinical Guidelines in Cross-Cultural Mental Health.* New York: John Wiley and Sons.

Conrad, P., & Schneider, J. W. (1992). In *Deviance and Medicalization: From Badness to Sickness.* Philadelphia: Temple University Press.

Culture clash: Working with a difficult patient. (1996). *American Journal of Nursing* 96(11), 58.

Devereux, G. (1980). *Basic Problems of Ethnopsychiatry.* Chicago: University of Chicago Press.

Dewit, D. J., Wister, A. V., & Burch, T. K. (1988). Physical distance and social contact between elders and their adult children. *Research on Aging, 10*(1), 56–79.

Diekelmann, N. (1991). The emancipatory power of the narrative. In R. H. Schaperow (Ed.). *Curriculum Revolution: Community Building and Activism* (pp. 41–62). New York: National League for Nursing Press. Pub. No. 15–2398.

Diekelmann, N. (1994). Nursing Institute for Heideggerian Hermeneutical Studies, University of Wisconsin-Madison.

Diekelmann, N. (1995). *Narrative Pedagogy: Caring, Dialogue, and Practice.* Advanced Nursing Institute for Heideggerian Hermeneutical Studies, University of Wisconsin-Madison.

DuBray, W. H. (1992). *Human Services and American Indians.* Minneapolis: West Publishing.

Dunst, C., Trivette, C., & Deal, A. (1988). *Enabling and Empowering Families.* Cambridge, MA: Brookline Books.

Durant, J., & Miller, J. (1988). *Laughing Matters: A Serious Look at Humor.* New York: John Wiley and Sons.

Eisenbruch, M. (1992). Toward a culturally sensitive DSM: Bereavement in Cambodian refugees and the traditional healer as taxonomist. *Journal of Nervous and Mental Disease, 180*(1), 8–10.

Escobar, J. I. (1987). Cross-cultural aspects of the somatization trait. *Hospital and Community Psychiatry, 38*(2), 174–180.

Essed, P. (1991). *Understanding Everyday Racism: An Interdisciplinary Theory.* CA: Sage.

Fabrega, H. (1989). An ethnomedical perspective of Anglo American psychiatry. *American Journal of Psychiatry, 146,* 588–596.

Ficarrotto, T. J. (1990). Racism, sexism, and erotophobia: Attitudes of heterosexuals towards homosexuals. *Journal of Homosexuality 19,* 111–116.

Foster, G. M., & Anderson, B. G. (1978). *Medical Anthropology.* New York: John Wiley and Sons.

Franks, F., & Faux, S. A. (1990). Depression, stress, mastery, and social resources in four ethnocultural women's groups. *Research in Nursing and Health, 13,* 283–292.

Fry, C. L. (1990). Cross-cultural comparison of aging. In K. F. Ferraro (Ed.), *Gerontology: Perspectives and Issues.* New York: Springer.

Gaines, A. D. (1992). *Ethnopsychiatry: The Cultural Construction of Professional and Folk Psychiatries.* Albany: State University of New York Press.

Geller, J. D. (1988). Racial bias in the evaluation of patients for psychotherapy. In L. Comas-Diaz & E. E. H. Griffith (Eds.), *Clinical Guidelines in Cross-Cultural Mental Health* (pp. 112–134). New York: John Wiley and Sons.

Giago, T. (1984). *Notes from Indian Country, Volume 1.* Pierre, SD: State Publishing Company.

Goleman, D., & Gurin, J. (1993). *Mind Body Medicine.* Yonkers, NY: Consumer Reports.

Goode, E. E. (1988, 21 March). How psychiatry forgets the mind. *U.S. News and World Report,* 56–58.

Goode, E. E. (1993, 15 February). The cultures of illness. *U.S. News and World Report,* 74–76.

Gorman, L. M., Sultan, D. F., & Raines, M. L. (1996). *Davis's Manual of Psychosocial Nursing for General Patient Care.* Philadelphia: F. A. Davis.

Harrison, P. (1997). Suicidal behavior. In W-S. Tseng & J. Streltzer (Eds.). *Culture and Psychopathology* (pp. 157–172). New York: Brunner/Mazel.

Hauenstein, E. J. (1997). A nursing practice paradigm for depressed rural women: The women's affective illness treatment program. *Archives of Psychiatric Nursing 1,* 37–45.

Helman, C. G. (1990). *Culture, Health and Illness.* London: Wright.

Henry, W. A. (1990, 9 April). Beyond the melting pot. *TIME,* pp. 28–29.

Hirayama, H. (1985–86). Public policies and services for the aged in Japan. *Journal of Gerontological Social Work, 9,* 39–52.

Ho, M. K. (1987). *Family Therapy with Ethnic Minorities.* Newbury Park, CA: Sage.

Hughes, C. (1990). Ethnopsychiatry. In T. M. Johnson and C. F. Sargent (Eds.), *Medical Anthropology: A Handbook of Theory and Method* (pp. 133–148). New York: Greenwood Press.

Jackson, J. J. (1990). Suicide trends of Blacks and Whites by sex and age. In D. S. Ruiz(Ed.), *Handbook of Mental Health and Mental Disorder among Black Americans* (pp. 95–109). New York: Greenwood Press.

Jalali, B. (1982). Iranian families. In M. McGoldrick, J. K. Pearce and J. Giordano (Eds.), *Ethnicity and Family Therapy* (pp. 289–309). New York: Guilford Press.

Jezewski, M. A. (1990). Culture brokering in migrant farm worker health care. *Western Journal of Nursing Research, 12,* 497–513.

Jezewski, M. A. (1993). Culture brokering as a model for advocacy. *Nursing and Health Care, 14*(2), 78–85.

Kavanagh, K. H. (1988). The cost of caring: Nursing on a psychiatric intensive care unit. *Human Organization, 47*(3), 242–251.

Kavanagh, K. H. (1991). Invisibility and selective avoidance: Gender and ethnicity in psychiatry and psychiatric nursing staff interaction. *Culture, Medicine and Psychiatry, 15,* 245–274.

Kavanagh, K. H., & Kennedy, P. H. (1992). *Promoting Cultural Diversity: Strategies for Health Care Professionals.* Newbury Park, CA: Sage.

Kiev, A. (1972). *Transcultural Psychiatry.* New York: Free Press.

Kim, Y. Y., & Gudykunst, W. B. (1988). *Cross-Cultural Adaptation: Current Approaches.* Newbury Park, CA: Sage.

Kleinman, A. (1982). The teaching of clinically applied anthropology on a psychiatric consultation liaison service. In N. J. Chrisman and T. W. Maretzki, (Eds.), *Clinically Applied Anthropology* (pp. 83–115). Dordrecht, Holland: Reidel.

Kleinman, A. (1988). *Rethinking Psychiatry: From Cultural Category to Personal Experience*. New York: Free Press.

Kleinman, A. (1991, 28 March). "The future psychiatry." Special Department of Psychiatry Grand Rounds, University of Maryland Medical System, Baltimore, MD.

Kluegel, J. R., & Smith, E. R. (1986). *Beliefs About Inequality: Americans' Views of What Is and What Ought to Be*. New York: Aldine de Gruyter.

Kuo, C-L., & Kavanagh, K. H. (1994). Chinese perspectives on culture and mental health. *Mental Health Nursing*, 15(6), 551–567.

LaFargue, J. (1985). Mediating between two views of illness. *Transcultural Nursing*, 7, 70–77.

Lee, J.-J. (1985–86). Asian American elderly: A neglected minority group. *Journal of Gerontological Social Work*, 9, 103–116.

Leininger, M. (1984). Transcultural interviewing and health assessment. In P. B. Pedersen, N. Sartorius, and A. J. Marsella (Eds.), *Mental Health Services: The Cross-Cultural Context* (pp. 109–133). Beverly Hills, CA: Sage.

Leininger, M. M. (1988). Leininger's theory of nursing: Cultural care diversity and universality. *Nursing Science Quarterly*, 1(4), 152–160.

Leininger, M. M. (1991). Ethnonursing: A research method with enablers to study the theory of culture care. In M. M. Leininger (Ed.), *Culture Care Diversity and Universality: A Theory of Nursing* (pp. 73–117). New York: National League for Nursing Press. Pub. No. 15–2402.

Levinson, D. (1989). *Family Violence in Cross-Cultural Perspective*. Newbury Park, Sage.

Lewis, Thomas. (1990). *Medicine Men: Oglala Sioux Healing*. University of Nebraska.

Lex, B. (1977). Voodoo death: New thoughts on an old explanation. In D. Landy (Ed.), *Culture, Disease and Healing: Studies in Medical Anthropology* (pp. 327–332). New York: Macmillan.

Lipson, J. G. (1996). Come all peoples of the earth. *Sigma Theta Tau International Reflections* Fourth Quarter, 9–10.

Lipson, J. G., & Steiger, N. J. (1996). *Self-care Nursing in a Multicultural Context*. Thousand Oaks, CA: Sage.

Littlewood, R. (1991, April). DSM-IV and culture: Is the classification valid? Paper presented at the NIMH/American Psychiatric Association meeting, Pittsburgh, PA.

Locke, D. C. (1992). *Increasing Multicultural Understanding: A Comprehensive Model*. Newbury Park CA: Sage.

Luna, L. J. (1989). Transcultural nursing care of Arab Muslims. *Journal of Transcultural Nursing*, 1(1), 22–26.

Lutzen, K. (1990). Moral sensing and ideological conflict. *Scandinavian Journal of the Caring Sciences*, 4(2), 69–76.

Manson, S. P., Walker, R. D., & Kivlahan, D. R. (1987). Psychiatric assessment and treatment of American Indians and Alaskan Natives. *Hospital and Community Psychiatry*, 38(2), 165–173.

Marmor, T. R. (1994). *Understanding Health Care Reform*. New Haven: Yale University Press.

Mason, T. (1997). Seclusion and the lunar cycles. *Journal of Psychosocial Nursing* 35(6), 14–18.

Matteson, P. S. (1995). *Teaching Nursing in the Neighborhoods: The Northeastern University Model*. New York: Springer.

McCubbin, H. I., & McCubbin, M. A. (1988). Topologies of resilient families: Emerging roles of social class and ethnicity. *Family Relations*, 37, 247–254.

McKenna, M. A. (1989). Transcultural perspectives in the nursing care of the elderly. In J. S. Boyle & M. M. Andrews (Eds.), *Transcultural Concepts in Nursing Care*. Glenview, IL: Scott, Foresman.

Meleis, A. I., Lipson, J. G., & Paul, S. M. (1992). Ethnicity and health among five Middle Eastern immigrant groups. *Nursing Research*, 41(2), 98–103.

Milio, N. (1970). *9226 Kercleval: The Storefront that Did Not Burn*. Ann Arbor: University of Michigan Press.

Mollica, R. F. (1983). From asylum to community. *New England Journal of Medicine*, 308(7), 367–373.

Moon, J.-H., & Pearl, J. H. (1991). Alienation of elderly Korean American immigrants as related to place of residence, gender, age, years of education, time in the U.S., living with or without children, and living with or without a spouse. *International Journal of Aging and Human Development*, 32(2), 115–124.

Morrison, E. F. (1990). The tradition of toughness: A study of nonprofessional nursing care in psychiatric settings. *Image*, 22(1), 32–38.

Moyers, B. (1993). *Healing and the Mind*. New York: Doubleday.

Myerhoff, B. G., & Simic, A. (Eds.). (1978). *Life's Careers—Aging: Cultural Variations on Growing Old*. Beverly Hills, CA: Sage.

Myers, L. J. (1990). Understanding family violence: An Afro-centric analysis based on optimal theory. In D. S. Ruiz (Ed.), *Handbook of Mental Health and Mental Disorder among Black Americans* (pp. 183–189). New York: Greenwood Press.

Neugeboren, J. (1997). *Imagining Robert (My Brother, Madness, and Survival): A Memoir*. New York: William Morrow and Company.

Nguyen, M. N., & Organista, K. C. (1997). Vietnam Amerasians: Assimilation and adjustment problems in the United States. *Journal of Multicultural Social Work*, 6(1/2), 77–91.

Oakley, L. D., & Potter, C. (1997). *Psychiatric Primary Care*. St. Louis: Mosby.

Oltmanns, T. F., & Maher, B. A. (1988). *Delusional Beliefs*. New York: John Wiley and Sons.

Ory, F. G., Simons, M., Verhulst, F. C., Leenders, F. R. H.; & Wolters, W. H. G. (1991). Children who cross cultures. *Social Science and Medicine*, 32(1), 29–34.

Parker, S. (1977). Eskimo, psychopathology in the context of Eskimo personality and culture. In D. Landy (Ed.), *Culture, disease and healing: Studies in Medical Anthropology* (pp. 349–358). New York: Macmillan.

Pedersen, P. (Ed.). (1985). *Handbook of Cross-Cultural Counseling and Therapy*. Westport, CT: Greenwood Press.

Pedersen, P. (Ed.). (1988). The three stages of multicultural development: Awareness, knowledge, and skill. In *A Handbook for Developing Multicultural Awareness* (pp. 3–18). Alexandria, VA: American Association for Counseling and Development.

Pesut, D. J. (1991). The art, science, and techniques of reframing in psychiatric mental health nursing. *Issues in Mental Health Nursing*, 12(9), 9–18.

Pinderhughes, E. (1982). Afro-American families and the victim system. In M. McGoldrick, J. K. Pearce, & J. Giordano (Eds.), *Ethnicity and Family Therapy* (pp. 108–122). New York: Guilford Press.

Poussaint, A. F. (1990). The mental health status of black Americans, 1983. In D. S. Ruiz (Ed.). *Handbook of Mental*

Health and Mental Disorder Among Black Americans (pp. 17–52). New York: Greenwood Press.

Remen, R. N. (1996). *Kitchen Table Wisdom: Stories That Heal.* New York: Riverhead Books.

Rempusheski, V. F. (1989). The role of ethnicity in elder care. *Nursing Clinics of North America, 24*(3), 717–724.

Rose, S. M., & Black, B. L. (1985). *Advocacy and Empowerment: Mental Health Care in the Community.* Boston: Routledge & Kegan Paul.

Rothenberg, P. S. (1988). *Racism and Sexism: An Integrated Study.* New York: St. Martin's Press.

Rubel, A. J. (1977). The Epidemiology of a folk illness. In D. Landy (Ed.), *Culture, Disease and Healing: Studies in Medical Anthropology* (pp. 119–129). New York: Macmillan.

Russell, D. (1997). An oral history project in mental health nursing. *Journal of Advanced Nursing, 26,* 489–495.

Ruiz, D. S. (Ed.). (1990). *Handbook of Mental Health and Mental Disorder Among Black Americans.* New York: Greenwood Press.

Sabatino, F. (1993, 20 May). Culture shock: Are U.S. hospitals ready? *Hospitals,* pp. 23–28.

Sanday, P. R., & Goodenough, R. G. (Eds.). (1990). *Beyond the Second Sex: New Directions in the Anthropology of Gender.* Philadelphia: University of Pennsylvania Press.

Sandhu, D. S. (1997). Psychocultural profiles of Asian and Pacific Islander Americans: Implications for counseling and psychotherapy. *Journal of Multicultural Counseling and Development 25,* 7–22.

Scheper-Hughes, N. (1978). Saints, scholars, and schizophrenics: Madness and badness in Western Ireland. *Medical Anthropology, 2,* 59–93

Scheper-Hughes, N. (1982). Recent works in cultural psychiatry. *Medical Anthropology Newsletter, 13*(3), 1–2, 6–11.

Scheper-Hughes, N. (Ed.). (1987). The cultural politics of child survival. *Child Survival* (pp. 1–29). Dordrecht, Holland: D. Reidel.

Schultz-Ross, R. A. (1997). Violent behavior. In W-S. Tseng & J. Streltzer (Eds.). *Culture and Psychopathology* (pp. 173–189). New York: Brunner/Mazel.

Secundy, M. G. (1992). *Trials, Tribulations, and Celebrations: African-American Perspectives on Health, Illness, Aging and Loss.* Yarmouth ME: Intercultural Press.

Seelye, H. N. (1993). *Teaching Culture: Strategies for Intercultural Communication.* Lincolnwood, IL: National Textbook Company.

Sherer, J. L. (1993, 20 May). Crossing cultures: Hospitals begin breaking down the barriers to care. *Hospitals,* 29–31.

Shon, S. P., & Ja, D. Y. (1982). Asian families. In M. McGoldrick, J. K. Pearce, & J. Giordano (Eds.), *Ethnicity and Family Therapy* (pp. 208–228). New York: Guilford Press.

Snow, L. F. (1977). Popular medicine in a black neighborhood. In E. H. Spicer (Ed.), *Ethnic Medicine in the Southwest* (pp. 19–95). Tucson, AZ: University of Arizona Press.

Snow, L. F. (1993). *Walkin' Over Medicine.* Boulder, CO: Westview.

Sokolovsky, J. (1985). Ethnicity, culture and aging: Do differences really make a difference? *Journal of Applied Gerontology 4*(1), 6–17.

Sokolovsky, J. (Ed.). (1990). *The Cultural Context of Aging: Worldwide Perspectives.* New York: Bergin & Garvey.

Stanley, S. (1993, February). Bringing mental health care to Russia. *American Nurse,* pp. 12, 14.

Steinhausen, H-C., Offer, D., Ostrov, E., & Howard, K. I. (1988). Transcultural comparisons of self-image in German and United States adolescents. *Journal of Youth and Adolescence, 17*(6), 515–520.

Stringer, E. T. (1996). *Action Research: A Handbook for Practitioners.* Thousand Oaks, CA: Sage.

Summergrad, P. (1991). General hospital impatient psychiatry in the 1990s: Problems and possibilities. *General Hospital Psychiatry, 13,* 79–82.

Takeshita, J. (1997). Psychosis. In W-S. Tseng & J. Streltzer (Eds.) *Culture and Psychopathology* (pp. 124–138) New York: Brunner/Mazel.

Thomas, R. R. (1991). *Beyond Race and Gender: Unleashing the Power of Your Total Work Force by Managing Diversity.* New York: American Management Association.

Tripp-Reimer, T. (1984). Cultural diversity in therapy. In C. M. Beck, R. P. Rawlins, and S. R. Williams (Eds.), *Mental Health-Psychiatric Nursing: A Holistic Life-Cycle Approach* (pp. 381–398). St. Louis: C. V. Mosby.

Tseng, W-S. (1997). Overview: Culture and psychopathology. In W-S. Tseng & J. Streltzer (Eds.). *Culture and Psychopathology* (pp. 1–27). New York: Brunner/Mazel.

Tseng, W-S., & Streltzer. J. (1997).Integration and conclusions. In W-S. Tseng & J. Streltzer (Eds.). *Culture and Psychopathology* (pp. 241–252). New York: Brunner/Mazel.

United States Department of Health and Human Services. (1991). *Healthy People 2000.* Arlington, VA: CACI Marketing Systems.

Uzzell, D. (1977). Susto revisited: Illness as strategic role. In D. Landy (Ed.). *Culture, Disease and Healing: Studies in Medical Anthropology* (pp. 402–408). New York: Macmillan.

Vogel, V. J. (1970). *American Indian Medicine.* Norman: University of Oklahoma.

Vontress, C. E., & Epp, L. R. (1997). Historical hostility in the African American client: Implications for counseling. *Journal of Multicultural Counseling and Development 25,* 170–184.

Wali, A. (1992). Multiculturalism: An anthropological perspective. *Report from the Institute for Philosophy and Public Policy* (University of Maryland College Park) *12*(1), 6–8.

Weidman, H. (1979). Falling out: A diagnostic and treatment problem viewed from a transcultural perspective. *Social Science and Medicine, B13*(2), 95–112.

Westermeyer, J. (1987). Clinical considerations in cross-cultural diagnosis. *Hospital and Community Psychiatry, 38*(2), 160–165.

Wilson, H. S., & Kneisl, C. R. (1983). *Psychiatric Nursing.* Reading, MA: Addison-Wesley.

Wood, J. B. (1989). Communicating with older adults in health care settings: cultural and ethnic considerations. *Educational Gerontology, 15,* 351–362.

World Health Organization. (1973). *The International Pilot Study in Schizophrenia.* Geneva, Switzerland: WHO.

Yap, P. M. (1977). The culture-bound reactive syndromes. In D. Landy (Ed.), *Culture, Disease and Healing: Studies in Medical Anthropology* (pp. 340–349). New York: Macmillan.

Young, J. C. (1988). Rationale for clinician self-disclosure and research agenda. *Image, 20*(4), 196–199.

Chapter 8

Trends in Health Care Delivery and Contributions of Transcultural Nursing

Patti Ludwig-Beymer

KEY TERMS

Acute Care
Capitated Payment
Community Assessment
Community Mapping
Community Partnership
Continuous Quality Improvement
Coping Strategies
Critical Care

Critical Care Family Needs
   Inventory (CCFNI)
Cultural Assessment
Culturally Congruent Care
Customer Focus
Emic
Ethnocentrism

Etic
Family Issues
Fee-for-Service Reimbursement
Hospital Acuity
Per Member per Month (PMPM)
Stress
Vulnerability

OBJECTIVES

1. Describe the role of transcultural nursing in mediating the stress of hospitalized patients and their families.
2. Explain the changes in acuity experienced in hospital settings.
3. Illustrate the need for hospitals to partner with communities to achieve their mission.
4. Categorize the opportunities for transcultural nurses to enhance community partnerships.
5. Explain the role of listening to the customers in achieving continuous quality improvement.
6. Identify the capacity of transcultural nurses to improve care under capitated health care financing.

This book primarily deals with the impact of culture in a variety of health care settings (such as the hospital and community), in complex patient care situations (such as pain management), and across the life span of individuals (for example, childhood and aging). This chapter, however, chronicles four major trends in health care delivery and outlines how the specialty of transcultural nursing may impact the delivery of care given these trends. The major trends are (1) increasing hospital acuity, (2) increasing community partnership, (3) continuous quality improvement, and (4) payment changes from fee-for-service to capitation.

Hospital Acuity

Hospital acuity is rising at an ever-increasing rate. A number of factors contribute to this rise. First, procedures and testing previously performed on hospitalized patients have moved to the outpatient setting. In addition, many less complex surgical cases are being performed in ambulatory surgery, with a recovery period of several hours rather than several days. Third, nonsurgical patients are staying in the hospital for shorter periods of time. To provide a few examples, clients are able to receive chemotherapy, total parenteral nutrition, and ventilator care at home and in other non-acute care settings. Last, advanced technology results in acutely ill hospitalized patients. For example, advanced technology and treatments allow neonates to survive at lower birth weights. All of these factors contribute to increased acuity during hospitalization. It is predicted that in the near future, all hospitalized patients will be comparable to today's "critical care" patients.

Technology in the hospital environment is also increasing at a rapid rate, bringing obvious advantages, such as ease and accuracy of monitoring physical conditions and faster treatment of critically ill patients. However, a major challenge accompanies this use of technology: non-physiologic needs may not be identified and met as needed. In addition, family members or others significant to the client may be subjected to high levels of stress when they visit these technological environments, which may affect the demands they make on nursing staff (Clifford, 1986).

Transcultural concepts have been largely ignored as an aspect of providing nursing care to acutely ill clients. The lack of integration between critical care nursing and transcultural nursing may be partially explained by the relatively recent development of both areas. The formation of large intensive care units with sophisticated and specialized equipment occurred in the early 1960s (Stanton, 1991). The field of transcultural nursing, although conceptualized in the mid-1950s, did not emerge until the later part of the 1960s (Leininger, 1978, 1991, & 1995). In addition, critical care nursing has historically placed much emphasis on technical skills, procedures, and knowledge of physical sciences. When patients and their families experience the crisis of hospitalization in a critical care area, the nurse spends much energy providing curative interventions and physical care, often with little time available to help the family deal with the crisis (Caine, 1991). Adherence to the scientific or biomedical health paradigm is strong in critical care nursing. However, although scientific knowledge and technical skills are essential for critical care nurses, alone they fail to provide sufficient background for the practice of professional nursing. Health and nursing services cannot be adequate, effective, or comprehensive in any setting unless cultural aspects of health and illness are considered (Leininger, 1978, 1991, & 1995).

Regardless of reasons, the lack of integration between acute nursing care and transcultural nursing care has serious implications for clients. The delivery of culturally sensitive and congruent care (as described in Chapter 1) is imperative for nurses in all settings. This concept is particularly important in the acute care setting, where the patient is especially vulnerable due to separation from family and significant others, separation from familiar references, and situation stress.

Vulnerability

When acutely ill and requiring hospitalization, the patient is separated from family and significant others for long periods of time. In addition, by defining a family member in white American kinship terms (generally nuclear), the hospital may be isolating clients from important support offered by extended family members and friends. Despite the high activity level, it is easy for patients and their family members to feel alone in a critical care unit. Patients who come from traditional extended families are accustomed to interacting with a variety of family members. They may find the isolation to be particularly distressing. This forced separation from their family increases patients' vulnerability.

Even when family members are present, they are often prevented from participating in the delivery of patient care because of the complexity and technical nature of care required (Resin and Meleis, 1986) or because they feel uncomfortable in such a place. Families may even fear touching the patient because of the many tubes and machines attached to their loved one. The inability to touch is particularly alienating for cultural groups who express caring through overt gestures such as touching and when members expect care to be delivered by family members.

A second cause of vulnerability in critically ill patients involves separation from familiar references. Concepts such as time may have a different meaning for critical care nurses and critically ill patients. The nurse may attempt to be reassuring by saying "I'll check back with you in a little while." However, the patient's sense of time may be distorted by the hospitalization experience, resulting in anxiety and concern. In addition to the time distortion that occurs in a critical care setting, there are also cultural differences in time expectation. For example, the client may wonder, "What is a 'little while'?" or "What if something happens to me before that time is up?" These distortions and differences should be clarified with patients and families on a routine basis. Nurses should also consider expectations surrounding the concept of time when working with family members of patients from diverse cultures as not all cultures are as precise and "clock oriented" as are acute care settings.

Another cause of separation from familiar references is restriction of familiar objects. To reduce the amount of clutter in the area and prevent safety hazards, many hospital units permit very few personal items. Instead, patients may be surrounded by items that have no meaning to them. Yet often a few items that have cultural meaning, such as photographs, mementos, or familiar clothing, would be of comfort to patients.

A third familiar reference that may be restricted is sleep. Hospitals are typically noisy, active places both day and night. Lights may shine continuously; the sounds of technical equipment, particularly shrill alarms, also make it difficult to sleep or rest. In addition, patients may be unaccustomed to sleeping alone, or in Western-style beds. Instead, patients of diverse cultural groups may be more comfortable sleeping with others in the same room or bed, or resting on mats on the floor.

Conversely, the patient may be used to sleeping alone or in a separate room and may find it disconcerting to share a large unit with several patients of mixed genders.

A third cause of vulnerability, affecting both acutely ill patients and their families, is stress. Literature about critical care addresses the nature and degree of stress experienced by patients and family members. However, cultural differences are not addressed. Pain, fear of death, isolation, loss, grief, sensory overload, sensory deprivation and many other factors contribute to the stress experienced in a critical care setting and they are expressed by culturally diverse patients and families in a variety of ways. Common hospital practices may be disturbing to many patients, especially to those from cultures other than the dominant Anglo-American culture. For example, patients may feel vulnerable when their care is provided by a caregiver of the opposite gender. The practice of "rounding," with lengthy case discussion by the bedside, may also result in a sense of vulnerability and embarrassment. This perception is worsened by isolation from family.

Perhaps the biggest factor in the development of stress is the unknown. Exposure to the hospital, where the patient observes strange procedures and hears unfamiliar words and noises, may result in culture shock. Certainly, the usual stress may be intensified by cultural differences. This is especially evident when the language of the patient is different from the language spoken by the health care providers, with communication in this situation quite difficult. Increased stress may even result in regression to a language spoken during childhood, a more safe and secure period. Patients who have not spoken their native language for years have reverted to that language while hospitalized for an acute illness or injury.

To complicate matters further, support for both patients and family members is often fragmented in critical care settings (Halm, 1990). Families must interact with a myriad of providers from many disciplines, with each person involved in only one aspect of the overall care. Concerned family members often lack one contact person to help them work through this fragmentation. Nurses are challenged to demonstrate cultural sensitivity and plan and deliver culturally congruent care to vulnerable acutely ill patients and their families.

Family Issues

Hospitalization for an acute illness is typically viewed as a crisis situation. Admission to the critical care unit causes distress for both patients and families. Most of the staff's energy is devoted to providing patient care, with little time left to help the family deal with the crisis. Yet the family has a tremendous influence on the sick member's immediate and long-term recovery. Considering the patient as a member of a family unit is essential when attempting to provide comprehensive and culturally congruent care. Critical care nurses must identify the specific needs of family members and intervene appropriately to meet these needs (Wooley, 1990). By providing support and care for the family, the family can be healthier, leading to better care for the critically ill patient.

Establishing relationships with families in critical care is an essential part of high-quality care. Critical care nurse–family relationships are important to the patient and family and also benefit the nurse. These relationships require negotiation and must take into account the needs of family and nurse. Possible barriers include limited time, perception that families are stressors, dysfunctional response styles, and premature judgment. Essential skills are trust, empathy, respect, warmth, sensitivity, and touching. In such a situation, the nurse needs both verbal and nonverbal skills (Artinian, 1991).

Numerous independent studies suggest that families of critically ill hospitalized patients have primary needs for assurance, proximity, and information (Hickey, 1990; Koller, 1991; Leske, 1991). Many of these studies have used the Critical Care Family Needs Inventory (CCFNI). The tool has established reliability and validity (Leske, 1988) and inventories five need areas: support, comfort, information, proximity, and assurance.

An early attempt to identify the needs of critical care family members was made by Molter (1979). In this research, the need for hope was the most important universal need identified by critical care family members. Other important needs included receiving adequate and honest information, and feeling that the hospital staff members were concerned about the patient. These needs were most often met by nurses, followed by physicians and other sources of support. The relatives perceived the role of the health professional to be patient, rather than family, focused.

These findings have been corroborated by other researchers (Engli & Kirsivali-Farmer, 1993; Leske, 1986; Norris & Grove, 1986). Additional research (Price, et. al., 1991) suggested critical care family members need honest, intelligible, and timely information and need to feel assured that their loved one is being cared for by competent and caring people. In this study, however, the need to feel there was hope had lesser importance. Similarly, when examining the immediate needs of families of neurologic/neurosurgical patients during the critical care period, Bernstein (1990) found that the most important needs were communication, honesty, and reassurance.

In a phenomenologic study, Titler, Cohen, and Craft (1991) identified six ways in which hospitalization in a critical care unit affected the family unit, including lack of communication among family members; protecting children from anxiety-provoking information; overriding threat, exemplified by feelings of vulnerability, uncertainty, intense emotions, and physical illness in children; disruption of normal home routines; changes in relationships; and role conflict.

Kreamer (1989) investigated coping strategies of critical care family members. Common coping strategies used by family members included seeking social support, positive reappraisal, playful problem solving, and self-controlling. Families tended to perceive their family members as more severely ill than objective measures indicated.

Koller (1991) found that the need to know the patient's prognosis was identified as most important by critical care family members. Although hope was the most commonly used method of coping, confronting and optimism were described as most useful and effective overall. Nursing interventions described by family members as helpful included the provision of information and emotional support, and the competence and manner of the nurse. This research fails to describe the cultural composition of subjects from whom data were collected. Thus, the applicability of these findings to culturally diverse families is unknown.

A limited amount of transcultural research has been conducted in this area. Coutu-Wakulczyk and Chartier (1990) used a translated version of the CCFNI with French-speaking critical care family members to begin to examine family needs in a

French-Canadian context. In this study, the most important needs identified by family members were honestly answered questions, assurance of best possible care, and hope. This research enhances the understanding of family needs in relation to culture. In a follow-up study conducted in both French and English, Rukholm, et al. (1991) found that situation anxiety and family needs were significantly related.

Nurses are only moderately accurate in their assessments of critical care family needs. Using the CCFNI, Kleinpell and Powers (1992) compared family and nurse perceptions of family needs and the degree to which the needs were met. Family members and nurses identified many similar important needs, including the need to have questions answered honestly, the need to be called at home about changes in the patient's condition, and the need to know why things were done for the patient. However, family members rated the need to (1) know the occupational identity of the staff members, (2) receive instructions of actions to take at the patient's bedside, and (3) have friends for support higher than did nurses, and family members indicated these needs were not being met.

When comparing family members' perceptions and nurses' assessments of the most and least important needs, Forrester, et al. (1990) detected statistically significant differences for 50 percent of the critical care family needs. Further, Murphy, et al. (1992) explored the relationship between the empathy of intensive care unit nurses and their ability to accurately assess the needs of critical care family members. Using the CCFNI, they found that the more empathetic the nurses were, the more accurately they were able to assess family member needs. Length of nursing experience negatively affected the nurse's ability to assess family members' needs accurately. Research also suggests that nurses' perceptions of critical care family needs were influenced by units worked, length of time practicing in critical care, educational preparation, and time in nursing (O'Malley, et al., 1991).

Reider's research (1989) suggested that satisfaction of family needs was not related to family adjustment. However, family coping, seeking spiritual support, and passive appraisal were positively related to family adjustment. Age of the family member and age of the patient were also related to family adjustment, with more difficult adjustments being noted for younger family members and pediatric patients. Trauma cases were associated with lower levels of family adjustment.

Critical care nurses can provide social support to family members through family assessment, counseling, referral, and support groups. Families must be an integral part of the hospitalization experience. Strategies that may be helpful in achieving this include formulating a staff-led family support group and family committee, instituting a family visitation contract, and developing nurse expertise in family care (Smith, et al., 1991). Although not empirically tested, it is generally believed that such support will influence the ability of family members to provide support to the patient and thereby influence a positive recovery from critical illness (Halm, 1992).

In a quasi-experimental study to examine the effectiveness of support groups for critical care family members, Halm (1990) found that subjects who attended a support group to share feelings and experiences in coping with illness had a statistically significant reduction in anxiety compared with subjects who received standard bedside support from nurses during visiting hours. These findings suggest that interventions may be helpful in reducing anxiety associated with the crisis of critical illness in the family system.

Conversely, Watson's (1991) research found no statistically significant differences in the extent to which family members perceived their needs as being met between a group receiving usual nursing interventions, a group receiving support interventions, and a group receiving informational interventions. As with research into the needs of family members of patients in critical care, the cultural composition of the intervention research subjects is unknown. The studies, while valuable, do little to advance our ability to work with culturally diverse patients and families. Yet there is a real need to create an environment for acutely ill patients and their family members that provides and allows for well-balanced, humanistic, and thoughtful patient care (Clement, 1988). To provide such care, critical care nurses must have the ability to address cultural needs of patients.

Implications for Nurses: Providing Culturally Congruent Care

When nurses do not understand the dynamics of a particular situation, a cycle of distrust may develop. The nurse may assist the patient and family members without understanding and taking into account their culture. Patients and family members, who may not understand the dominant culture, may begin to feel stressed, estranged, and vulnerable, and may withdraw or lash out. The nurse may become hurt and angry when the care is not well received or appreciated, Thus, a cycle of distrust and antagonism develops.

However, misconceptions, inaccurate perceptions, distrust and antagonism need not occur with individuals from different cultures. If nurses acknowledge cultural differences and incorporate cultural sensitivity into their practice of critical care nursing, patients and their families may experience increased well-being. Assessment skills may be honed to ensure an adequate understanding of the patient so that appropriate care may be delivered. In addition, practices may be modified and delivered in a way that is compatible with the patient's culture. Two cases are described below to illustrate these points.

Cultural Assessment

Most practicing nurses provide care to some people whose cultural beliefs and values are different from their own. It is unrealistic to expect any nurse to have full knowledge of the beliefs, lifestyles, and health practices of the many cultural groups for whom she or he provides care. However, in order to provide nursing care that is congruent with the patient's own lifestyle and cultural values, the nurse must incorporate transcultural concepts into nursing practice. The critical care nurse, who must remain technically competent, is no exception. Transcultural concepts should not replace other aspects of nursing care. Instead, these concepts should be integrated into the everyday practice of critical care nursing. The nursing assessment provides an ideal entry point for transcultural concepts.

Several parts of the nursing assessment process used in critical care settings are meaningless when taken out of cultural context. This is particularly true for a neurologic assessment, which cannot be interpreted without some knowledge of the patient's culture. Consider the following example:

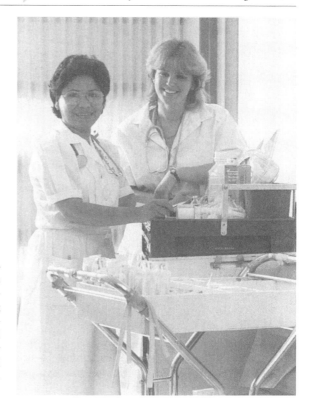

Incorporating individuals with a variety of racial, ethnic, and cultural backgrounds in the planning of care may facilitate the administration of culturally specific and appropriate care. (Reprinted by permission of Lutheran General Health System, Parkridge, Illinois.)

CASE STUDY 8.1

Mrs. Christiansen, an elderly woman who appears to fit within the dominant culture, is admitted to the intensive care unit after a craniotomy. A thorough neurologic assessment is a high priority. As part of the assessment to determine level of consciousness, the nurse asks Mrs. Christiansen, "Who's the president?"

The nurse is surprised when Mrs. Christiansen responds with an unfamiliar name. The nurse repeats the question and is further concerned when Mrs. Christiansen's curt response is the same. "Furthermore," Mrs. Christiansen indignantly adds, "Everyone knows that."

Upon investigation, the nurse learns that the name mentioned by Mrs. Christiansen is that of the president of the Mormon Church. Mrs. Christiansen is a Mormon (member of the Church of Jesus Christ of Latter Day Saints), and she has responded from her primary field of reference. The president of her church is far more important in her daily life than is the President of the United States.

Mrs. Christiansen's response indicates considerable mental awareness and is the most correct and culturally specific answer for her. However, if the nurse had not recognized the cultural values held by Mrs. Christiansen, the assessment would have been incorrect and might even have been used for unwarranted treatment.

In this example, both the nurse and the patient demonstrate ethnocentricism. Because the patient looks the same and speaks the same language as the nurse, the nurse assumes that the patient's frame of reference is the same as her own. The possibility of a subculture is not considered. At the same time, the client assumes that her religion is known and understood by the nurse.

Patients and families benefit from cultural sensitivity and the provision of culturally congruent care in many ways. The following case study demonstrates the importance of understanding family roles when providing culturally congruent care in an acute care setting. In addition, this case emphasizes the need for an open attitude and a willingness to ask questions rather than making false assumptions.

CASE STUDY 8.2

Mrs. Trudeau, a 42-year-old woman from Trinidad, was in the terminal stages of leukemia. Because of her need for intensive care, she was placed on a step-down unit. Although her husband visited daily with clean nightgowns and food from home, he failed to offer emotional support and solace to his wife.

The nurse staff was appalled and had difficulty interacting with Mr. Trudeau. In fact, some nurses had difficulty even being polite to him. Yet Mrs. Trudeau, although depressed, did not seem concerned by what the staff perceived as a lack of support.

Finally, a nurse asked Mrs. Trudeau about her husband's behavior. Mrs. Trudeau explained that in their culture, his behavior was quite appropriate. He was expected to provide physically for her, but emotional support was to come from female relatives, particularly sisters.

Because no sisters were present to provide emotional support, Mrs. Trudeau felt isolated. Nursing staff and hospital volunteers became surrogate sisters and provided much support to Mrs. Trudeau. With an understanding of the cultural dynamics, the staff members were also able to support Mr. Trudeau during his wife's illness and after her death.

This example demonstrates the serious consequences of judging without understanding. In an ethnocentric manner, nurses assumed that they understood the dynamics of the situation. In addition, they sent a paternalistic message to the Trudeaus: "We know what's best for you." This was communicated to Mr. Trudeau through their avoidance of him when he visited his wife. Perhaps through behavior modification, the nurses hoped to moderate what they considered to be a negative behavior.

Fortunately, the behavior was questioned by a nurse. Cultural variations in the husband-wife role were acknowledged and addressed. Rather than imposing the roles advocated by the dominant society, the nurses accepted the roles used by the Trudeaus. Mr. Trudeau's visits were welcomed and emotional support was provided to Mrs. Trudeau by female nurses and volunteers, addressing the culturally specific need for female support.

Acuity Summary

As increasingly critically ill patients are hospitalized, health care must learn the lessons experienced in critical care units. Today's critical care environment is some-times viewed as contrary to the humane treatment of critically ill patients and their families. For patients and their family members, hospitalization is a frightening and dehumanizing experience as they are confronted with stressors that disrupt normal family functioning. The nurse is the pivotal person to positively affect family coping (Kupferschmid, et al., 1991).

To diminish the negative aspects of both the acute illness and the environment, specific strategies to foster more culturally appropriate care are needed. Transcultural concepts can facilitate the shift, creating an environment where healing and recovery are possible. It is undesirable for nurses to stereotype based on culture or use a "cookbook" approach when dealing with people of different cultures. However, a knowledge of the general concepts presented in this text will assist the nurse in caring for people from diverse cultures. Within critical care practice, nurses must begin by recognizing their own beliefs and values. Incorporating a cultural assessment into routine nursing practice is essential. Modifying nursing care practices to fit patients' special values and health needs must also be accomplished. Only in this fashion will professional nursing care be provided to vulnerable critically ill patients and their families.

Community Partnerships

At the same time that hospitals are experiencing increased acuity, they are also reaffirming their intent to partner with communities (Pelfrey & Theisen, 1993). Hospitals are clearly stating their mission to improve the health of the communities they serve. Historically, hospitals have fulfilled this mission through charity care, health care professional education and research, community education programming, and community outreach (Pelfrey & Theisen, 1993). However, there is growing recognition that true improvements in the health of a community require the focused efforts of the entire community. Such improvement may only occur in partnerships with community members and other community organizations. The Healthy Communities Project, as envisioned by Health Care Forum and others, is one example of this trend in health care.

Types of Partnering

To explain community partnerships in part, examples will be used from Advocate Health Care, an Integrated Delivery System in the Chicago metropolitan area. Advocate Health Care consists of eight hospitals, home health, extended care, physician medical groups, and physician-hospital organizations. Personnel at each hospital have collaborated with surrounding communities to conduct community health assessments. In community mapping, staff collect a variety of data including demographics, health status, community resources, barriers, and enablers. Both strengths and needs are identified from the perspective of the community. All of these data are then used collaboratively with communities to set priorities (see Chapter 10 for additional detail on community assessment).

To conduct such community assessments requires cultural awareness and sensitivity. To interpret the data requires knowledge of the cultural dimensions to health and illness. To use the data to develop and implement programs in conjunction with the community requires the ability to plan and implement culturally congruent care. Data from these assessments have been used to set priorities and guide the planning and implementation of key initiatives. These initiatives are most well accepted when they are sponsored by a variety of community organizations, not just by a hospital.

After priorities are set, hospital personnel are partnering with schools and the health department to establish school-based programs. In addition, hospital personnel are partnering with a variety of religious denominations to provide congregationally based programs, such as parish nursing services and congregational health services. To enhance disease prevention, hospital personnel are working with local health departments to provide immunization programs and with youth groups, schools and churches to provide health fairs and career mentoring. Hospital personnel are working with physicians and communities to implement the Healthy Steps for Young Children program, sponsored by the Commonwealth Fund.

This 3-year demonstration program offers mothers and fathers with young children primary health care, sequential in-home visits, periodic developmental assessments, a free parental advice line, books, pamphlets, videos and other materials, support groups, and information about and access to available community services. It is being implemented at pediatric sites linked with three Advocate Health Care hospitals. Last, to address specific disease conditions, hospital personnel are partnering with appropriate personnel from community agencies. For example, partnerships between individuals from hospitals, the Metropolitan Chicago American Lung Association, the Chicago Asthma Consortium, and schools are designed to provide better care for children with asthma.

By using the assessment of the communities served by Lutheran General Hospital, one of Advocate Health Care's hospitals, and analyzing data from clinical practice, staff identified that Hispanics make up an increasing proportion of the population, and are the most frequently underserved population. As a result, a family practice physician initiated the idea for a community center for health and empowerment. A coalition comprised of individuals from health care, social services, health care agencies, schools, police, churches, businesses, city government, and other community services also identified the Hispanic community as underserved. This group provided an etic, or outsider, view of the Hispanic community.

To provide a local or emic (insider) view, community members worked with health care personnel to design and conduct a door-to-door community assessment. As described elsewhere (Ludwig-Beymer, et al., 1996), Leininger's Theory of Cultural Diversity and Universality served to guide the assessment. The steps in the assessment are summarized in Table 8–1. The community made key decisions, including selecting the site for the center, choosing the name for the center, and establishing a sliding scale for fees. The bilingual primary care center was opened in July 1995.

In addition to primary health care services, clients may also access the WIC (Women-Infant-Children) program on site, run by the county health department. A salaried community outreach worker coordinates the community empowerment program. In collaboration with businesses, churches, and city services, community members have undergone training in group work and priority setting. Activities for youth were identified as concerns on the community assessment. As a result, community members and center personnel have actively partnered with the Park District, schools, churches and the police to provide recreational activities for youth. The community also uses this as an opportunity to celebrate their cultural heritage. Health

TABLE 8-1

Steps in the Community Assessment Used at Genesis Center of Health and Empowerment

1. Conduct focus groups to identify common community issues
    −Community members explore values, needs, and priorities
2. Develop a questionnaire of structured interview guide based on the focus group results
    −Each item is evaluated on two dimensions: importance of the issue and satisfaction with the current status
3. Administer the interview guide to community members
    −Pilot the tool and revise as needed
    −Train community members to serve as interviewers
    −Administer the guide to a broad sample of the community
4. Analyze the data
    −Interpret the data based on transcultural understanding of the community
    −Solicit input from community interviewers
5. Share the results with the community
    −Conduct public hearings in which community members discuss the results and identify strategies for preserving strengths and remediating needs
    −Organize action committees to address strengths and needs
    −Share results with other community agencies
    −Prepare final report and disseminate throughout the community

promotion materials and activities are also provided through collaboration. For example, a health fair for seniors was provided in partnership with the health department and the park district.

Transcultural Nursing Implications

Transcultural nurses can and should play an active role in healthy community projects and community partnerships because they possess the necessary knowledge and

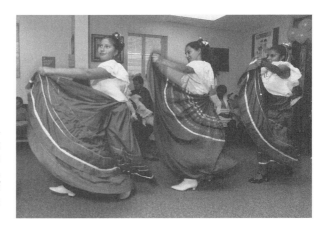

By active partnering, youth are able to participate in native music and dance exhibitions. (Reprinted by permission of Advocate Health Care, Oak Brook, IL.)

skill sets. In particular, the transcultural nurse brings sensitivity and insight to the assessment process. In addition, programs must be planned in conjunction with nurses who understand the need and the way to deliver culturally congruent care. The Center described above exemplifies the type of care possible in an environment in which personnel insist upon the delivery of culturally congruent health care. Additional aspects of the Center are discussed in the next section of this chapter.

Continuous Quality Improvement

Everywhere in health care, the concept of quality is being emphasized. Whether the term is quality management, continuous quality improvement, quality deployment, total quality management, or just quality, the concept is ever-present in health care. Continuous Quality Improvement (CQI) is a philosophy that involves a never ending cycle of continuous improvements in quality (Deming, 1986). This new perception of quality is different from the previous view of quality assurance (QA). Traditionally, QA looked at quality in terms of standards. When standards were not met (or thresholds were not reached), action was taken with the individuals deemed responsible for the failures. On the other hand, CQI looks at quality as a dynamic phenomenon. Rather than blaming individuals, CQI looks at processes to determine why a process is producing outcomes that do not meet or exceed customer expectations. Instead of identifying quality deficiencies, the new quality strives to continually improve the quality of health care products and services.

CQI is grounded in three basic principles: (1) it is customer focused, (2) it analyzes the processes that customers experience, and (3) it uses data to make decisions (Carey & Lloyd, 1995). CQI occurs when all three of these concepts come together on a daily basis. Pursuit of only one or two of these principles will cause organizations to fall short of the true potential of CQI.

CQI begins with listening to the needs and wants of the "customer." In the past, health care professionals often forgot the importance of the customer, believing only they (and not the patients) could understand and appreciate the complexities of the health care industry. However, the health care industry is increasingly coming to understand that customers can and should help to define quality and set the expectations for performance. While customers may not know the specifics of how technical dimensions of care are delivered, they can certainly identify how they feel about the ways in which they were treated and the outcomes they experienced.

After listening to the customers and determining what they want, need or expect, the next step is to gain an understanding of the processes in place that will either delight or repel the customers. One of the most frequently used tools to assist in this stage of CQI is the flowchart. By using a flowchart of the current process, nurses gain a deeper appreciation for the complexity of the process and identify opportunities for improvement. Nurses must understand the processes in place and comprehend which components of the process are having the greatest influence on the customers.

For example, the processes in place for accessing care are often complex and time-consuming to negotiate. These processes are particularly difficult for non-English speaking individuals. By using a flowchart what the client experiences, the nurse

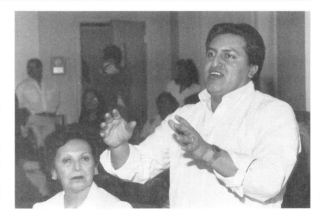

Community meetings provide a forum for listening to what the customers—community members—need and want. Here, a community member discusses the results of community assessment. (Reprinted by permission of Advocate Health Care, Oak Brook, IL.)

becomes aware of barriers to care. Culturally sensitive nurses must help streamline these processes to decrease the barriers to access to health care.

The final CQI principle is that data are needed for making good decisions. A criticism of the health care profession has been that decision making is often driven by anecdotes rather than data. Organizations embracing CQI rely on current data to evaluate the processes delivering products or services to customers.

To describe the process of listening more clearly, consider the center described earlier. The center was established in collaboration with the community it seeks to serve. Researchers and staff members listened carefully to the concerns of Hispanic community members and planned the health center accordingly. This was accomplished both formally and informally. Formally, the center sponsored a community assessment. The assessment process involved two focus groups, 15 community interviewers, and 220 door-to-door interviews. In addition, five meetings, attended by 180 community members, were held to report the findings to community members and solicit their input into the etiology and retention of strengths or resolution of needs. As a result, numerous task forces have been formed to preserve strengths or mediate needs. Less formally, the staff listen attentively to individuals who use the center, for both medical care and social support. The stories they hear are shared with other staff members and the center's director at regularly scheduled staff meetings.

These examples illustrate the eagerness of personnel at the center to understand the local or emic perspective of the people they serve. It must go beyond listening, however. The emic perspective must be used to tailor the delivery of health care. In addition, the center also needs to demonstrate that it is making a difference in the lives of community members it serves. One way it is demonstrating this is through the use of a standard patient satisfaction survey, which has been administered to clients receiving care in 225 physician offices nationwide. Using the Spanish version, 141 patients completed the survey at the Center. Patient satisfaction with care delivered at the Center was compared with overall satisfaction in the reference data base (225 physician offices). The survey results suggest that the Center's patients view the quality of care they receive positively (see Table 8–2).

TABLE 8-2
Genesis Center of Health and Empowerment Patient Satisfaction

Quality Scale/Subscale	Genesis Center of Health and Empowerment (n = 141 patients)	Medical Group Norms (n = 225 physician offices)
Composite quality (weighted average)	86.5*	80.4
Satisfaction subscales		
Physician care	85.9*	80.3
Nursing care	89.3*	80.3
Front office	88.0*	80.3
Accessibility	78.9	72.0
Testing services	81.7	79.4
Facility	85.4*	76.0
Billing	82.2*	72.9
Single-item questions		
How would you rate doctor's instructions about medications and follow-up?	87*	82
How would you rate doctor's advice on avoiding illness/staying healthy?	88*	76
How would you rate the outcome of your medical care?	86*	77
How would you rate the nurse's personal manner?	91*	84
How would you rate how well the nurse answered your questions?	89*	80
How would you rate the courtesy of the office receptionist?	90*	82
How would you rate the comfort of the waiting area?	89*	79
How would you rate the availability of the doctor to talk on the phone?	80**	55
How would you rate the availability of the nurse to talk on the phone?	83*	74
How would you rate the reasonableness of fees?	80*	63
How would you rate the convenience of the location of doctor's office?	85*	78
How would you rate the respect shown for your privacy?	91*	86
How would you rate the cleanliness of the examination room?	91*	86

*Genesis is one standard deviation higher than the medical group norms.
**Genesis is two standard deviations higher than the medical group norms.

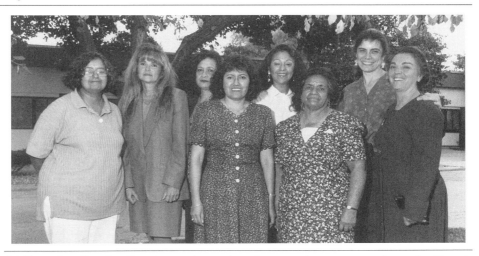

A bilingual staff makes listening to the needs and wants of customers easier at the Genesis Center. (Reprinted by permission of Advocate Health Care, Oak Brook, IL.)

Transcultural Nursing Implications

The data that come from listening to the customer provide clear messages about the expectations of those served. Transcultural nurses have a long history of listening to people; such listening occurs whenever the emic view of the situation is elicited. Transcultural nurses avoid imposing the etic, or outsider, view on a cultural group. Instead, the research methodologies used by transcultural nurses help explicate meaning for the cultural groups studied and served. This is a step in the journey of truly listening to the customer, and can benefit the customer as well as the health care system. Transcultural nurses also apply what they learn in their research. By applying research findings, culturally congruent care is provided.

Do listening, designing culturally appropriate care, and delivering that care really make a difference? According to the patient satisfaction data, satisfaction with the care provided at the center is significantly greater than patient satisfaction in other office settings. The culturally congruent care delivered at the center explains at least part of this level of satisfaction. Investigation into the impact of culturally appropriate care on functional status and use of health care resources is currently under way, with positive preliminary results.

Payment Changes From Fee-for-Service to Capitation

Most people in the Unites States have some form of private or public health insurance, although the coverage may be limited. About 80 percent of those in the U.S. carry private health insurance. In Canada, nearly all people are covered by provincial government health insurance. Additional coverage through private insurers is also available.

Private health insurance in the U.S. is offered mainly by insurance companies, medical service plans, health maintenance organizations (HMOs), and employers.

Many companies that sell health insurance policies provide cash benefits to the insured person. A cash benefit is a fixed dollar amount for each medical expense or day of hospitalization. If the cost of the service is greater than the cash benefit, the policyholder must pay the balance. Medical service plans pay service benefits, which is a direct payment to the hospital or physician that provided the medical care. Payments are limited to "usual and customary charges," the average cost of a particular medical service in the area in which the insured person lives. HMOs provide nearly complete health care services for a prepaid monthly or yearly fee. Such services include preventive care, checkups, emergency services and hospitalization. Members may use only physicians and hospitals approved by the HMO (Ellwood, 1994). Finally, employers may pay for the health care costs of their employees rather than purchase insurance. In this way, companies can design benefit plans to meet the needs of their employees. Many larger companies have made these arrangements. Health care coverage in the U.S. is outlined in Table 8–3.

Changing Financial Incentives

As financial incentives in health care change, it is becoming increasingly important to keep people well rather than treating them after an illness has occurred. Traditionally, insurance companies, medical service plans, and employers provided fee-for-service reimbursement. Under this payment system, physicians, hospitals, and other providers were reimbursed based on the volume and type of care they provided. There was little incentive to minimize the number of tests or procedures or hospital lengths of stay, and abuses of the payment system were prevalent. More care was viewed as better; it resulted in higher reimbursements to providers and in well-tested clients.

However, capitation (through managed care) is becoming increasingly prevalent today. HMOs control costs partly by selecting cost-effective physicians and hospitals and by emphasizing preventive care. They also reduce costs by substituting outpatient care for inpatient care when appropriate and by reviewing the need for hospitalization. Under a capitated system, physicians, hospitals and other providers are prospectively paid a fixed amount of money, typically referred to as "per member per month" or "PMPM." This prospective payment must be used to provide whatever care is needed for the individual within the given time period. Abuses of this payment system may also occur; for example, less than optimal care may be delivered if providers deny

TABLE 8-3
Health Care Coverage for Persons Younger than Age 65 in the United States

Insurance Status	Percentage
Employer-provided health insurance, 1994	64.5
Full-time nonelderly workers without health insurance, 1994	17.3
Medicaid	12.6
Other private insurance	7.2
Other public insurance	3.7

Data source: McCloskey, A. H., Holahan, D., Brangan, N. et al. (1996). *Reforming the health care system: State profiles 1996.* Washington, D.C.: American Association of Retired Persons.

needed services in order to preserve dollars. However, capitated payments do align incentives to keep people healthy rather than allowing illness to progress.

A less restrictive type of managed care is available through preferred provider organizations (PPOs). PPOs consist of doctors and hospitals offering consumers effective, economic health care. PPO consumers pay lower than normal fees by using "preferred" doctors and hospitals. Consumers may elect to use physicians and hospitals not in the network but must pay the difference between the discounted fee provided to in-network providers and the higher fee of non-participating physicians and hospitals.

HMOs and PPOs are becoming increasingly available. According to the HMO/PPO Directory (1996), there are over 1400 HMO and PPO plans in the United States. Within the U.S., the number of people who belong to HMOs has increased from 3.5 million in 1971 to more than 46 million in 1995 (U.S. Department of Commerce; Economics and Statistics Administration; Bureau of the Census, 1996). HMO enrollment varies considerably across the nation, from highs of 44.8 percent and 40.3 percent in Oregon and California respectively, to lows of 1.2 percent in Mississippi and North Dakota. Even individuals covered by Medicare and Medicaid are choosing capitated programs. Managed care experience with older adults is fairly new. As recently as 1980, there were only a few HMOs contracting with Health Care Financing Administration (HCFA) to provide Medicare services. That number has now grown dramatically. Several studies suggest that the quality of care in HMOs is similar to that of fee-for-service care (Wagner, 1996). Enrollment in capitated systems is summarized in Table 8–4.

Transcultural Nursing Implications

What role may transcultural nurses play in this evolving payment structure? Implications for research and practice will be identified. First, transcultural nurses are in an ideal position to help health care consumers understand the implications of the changing health care financing. Much information is available in print and on the Internet to assist nurses in this role. Health care consumers need to understand their insurance options. The culturally sensitive nurse can help the consumer identify positive and negative aspects of each health plan option, within the context of the consumer's family and culture.

In addition, transcultural nurses can help the health system understand health care consumers. For example, transcultural nurses have identified various types of

---

TABLE 8-4
Managed Care Enrollment in the United States

Enrollment	Percentage
Enrollment in HMOs (in 1996)	22
Enrollment in HMOs with point-of-service option (in 1995)	65.2
Medicare beneficiaries enrolled in prepaid health plans (in 1996)	11.5
Medicaid beneficiaries enrolled in managed care plans (in 1995)	28.4

Data source: McCloskey, A. H., Holahan, D., Brangan, N. et al. (1996). *Reforming the health care system: State profiles 1996.* Washington, D.C.: American Association of Retired Persons.

subcultures, such as the subculture of the homeless. These findings must be shared with insurers and providers to better reach these particular groups.

In addition to understanding cultural groups more clearly, transcultural nurses can also assist in modifying the delivery of care to a variety of cultural groups. It is well known that the meaning of health and illness is different for various cultural groups. For example, the areas of self-help and patient empowerment have white middle class origins. Further research is needed in these areas. In addition, this research must be applied in practice. Based on research, culturally congruent health care must be fostered. Similarly, there is a need for further research into the practices cultural groups employ for staying well. Again, this research must be used to provide health care to these groups of people. Last, research to understand the cultural factors that influence care during and after illness, while impressive, has only begun to scratch the surface. More research is needed in this arena, and the findings must be applied to the provision of culturally congruent health care for ill and recovering individuals.

Challenges

Increased hospital acuity, increasing community partnerships, CQI, and payment changes from fee-for-service to capitation: these four trends in health care represent opportunities for nurses versed in transcultural nursing to take leadership positions in health care to improve care for clients of all cultures. However, in order to hold legitimate places in improving care, hospitals, communities, and other sites of care must understand the skill sets transcultural nurses bring to the table. In addition, they must understand the impact that delivering culturally congruent care has on patient outcomes and corporate finance.

Thus, both qualitative and quantitative data will be needed to document the contributions made by transcultural nurses. Qualitative data will continue to give voice to the emic view of the cultural group. Qualitative study results will have a great impact on the cultural group itself, the community, and those planning innovative programs to deliver culturally competent care. Health care system administrators, on the other hand, will be more rapidly convinced by quantitative data. The administrators will require outcomes data, including clinical quality, functional status, patient satisfaction, and resource utilization data. This represents an opportunity to demonstrate how the provision of culturally congruent care by transcultural nursing has and will shape health care for the next millennium.

Review Questions

1. How is acuity changing in hospitals? What are the implications for patients, families, and nurses?
2. What roles may transculturally prepared nurses play in assisting healthy community programs?
3. How might listening to customers to continually improve care processes impact culturally diverse groups? What special skills are needed to foster accurate and timely listening?
4. How might transcultural nurses improve care under capitated health care payments?

Learning Activities to Promote Critical Thinking

Visit a hospital and arrange for a tour of a critical care unit.

1. Talk to the nurses about how acuity has changed in their units. Ask the nurses if they provide care to people from a variety of cultures. Ask how a cultural assessment is included in the care they provide. Find out how they obtain an interpreter if needed.
2. Observe a critical care unit. What aspects of the environment are most pleasing or disturbing for you? How do you believe your culture influences your response to the unit? What are the visiting hours of the unit? How might these hours affect families from a variety of cultures?
3. Spend some time in the family waiting area. Talk to several family members. What do they view as their biggest need while their family member is acutely ill? What assistance for coping are they receiving and from whom? What additional support would they like to receive? How do these responses vary by cultural group?

Select a community you live in or know.

1. Read a community newsletter distributed by a local hospital. What groups are identified in the newsletter? How is the hospital partnering with these groups?
2. Based on your knowledge of the community, what partnerships might be important? What cultural groups may be omitted from these partnerships?
3. Consider a prevalent disease condition in this community. How might a quality improvement effort be put in place to bring together all the pertinent stakeholders for this condition? How might health care agencies better partner with community members to improve management of this condition?
4. Talk to 10 community members about their health insurance. How many of them are enrolled in a Health Maintenance Organization (HMO), meaning their providers are being paid on a per member per month (PMPM) basis? What services would they like to see enhanced in their health plan?

Acknowledgments

Sincere thanks to Advocate Health Care, Lutheran General Hospital and Genesis Center of Health and Empowerment for sharing their efforts to meet the challenges inherent in the health care trends outlined in this chapter.

References

Artinian, N. T. (1991). Strengthening nurse-family relationships in critical care. *AACN Clinical Issues in Critical Care Nursing, 2*(2), 269–275.

Bernstein, L. P. (1990). Family-centered care of the critically ill neurologic patient. *Critical Care Nursing Clinics of North America, 2*(1), 41–50.

Caine, R. M. (1991). Incorporating CARE into caring for families in crisis. *AACN Clinical Issues in Critical Care Nursing, 2*(2), 236–241.

Carey, R., & Lloyd, R. (1995). *Measuring Quality Improvement in Health Care: A Guide to Statistical Process Control Applications.* New York, New York: Quality Resources

Clement, J. M. (1988). The need for and effects of touch in ICU patients. In B. S. Heater & B. AuBuchon. *Controversies in Critical Care Nursing* (Eds.). Rockville, MD: Aspen Publishers, Inc.

Clifford, C. (1986). Patients, relatives and nurses in a technological environment. *Intensive Care Nursing, 2*(2), 67–72.

Coutu-Wakulczyk, G., & Chartier, L. (1990). French validation of the critical care family needs inventory. *Heart & Lung, 19*(2), 192–196.

Dailey, L. (1984). The perceived immediate needs of families with relatives in the I intensive care setting. *Heart & Lung, 8*, 332–329.

Deming, W. E. (1986). *Out of Crisis*. Cambridge, MA: Massachusetts Institute of Technology.

Ellwood, P. M., Jr. (1994). Health Care Plans in *Information Finder* (TM). Chicago, IL: World Book, Inc.

Engli, M., & Kirsivali-Farmer, K. (1993). Needs of family members of critically ill patients with and without acute brain injury. *Journal of Neuroscience Nursing, 25*(2), 78–85.

Forrester, D. A., Murphy, P. A., Price, D. M., & Monaghan, J. F. (1990). Critical care family needs: Nurse-family member confederate pairs. *Heart & Lung, 19*(6), 655–661.

Halm, M. A. (1990). Effects of support groups on anxiety of family members during critical illness, *Heart & Lung, 19*(1), 62–71.

Halm, M. A. (1992). Support and reassurance needs: Strategies for practice. *Critical Care Nursing Clinics of North America, 4*(4), 633–643.

Hickey, M. (1990). What are the needs of families of critically ill patients? A review of the literature since 1976. *Heart & Lung, 19*(4), 401–415.

Kleinpell, R. M., & Powers, M. J. (1992). Needs of family members of intensive care unit patients. *Applied Nursing Research, 5*(1), 2–8.

Koller, P. A. (1991). The family needs and coping strategies during illness crisis. *AACN Clinical Issues in Critical Care Nursing, 2*(2), 338–345.

Kreamer, C. L. (1989). *The Relationship of Family Functioning, Family Demographics, and Severity of Illness to Family Coping with the Crisis of Critical Illness*. Unpublished Doctoral Dissertation: The University of Texas at Austin.

Kupferschmid, B. J., Briones, T. L., Dawson, C., & Drongowski, C. (1991). Families: A link or liability? *AACN Clinical Issues in Critical Care Nursing, 2*(2), 252–257.

Leininger, M. (1978). *Transcultural Nursing: Concepts, Theories and Practices*. New York: John Wiley & Sons.

Leininger, M. M. (1991). *Culture Care Diversity and Universality: A Theory of Nursing*. New York: National League for Nursing Press.

Leininger, M. (1995). *Transcultural Nursing: Concepts, Theories and Practices* (2nd Ed). New York: McGraw-Hill Inc.

Leske, J. S. (1986). Needs of relatives of critically ill patients: A follow-up. *Heart & Lung, 15*(2), 189–193.

Leske, J. S. (1988). *Selected Psychometric Properties of the Critical Care Family Needs Inventory*. Unpublished Doctoral Dissertation: The University of Wisconsin, Milwaukee.

Leske, J. S. (1991). Overview of family needs after critical illness: From assessment to intervention. *AACN Clinical Issues in Critical Care Nursing, 2*(2), 220–228.

Ludwig-Beymer, P., Blankemeier, J. R., Casas-Byots, C., & Suarez-Balcazar, Y. (1996). Community Assessment in a Suburban Hispanic Community: A Description of Methods. *Journal of Transcultural Nursing, 8*(1): 19–27.

McCloskey, A. H., Holahan, D., Brangan, N., & Yee, E. (1996). *Reforming the Health Care System: State Profiles 1996*. Washington DC: American Association of Retired Persons.

Medical Economics (1996). *HMO/PPO Directory 1997*. Montvale, NJ: Medical Economics Company.

Molter, N. C. (1979). Needs of relatives of critically ill patients: A descriptive study. *Heart & Lung, 8*(2), 332–339.

Murphy, P. A., Forrester, D. A., Price, D. M., & Monaghan, J. F. (1992). Empathy of intensive care nurses and critical care family needs assessment. *Heart & Lung, 21*(1), 25–30.

Norris, L. O., & Grove, S. (1986). Investigation of selected psychosocial needs of family members of critically ill adult patients. *Heart & Lung, 15*(2), 194–199.

O'Malley, P., Favaloro, R., Anderson, B., Anderson, M. L., Siewe, S., Benson-Landau, M., Deane, D., Feeney, J., Gmeiner, J., Keefer, N., Mains, J., & Riddle, K. (1991). Critical care nurse perceptions of family needs. *Heart & Lung, 20*(2), 189–201.

Pelfrey, S., & Theisen, B. A. (1993). Valuing the community benefits provided by nonprofit hospitals. *Journal of Neuroscience Nursing, 23*(6), 16–21.

Price, D. M., Forrester, D. A., Murphy, P. A., & Monaghan, J. F. (1991). Critical care family needs in an urban teaching medical center. *Heart & Lung, 20*(2), 183–188.

Reider, J. A. (1989). *The Relationship of Family Needs, Satisfaction and Family Coping Strategies to Family Adjustment During the Critical Illness of a Family Member*. Unpublished Doctoral Dissertation: The Catholic University of America.

Reizian, A., & Meleis, A. I. (1986). Arab-Americans' perceptions of and responses to pain. *Critical Care Nurse, 6*(6), 30–37.

Rukholm, E., Bailey, P., Coutu-Wakulczyk, G., & Bailey, W. B. (1991). Needs and anxiety levels in relatives of intensive care unit patients. *Journal of Advanced Nursing, 16*(8), 920–928.

Scherkenbach, W. W. (1991). *Deming's Road to Continual Improvement*. Knoxville, TN: SPC Press.

Skoner, M. M. (1989). Culture and the meaning of illness. In C. Malloy and J. Hartshorn, *Acute Care Nursing in the Home. A Holistic Approach*. Philadelphia: J.B. Lippincott.

Smith, K., Kupferschmid, B. J., Dawson, C., & Briones, T. L. (1991). A family-centers critical care unit. *AACN Clinical Issues in Critical Care Nursing, 2*(2), 258–268.

Stanton, D. J. (1991). The psychological impact of intensive therapy: The role of nurses. *Intensive Care Nursing, 7*(4), 230–235.

Titler, M. G., Cohen, M. Z., & Craft, M. J. (1991). Impact of adult critical care hospitalization: Perceptions of patients, spouses, children, and nurses. *Heart & Lung, 20*(2), 174–182.

U.S. Department of Commerce; Economics and Statistics Administration; Bureau of the Census (1996). *Statistical Abstract of the United States 1996* (16th Ed). Lanham, MD: Bernan Press.

Wagner, E. H. (1996). The promise and performance of HMOs in improving outcomes in older adults. *Journal of American Geriatrics Society, 44*, 1251–1257.

Watson, L. A. (1991). *Comparison of the Effects of Usual, Support, and Informational Nursing Interventions of the Extent to Which Families of Critically Ill Patients Perceive Their Needs Were Met*. Unpublished Doctoral Dissertation, The University of Alabama at Birmingham.

Wooley, N. (1990). Crisis theory: A paradigm of effective intervention with families of critically ill people. *Journal of Advanced Nursing, 15*(12), 1402–1408.

Transcultural Aspects of Pain

Patti Ludwig-Beymer

KEY TERMS

Acupressure
Acupuncture
Autogenic Training
Benson's Relaxation Response
Biofeedback
Cutaneous Stimulation
Distraction
Herbal Remedies
Hypnosis
Imagery

Nurse Client Relationship
Nurse Competence
Nursing Subculture
Pain
Pain Assessment
Pain Expressions
Pain Interpretation
Pain Threshold
Pain Tolerance
Pain Tolerance—Encouraged

Personal Attitude
Progressive Relaxation
Relaxation Techniques
Religious Rituals
Sensation Threshold
Silent Suffering
Therapeutic Touch
Transcendental Meditation
Yoga

OBJECTIVES

1. Analyze the components responsible for pain perception.
2. Identify the universal aspects of the pain experience.
3. Compare and contrast expressions of pain by culture, gender, and type of pain.
4. Describe the views and attitudes about pain held by the subculture of nursing.
5. Explain the rationale for nurses to identify their personal attitudes toward pain
6. Illustrate the steps used in establishing a relationship with individuals experiencing pain.
7. Compare and contrast alternative practices in pain management.

Pain, a universally recognized phenomenon, is an important area of consideration in nursing practice. Chronic pain is now considered to be the most frequent cause of disability in the U.S. and in other industrialized nations. Chronic pain has often been mismanaged and has resulted in significant amounts of medical expense, lost work hours, and law suits (Encandela, 1993). Pain is the most frequent and compelling reason for seeking health care (Kim, 1980) and is a common result of many diagnostic, surgical, and treatment procedures. The elderly are at special risk for pain. One study found that 51 percent of nursing home residents reported pain on a daily basis (Ferrell & Ferrell, 1990) while other research reported that approximately 70 percent of elderly people living in the community experience some degree of pain on a regular basis (Crook, Rideout & Brown, 1984; Roy & Thomas, 1986; Sorkin, Rudy, Hanlon, Turk, & Steig, 1990). The management of pain is particularly important in nursing because nurses often encounter people either experiencing or anticipating pain. Also, pain management has traditionally been a nursing responsibility. Thus, nurses are in an ideal position to assess pain and to take action to alleviate it.

Pain is a very private experience and is influenced by cultural heritage. Culture has long been recognized in nursing practice and research as a factor that influences a person's expression of and reaction to pain (Villarruel & de Montellano, 1992). Expectations, manifestations and management of pain are embedded in a cultural context. The definition of pain, like that of health or illness, is culturally influenced. Thus, understanding culture is critical when dealing with clients in pain.

Definition of Pain

Definitions of pain are quite diverse, partly because of the complex nature of pain and partly because of the many different existing perspectives on pain. The term pain is derived from the Greek word for penalty, which helps explain the long association between pain and punishment in Judeo-Christian thought. The medical profession has dominated our understanding of pain since the late 1800s. Consequently, pain has come to be defined as a sensation associated with real or potential tissue damage involving chemical disturbances along neurologic pathways (Morris, 1991). The national guidelines on acute pain management define pain as an unpleasant sensory and emotional experience arising from actual or potential tissue damage or described in terms of such damage (U.S. Department of Health and Human Services, 1992). Yet pain is much more variable and modifiable than previously believed. Variations within and among people and cultures have been identified. Stimuli that would produce intolerable pain in one person may be embraced by another. For example, in some cultures, initiation rites and other rituals involve procedures generally associated with severe pain. However, participants reportedly feel little or no pain (Melzack & Wall, 1983).

Pain perception, then cannot be defined simply in terms of particular kinds of stimuli. Rather, pain is a highly personal experience, depending on cultural learning, the meaning of the situation, and other factors unique to the individual. Perhaps the most comprehensive definition of pain has been proposed by McCaffery (1979): "Pain is whatever the experiencing person says it is, existing whenever he says it does." The meaning of painful stimuli for individuals, the way individuals define their situation, and the impact of previous personal experiences help determine the experience of pain.

Measurement of Pain

In terms of pain measurement, it is generally believed that humans normally experience similar sensation thresholds. However, pain perception thresholds, pain tolerance, and encouraged pain tolerance may vary considerably among individuals. Sensation threshold, pain threshold, pain tolerance and encouraged pain tolerance are defined with related research results presented below.

Sensation Threshold

Sensation threshold refers to the lowest stimulus that results in tingling or warmth. Research suggests that most people, regardless of cultural background, have a uniform sensation threshold. For example Sternbach and Tursky (1965) measured sensation threshold in American-born women from Irish, Italian, Jewish, and Old American (defined as third-generation Americans) ethnic groups. They found no differences in the amount of stimulation needed to produce a detectable sensation.

Pain Threshold

Pain threshold refers to the point at which the individual reports that a stimulus is painful. Cultural background appears to have some effect on this measure of pain. For example, Hardy, Wolff, and Goodell (1952) found that levels of heat reported as painful by people of Mediterranean origin were described merely as warm by Northern Europeans. Clark and Clark (1980) used electric shock to measure pain. They found that Nepalese porters and Western guests were equally sensitive to electric shock. However, the Nepalese required higher intensities before describing the stimuli as painful.

Pain Tolerance

Pain tolerance is the point at which the individual withdraws or asks to have the stimulus stopped. Cultural background appears to have a strong effect on pain tolerance levels. A number of studies examining pain thresholds have been conducted, and several studies have compared pain responses across racial groups, with mixed results. Chapman and Jones (1944) compared pain responses of Southern African Americans, Northern European Americans, Russian Jewish Americans and Italian Americans using radiant heat technique. They found that Northern European Americans had the highest pain perception threshold and pain reaction threshold. Italian Americans tended to vocalize their pain while African Americans did not verbally express their pain.

Meehan, Stoll, and Hardy (1954) compared Alaskan Indians, Eskimos, and Anglo Americans using radiant heat technique. They found that whites had the highest and Eskimos the lowest pain thresholds, but the results were not statistically significant. Last, Merskey and Spear (1964) compared white and black medical students in England. When they inflicted pain through a pressure algometer, they found no statistically significant differences between the two groups in pain threshold or reaction time.

Researchers have also looked at pain responses in persons of various religions backgrounds. Lambert, Libman, and Poser (1960) found no significant differences between pressure pain in Jewish and Protestant groups. Poser (1963, cited by Wolff & Langley, 1977) also found no differences between Jewish and Roman Catholic groups in Canada.

The generalizability of these findings to clinical settings is questionable. It is unlikely that individuals experiencing pain due to illness or injury will respond in the same manner as people experiencing short episodes of controllable pain induced in a laboratory setting. However, the studies do provide some support for the idea that attitudinal factors influence the pain responses of various cultural groups.

Differences in pain tolerance may reflect different attitudes toward pain. For example, in clinical studies, Zola (1966) and Zborowski (1969) found major cultural differences in tolerance of pain. Yet clinical pharmacologic studies generally neglect cultural and psychosocial effects on pain, such as culture group membership, socioeconomic status, and treatment expectations. Too often, health care providers are interested in the physical and somatic basis of pain to the exclusion of psychological and cultural components.

Encouraged Pain Tolerance

Encouraged pain tolerance is the amount of painful stimuli an individual accepts when encouraged to tolerate increasingly higher levels of stimulation. Again, cultural differences have been documented. Early anthropological studies remarked on the large amount of pain tolerated by members of the so-called primitive tribes. Wissler (1921), for example, described the Sun Dance "self-torture" ceremonies of the North American Plains Indians. Each participating young man had incisions made in his chest; skewers were then passed through the incisions and attached to the top of the sacred Sun Dance pole. As part of the ceremony, the man danced until his skin was torn from the skewers. The elders then inspected the wounds, cut away any dangling skin and ended the ceremony. As a result of participating in this ceremony, the man gained esteem and was admitted into the band of warriors.

Clearly, the situation described above was very painful; there is no reason to believe that these young men were physiologically different from anyone else. However, they somehow modified and tolerated the pain because the ceremony was accepted and encouraged by the culture. The euphoria of progressing to warrior, the increased esteem obtained, the trust of the elders, and many other factors appear to have altered the experience of pain.

As described above, pain perception thresholds, pain tolerance, and encouraged pain tolerance vary. Culture is one variable that influences the perception and toleration of pain. Because other factors also play a role in pain perception, the nurse should not expect all clients to react in the same fashion to painful stimuli.

Expressions of Pain

In addition to expecting variations in pain perception and tolerance, the nurse should also expect variations in the expression of pain. According to Festinger's (1954) theory of social comparisons, everyone wants to test the validity of his or her judgments and opinions of the outside world. Individuals tend to turn to their social environments for validation of their experiences. Since pain is a private, ambiguous situation, comparisons with others in the culture group helps determine what reactions are appropriate.

A first important comparison group is the family, which transmits cultural norms to children. For example, in their study of adult fears of dental care, Shoben and Borland (1954) found that the experiences and attitudes of one's family were the most important factors determining whether one would react with anxiety to dental treatment, avoid it for a long time, or be uncooperative in the dental chair.

In addition to family influence, it has long been recognized that emotional factors abate the severity of pain or abolish it entirely, even in cases of extensive physical injury. Beecher (1956), for example, found that wounded soldiers, for whom a wound meant an honorable release from danger, were less in need of analgesics that civilians with comparable wounds, for whom a wound represented a largely unwelcome disturbance in their normal lives.

Perhaps the greatest contribution to our understanding of cultural responses to pain and the subjective nature of the pain experience has been made by Zborowski (1952, 1969). An anthropologist, Zborowski studied 103 patients on a Veteran's Administration Hospital medical-surgical unit using a variety of qualitative methods including questionnaires, unstructured interviews, and direct observations. Data were collected from four cultural groups: Irish Americans, Italian Americans, Jewish Americans and Old Americans.

Zborowski compared pain interpretation, significance of pain, and other specific aspects of the pain experience, such as intensity, duration, and quality across the four cultural groups. He found that Irish Americans had difficulty describing and talking about pain, showed little emotion with pain, de-emphasized the pain, and withdrew socially when experiencing pain. Italian Americans were expressive in their pain and preferred the company of others when in pain. They tended to request immediate pain relief by any means possible and were generally happy when the pain was relieved. Like the Italian Americans, the Jewish Americans preferred company while in pain, sought relief from pain. and freely expressed their pain through crying, moaning and complaining. However, the Jewish American men were skeptical and suspicious of the pain, and were concerned about the implications of the pain. The "Old-Americans" were precise in defining pain, displayed little emotion, and preferred to withdraw socially when in pain.

Zborowski suggested that patterned attitudes toward pain behavior exist in every culture. Appropriate and inappropriate expressions of pain are thus culturally prescribed. Zborowski maintained that cultural traditions dictate whether to expect and tolerate pain in certain situations as well as how to behave during a painful experience. In addition, cultural groups expect individuals to conform to these culturally prescribed rules and norms. Despite some methodological flaws, Zborowski's research remains the classic study of cross-cultural pain responses.

More recent studies have substantiated Zborowski's findings. Zola (1983) compared Italian-American and Irish American men and women experiencing pain. The findings indicated that the Irish Americans tended to deny pain. Italian Americans tended to admit to pain and presented significantly more symptoms than the Irish Americans. Cluster analysis revealed that the variable most consistently correlated with pain response and illness behavior was the individual's cultural background.

Abu-Saad (1984) studied Arab American, Asian American and Latin American children. Descriptors of pain varied by cultural group. Arab American children used words such as sore, uncomfortable, and tingling to describe the pain. Asian children described the pain as scary, paralyzing and cold. Latin American children used words such as hitting, terrible, and sickening to describe pain. Children from all three cultures agreed that when in pain they felt miserable or awful and scared. Arab American and Latin American children frequently indicated "feeling sick to their stomach" when experiencing pain while Asian American children felt "like being lost." Arab American and Asian American children often reported feeling nervous, embarrassed, or angry when in pain, while Latin American children reported feeling bad when in pain.

Other researchers have examined pain responses in a variety of cultural groups with conflicting results. In a study of episiotomy pain, Flannery, Sos, and McGovern (1981) reported no significant differences in pain response between African American, Anglo-Saxon Protestant-American, Irish American, Italian American, and Jewish American women. Weisenberg, Kreindler, Schachat, and Werboff (1975) compared pain anxiety and pain attitudes in African American, Anglo American and Puerto Rican dental patients. Although no significance between-group differences were noted in the amount of pain or the number and types of symptoms experienced, anxiety levels were significantly different. Puerto Rican patients were more anxious than the other two groups and preferred to deny, eliminate or not deal with the pain. The Anglo Americans reported less anxiety and were most willing to face and deal with the pain.

Perkoff and Strand (1973) identified variations in the presentation of symptoms of acute myocardial infarction. White men were more likely to report chest pain, whereas black men were more likely to describe dyspnea. Studying patients after acute myocardial infarction, Neill (1993) found no statistically significant differences in sensory, affective, evaluative or pain intensity measures among Yankee, Irish, Italian, Jewish, and black men. However, black men in the study were more likely to present with shortness of breath than were men from the other groups.

Rather than comparing cultures, several studies have examined a single cultural group. Calatrella (1980) found that Mexican Americans rarely acknowledge signs and symptoms of pain because they consider lack of stamina a sign of weakness. However, these individuals may moan while in pain, because this is seen as an acceptable expression of pain and may be used in an attempt to relieve the pain. Balin (1988) also found that pregnant women who became identified with the subcultures of expecting or new mothers tended to find support within these groups to express actual pain or fears related to labor.

Reizian and Meleis (1986) found that Arab Americans had a present-time orientation to pain similar to Zborowski's findings with Italian Americans. The Arab Americans tended to focus on the immediacy of the pain. Pain was viewed as unpleasant, to be avoided, or controlled at all costs. Responses were private and reserved for immediate family members, with families often overseeing and making decisions about the care. When responses were shared with family but not with health care professionals, conflicts could arise. In addition, different pain episodes resulted in different responses. Some pain, such as labor pain, induced loud moans, groans and screams. Arab Americans often used metaphors and analogies to describe pain.

Researchers suggest that gender plays a role in shaping an individual's response to pain (Kleinman, 1988; Lawlis, Achterberg, Kenner, & Kopetz, 1984). Their research suggests that women tend to express distress and strain related to pain more openly and more often than men. Encandela's (1993) research on pain experiences in life care retirement communities also suggests that women express pain more freely than men, and report that they talk about pain more frequently with friends and health professionals. Women also report encountering pain, most often menstrual pain and labor pain, at earlier ages than men. As a result, women may be more familiar with pain and come to expect it as an inevitable part of life.

Hilbert (1984) found that many chronic pain sufferers experience social isolation because of the inadequacy of cultural resources to help them understand and express their pain. He reported that these individuals often concealed their pain and their pain management techniques. Kotarba (1983) researched chronic pain sufferers and found that they viewed their conditions primarily as a personal problem rather than a medical problem. As such, their pain took on a variety of meanings related to feelings of hope, fear, and trust. These meanings found expression within the cultural context of the research participants. For example, strongly religious people found meaning and expression for their pain through religious doctrines. Similarly, Ohnuki-Tierney (1984) found that in contemporary Japan, the Japanese have drawn upon traditional sacred symbolism to construe meanings for pain. For example, abdominal pain may indicate a spiritual imbalance since the abdomen is thought to be the seat of the soul among many Japanese.

Although these studies are interesting, it is important to emphasize the great variation within cultures. Differences exist among individuals in any culture in terms of pain perception and expression. Nurses should avoid stereotyping or assuming that an individual will respond to pain in a certain way based on culture.

Nursing Subculture: Views And Attitudes About Pain

Although the population of the United States is composed of people whose ancestors immigrated from many counties, social customs and practices in society at large and particularly in health care have been dominated by white Anglo Saxon Protestants. Regardless of their ethnic backgrounds, most individuals have been somewhat influenced by these dominant values and beliefs.

Silent suffering is probably the most valued response to pain in the United States (McCaffery, 1979). The majority of nurses in the United States are white, middle-class women who have been socialized to believe that self-control is better than open displays of strong feelings. It has been suggested that nurses as a subculture may be socialized, even more than most individuals, to place a high value on self-control in response to pain. One explanation for this is that nurses, because of the nature of their professional activities, must learn to control their feelings and function well under pressure and thus expect the same behavior from others (Benoliel & Crowley, 1974).

Research studies support the belief that these values are internalized by nurses. In a study of 52 white nurses, Acheson (1988) found that the nurses reported their own behavior while experiencing pain as "stoic" and "non-verbal." Further, they indicated a minimal use of analgesics when personally experiencing pain.

Partly as a result of the nursing subculture, nurses often expect people to be objective about the very subjective experience of pain. In clinical practice, nurses may expect a person experiencing pain to report it and give a detailed description of it, but to display few emotional responses to the pain. When in pain, nurses expect people to stay calm and avoid complaining, screaming, and crying.

In addition, nurses may deny the pain that they observe in others. In a study of the biases of health care professionals, Baer, Davitz, and Lieb (1970) found that social workers tend to infer the greatest degree of pain, whereas physicians and nurse infer less pain. The researchers speculated that individuals who are in frequent contact with people in pain may protect themselves from becoming overwhelmed by denying the pain.

Davitz and Davitz (1981), who have extensively studied nursing attitudes toward pain, found that ethnic background of the client is an important determinant for inference of suffering due to both physical and psychological distress by United States nurses. Nurses viewed Jewish and Spanish clients as suffering most and Oriental, Anglo Saxon and Germanic clients as suffering least. In addition, Davitz and Davitz found that nurses who inferred relatively greater client pain tended to report their own experiences as more painful than nurses who inferred less client pain. In general, United States nurses with Eastern European, Southern European or African backgrounds tended to infer greater suffering than did nurses with Northern European backgrounds. Years of experience, current position, and area of practice were unrelated to inferences of suffering.

In a larger study, Davitz and Davitz examined the relationship between the degree of client suffering inferred by the nurse and the national background of the nurse. The researchers collected data from nurses in Belgium, England, India, Israel, Japan, Korea, Nepal, Nigeria, Puerto Rico, Taiwan, Thailand, Uganda, and the United States. Nurses were asked to infer physical and psychological pain for clients described in brief case studies. Analysis of the data from all 13 countries confirmed the assumption that attitudes are in part socially learned responses. Nurses from these cultures differed markedly. Korean nurses inferred the highest level of psychological distress, followed by Puerto Rican and Ugandan nurses; Nepalese, Taiwanese and Belgian nurses inferred the least amount of psychological distress. Korean nurses also inferred the greatest amount of physical pain, followed by Japanese and Indian nurses; nurses from Belgium, the United States, and England inferred the least amount of physical pain.

In a separate study, Acheson (1988) found that nurses' inferences of client suffering varied by the client's culture. Using vignettes that described American Indian, Southeast Asian, White American, and Mexican American clients, nurses were asked to infer physical pain, psychological distress, and intervention choices. Nurses tended to infer the greatest physical pain for Southeast Asian clients, followed closely by Mexican American clients. Inference of pain for American Indians and white American clients were identical. In addition, a statistically significant relationship was found between the level of pain inferred and the choice of intervention.

These findings provide dramatic support for the belief that one's perspective is important in making inferences about another person's experiences and that culture constitutes an important part of one's perspective. Significant differences in nurse perceptions were found in these studies. Perception is a crucial component of pain assessment and forms the basis of subsequent decisions about pain management.

According to McCaffery and Ferrell (1992), undertreatment of pain has been identified as a problem for over 20 years. The Agency for Health Care Policy and Research issued guidelines related to acute pain management in "recognition of the widespread inadequacy of pain management" (U.S. Department of Health and Human Services, 1992, page 4). Even the lay press describes the Unites States culture as one "that prizes the stiff upper lip: no pain, no gain" (Allis, 1992, page 61).

Several studies (Cohen, 1980; Jacox, 1979; Teske, Daut, & Cleeland, 1983) suggest that nurses' perception of pain does not coincide with the patients' resulting in increased suffering for patients. Rankin and Snider (1984) found that 58 percent of nurses have the goal of reducing rather than eliminating pain. Sixty-seven percent of the patients in the study continued to have moderate pain despite interventions. Dudley and Holme (1984) found that nurses tended to infer a greater degree of psychological distress than physical distress from pain. This may lead to inappropriate interventions, such as psychological support without other pain interventions. Client dissatisfaction with pain control has also been documented in research conducted in Kenya (Ngugi, 1986).

In addition, administration of analgesia may differ by cultural group, with medications withheld from less vocal clients. For example, Streltzer and Wade (1981) studied postcholecystectomy pain in whites, Hawaiians, and Asians. They found that nurses limited the amount of analgesia given to all groups, with significantly fewer analgesics given to Japanese, Filipino, and Chinese patients, the least vocal group in this study.

According to research on hospice care, this tendency to undermedicate is not restricted to the United States. Studies typically show that 75 percent to 90 percent of cancer pain in terminally ill patients is well controlled using the World Health Organization approach, with mean medication doses as high as 30 mg of morphine every 4 hours. However, appropriate doses are often not used. A study of treatment of cancer pain in Germany found that only 322 of 16,630 cancer patients received strong opiates, that adjuvant therapy was rarely used, and that treatment for breakthrough pain was rarely given. Health care professionals may be concerned about addiction and respiratory depression or may think that morphine is a drug only for those actively dying. Similar beliefs exist among patients and family members. For example, a study in Poland identified common lay morphine myths including that it is only to be given in the very last stages of disease, that it will cause addiction, and that if it is used too early, there will be nothing stronger to use with which to relieve pain . The barriers to effective palliative care appear to be similar worldwide (Rhymes, 1996).

Applying Transcultural Nursing Concepts To People In Pain

Although it is beyond the scope of this chapter to present all of the various pain management techniques, five helpful strategies for dealing with the client in pain are described below: identifying personal attitudes; establishing an open relationship; establishing nurse competence; assessing pain; and clarifying responsibility. Transcultural concepts are integrated into these strategies. When these strategies are not employed, culturally insensitive care may be the result, as summarized in Table 9–1.

Identifying Personal Attitudes

Nurses bring their own attitudes about pain to each client interaction (Douglas, 1991). To have empathy for others, nurses must understand and confront their own personal beliefs (Martinelli, 1987) about pain and suffering. Each nurse must confront her or his own beliefs; therefore, it is helpful for individual nurses to identify how they

TABLE 9-1

A Case Study

	Culturally Insensitive	Culturally Congruent
History	Mr. Varrow is a 45-year-old man admitted to the hospital with abdominal pain.	Mr. Varrow is a 45-year-old man admitted to the hospital with abdominal pain.
Nursing Assessment	Ms. Smith, the nurse assigned to Mr. Varrow, attempts to perform her admission assessment. Mr. Varrow begins to moan and cry. Ms. Smith is both uncomfortable and annoyed with Mr. Varrow's behavior. She leaves the room abruptly, stating "I'll be back later to do your assessment."	Ms. Smith, the nurse assigned to Mr. Varrow, enters his room and introduces herself. She explains she will be asking a few questions that will make his hospitalization more comfortable. Mr. Varrow begins to cry and moan. Ms. Smith states "I know you're in pain and this is difficult for you." Mr. Varrow states, "It hurts so much, but I'll try to cooperate." The nurse assesses Mr. Varrow's abdomen and then asks Mr. Varrow how he would handle this pain at home.
Client Reaction	Mr. Varrow is unaware of why the nurse has become so irritated with him. He does not like to be left alone and would prefer some distraction from the pain. As Ms. Smith's absence lengthens, Mr. Varrow begins to feel anxious, abandoned, hurt, and angry. He wonders if anyone will take care of him.	Mr. Varrow indicates, "My wife would make me some herbal tea. It helps to calm me down. Then she would sit with me." Since the nurse knows that Mr. Varrow is permitted a liquid diet, she encourages him to call his wife and have her bring some tea from home. Mrs. Varrow is pleased to participate in the care. Later, after his tea, Ms. Smith talks to Mr. Varrow about his condition. Mr. Varrow is more relaxed, and Ms. Smith completes her assessment. As she leaves the room, she hears Mr. Varrow whisper to his wife, "I think I'll be all right here."
Analysis	The nurse expects the client to respond to pain in a stoic manner. When it becomes obvious that the client will not behave in the expected way, the nurse is uncomfortable and retreats from the situation. The client is abandoned to handle his pain alone. A negative nurse–client relationship has been established. The client may lose faith in the nurse and the health system in general and may reject the care offered by the nurse.	The nurse accepts the client and his expression of pain. She doesn't embarrass or demean him as a result of his response. As a result, some of his anxiety is alleviated, possibly decreasing pain perception. The nurse encourages family involvement and herbal tea, two strategies that have been used by the client at home. These strategies make the hospital environment more tolerable for the client and foster a relationship of trust between client and nurse. As a result, the client feels cared for rather than abandoned.

view, express and manage their own pain. Nurses must also identify beliefs they have regarding client expression of pain. Learner activities at the end of this chapter will assist nurses in this process. For example, is a nurse truly nonjudgmental or does the nurse prefer the patient to express pain stoically? Identifying personal cultural beliefs is the first step in recognizing how these beliefs may interfere with truly therapeutic nurse–client relationships.

Establishing an Open Nurse–Client Relationship

The relationship between the person in pain and the health care provider is always colored by the issue of power and powerlessness (Encandela, 1993). Because pain is a wholly subjective experience that cannot be proven or verified, people in pain are at the mercy of the health care provider with whom they chose to disclose information about their pain. The health care provider may decide to believe or disbelieve the person's account of pain, ignore it completely, or intentionally or inadvertently make it worse.

Thus, it is important to establish an effective and supportive nurse–client relationship. The quality of the relationship may be as important as the pain-relieving skills used. The nurse should strive to create a relationship with the client that is characterized by genuineness, empathy, warmth, and respect. These caring behaviors constitute the essence of transcultural nursing. A positive relationship incorporates respect for the client and avoidance of stereotyping.

Respect Clients as Individuals
It is essential for nurses to respect clients as unique individuals. Recognition that culture is an important aspect of individuality is also critical. For example, nurses must recognize that clients hold a variety of beliefs about pain. In addition to recognizing the existence of different perspectives on pain, nurses must acknowledge that clients are entitled to their own belief systems.

Respect the Client's Response to Pain
Although personal values and cultural expectations differ, nurses must accept the rights of clients to respond to pain in the way they deem appropriate. Clients should never be made to feel ashamed of their responses to pain, even if the responses are not congruent with what nurses consider typical. Nurses need to remember there are a wide variety of pain expressions, with none of the expressions being inherently good or bad.

The nurse who is aware of cultural differences and understands clients in terms of cultural backgrounds will respond effectively and appropriately to their needs. Such a nurse will not be disturbed by the emotional expressiveness of a client whose culture expects and encourages open expression of pain. Similarly, the sensitive nurse will not mistake the stoic attitude of a client from another culture for lack of pain.

Never Stereotype a Person Based on Culture
Culture should never be used as a basis to stereotype an individual. Intragroup differences in pain perception and expression have been well documented in pain

research (Wolff and Langley, 1977). When providing care, the nurse should take into account many aspects of the experience, including the pain itself, the client's culture, the psychological aspects of the situation, and additional needs of the client. There are a wide variety of expressions of pain within each culture, and nurses must anticipate and accept these variations.

Nurse Competence

Benoliel and Crowley (1974) describe the importance of establishing nurse competence to clients. Clients should feel comfortable with both the technical and interpersonal skills of nurses. The way nurses present themselves and their care may greatly influence their reception. For example, Neufeld (1970) reported that the status of the person suggesting that a treatment will be effective influences the extent to which subjects believe the suggestion. In Neufeld's research, hypothetical treatments supposedly endorsed by ninth-grade students and by nurses' aides were found to be much less effective in increasing pain tolerance than the same endorsements supposedly given by physicians.

Part of establishing interpersonal competence involves being available to the client who is experiencing pain. This may involve staying with the client, providing privacy to the client or using ordinary touch as an adjunct to pain relief. Research suggests that nurses often provide "instrumental touch," such as dressing changes and technology-related touch. However, "caring touch" is essential for comforting clients, generating warmth, decreasing anxiety, diminishing pain, and creating a bond (Mulaik et al., 1991).

In addition, nurses should not assume that they are the only people available to clients in pain. Discussions with the client and family, and involvement of family members in the care may be helpful (Gropper, 1990). Friends, volunteers, and other health care providers may also be used to provide care. The ideal caregiver is at least partially determined by culture. For example, a member of a particular culture may prefer a caregiver of the same gender. These restrictions should be respected and honored as much as possible.

Assessing Pain

Nurses obtain the most useful results when they approach pain assessment not as a task but as an important interaction with the client (Thiederman, 1989). It is essential for nurses to believe clients when they say they are in pain. The single most reliable indicator of the existence and intensity of pain is self-report (National Institute of Health, 1987). In practice, however, nurses tend to use other, less reliable measures for assessing pain. For example, in one study, five of the six top factors identified by nurses as useful in assessing the patient's degree of suffering were found to be influenced by culture. These factors include facial expression, position and movement, vocalization, request for relief, and verbalization. The danger in using these measures alone is that clients who do not exhibit expected signs of distress may be overlooked by nurses (Oberst, 1978). Neither vital signs nor behavior can substitute for a self-report (Beyer, McGrath & Berde, 1990).

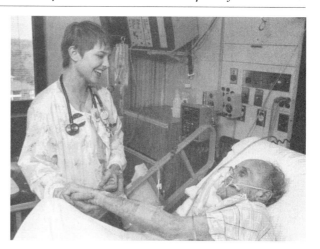

Caring touch helps to create a bond between client and nurse and provides comfort to the client. (Reprinted by permission of William Arnold, MD, Lutheran General Health System, Parkridge, Illinois.)

When people in pain realize that the existence of their pain is not believed by others, they experience stress and increased pain intensity. Nurses need to try to understand how the client is experiencing pain and convey that understanding to the client. Since the word pain has so many different meanings and refers to such a variety of sensations, clarifying clients' experience of pain will be helpful for both nurses and clients.

Assessing pain in the elderly presents additional challenges. There are specific biologic and psychosocial factors that influence elderly people's perceptions and experience of pain (Melding, 1991). In addition, elderly people hold misconceptions about pain, including the belief that pain is a normal part of aging and should be tolerated, staff are too busy to hear complaints of their pain, and telling nurses about pain may result in further testing and expenses (Herr & Mobily, 1991; Hofland, 1992; Witte, 1989). Additional research suggests three major themes in the perception of pain in the elderly: resignation to pain, ambivalence about the benefits of pain relief, and reluctance to express pain (Yates, Dewar, & Fentiman, 1995).

Despite these challenges, the nurse is responsible for knowing the person's pain history and established coping mechanisms (Copp, 1990). A variety of pain assessment tools have been developed and summarized (U.S. Department of Health and Human Services, 1992). Although they have different formats, they are meant to assess the same type of information. Cultural influences on pain (as described in Chapter 2) must always be a component of pain assessment.

The assessment of pain has three major objectives. First, it allows the nurse to understand what the client is experiencing. Second, it evaluates the effect the experience of pain is having on the client. Third, it sometimes allows for a determination of the physical nature of the phenomenon that has resulted in the pain (Fagerhaugh & Strauss, 1977). The first two objectives are described in the next section. The third objective falls primarily within the domain of medicine rather than nursing and is therefore not addressed.

Understanding the Experience

To understand what the client is experiencing, the nurse seeks information about the location, duration, intensity, and type of sensation. The main task is to facilitate communication about what is being experienced. Many clients are able to use numbers to describe and rank their pain. Other clients may use poker chips, drawings, or words to describe their pain (Tesler, Savedra, Holzemer, et al. 1991).

The nurse must remember that pain expressions will vary among clients and even with the same client in different situation. For example, stress resulting from fear of cancer may result in an increased expression of pain. Variations must also be acknowledged within cultures.

Clients experiencing chronic pain may display less intense nonverbal behavior relative to the pain they feel than clients experiencing acute pain. The absence of nonverbal pain behaviors such as grimacing and squinting, however, does not signify the absence of pain (Teske, Daut, & Cleeland, 1983). In addition, the nurse must remember that pain expressions will vary among clients and even with the same client in different situations. Variations must also be acknowledged within cultures.

Evaluating the Effect

Often the most difficult aspect of pain assessment is evaluating the effect the experience is having on the client. At the most fundamental level, the nurse should avoid dictating to clients what effect the pain "should" be having on them. Instead, the meaning of the experience should come from the clients.

An assessment of actual responses to pain should include gathering data on what a particular behavior means. For example, although Mexican American women in pain may moan, the crying out with pain does not necessarily indicate that the pain is severe, the woman is out of control, or that the nurse should intervene. Instead, it may be used to express and relieve discomfort (Calvillo & Flaskerud, 1991).

A baseline understanding of the client and his or her response to pain is essential. The nurse needs to assess the type of interventions desired by the client. For example, does the client want traditional interventions, nurturing behaviors, psychological support, physical interventions, or a combination of these interventions? The role of the family or social support network in providing these interventions should also be assessed (Calvillo & Flaskerud, 1991). Children, too, should be asked about their preferred coping strategies for managing pain (Abu-Saad, 1984).

Clarifying Responsibility

Responsibilities in pain relief should always be clarified with clients so that they know what they can do to achieve relief. For example, a member of a particular cultural group may consider it inappropriate to complain of pain. The client may need permission to request pain relief. A simple statement such as "please tell me when your pain returns" may be all that is needed. This will allow the client to feel in control of the situation and involved in pain management. In addition, the nurse should assess how the client ordinarily copes with pain. This will identify some potentially effective therapeutic techniques, outlined later in this chapter. Above all, the nurse must be open to alternative forms of treatment.

Nurse–client collaboration is essential in pain management. Too often, nurses approach a situation as if they had all the answers. Clearly, this attitude is not helpful. Instead, the client should be involved, actively setting goals. The client should not be left alone to manage the situation. Similarly, the client should not be managed by the health team, without his or her input. Instead, health professionals and clients should work together to meet the challenge of pain.

Alternative Practices

A number of practices have been used for centuries in the management of pain. Unfortunately, the predominant biomedical system has adapted very few of these techniques, often restricting its practice to medication and biostimulation techniques. On a positive note, the National Institute of Health has created an Office of Alternative Medicine and is funding research projects to test the effectiveness and efficacy of these nontraditional treatments (National Institute of Health, 1993). Research suggests that unconventional medicine is currently being used by 34 percent of the population in the United States (Eisenberg et al., 1993). The topic of alternative therapies is also receiving increased attention in nursing practice and literature (Andreola, Steefel & O'Sullivan, 1993). Even Time Magazine is writing about natural healing and the use of herbs to treat pain (Kluger, 1997).

This section is not designed to prepare the nurse to deliver the alternative practices described. Instead, it is meant to sensitize the nurse to the many options available to clients. In addition, the nurse and the client may choose together to use some of the techniques described below and summarized in Table 9–2, including relaxation

TABLE 9-2
Alternative Methods of Pain Control

Relaxation Techniques	Reduce stress and promote a sense of well-being
Benson's relaxation response	
Transcendental meditation	
Autogenic training	
Progressive relaxation	
Hypnosis	
Yoga	
Distraction	Shields individual from pain
Imagery	Decreases intensity of pain
Cutaneous stimulation	Reduces intensity of pain
Therapeutic touch	Stimulates client's healing potential
Herbal remedies	Nourishes body with natural ingredients
Religious Rituals	Promote healing of whole person
Biofeedback	Provides client with information about bodily function
Acupuncture/Acupressure	
Acupuncture	Intercepts life energy (*ch'i*) at acupoints
Acupressure	Massages at acupoints

techniques, distraction, imagery, cutaneous stimulation, therapeutic touch, herbal remedies, religious rituals, biofeedback, and acupuncture or pressure.

Relaxation Techniques

Many relaxation techniques have been demonstrated to result in physiologic changes. These changes act to reduce the damaging effects of stress and promote a sense of physical, mental, and spiritual well-being. Some of the relaxation methods most widely taught include Benson's relaxation response, transcendental meditation, autogenic training, progressive relaxation, hypnotic suggestion, and yoga. All of these techniques result in an altered state of consciousness and produce a decrease in sympathetic nervous system activity. Each technique requires a calm and quiet environment, a comfortable position, a mental device or image (such as a mantra sound), and a willingness to let relaxation happen.

Benson's Relaxation Response

This relation technique is a simple procedure that does not require a change in lifestyle. The method was developed by Harold Benson (1976). Relaxation is achieved through six basic steps: sit quietly; close eyes; deeply relax all muscles; breathe through nose; continue for 20 minutes; allow relaxation to occur at its own pace.

Transcendental Meditation

This type of meditation was originally developed by the Maharishi Mahesh Yogi, an Indian scholar and teacher. The technique, which is taught individually, involves the use of a specific mantra during the meditation.

Autogenic Training

Autogenic training emphasizes passive attention to the body. The training, which was first recognized within the biomedical model in 1910, incorporates elements of hypnotism, spiritualism, and various yogic disciplines. Luthe and Schultz (1970) have written a handbook that includes a training system of meditative exercises. This form of systematized relaxation training has been used with some success to treat pain.

Progressive Relaxation

Progressive relaxation, originated by Jacobson (1964), is probably the most widely used relaxation technique today. The method teaches the client to concentrate on various gross muscle groups in the body by first tensing and then relaxing each group.

Hypnosis

This technique was introduced into Western medical practice in the 18th century by Mesmer. A hypnotic state may be induced either by a hypnotist or by the client (autohypnosis). Hypnosis is based on the power of suggestion and the process of focusing attention. It has been used as an adjunct to other pain-relieving therapies and has been found to be helpful in dentistry, surgery, and childbirth as well as malignancies. Although hypnosis cannot change organic lesions that are causing pain, it can be used to reduce the discomfort of a wide range of conditions.

Yoga

Yoga techniques have been employed within the Hindu culture for thousands of years. Yoga involves the practice of both physical exercise (hatha yoga) and meditation (raja yoga). The correct performance of yoga results in deep relaxation without drowsiness or sleep.

All of these techniques may be clinically useful, especially in conditions caused by sympathetic nervous system activity. The interventions have been particularly helpful in the management of pain such as migraine headache.

Distraction

Distraction from pain is a kind of sensory shielding in which one is protected from the pain sensation by focusing on and increasing the clarity of sensations unrelated to the pain. Most nurses are probably not aware of the extent to which clients use distraction because clients do not readily share this information with the health care team. Research conducted in Kenya suggests that 59 percent of clients engage in diversional activities to assist their coping with pain (Ngugi, 1986). Like pain, research suggests that distraction techniques may also be a cultural phenomenon (Zadinsky & Boyle, 1996)

Although some nurses believe that "real" pain cannot be relieved by distraction, clinical and research findings suggest that distraction may be a potent method of pain relief, usually by increasing the client's tolerance for pain (McCaffery, 1990; Miller, Hickman & Lemasters, 1992). Distraction techniques include watching television, listening to music, reading, telling jokes, walking, playing with pets, crocheting, doing housework, interacting with children, and getting out of the house (Zadinsky & Boyle, 1996). Distraction appears to place the pain at the periphery of awareness. The pain is no longer the center of attention, although it still exists. When clients use distraction, they can at least partially avoid thinking about the pain.

Imagery

Imagery techniques for physical healing date back hundreds of years (Samuels & Samuels, 1975). In health care, guided imagery has been used for pain relief. Guided imagery involves using one's imagination to develop sensory images that decrease the intensity of pain or that become a nonpainful or pleasant substitute for pain. During guided imagery the client is alert, concentrating intensely, and imagining sensory images (McCaffery, 1979). Research suggests that pleasant imagery can effectively reduce the perception of postsurgical pain (Daake & Gueldner, 1993). Music therapy is being used with increased frequency to augment imagery and other relaxation techniques (Coverston, 1993).

Cutaneous Stimulation

Cutaneous stimulation reduces the intensity of pain or makes the pain more bearable. Types of cutaneous stimulation for pain relief include massage and pressure, vibration, heat or cold application, topical application, and Transcutaneous Electrical Nerve

Stimulation (TENS). Stimulation need not be applied directly to the painful site to be effective (McCaffery, 1990)

Therapeutic Touch

Therapeutic touch is derived from the ancient art of laying-on of hands but has no religious basis. According to Kreiger (1975, 1981), it is a conscious, intentional act that involves an actual energy transfer from the nurse-healer to the client to stimulate the client's own healing potential. It may be employed for a variety of problems, including pain. Research has documented the effectiveness of therapeutic touch in reducing tension headache pain (Keller & Bzdek, 1986).

Herbal Remedies

Herbalism, a specialty in the area of naturopathy, involves the belief that the body is nourished by natural ingredients. Further, proponents of herbalism believe the even if the body is exposed to disease-causing organisms, it can be strengthened through natural living, including exercise, fresh air, medication, and the use of unrefined foods. Herbal treatments have been used in China since at least 3000 BC, and over 700 herbs were used for healing in Egypt in 1550 BC (Moore, Van Arsdale, Glittenberg, & Aldrich, 1980). Although adherence to herbalism diminished in the West, interest is currently increasing, as exemplified by the popularity of herbal teas.

The nurse should be sensitive to the desire of clients to use natural substances to enhance their health, cure their disease, or relieve their pain. Many of the herbs used have a physiologic effect and may result in comfort for the client who is experiencing pain.

Religious Rituals

Nurses deal with a variety of religious rituals daily. For example, Catholic clients in pain may wish to pray the rosary or attend mass whereas Jewish clients experiencing pain may ask to speak to a rabbi. Clients of many Christian denominations may actively seek healing through prayer and other rituals. Christianity has included the notion of healing through divine intervention since its inception.

In addition to recognizing Western religious rituals, nurses must be sensitive to non-Western religious rituals. A religious ritual for the purpose of healing or pain relief, for example, may be conducted by a shaman. In this context, the illness or pain is viewed as a disorder of the total person, involving all parts of the individual as well as relationships to others. The shaman focuses on strengthening or stimulating the client's own natural healing powers. The ritual typically includes the shaman, the client, family members, and other members of the cultural group. The client is the focus of the group, with attention and resources devoted to him or her. Thus, the healing ritual may improve the client's sense of self-worth (Frank, 1974).

Clients should be encouraged to use their religious practices as they desire to help in pain management. In addition, privacy should be provided. For example, the client may require a private room for a religious ritual, and this need should be respected. Various amulets and charms should also be respected and incorporated into the care provided.

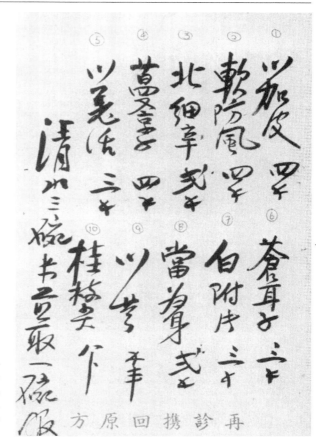

Herbal remedies are being used to enhance health, cure disease, and relieve pain. Above is a Chinese herbal prescription to treat some symptoms of lupus.

Biofeedback

Biofeedback comprises a wide variety of techniques that use instrumentation to provide a client with information about changes in bodily functions of which the person is usually unaware. Clients are taught to manipulate and control their degree of relaxation and tension by way of biofeedback training using electroencephalography (EEG) or electromyogram muscle potential (EMG). Since these methods give precise feedback information immediately and continuously, they are often an effective way to reduce tension.

Acupuncture/Acupressure

Acupuncture

Acupuncture, believed to have been practiced for at least 3000 years, is a method of preventing, diagnosing, and treating pain and disease by the skilled insertion of special needles into the body at designated locations and at various depths and angles. According to Chinese thought, life energy, or *ch'i*, constantly flows and energizes

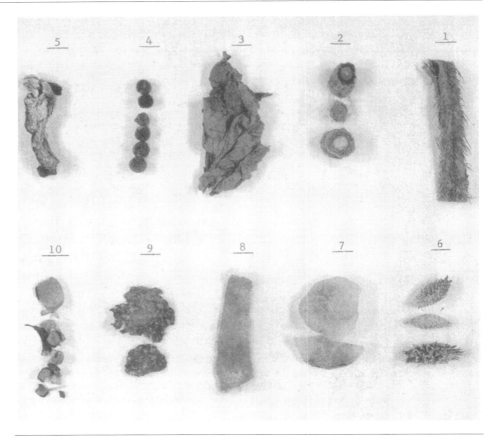

Above are the 10 herbs named in the prescription on the previous page. The client brews the herbs into a tea and then drinks it on an empty stomach.

humans through a pattern known as meridians. *Ch'i* may be intercepted at various acupoints throughout the body.

Acupuncture has been used as an alternative to other forms of analgesia for many minor surgical procedures in China. It has also been used in the treatment of pain in a variety of other countries. There are no simple explanations for the mechanisms that underlie the analgesia-producing effects of acupuncture. However, research has documented the release of endorphins into the vascular system during acupuncture, contributing to pain relief (O'Sullivan, 1993). Acupuncture and acupressure have been used to manage various types of pain, including labor (Beal, 1992).

Acupressure
Acupressure involves a deep-pressure massage of the appropriate acupoints. Self-help books are available to teach clients this technique (Chan, 1974; Kurland, 1977; Thie, 1973; Warren, 1976).

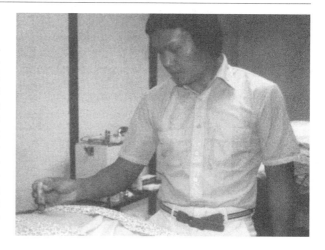

Traditionally a Chinese practice, acupuncture has gained acceptance in the United States and Canada. Research reveals that the procedure produces an analgesic effect because it causes the release of enkephalin, a naturally occurring endorphin that has opiate-like effects. The practitioner shown here is using moxibustion (heat) to enhance the therapeutic effects of acupuncture.

As seen in this brief overview, a number of alternative practices may be used to assist clients in the management of pain. Some practices involve only the nurse and the client. Other techniques involve different types of healers, family members and significant others. Nurses who are familiar with these techniques will feel more comfortable suggesting, observing, participating in or performing a variety of healing practices. An example of using some of these practices to provide culturally congruent care is presented in Table 9-1.

Summary

Pain has been experienced throughout the ages. Sophisticated pharmacologic interventions do not necessarily relieve pain, which people define, express, cope with, and manage in a variety of ways. Culture is a major influence in this process. Culture helps determine the innermost feelings of the individual. According to Mead, the behavior of an individual may only be understood in terms of the behavior of the whole social group of which he or she is a member (Mead, 1934). To examine the phenomenon of pain in its entirety, a model of pain is needed. Such a model would build in physical, psychological, social, and cultural factors, which interact and define the pain experience for individuals (Encandela, 1993).

Nurses practicing in the United States come in contact with people from a variety of cultural backgrounds. In addition, nurses encounter clients experiencing pain in virtually every clinical setting. Recognizing cultural differences in beliefs about pain and suffering can prevent misunderstandings and lead to more sensitive, effective, and professional care.

Review Questions

1. How is pain defined?
2. How does pain tolerance differ from pain threshold?

3. How does the expression of pain vary by culture? By gender? By type of pain?
4. How does the nursing subculture view pain? What are their typical expectations for expressions of pain by others?
5. What techniques may appropriately be used for assessing pain? How may the nurse demonstrate her or his competence to clients and families?
6. What alternative practices may be used by clients experiencing pain? How may nurses support these practices?

Learning Activities to Promote Critical Thinking

1. Think about the last time you experienced pain. Describe it. How intense was the pain? What do you think caused the pain? Did you want others to know about it? How did you respond to the pain? Did you want to be alone or with other people? What treatments did you use for the pain? Did you worry about the pain?
2. Ask five of your friends or relatives what treatments they use when they have a headache. Be sure to ask about folk remedies, and who taught them to use a particular treatment. Identify similarities and differences with the treatments you use.
3. Think about one of the clients in pain for whom you have provided care. How did that client respond to pain? How did you help the client? How would you modify your practice based on what you've learned in this chapter?
4. Identify three times you have encouraged (or have seen others encourage) a client to accept more pain. What words were used? How was family involved? What was the ultimate outcome? Did you realize you were applying principles of encouraged pain tolerance?
5. Select several clients with different cultural backgrounds. Assess their pain using several different techniques. Which technique is most helpful? Are your clients able to use numbers to describe their pain? Can they draw pictures or use colors to describe their pain? What words do they use to describe their pain?

References

Abu-Saad, H. (1984). Cultural group indicators of pain in children. *Maternal–Child Nursing Journal, 13*, 187–196.

Acheson, E. S. (1988). *Nurses' Inferences of Pain and the Decision to Intervene for Culturally Different Patients*. University of Texas at Austin, Dissertation.

Allis, S. (October 19, 1992). Less Pain, More Gain. *Time*, 61–64.

Andreola, N. M., Steefel, L., & O'Sullivan, C. (1993). A different way: A look at alternative therapies. *Nursing Spectrum, 6*(18):7–9.

Baer, E., Davitz, L. J., & Lieb, R. (1970). Inferences of physical pain and psychological distress in relation to verbal and nonverbal patient communication. *Nursing Research, 19*, 388.

Balin, J. (1988). The sacred dimensions of pregnancy and birth. *Qualitative Sociology, 11*, 257–301.

Beal, M. W. (1992). Acupuncture and related treatment modalities. Part II: Applications to antepartal and intrapartal care. *Journal of Nurse-Midwifery, 37*(4), 260–268.

Beecher, H. K. (1956). Relationship of wound to pain experienced. *JAMA, 161*, 1609.

Benoliel, J. Q., & Crowley, D.M. (1974). *The Patient in Pain: New Concepts*. New York: American Cancer Society.

Benson, H. (1976). *The Relaxation Response*. New York: Avon Books.

Beyer, J. E., McGrath, P. J., & Berde, C. V. (1990). Discordance between self-report and behavioral pain measures in children age 3–7 years after surgery. *Journal of Pain and Symptom Management, 5,* 350–356.

Calatrella, R. L. (1980). The Hispanic concept of illness: An obstacle to effective health care management? *Behavioral Medicine, 7*(11), 23–28.

Calvillo, E. R., & Flaskerud, J. H. (1991). Review of literature on culture and pain of adults with focus on Mexican-Americans. *Journal of Transcultural Nursing, 2*(2), 16–23.

Chan, P. (1974). *Finger Acupressure.* Los Angeles: Price/Stern/Sloan Publishers, Inc.

Chapman, W. P., & Jones, C. (1994). Variations in cutaneous and visceral pain sensitivity in normal control subjects. *Journal of Clinical Investigations, 23,* 81–91.

Clark, W. C., & Clark, S.B. (1980). Pain responses in Nepalese porters. *Science, 209,* 410–412.

Cohen, F. L. (1980). Postsurgical pain relief: Patients' status and nurses' medication choices. *Pain, 9*(1), 265–274.

Copp, L. A. (August, 1990). The spectrum of suffering. *American Journal of Nursing,* 35–39.

Coverston, C. (1993). The therapeutic use of music during childbirth. *Pro Re Nata,* Utah Nurses Association, *2*(3), 14.

Crook, J., Rideout, E., & Brown, G. (1984). The prevalence of pain complaints in a general population. *Pain, 18,* 299–314.

Daake, D. R., & Gueldner, S.H. (1993). The use of imagery instruction as a measure to control postsurgical pain. *Search* (Center for Nursing Research, College of Nursing, Medical University of South Carolina, *16*(2), 4–6.

Davitz, L. J., & Davitz, J. R. (1975). How do nurses feel when patients suffer? *American Journal of Nursing, 75,* 1505.

Davitz, J. R., & Davitz, L. J. (1981). *Influences of Patients' Pain and Psychological Distress.* New York: Springer-Verlag.

Douglas, M. K. (1991). Cultural diversity in the response to pain. In K. A. Puntillo (Ed.), *Pain in the Critically Ill.* Gaithersburg, MD: Aspen Publishers, Inc.

Dudley, S. R., & Holm, K. (1984). Assessment of the pain experience in relation to selected nurse characteristics. *Pain, 18*(2), 179–186.

Eisenberg, D. M., Kessler, R. C., Foster, C., Norlock, F. E., Calkins, D. R., & Delbanco, T. L. (1993). Unconventional medicine in the United States. Prevalence, costs, and patterns of use. *New England Journal of Medicine, 328*(4), 246–252.

Encandela, J. A. (1993) Social science and the study of pain since Zborowski: A need for a new agenda. *Social Science Medicine, 36*(6), 783–791.

Fagerhaugh, S. Y., & Strauss, A. (1977). *Politics of Pain Management: Staff-Patient Interactions.* Menlo Park, CA: Addison-Wesley.

Ferrell, B. R., & Ferrell, B. A. (1990). Easing the pain. *Geriatric Nursing, 11,* 175–178.

Festinger, L. (1954). A theory of social comparison processes. *Human Relations, 7,* 117–140.

Flannery, R. B., Sos, J., & McGovern, P. (1981). Ethnicity as a factor in the expression of pain. *Psychosomatics, 22,* 39–50.

Frank, J. D. (1974). *Persuasion and Healing.* New York: Schocken Books.

Gropper, E. I. (1990). Your Jewish patients in pain. *Advancing Clinical Care, 5*(5), 39–40.

Hardy, J. D., Wolff, H. G., & Goodell, H. (1952). *Pain Sensations and Reactions.* Baltimore: Williams & Wilkins.

Herr, K. A., & Mobily, P. R. (1991). Complexities of pain assessment in the elderly: Clinical considerations. *Journal of Gerontological Nursing, 17,* 12–19, 44–45.

Hilbert, R. A. (1984). The acultural dimensions of chronic pain: Flawed reality construction and the problem of meaning. *Social Problems., 31:* 365–378.

Hofland, S. L. (1992). Elder beliefs: blocks to pain management. *Journal of Gerontological Nursing, 18,* 19–24, 39–40.

Jacobson, E. (1964). *Self-Operations Control: A Manual of Tension Control.* Chicago: National Foundation for Progressive Relaxation.

Jacox, A. K. (1979). Assessing pain. *American Journal of Nursing, 79*(5), 859–900.

Keller, E., & Bzdek, V.M. (1986). Effects of therapeutic touch on tension headache pain. *Nursing Research, 35*(2), 101–105.

Kim, S. (1980). Pain: Theory, research and nursing practice. *Advances in Nursing Science, 2,* 43–59.

Kleinman, A. (1988). *The Illness Narratives.* New York: Basic Books.

Kluger, J. (May 12, 1997). Mr. Natural. *Time Magazine,* 68–75.

Kot, P. A. (1976). The physiology of TM. *American Family Physician, 14,* 155.

Kotarba, J. (1983). *Chronic Pain: Its Social Dimension.* Beverly Hills, CA: Sage.

Krieger, D. (1975). Therapeutic Touch: The Imprimatur of Nursing. *American Journal of Nursing, 75,* 784.

Krieger, D. (1981). *Foundations of Holistic Health Nursing Practices: The Renaissance Nurse.* Philadelphia: J.B. Lippincott.

Kurland, H. D. (1977). *Quick Headache Relief Without Drugs.* New York: Ballantine Books.

Lambert, W. E., Libman, E., & Poser, E. G. (1960). The effect of increased salience of a membership group on pain tolerance. *Journal of Personality, 38,* 350–357.

Lawlis, G. G., Achterberg, J., Kenner, L., & Kopetz, K. (1984). Ethnic and sex differences in response to clinical and induced pain in chronic spinal pain patients. *Spine, 9,* 751–754.

Leininger, M. M. (1991). *Cultural Care Diversity and Universality: A Theory of Nursing.* New York: National League for Nursing.

Luthe, W., & Schultz, J. H. (1970). *Autogenic Therapy: Medical Applications.* New York: Grune & Stratton.

McCaffery, M., & Ferrell, B. R. (August, 1992). Does the gender gap affect your pain-control decisions? *Nursing,* 48–51.

McCaffery, M. (1979). *Nursing Management of the Patient with Pain,* (2nd Ed.). Philadelphia: J.B. Lippincott.

McCaffery, M. (1990). Nursing approaches to nonpharmacological pain control. *International Journal of Nursing Studies, 27*(1), 1–5.

McMahon, M. A., & Miller, P. (1978). Pain response: The influence of psychosocial- cultural factors. *Nursing Forum, 17*(1), 58.

Marks, R. G. (1979). Intractable headache? Biofeedback could be a solution. *RN, 42,* 73.

Martinelli, A. M. (1987). Pain and ethnicity. *AORN Journal, 46*(2), 273–281.

Mead, G. (1934). Mind, Self and Society. Chicago, IL: University of Chicago Press.

Meehan, J. P., & Stoll, A. M. (1954). Cutaneous pain threshold in Native Alaskan, Indian and Eskimo. *Journal of Applied Psychology, 6*, 297–400.

Melding, P. S. (1991). Is there such a thing as geriatric pain? *Pain, 46*, 119–121.

Melzack, R., & Wall, P.D. (1983). *The Challenge of Pain*. New York: Basic Books.

Mersky, H., & Spear, F.G. (1964). The reliability of the pressure algometer. *British Journal of Social and Clinical Psychology, 3*, 130–136.

Miller, A. C., Hickman, L. C., & Lemasters, G. K. (1992). A distraction technique for control of burn pain. *Journal of Burn Care and Rehabilitation, 13*(5), 576–580.

Moore, L. G., Van Arsdale, P. W., Glittenberg, J. E., & Aldrich, R.A. (1980). *The Biocultural Basis of Health*. Prospect Heights, IL: Waveland Press.

Morris, D. (1991). *The Culture of Pain*. Berkeley, CA: University of California Press.

Mulaik, J. S., Megenity, J. S., Cannon, R. B., Chance, K. S., Cannella, K. S., Garland, L. M., & Gilead, M. P. (1991). Patients' perception of nurses' use of touch. *Western Journal of Nursing Research, 13*(3), 306–323.

National Institute of Health (1993). Exploratory Grants for Alternative Medicine. In *National Institute of Health Guide for Grants and Contract, 22*(12).

National Institute of Health (1987). The integrated approach to the management of pain. *Journal of Pain and Symptom Management, 2*, 35–44.

Neill, K. M. (1993). Ethnic pain styles in acute myocardial infarction. *Western Journal of Nursing Research, 15*(5), 531–547.

Neufeld, R. W. J. (1970). The effect of experimentally altering cognitive appraisals on pain tolerance. *Psychonomic Science, 2*, 106.

Ngugi, E. N. (1986). Pain—An African perspective. *Nursing Practice, 1*(3), 169–176.

Oberst, M. (1978). Nurses' inferences of suffering: The effects of nurse-patient similarity and verbalization of distress. In M. Nelson (Ed.), *Clinical Perspectives in Nursing Research*. New York: Teachers College Press.

Ohnuki-Tierney, E. (1984). *Illness and Culture in Contemporary Japan*. Cambridge: Cambridge University Press.

O'Sullivan, C. (1993). Profile of a nurse acupuncturist. *The Nursing Spectrum, 6*(18), 9.

Pearson, B. D. (1987). Pain control: an experiment with imagery. *Geriatric Nursing, 8*(1), 28–30.

Perkoff, G. T., & Strand, M. (1973). Race and presenting complaints in myocardial infarction. *American Heart Journal, 85*(5), 716–717.

Putt, A. M. (1979). A biofeedback service by nurses. *American Journal of Nursing, 79*(1), 88–89.

Rankin, M. A., & Snider, B. (1984). Nurses' perception of cancer patients' pain. *Cancer Nursing, 7*(2), 149–155.

Reizian, A., & Meleis, A. I. (1986). Arab-Americans' perceptions of and responses to pain. *Critical Care Nurse, 6*(6), 30–37.

Rhymes, J. A. (1996). Barriers to effective palliative care of terminal patients. *Clinics in Geriatric Medicine, 12*(2), 407–416.

Roy, R., & Thomas, M. (1986). A survey of chronic pain in an elderly population. *Canadian Family Physician, 32*, 513–516.

Samuels, M., & Samuels, N. (1975). *Seeing with the Mind's Eye: The History, Techniques and Uses of Visualization*. New York: Random House.

Shoben, E. J., & Borland, L. (1954). An empirical study of the etiology of dental fears. *Journal of Clinical Psychology, 10*, 171–174.

Sorkin, B. A., Rudy, T. E., Hanlon, R. B., Turk, D. C., & Steig, R. L. (1990). Chronic pain in older and younger patients: Differences are less important than similarities. *Journal of Gerontology, 45*, 64–68.

Sternbach, R. A., & Tursky, B. (1965). Ethnic differences among housewives in psychophysical and skin potential responses to electric shock. *Psychophysiology, 1*, 241–246.

Streltzer, J., & Wade, T. C. (1981). The influence of cultural group on the undertreatment of postoperative pain. *Psychosomatic Medicine, 43*(5), 397–403.

Teske, K., Daut, R. L., & Cleeland, C.S. (1983). Relationship between nurses' observation and patients' self-reports of pain. *Pain, 16*, 289–296.

Tesler, M. D., Savedra, M. C., Holzemer, W. L., Wilkie, D. J., Ward, J. A., & Paul, S. M. (1991). The word-graphic rating scale as a measure of children's and adolescents' pain intensity. *Research in Nursing and Health, 14*, 361–371.

Thie, J. (1973). *Touch for Health*. Marina Del Ray, CA: De Vorss and Co., Publishers.

Thiederman, S. (June, 1989). Stoic or shouter, the pain is real. *RN*, 49–50.

U.S. Department of Health and Human Services (February, 1992). *Acute Pain Management: Operative or Medical Procedures and Trauma*. Rockville, MD: Agency for Health Care Policy and Research, Public Health Service, U.S. Department of Health and Human Services.

Villarruel, A. M., & de Montellano, B. O. (1992). Culture and pain: A Mesoamerican perspective. *Advances in Nursing Science, 15*(1), 21–32.

Warren, F. (1976). *Freedom from Pain through Acupressure*. New York: Frederick Fell Publishers, Inc.

Weisenberg, M. (1975). Cultural influences on pain perception. In M. Weisenberg (Ed.). *Pain: Clinical and Experimental Perspective* (pp. 141–143). St. Louis: C.V. Mosby.

Weisenberg, M., Kreindler, M. L., Schachat, R., & Werboff, J. (1975). Pain: Anxiety and attitudes in Black, White and Puerto Rican patients. *Psychosomatic Medicine, 37*, 123–135.

Witte, M. (1989). Pain control. *Journal of Gerontological Nursing, 15*, 32–37, 40–41.

Wissler, C. (1921). The sun dance of the Blackfoot Indians. *American Museum of Natural History Anthropology Papers, 16*, 223–270.

Wolff, B. B., & Langley, S. (1977). Cultural factors and the response to pain. *Culture, Disease, and Healing*. New York: MacMillan Publishing Co., Inc.

Yates, P., Dewar, A., & Fentiman, B. (1995). Pain: The view of elderly people living in long-term residential care settings. *Journal of Advanced Nursing, 21*: 667–674.

Zadinsky, J. K., & Boyle, J. S. (1996). Experiences of women with chronic pelvic pain. *Health Care for Women International, 17*, 223–232.

Zborowski, M. (1952). Cultural components in response to pain. *Journal of Social Issues, 8*, 16–30.

Zborowski, M. (1969). *People in Pain*. San Francisco: Jossey-Bass.

Zola, I. K. (1966). Culture and symptoms: an analysis of patients' presenting complaints. *American Sociological Review, 31*, 615–630.

Zola, I. K. (1983). *Socio-Medical Inquiries: Recollections, Reflections and Reconsideration*. Philadelphia: Temple University Press.

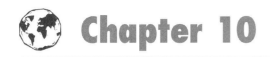

Chapter 10

Culture, Family and Community

Joyceen S. Boyle

OBJECTIVES

1. Use cultural concepts to provide care to families, communities and aggregates.
2. Explore interactions of *community* and *culture*
3. Analyze how cultural factors influence health and illness of groups.
4. Critically evaluate potential health problems and solutions in refugee and immigrant populations.
5. Assess factors that influence the health of diverse groups within the community.

An understanding of culture and cultural concepts enhances the nurse's knowledge and facilitates culturally competent nursing care in community settings. Currently, many nurses practice in community settings with clients from a wide variety of cultural backgrounds, and it is expected that this trend will only increase with more nurses moving from acute care institutions to community settings. Trends in our health care delivery system as well as an increased emphasis on health promotion have influenced nurses to make changes in their nursing practice. Concepts such as partnership, collaboration, empowerment and facilitation now form the basis for nursing practice with individuals, families and aggregates in the community. However, a word of caution is in order. Just because services are provided in a community setting does not mean they are community-based. Community-based services " require active involvement of clients and communities in assessing the needs for care, designing service programs, implementing interventions, and evaluating outcomes" (National Institute of Nursing Research, 1995, p. 2).

Community-based services are built on collaboration and partnerships between community leaders, consumers and providers. When community residents are involved as partners, community-based services are more likely to be responsive to locally defined needs, are better utilized, and are sustained through local action. Federal and state agencies as well as private foundations are increasingly requiring broad-based public and private collaboration and partnerships as prerequisites for funding of community-based services (Flynn, 1997; National Institute of Nursing Research, 1995). Community-based services are organizations that are complex and often fragile; they require a high level of nursing knowledge and skills in working and relating to different individuals and groups. In many instances, the complexity is increased when clients and their families come from diverse cultures. Nurses must understand how to help persons from various cultures work with community leaders and health providers to form partnerships that are responsive and can structure health care in ways that are culturally sensitive.

In this chapter, the terms *community nursing* and *community health nursing* are used interchangeably. Whether the nurse is employed as a community health nurse in a health department or practices in a community-based setting, the ability to provide culturally competent care is necessary. The practice of nursing in a community setting requires that nurses be comfortable with clients from diverse cultures and the broader socioeconomic context in which they live. In the current health care climate of economic restraints, the health care industry has focused on cost effectiveness but such a focus is tempered with positive outcomes. Care that is not congruent with the client's value system is likely to increase cost of care as the quality has been compromised. Furthermore, members of diverse cultural groups, such as officially designated U.S. minority groups, tend to experience more health problems than the general population. This was the impetus for targeting the four ethnic minority groups in *Healthy People 2000* (1991), as cultural diversity must be respected and taken into account by health care professionals.

Culturally Appropriate Nursing Care in Community Settings

The use of cultural knowledge in community nursing practice begins with a careful assessment of clients and families in their home environment. Cultural data that have implications for care are selected from the client, family and the environment during the assessment phase and discussed with the family so that mutually shared nursing goals can be developed. Clark (1996) suggested that there are four basic principles of cultural assessment. First, all cultures must be viewed in the context in which they have developed. Cultural practices develop as a "logical" or understandable response to a particular human problem, and the setting as well as the problem must be considered. This is one of the reasons why environmental or contextual data are so important. Second, the underlying premises of the behavior must be examined. For example, the Hispanic client's refusal to take a "hot" medication with a cold liquid is understandable if the nurse is aware that many Hispanic patients adhere to hot/ cold theories of illness causation. Third, the meaning and purpose of the behavior must be interpreted within the context of the specific culture. An example would be the close relationship that is often seen in Hispanic cultures between a mother and son; such an intense relationship might be viewed as abnormal in European American families. Finally, there is such a phenomenon as intracultural variation. Not every member of a cultural group displays all of the behaviors that we associate with that group. For instance, not every Hispanic client will adhere to hot/cold theories of illness or not every Hispanic mother will have a close personal relationship with a son. It is only by careful appraisal of the assessment data and validation of the nurse's assessment with the client and family that culturally competent care can be provided.

Of particular challenge to community nurses is the fact that they frequently encounter clients and families who must change behaviors and living patterns to maintain health or to promote wellness. Nursing interventions based on cultural knowledge help clients and families adjust more easily and assist nurses to work effectively and comfortably with all clients, especially those from different cultural backgrounds. An appreciation of cultural factors enhances family support of the client and the family's acceptance of nursing goals that have been developed collaboratively with the client and family.

Cultural data are important in the care of all clients; however, in community nursing, they are a prerequisite to successful nursing interventions. Community nursing is practiced in a community setting, often in the home of the client, and frequently requires more active participation on the part of the client and family. Usually, the client and family must make basic changes in their lifestyle, such as changes in diet and exercise patterns. Cultural competence requires that the nurse understand the family lifestyle, the family value system, as well as health and illness behaviors. This competency assists the client and family to plan and cope with changes in activities of daily living. Nurses often monitor clients with chronic diseases over a long period of time, and the nursing interventions must include aspects of counseling and education as well as anticipatory guidance directed toward helping clients and families adjust to what may be lifelong conditions. Nursing care must take account of the diverse cultural factors that will motivate clients to make successful changes in behavior, as improvement in health status requires lifestyle and behavioral modifications.

Transcultural nursing practice improves the health of the community as well as the health of individual clients and families. Additional considerations of the nurse who is involved in community-focused planning are the health needs of populations at risk. Special at-risk groups can be found in all communities—the homeless, the poor, persons with HIV disease and/or tuberculosis, pregnant women, infants and children and elderly are groups at risk for decreased health status. From a community standpoint, an understanding of culture and cultural concepts will increase the skill and abilities of the nurse to work with diverse groups within the community. Identification of high-risk groups and appropriate community-based strategies to reduce health risk requires considerable knowledge about cultural and ethnic groups and their place within the community. Nurses who have knowledge of and an ability to work with diverse cultures are able to devise effective community interventions to reduce risks that are consistent with the community, group and individual values of community members.

A Transcultural Framework

A distinguishing and important aspect of community nursing practice is the nursing focus on the community as the client (Clark, 1996; Stanhope & Lancaster, 1996). Effective community health nursing practice must reflect accurate knowledge of the

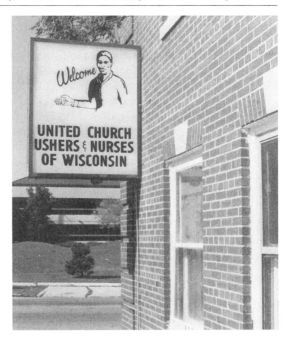

Some African American churches are organized to meet health, social and emotional needs of church members.

causes and distribution of health problems and of effective interventions that are congruent with the values and goals of the community. An epidemiologic model is used by the community nurse to collect, organize and analyze information about high risk groups that are encountered in community practice. An epidemiologic model emphasizes human biology, environment, lifestyle and the health care system; however, with modifications, the nurse can use this model to collect cultural data that influences health of the community (Clark, 1996). The epidemiologic model focuses on the community or on aggregate groups rather than individuals or families. Using a cultural overlay with the epidemiologic model enhances nurse–community interactions in the numerous ways:

1. A transcultural framework for nursing care helps the nurse to identify subcultures within the larger community and to devise community-based interventions that are specific to community health and nursing needs. In the multicultural society of the United States, it is common to speak of "the black community" or "the Hispanic community". We also speak more broadly of "the immigrant community" or "the drug community." A cultural focus allows this variety and facilitates data collection about specific groups based on their health risks. A cultural or epidemiologic framework facilitates a view of the community as a complex collective yet allows for diversity within the whole as well. Interventions that are successful in one subgroup may fail with another subgroup of the same community, and often the failure can be attributed to cultural differences.

2. Transcultural concepts often are useful in identifying and analyzing vari-

ous components of the community such as the social structure and religious and political systems. A cultural approach allows the nurse to identify cultural health care systems that are made up of individuals who experience illness as well as those who provide care for them. Anderson and MacFarlane (1996) suggest that each cultural health care system can have as many as three recognized sectors, most commonly referred to as popular, folk, and professional. We often forget that alternative systems and alternative therapies exist side by side with the professional system. How individuals organize themselves to meet group and individual needs is important information for community nurses. An assessment of whether social institutions such as churches and to meet health, social and emotional needs of church members. schools, as well as the health and political system, are responsive to the needs of all citizens and sometimes pinpoints critical needs and identifies gaps in care. Cultural traditions within a community often determine the structure of community support systems as well as how resources are organized and distributed.

3. A transcultural framework is essential to the community nurse's identification of the values and cultural norms of a community. Although values are universal features of all cultures, the types and expressions vary widely even within the same community. Values often serve as the foundation for a community's acceptance and use of health resources or a group's participation in community-based intervention programs to promote health and wellness. Just as nurses share data and collaborate with clients and families to establish mutually acceptable goals for nursing care, the community nurse works with the community or aggregates within the community to plan community-focused health programs. In addition to forming partnerships with communities, the community nurse considers the influences of social, economic, ecological and political issues. Many if not all community health issues are directly and profoundly affected by larger policy issues. These larger policy issues are, in turn, influenced by the wider national culture.

Cultural Issues in Community Nursing Practice

The material presented in this section will assist nurses to be aware of cultural factors that affect health, illness, and the practice of nursing in community settings. A number of other cultural assessment tools or guides are available that provide comprehensive frameworks to guide the nurse in the assessment of cultural factors in the care of individuals, families, and groups (Stanhope & Lancaster, 1996; Spector, 1996). The majority of cultural assessment guides are oriented to individuals and occasionally to families. Only a few have the comprehensive view necessary for assessing cultural factors for intervention at the community level. Because individual clients and their families compose larger communities, nurses who work in community settings must understand cultural issues as they relate to both individuals and families as well as communities.

Cultural Views of Individuals and Families

When assessing individuals and families, the community health nurse should carefully examine the following:

1. Family roles, typical family households and structure, and dynamics in the family, particularly communication patterns and decision making
2. Health beliefs and practices related to disease causation, treatment of illness, and the use of indigenous healers or folk practitioners and other alternative therapies
3. Patterns of daily living, including work and leisure activities
4. Social networks, including friends, neighbors, kin and significant others, and how they influence health and illness
5. Ethnic, cultural, or national identity of client and family, e.g., identification with a particular group, including language
6. Nutritional practices and how they relate to cultural factors and health
7. Religious preferences and influences on well-being, health maintenance, and illness, as well as the impact religion might have on daily living and taboos arising from religious beliefs that might influence health status or care
8. Culturally appropriate behavior styles, including what is manifested during anger, competition, and cooperation, as well as relationships with health professionals, relationships between genders, and relations with groups in the community

A cultural assessment of individuals and families includes all the preceding factors. This list is by no means exhaustive; rather, it is presented as a guide for community nurses as they assess cultural aspects of individuals and families.

Role of the Family in Transmitting Cultural Beliefs and Practices: A Context for Health and Illness

Cultural values shape human health behaviors and determine what individuals will do to maintain their health status, how they will care for themselves and others who become ill, and where and from whom they will seek health care. Families have an important role in the transmission of cultural values and learned behaviors that relate to both health and illness. It is in the family context that individuals learn basic ways to stay healthy and to ensure the well-being of one's self and family members.

One of the commonalties shared by members of functioning families is a concern for the health and wellness of each individual within the family, since the family has the primary responsibility for meeting the health needs of its members. The community nurse not only must assess the health of each family member but also must define how well the family can meet family health needs. Just how well families function in relation to this will determine how, when, and where interventions will take place, by whom, and what the specific approach will be to the family. A cultural orientation assists the nurse in understanding cultural values and interactions, the roles that family members assume, as well as the support system available to the family to help them when health problems are identified.

The family is usually a person's most important social unit and provides the social context within which illness occurs and is resolved and within which health promotion and maintenance occur. Most traditional health beliefs and practices promote the health of the family because they are generally family and socially oriented. Frequently, traditional beliefs and practices reinforce family cohesion. Some values are more central and influential than others, and given a competing set of demands, it is these central values that will typically determine a family's priorities. In families that adhere to traditional cultural values, the family needs and goals often will take precedence over individual needs and goals (Friedman & Ferguson-Marshalleck, 1996). A community health nurse can recognize and use the family's role in promoting and maintaining health. This requires an appreciation of the family context in health and illness and how this varies among diverse cultures.

Cultural Diversity Within Communities

The United States has many diverse cultures as a result of the history of immigration by a variety of cultural and ethnic groups to this country as well as the indigenous populations of Native Americans and Hawaiians. According to the U.S. Census Bureau, 24.5 million people—nearly one in every 10 people in the United States was born in another country (U.S. Bureau of the Census, 1992). Although broad cultural values are shared by most people in this country, a rich diversity of cultural orientations does exist, including those with considerable variations in health and illness practices.

Subcultures in the United States
Subcultures are fairly large aggregates of people, who, although members of a larger cultural group, have shared characteristics that are not common to all members of the culture and that enable the subculture to be thought of as a distinguishable group (Saunders, 1954). Many newcomers are actually relatives of U.S. citizens or they are new immigrants, adding numbers to the original subculture. Obviously, there can be diversity within each subculture also. Hispanic culture as a group includes Mexican Americans, Puerto Ricans, Cubans, and Central and South Americans, and there is diversity within each of these groups as well.

Certain geographic areas of the country such as Appalachia can be singled out as subcultures. Persons born and reared in the South or in New York City often can be identified by their language and mannerisms as members of a distinct subculture. We used to believe that the United States had a "melting pot" culture in which new arrivals gave up their former language, customs, and values to become Americans. It is now agreed that the "melting pot" notion may not be an appropriate analogy, at least not for everyone.

Refugee and Immigrant Populations
Immigrants are those persons who voluntarily and legally immigrate to the United States to live. Immigrants come of their own choice and most plan to eventually become citizens of the United States. Of course, many persons come to the United States illegally also. Although terms differ for these persons, usually they are referred to as "illegal immigrants." Research Application 10-1 discusses health issues and problems encountered by Afghan refugee women. Refugee is a special term that is

Research Application 10-1

Afghan Women's Health

Lipson, J. G., Hosseini, M. A., Kabir, S., Omidian, P. A., & Edmonston, F. (1995). Health issues among Afghan women in California. *Health Care for Women International* 16 (4), 279–286.

Afghan citizens began leaving their war-torn country in 1979. Afghans remain among the world's largest refugee population with Northern California being home to some 20,000 refugees. Afghan culture is strongly patriarchal even in the United States and this has caused considerable family conflict for young women. Women face problems with access to health care because of cultural emphasis on modesty; their care is complicated by their lower status and men's gatekeeping. Older women avoid preventive care such as mammograms and Pap smears because of embarrassment. Lack of health education is especially problematic; many older Afghan women have little or no formal education. The problem of wife abuse is of much concern in this population. Health education can be accomplished in a culturally sensitive and appropriate manner.

Clinical Application

- Afghan women will be more comfortable with female providers, i.e., female nurse practitioners, physician assistants, or physicians.

- Nurses who are culturally competent can interpret mainstream health culture to Afghans and Afghan culture to health care providers.

- Health education can be successful if presented appropriately. It can best be accomplished in small groups of women who know each other, meeting face to face, teaching in their own language. It is important to have plenty of pictures and time to ask questions as well as to socialize, perhaps over a cup of tea.

- Sex education in the schools is more culturally acceptable if it is conducted privately and separate classes are held for boys and girls. Parents' permission for their children to attend the classes is important and an Afghan adult should be present.

- Wife battering is an extremely sensitive issue in this patriarchal society where men consider it their right and duty to physically discipline their wives. Health care professionals must approach this problem with considerable caution and sensitivity. Afghan women who advocate for other women should be sought for advice on how to approach this concern.

used for groups of persons who come to this country under special legal processes usually requiring congressional action. By definition, refugees are those persons escaping persecution based on race, religion, nationality, or political stance (Scanlan, 1983).

The most well-known group of refugees were those persons who came to the United States from Southeast Asia after the Vietnam War. Most often refugees are fleeing war, famine and other social upheavals. They are fleeing for their lives and safety rather than personally choosing to leave their homeland. The term "refugee" and the status of an individual who is a refugee has a legal meaning and designation that differs from ordinary immigrants. Another classification of newcomers is that of "asylee"—those persons who come to this country seeking political asylum from some sort of persecution in their home country. These various types of classification—

immigrant, refugee, asylee or illegal immigrant—often determine the rights, for example, the granting of work permits, or the types of social and health services that newcomers may access.

The United States has grown and achieved its success as a nation of immigrants and foreigners. Immigration is a continuing phenomenon in the United States; for example, Spector (1996) pointed out that foreign born residents accounted for 8.7 percent of the population in the United States in 1994. In 1994, over 6 million persons came to the United States from Mexico; the Philippines was next in terms of immigrants with 1 million persons coming to the United States (U.S. Bureau of the Census, 1992). Many recent immigrants and refugees are unacculturated to prevailing American norms of health beliefs or behaviors. Many arrive with scant economic resources and must learn English and become economically self-sufficient as quickly as possible. Certain factors such as settlement patterns or living near friends or family, communication networks, social class, and education have helped many immigrants maintain their cultural traditions. Meleis (1997) noted that such communities provide support for newcomers and opportunities for cultural continuity. At the same time, belonging to such a community tends to set immigrants and refugees apart and isolate them from the larger community. For example, newcomers from Mexico realize that they need to learn English to get better jobs, but they often join expanding Latino communities where only Spanish is spoken by the residents. Learning English well enough to obtain employment in the English speaking world is difficult.

In addition to the legal entrance of immigrants and refugees, many other persons seeking political asylum have entered the United States from all over the world. Often, those seeking asylum or those who enter the country both legally and illegally are at considerable risk for health and social problems (Aroian, 1993). In addition to language and employment barriers, they have few economic resources; some have experienced rapid change and traumatic life events, their coping abilities have been overwhelmed, and there are few resources available to assist them. Immigrants in general, whether they are here legally or illegally, have special health risks.

Demographics and Health Care

During the 21st century, the United States and Canada will face enormous demographic, social and culture change. North America is becoming more diverse, not less so, and thus it is incumbent on nurses to be prepared to respond appropriately. Since the 1960s and 1970s, there has been a steady growth in cultural diversity in the United States. Currently, more than one resident in four is nonwhite or of Hispanic origin (U.S. Bureau of the Census, 1992). The health status of individuals in the United States differs dramatically across cultural groups and social classes. Major indicators such as morbidity and mortality rates for adults as well as infants show that the health status of minority Americans in the U.S. compared with white Americans is substantially worse. The same holds true for social class difference; health status is worse among those who live in poverty. Lack of economic resources predisposes individuals, families and communities to major difficulties in accessing appropriate health care. Thus, community nurses must assess groups within the community in a very sensitive manner; often those characteristics that we assume are related to the group's culture may be due to poverty instead.

Maintenance of Traditional Values and Practices

An important aspect of transcultural nursing is the collection of cultural data and the assessment of traditional values and practices and how they are maintained over time. The processes of assimilation and acculturation can be briefly defined as those ways in which individuals and cultural groups adopt and change over time. Yet, at the same time, both individuals and groups may be resistive to some changes and retain many traditional cultural traits. Hispanics are the largest cultural/ethnic group in the U.S. and there are several large American cities where Hispanics comprise large percentages of the population. Obviously, in these ethnic communities, it is easier to speak Spanish and to maintain other traditional cultural practices. Because traditional health beliefs and practices influence health and wellness, it is important for the nurse to understand the degree to which clients, families and communities adhere to traditional health values and how nursing practice should reflect these values. Spector (1996) suggested that a person's health care and behavior during illness may well have roots in that person's traditional belief system. Unless community health nurses understand traditional health beliefs and practices of their clients and communities, they may intervene at the wrong time or in an inappropriate way.

A number of factors influence the likelihood that clients, families and communities will maintain traditional health beliefs and practices. For example, the length of time that a person lives in the United States will influence factors such as language and use of media such as radio and television. The ability to speak English and to communicate with members of the majority culture is crucial to acculturation. The size of the ethnic or cultural group is also important, as obviously if the group is small, individuals from that group are more likely to be exposed to outsiders and will not spend all of their time within their own group or community.

Generally, children acculturate more quickly as they are exposed to other through schooling and learn cultural characteristics through association with others. The necessity of working outside of the household often exposes women from traditional cultures to others of the majority culture; thus they learn English more quickly than if they remain isolated at home. As individuals from other cultures seek health care in this country, they become familiar with our health care system. This does not mean that they comply with all health advice by any means, but contact with the system decreases anxiety and confusion, and individuals are more likely to seek care again. In addition, if individuals or groups have distinguishing ethnic characteristics such as skin color, they may be more isolated because of discrimination and thus retain traditional values, beliefs and practices over a longer period of time.

Some factors that influence the likelihood that clients, families and communities will maintain traditional health beliefs and practices are shown in Box 10-1.

Access to Health and Nursing Care for Diverse Cultural Groups

Diverse cultural groups, especially those who are poor, face special problems in accessing health and nursing care. Access to care is often determined by economic and geographic factors. Community nurses who focus on care of aggregates face the challenge of promoting the health of populations with new causes of mortality (such

Box 10-1 *Factors Influencing Traditional Beliefs and Practices*

1. The length of time in the United States.
2. The size of the ethnic or cultural group with which an individual identifies and interacts.
3. Age of the individual. As a general rule, children acculturate more rapidly than adults or seniors.
4. The ability to speak English and communicate with members of the majority culture.
5. Economic and education status. For example, if the family economic situation necessitates that a Salvadoran woman work outside the home, she may learn English more quickly than if she remains within the household and just speaks Spanish with her family members.
6. Health status of family members. If individuals and their families seek health care in this country, they begin to "learn the system," so to speak. This does not mean that they comply with all health advice by any means, but contacts with the system should decrease anxiety and confusion.
7. Individuals and groups who have distinguishing ethnic characteristics, such as skin color, may be more isolated because of discrimination and thus may retain traditional values related to health beliefs and behavior.

as HIV disease) and underserved populations who are more likely to experience health problems. Certain cultural groups have faced discrimination and poverty, and their ability to access care has been compromised. Sensitivity to cultural factors has often been lacking in the health care of traditional communities or identified minority groups.

Besides economic status and discriminatory factors that limit access to care, geographic location plays an important role. Many rural areas lack medical personnel and the variety of health facilities and services that are available to urban populations. For example, Native Americans, living in sparsely settled and isolated reservations in the western part of the United States must travel long distances over primitive roads to obtain health care services. Many individuals from culturally diverse backgrounds seek the services of health professionals who speak their language. When this is not possible, they are reluctant to seek care or may not understand the importance of following medical advice.

Another common and rather significant factor that limits access to health services is a lack of understanding on the part of clients of how to use health resources; this lack of understanding may be due in part to cultural factors. Often this lack of understanding means that members of diverse cultural groups are less able to adequately cope with health problems than other members of the community. Nurses can develop a sensitivity to diverse groups within communities and reach out to them with culturally specific health programs. Some important factors that nurses must take into account for culturally appropriate community-based care are shown in Box 10-2.

The need for nurses to be sensitive toward culturally different clients is increasing as we become more aware of the complex interactions between health care providers and clients and how these interactions might affect the client's health. The community

---

Box 10-2 *Factors to Consider in the Nursing Care of Culturally Diverse Groups*

1. Lack of employment opportunities and finances for health care services
2. Different traditional belief systems as well as different norm and values
3. The lack of cultural sensitivity on the part of social service and health care workers
4. Lack of bilingual personnel or staff members or the lack of interpreters to assist clients and providers
5. Rapid changes in the U.S. health care system where clients are "lost" in the gaps between agencies and services
6. Inconvenient locations or hours that preclude clients from accessing care
7. A lack of understanding, trust, and commitment on the part of health care providers

---

health nurse must be able to identify and meet the cultural needs of clients and families; in addition, nurses must take into account social and cultural factors on a community level as well in order to respect cultural values, mobilize local resources, and develop culturally appropriate health programs and services.

Community Nursing Interventions: Cultural Knowledge in Health Maintenance and Health Promotion

Leininger (1978, 1995) suggested that cultural groups have their own culturally defined ways of maintaining and promoting health. Pender (1987) suggested that "health promoting behaviors can be understood only by considering persons within their social, cultural, and environmental contexts" (p. 16). Community nurses who have direct access to clients in the context of their daily lives should be especially aware of the importance of cultural knowledge in promoting and maintaining health. The range of cultural influences on health maintenance and promotion is considerable. Major cultural issues and considerations must be addressed before health maintenance and promotion programs are implemented for culturally diverse groups.

First, it is very important to involve local community leaders who are members of the cultural group being targeted to promote acceptance of health promotion programs. An example might be a pastor of an African American Church in the rural south. Be sensitive to cultural differences in leadership styles also. For example, the pastor may not speak in favor of the health education program from his/her pulpit but might choose instead to work through more informal networks.

Second, involve family members, churches, employers and community worksites in supporting your health education program by using networks that already exist. An example would be establishing a health education program about mammography and breast self-exams at a worksite that employs mostly women. A display could be set up in the cafeteria/dining room or other accessible site. Women could peruse the educational material during breaks or after lunch.

Third, health messages are more readily accepted if they do not conflict with existing cultural beliefs. If the nurse plans to talk about prevention of teenage pregnancy to mothers and daughters at a local conservative church, discuss your plans prior to the educational intervention with some of the mothers and the pastor and ask for ways to strengthen the church's support of abstinence programs. This is not the appropriate time to focus on contraception methods. Be sensitive to religious values of the group.

Fourth, language barriers and cultural differences are a very real problem in many larger U.S. cities. Use local volunteers to disseminate messages in their own language and to help organize and present information that is culturally appropriate and understood by community members. As a health professional do not be afraid to ask for help and suggestions. Make it a point to find educational material such as brochures or videos in the appropriate language.

Last of all, sensitivity is essential to meeting health needs that exist within diverse cultural groups. For example, HIV disease is spreading rapidly in some Hispanic and African American populations. HIV disease is associated with intravenous drug use, violence and the spread of crack cocaine. In addition, the root causes of poverty and unemployment should be examined and programs that improve overall economic status of culturally diverse communities should be developed. Culturally relevant treatment programs should be implemented. Many minority women who seek treatment programs for their cocaine addiction encounter barriers that seem insurmountable. Treatment programs are not available in many areas, and child care facilities are not provided, even in day treatment programs. Thus, a young mother living in a rural area with children would not be able to find a treatment center that meets her needs. If she seeks admittance to a residential treatment program, she might have to agree to place her children in foster care.

Family Systems

Because the family is the basic social unit, it provides the context in which health promotion and maintenance are defined and carried out by family members within culturally diverse communities. The nurse can recognize and use the family's role in altering the health status of a family member and in supporting lifestyle changes. This requires an appreciation of the role of the family in diverse culture groups. African American families, for example, may demonstrate interchangeable roles for males and females, extended ties across generations, and strong social support systems including the African American church, all of which can be tapped by a community health nurse to activate health and wellness in families (Andrews & Bolin, 1993; Spector, 1996; Boyle, Ferrell, Hodnicki & Muller, 1996).

Coping Behaviors

Culturally diverse clients often have distinct behaviors to cope with illness as well as to maintain and promote health. These behaviors may be traced to the health-illness paradigms that were discussed earlier in Chapter 2. Beliefs about hot and cold, yin and yang, harmony and balance may underlie actions to prevent disease and to maintain health. Community nurses who understand cultural values and beliefs of clients can assess clients' understanding of health and illness; these assessment data serve as the basis for planning health guidance and teaching strategies that focus on incorporating cultural beliefs and practices in the nursing care plan. It seems likely that clients in the process of coping with illness and seeking help may involve a network of persons, ranging from family members and select laypersons to health professionals.

Lifestyle Practices

Cultural influences have a significant impact on such health-promoting factors as diet, exercise, and stress management. Community health nurses should assess the implications of diet planning and teaching to clients and family members who adhere to culturally prescribed practices concerning foods. There are particular food preferences that some cultural groups believe maintain or promote health. Certain foods often are restricted during an illness episode, just as there are "sick foods"—those special dishes served to an ill person such as the proverbial chicken soup. Cultural preferences determine the style of food preparation and consumption, frequency of eating, time of eating, and eating utensils. Milk is not always considered a suitable source of protein for Native Americans, Hispanics, African Americans and some Asians due to their relatively high incidence of lactose intolerance.

Nurses who work with culturally different clients must evaluate patterns of daily living as well as culturally prescribed activities prior to suggesting forms of physical activity or exercise to clients. Exercise is often defined in terms of white middle-class values. Not everyone has access to the tennis court at a local country club; in addition, many individuals would not feel comfortable in such surroundings or in aerobics classes regardless of the setting. Although stereotyping is possible, some African American men might feel more comfortable playing basketball ball after work. Tribal dancing has become popular on some reservations for Native Americans. Helping clients plan physical activities that are culturally acceptable is only the first step in implementing a program of physical activity.

Another aspect of lifestyle that is important to understand in order to successfully promote health and wellness is the manner in which culturally different clients manage stress. Stress management is learned from childhood through our parents, our social group, and our cultural group. Smoking and/or chewing tobacco often are ways that individuals use to manage stress. Persons who choose to smoke greatly increase the risk of the development of heart disease and cancer. Current debates rage about smoking in public places and the use of tobacco.

In addition, environmental tobacco smoke, that is, smoke that nonsmokers are exposed to from smokers, poses a risk of lung cancer and asthma to the nonsmoker (Cookfair, 1996, p. 656). The use and abuse of alcoholic beverages are also related to lifestyle practices. Often families coping with multiple stressors feel overwhelmed with the challenges of everyday living and individuals within families develop dysfunctional ways of coping such as alcohol abuse and domestic violence. Although many of these lifestyle practices are not associated with a group's culture per se, they are often found in groups that do not have appropriate options and/or alternatives, who are poor and unable to access employment and educational opportunities.

Many cultural groups tend to express psychological distress through somatic symptoms, and some studies have found that women are at high risk for depression and somatic complaints. Depressed women report more physical complaints, increased disability, increased functional limitations, and increased use of health care services than non depressed women (Betrus, Elmore & Hamilton, 1995). Indeed, for many

TABLE 10-1

Components of the Cultural Assessment

Cultural Component	Description
Family and kinship systems	Is the family nuclear, extended, or "blended"? Do family members live nearby? What are the communication patterns among family members? What is the role and status of individual family members? By age and gender?
Social life	What is the daily routine of the group? What are the important life cycle events such as birth, marriage, death, etc.? How are the educational systems organized? What are the social problems experienced by the group? How does the social environment contribute to a sense of belonging? What are the group's social interaction patterns? What are its commonly prescribed nutritional practices?
Political systems	Which factors in the political system influence the way the group perceives its status vis-à-vis the dominant culture, i.e., laws, justice, and "cultural heros?" How does economic system influence control of resources such as land, water, housing, jobs, and opportunities?
Language and traditions	Are there differences in dialects or language spoken between health care professionals and the cultural group? How do major cultural traditions of history, art, drama, etc., influence the cultural identity of the group? What are the common language patterns in regards to verbal and nonverbal communication? How is the use of personal space related to communication?
World view, value orientations, and cultural norms	What are the major cultural values about the relationships of humans to nature and to one another? How can the groups' ethical beliefs be described? What are the norms and standards of behavior (authority, responsibility, dependability, and competition)? What are the cultural attitudes about time, work, and leisure?
Religion	What are the religious beliefs and practices of the group? How do they relate to health practices? What are the rituals and taboos surrounding major life events such as birth and death?
Health beliefs and practices	What are the group's attitudes and beliefs regarding health and illness? Does the cultural group seek care from indigenous health (or folk) practitioners? Who makes decisions about health care? Are there biologic variations that are important to the health of this group?

immigrants and refugees, stress-related disorders such as Post Traumatic Stress Disorder are relatively common. The presence of large numbers of families with altered family processes and unhealthy lifestyles within the community may create problems for all members of the larger community or society. The nurse who works in community settings will frequently encounter these families and is in an ideal position to care for them, to act as their advocate, to refer them to appropriate care, and in effect, to improve the health of the community at large.

The nurse may find that in some cultural groups such as Mexican Americans, traditional healers can be helpful for those persons who suffer from some emotional or psychological disorders. In addition, health professional such as physicians, dentists, nurse practitioners and others may be more acceptable if they share the same ethnic heritage as the client. In some aggregate ethnic settings, such as Chinatown in San Francisco, there are practitioners of Chinese traditional medicine as well as Western medicine, acupuncturists, neighborhood pharmacies and herbalists, which are available to meet the diverse needs of that particular neighborhood.

Assessment of Culturally Diverse Communities

A cultural assessment may be directed toward individual clients to assess their cultural needs (Leininger, 1991) (see also Chapter 2). Individual cultural assessments are accomplished through the use of a systematic process. In community health nursing, the community is considered the client, and several schema have been proposed to help nurses assess the community (Clark, 1996; Lancaster, Lowry & Martin, 1996). A community nursing assessment requires gathering relevant data, interpreting the data base (including problem analysis and prioritization), and identifying and implementing intervention activities for community health (Goeppinger & Schuster, 1992). Although the community nursing assessment focuses on a broader goal, such as an improvement in the health status of a group of people, an important factor to remember is that it is the characteristics of people that give every community its uniqueness. These common characteristics that influence norms, values, religious practices, educational aspirations, and health and illness behavior are frequently determined by shared cultural experiences. Thus adding the cultural component to a community nursing assessment strengthens the assessment base.

Components of the Cultural Assessment

Orque (1983) developed an ethnic/cultural system framework to assess components of clients' cultural profiles. Leininger (1978) presented assessment domains within which to seek data to understand culture. Later, Leininger (1991) developed a tool to assess clients cultural patterns by broadly looking at lifeways. Inherent in most definitions of culture is the notion of *shared* cultural backgrounds or a *way of life* or *world view*. Thus the concept of culture may be more easily applied to a community or group of persons than to an individual. An overview of selected cultural components is presented in Table 10-1. These components can be used to assess diverse cultural groups within a community.

An Overview of a Cultural Assessment: Native American (Navajo)

Family and Kinship Systems

Often an extended family that consists of an older woman and her husband and unmarried children, together with married daughters and their husbands and unmarried children.

The Navajo (or other Native Americans) have many unique categories of relatives.

Descent is traced through the mother.

Head of household is the husband, although the wife has a voice in decision making.

Children are highly valued and are given responsibilities to make decisions about themselves.

There is prestige with age as long as the elderly person can function independently.

Social Life

The earth and nature are valued; the individual should be in harmony with nature; this thought is interwoven with daily activities. Cooperation with others rather than competition is a cultural value.

Life-cycle events are marked by special rituals; for example, the blessing way takes place shortly after the birth of a child.

Like many other indigenous people, the Navajo suffer high rates of alcoholism, suicide, domestic violence and homicide. Currently, abuse of drugs and HIV disease are becoming more common.

Tribal and family ties are strong and contribute to a sense of belonging to a social group.

Educational opportunities are often limited because of an inferior school system.

Diet is often high in carbohydrates and fats; staple foods are corn, mutton, and fried bread.

Political Systems

The system of tribal government was imposed by whites.

Poverty and high rates of unemployment are overriding concerns.

The extended family has an economic as well as a social function.

Control of resources (land, water) has been problematic given the role of the U.S. Government.

Improving housing, sanitation, and work opportunities are major goals.

A major problem is that of making deteriorated lands productive in an underpopulated region.

Language and Traditions

Most of the younger Navajo speak English. Reading, writing, and speaking English are taught in all the schools. Many elderly Navajo speak little or no English.

There are many homonyms in the Navajo language, words that have identical sounds but different meanings. The Navajo language is very specific.

Periods of silence during communication show respect.

Nonverbal communication is a high art form among the Navajo and silence is highly respected. There may be little eye contact. Direct and prolonged eye contact is considered extremely rude and intrusive.

There is a lack of need for personal space.

The group has a history of oppression from the white dominant group.

The "Long Walk" (a forced move of 300 miles to Ft. Sumner in 1863) was a major calamity for the Navajo and remains a poignant chapter in cultural history that enforces Native American culture and identity.

World View, Value Orientations, and Cultural Norms

The basic nature of human beings is neither good nor bad; both qualities exist in each person.

Nature is more powerful than human beings.

Individual success is not valued as highly as providing security to the extended family.

The traditional Navajo views on the relationship of human beings with other human beings are both individualistic and collateral.

The integrity of the individual must be respected. There is respect for the choice of an individual (even a child's decision is respected).

There is also pressure for a Navajo to consider the extended family's welfare when making decisions.

Time orientations are not strict; work and productivity are valued.

Religious Ideology

Religion enters every phase of the traditional Navajo life, and an important emphasis is on curing illness.

There are many important Navajo ceremonies that may be used with illness; theology and medicine are difficult to separate in traditional Navajo culture.

Earth and nature are a part of the Navajo's cosmology, and health is viewed as harmony with the universe.

Many Native Americans, including some Navajo, are members of the Native American Church.

Peyote may be used in religious curing rituals to restore natural harmony. Peyote ceremonies may be conducted by special medicine men known as "Roadmen" who charge for their services.

Witchcraft may be practiced by certain individuals who are able to cause sickness in others.

Health Beliefs and Practices

Health is a reflection of a correct relationship between human beings and the environment. Health is associated with good, blessing, and beauty, all that is valued in life.

All ailments, both physical and mental, are believed to have supernatural aspects. The Navajo frequently use both their traditional health care system, including traditional health care practitioners, and the modern health care system.

There are two major types of traditional health care practitioners; the first is the diviner or diagnostician. Different methods, such as star gazing or hand trembling, are used to identify the cause of an illness. Then, once the cause of the illness is determined, the individual seeks the second kind of practitioner, the singer, who provides the treatment that counters the cause of disease and restores harmony.

Different types of ceremonials as well as herbal medicines and traditional remedies may be used. Infants are placed in cradleboards that have both traditional and religious significance.

Cornmeal may be used in healing ceremonies.

Women herbalists may prescribe herbs for specific and general reasons.

Health Concerns

Unintentional injuries and violence reflect the combined efforts of living conditions, environment and behavior. All told, unintentional injuries, homicides and suicides account for 25 percent of the deaths among the service population of the Indian Health Service (Rhoades, Hammond, Welty, Handler & Amler, 1987).

Heart disease is the leading cause of death among Native Americans, with a mortality rate of 393 per 100,000 population (Clark, 1996).

Obesity, hypertension and diabetes are also health concerns in Native American groups.

The rate of fetal alcohol syndrome is six times that of other Americans. Alcohol related mortality is four times that of the nation as a whole, and traumatic injury related to alcohol and substance abuse is a leading cause of death (U.S. Department Of Health and Human Services, 1993).

Diarrheal diseases contribute to a postneonatal death rate that is more than twice that of the general population (Rhodes, Hammond, Welty, Handler & Amler, 1987). Mortality in adults from infectious diseases is twice that of the general population and tuberculosis remains a pressing health problem (Centers for Disease Control and Prevention, 1992).

Reservations remain poor and often are geographically isolated. Geographical access to health care is of concern.

(Adapted from Phillips & Lobar, 1990; Boyle, Szymanski, & Szymanski, 1993; Huttlinger & Tanner, 1994; Bell, 1994; Clark, 1996; Kluckhohn & Leighton, 1974.)

Using Cultural Knowledge in Primary, Secondary and Tertiary Preventive Programs

Nurses working in community settings use health-related concepts that are identified with the practice of community health nursing. Concepts such as *community as client* or *population-focused practice* were discussed briefly in the first sections of this chapter. Another concept of importance to community nurses is that of *levels of prevention*. Preventive care, consisting of primary, secondary, and tertiary activities, is directed toward high-risk groups or aggregates within a community setting. *Primary prevention* is comprised of those activities that prevent the occurrence of an illness, a disease, or a health risk. The preventive actions takes place before the disease or illness occurs.

Secondary prevention involves the early diagnosis and appropriate treatment of a condition or disease. *Tertiary prevention* focuses on rehabilitation and the prevention of recurrences or complications. The major aim of community-based preventive programs is to reduce the risk for the population at large rather than prevent illnesses in specific individuals. As long as preventive actions are directed toward a given population rather than toward individuals, there is a chance of altering the general balance of forces so that although not all will benefit, many will have a chance to avoid illness. This last section of this chapter discusses the use of cultural knowledge to plan community nursing interventions for diverse cultural groups at the primary, secondary and tertiary levels of prevention.

Primary Prevention: Prenatal Services in a Mexican American Community

For some time now, it has been recognized that adequate prenatal care helps to reduce infant mortality. With this in mind, public health agencies have tried to improve maternal and infant services to high-risk populations. In the 1980s, a special government report on minority health reported that only 58 percent of Mexican American mothers begin prenatal care in the first trimester, less than that for African Americans or non-Hispanic women (Heckler, 1985a). The neonatal mortality rate appeared good for Mexican American babies, but there was a concern that the rate is artificially low due to underreporting (Heckler, 1985a; 1985b). Risk factors of pregnancy include age (both extremes), parity, and low socioeconomic status.

Many women of Mexican American origin fall in these categories; a high-risk group of great concern is the pregnant adolescent. A program of primary prevention would focus on preventing infant mortality and other health problems in Mexican American mothers and their infants. Nursing care must be broadly focused, providing some specific services but also helping clients access other resources in the community. Information can be provided through media campaigns that can be geared to the Mexican American community, informing women of available services and how to access them. Culturally related factors that might prevent Mexican American women from obtaining care early in their pregnancies would include the factors discussed below.

Access to Care

There are various reasons why Mexican Americans might not seek care during pregnancy. Cost is often a factor, and in many areas of the country, Mexican Americans have tended to belong to poorer socioeconomic groups (Heckler, 1985a, 1985b). The community health nurse can provide information about community resources and help clients access care early in pregnancy by referral to appropriate agencies. Many states now provide programs that provide funds and services for low-income pregnant women.

Cultural Views About Modesty

Any prenatal program that serves Mexican American women may be underutilized unless consideration is given to some Mexican American women's extreme modesty and resistance to examinations by male health care providers. The use of female nurse-practitioners and midwives is ideal for this population. In addition, some consideration should be given to incorporation of the traditional *parteras* (lay midwives) into the preventive educational services if deemed appropriate.

Language Barriers

It is absolutely essential in a prenatal program for a Mexican American population that the majority of health care professionals in the program be bilingual. If this is impossible, interpreters must be employed to facilitate the professional services. All prenatal classes should be offered in Spanish and English. This sometimes means that two classes must be offered concurrently; many Mexican American women speak predominantly either Spanish and English and would choose the class where they could understand the language. The availability of health education material in Spanish is critical to reinforce teaching and anticipatory guidance.

Cultural Views of Motherhood and Pregnancy

There is some evidence to indicate that women of Mexican American culture may adhere to different value orientations and cultural views of motherhood and pregnancy than those found in mainstream American culture (White, 1985; Burk, Wieser & Keegan, 1995). The Mexican American culture traditionally values motherhood, and young women are encouraged to prepare themselves for this role. In most traditional cultures, motherhood is the appropriately defined role for women, and there are few alternatives. White (1985) found that pregnant Mexican American women viewed their growing body as feminine, softening, and beautiful. Community health nurses are in important positions to help pregnant women prepare for motherhood and associated responsibilities. Understanding and reinforcing the approved cultural views of pregnancy may be helpful for clients in that trust and mutual goal setting can develop more rapidly.

Traditional Pregnancy-Related Folk Beliefs of Mexican Americans

Many Mexican Americans adhere to traditional beliefs and practices related to pregnancy and childbirth. Additionally, children are greatly valued and desired soon after marriage. Like many other cultures, Mexican Americans consider pregnancy, birth, and the immediate postpartum period as a time of great vulnerability for women and their newborns. Some traditional beliefs and practices related to pregnancy and childbirth are shown in Box 10-3.

Changing High-Risk Behaviors in Pregnant Mexican American Women

Certain high-risk behaviors during pregnancy, such as smoking, using drugs, alcohol consumption, and poor nutritional habits, should be targeted by the community health nurse for change. Although there is no set rule of thumb, a Mexican American mother-to-be may respond to suggestions for change if she is convinced that her behavior will cause harm to her baby. Family and social support groups found in Mexican American culture also can be helpful and supportive to expectant mothers wanting to make lifestyle changes. Some researchers have found pregnant Latin women will attempt to stop smoking and be successful with the help, support and assistance of their families. Research Application 10-2 provides an example and offers clinical applications for nursing practice.

Box 10-3 *Selected Beliefs and Practices of Pregnancy and Childbirth in Traditional Mexican American Culture*

- Avoid strong emotions such as anger and fear during pregnancy.
- Cool air is dangerous during pregnancy and should be avoided.
- Bathe often during pregnancy; be active so that the baby will not grow too big and hinder delivery.
- Eat a nutritious diet; "give in" to food cravings.
- Massage is helpful to place the baby in the right position for birth.
- Don't raise your arms above your head or sit with your legs crossed during pregnancy because it will cause knots in the umbilical cord.
- Moonlight should be avoided during pregnancy, especially during an eclipse, because it will cause a birth defect.
- After delivery, a 40-day period known as *la dieta* or *cuarentena* is observed. Activities and certain foods are restricted.
- Chamomile tea will relieve nausea and vomiting in pregnancy.
- Heartburn can be treated with baking soda.
- Laxatives and purges may be used to "clean" the intestinal tract.

Research Application 10-2

Cigarette Smoking and Pregnant Latinas

Pletsch, P. K., & Johnson, M. A. (1996). The cigarette smoking experiences of pregnant Latinas in the United States. *Health Care for Women International, 17,* 549–562.

Since cigarette smoking is harmful to pregnant women and their babies, most pregnant women make some smoking changes through cessation or reduced smoking. This study described cigarette smoking and smoking cessation experiences of pregnant Latinas who participated in focus groups. Smoking was described as a personal resource to deal with stress and as a social activity that facilitated interactions with family and friends. Many women described concern for their babies related to their smoking. The women related that the men in their lives disapproved of women smoking. Although the addictive properties of cigarette smoking impeded the cessation process, women reported that the support of others was a key element for success. Examination of the data in the context of cultural values revealed family involvement in Latinas' smoking behavior during pregnancy as powerful, unique, relevant, and consistent with the cultural values of allocentrism and familism. This finding provides a substantive base from which smoking cessation programs, tailored for pregnant Latinas, can be developed and implemented.

Clinical Application

- Involve family members such as mothers, sisters, and husbands in smoking cessation programs as they provide important support to Hispanic women.

- Smoking cessation messages and educational programs in Hispanic cultures should be targeted to families rather than individuals.

- Pregnancy is a time when many women are concerned for their babies' health and will be more committed to quit smoking.

Prenatal services should go beyond the birth of the baby to include information about breast-feeding and family planning services. Traditionally, it has been assumed by some health professionals that family planning services would not be accepted in a Mexican American population because of religious opposition and *machismo*—the need of the male to prove his manhood by having children or the belief in the biologic superiority of men. However, it may be that Mexican American men as well as women are interested in family planning and are concerned about the number of children that they can support. This is an issue that should be validated with individual clients and their spouses.

Strategies for promoting breast-feeding should be identified and encouraged. For example, educational levels, family experiences with breast-feeding, husband's attitude, the need to return to work, and feelings of embarrassment have been associated with infant feeding choices among Mexican American women (Young & Kaufman, 1988). These factors need to be explored with individual women in order to help them make choices best suited for them and their babies.

Mexican American Cultural Networks

Traditionally, the family is very important in Mexican American culture, and nursing care should be family focused. Ties often go beyond the family to a wide network of kin. Bauwens and Anderson (1992) observed that a Mexican American is expected to turn first to the family for help; if preventive services are to be effective, they must tap these kinds of cultural networks to ensure the support of community residents in preventive programs in their neighborhoods that involve family members, neighbors, or friends.

Secondary Levels of Prevention: Type II Diabetes and Native Americans

Non–insulin-dependent diabetes (NIDD), or type II diabetes, is seen commonly among some Native Americans, and certain tribes have extremely high rates of the disease. By all accounts, the high rate of diabetes in Native American groups is a leading health concern.

Cultural Views of Diabetes

The reasons for the epidemic of type II diabetes among some Native Americans are not clear. It is believed that some Native American tribes have an underlying genetic propensity for the disease that is triggered by changes in dietary practices, a sedentary lifestyle, and increasing obesity (Neel, 1962; West, 1978). These factors have been complicated by social conditions such as poverty as well as problems of compliance or lack of adherence to medical regimens (Huse, Oster, Kildeen, Lurey & Coldez, 1989).

Because of the high rate of diabetes on some reservations, numerous secondary preventive services that focus on early diagnosis and treatment have been instigated. Many of these secondary prevention programs have been modeled after programs that have been successful with white middle-class Americans. Culturally related factors that could influence the success of secondary preventive programs for diabetes among some Native Americans are shown in Box 10-4. Readers are cautioned that validation of beliefs and practices should always take place with individual clients and families, and stereotyping (thinking that all Native Americans are the same) should be avoided.

Box 10-4 *Beliefs and Practices Related to Diabetes Found in Some Native Americans*

Nutritional Practices

- Diets high in calories, carbohydrates, and fats.
- Sharing communal meals is a common and valued cultural practice.
- High incidence of obesity in some groups.
- Food preparation often adds fats and calories.
- Snack foods (potato chips, carbonated beverages, prepackaged pastries) are common.
- High intake of alcohol serious compromises the treatment of diabetes.

Activity Levels/Fitness Practices

- Sedentary lifestyles have become common.
- Many reservations lack recreational facilities.
- Formal exercise activities are associated with the white man's culture and are not thought to be appropriate for Native Americans.

Beliefs and Values Related to Diabetes

- Ideal body image favors a heavier physique, and weight gain is considered normal; thinness is a cause for worry and concern.
- Concept of "control of one's body," i.e., weight, glucose levels, blood pressure, may conflict with values and norms of Native American culture. For example, Native American clients may be uncomfortable with comparison of individual performance against others or against the norms and standards of biomedical care.
- Many Native Americans are uncomfortable with the discussion of "private body functions" such as providing urine samples or blood testing in a public situation.
- Illness is a personal and unpleasant topic, and Native American clients may be uncomfortable when asked to talk about it.
- Diabetes is a white man's disease; Native Americans did not have diabetes until the white man came.
- The term *diabetic* may be offensive to some, and the label *diabetic clinic* might discourage clients from seeking health care services.
- White health professionals may be viewed with some suspicion and distrust given the past history of cultural contact between whites and Native Americans.
- Because diabetes is so common in some tribal groups, there is a fatalism about developing the disease, especially if a family member already has diabetes.
- Beliefs and health practices surrounding diabetes may vary according to Native American tribe.

Culturally Appropriate Nursing Interventions at the Secondary Level of Prevention

Nursing interventions at the secondary level of prevention should focus on the implementation of healthful lifestyle changes that ultimately will decrease the complications of diabetes. Most of these are related to what health professionals call *diet* and *exercise*, but what is appropriate for Native American culture is an emphasis on *health* and a *healthy lifestyle*.

Emphasize health and a healthy lifestyle rather than negative factors such as control of diabetes, prevention of complications, weight reduction, and exercise. The choice of words, as well as the emphasis, is important. For example, when teaching the client and family about diabetic diets, the nurse can substitute the word *nutrition* for *diet*, thus removing the negative perceptions and leading to a nursing plan that emphasizes substitution rather than deprivation. *Substituting* fruits for candy bars and packaged pastries, whole grains for potato chips or doughnuts, and vegetables for sugared snacks will improve nutritional status and lead to a healthier lifestyle. Special traditional foods, even fried bread, can be eaten on special occasions, and other types of bread can be substituted during regular meals.

Health education can be oriented toward individual clients and directed toward the family rather than provided in an impersonal clinic situation. Physical activities that are culturally congruent can be encouraged, and again, the value of health and a healthy lifestyle should be stressed over exercise and weight reduction. Physical activities that are congruent with overall lifestyle and cultural context will be easier to incorporate into daily living situations.

Family and Community Support for Programs of Secondary Prevention

Usually, the Native American family system is an extended family that includes several households of closely related kin. Family members become exceedingly important during times of crisis, since they are a source of support, comfort, assistance, and strength. The importance of cultural ties with kin and other members of the reservation community always must be considered in planning for early diagnosis and treatment programs. It is in this context (family and community) that clients are encouraged and supported not only to seek care but also to instigate lifestyle changes that are congruent with cultural practices and that will enhance the health status of all members of the family and, ultimately, the tribal community.

Tertiary Levels of Prevention: Hypertension and African Americans

Significance of the Problem

African Americans are a highly heterogeneous group and display considerable variation in health beliefs and behaviors. For the most part, this section will discuss a more traditional, rural African American culture, and the reader is advised to validate beliefs and behaviors with individual clients and communities.

Hypertension is a major risk factor for heart disease and stroke. Mean blood pressure levels are higher in African Americans than in European Americans, with a marked excess in African Americans. A decade ago, in a government study on minority health, Heckler (1985a) stated that "hypertensive blacks were at least as likely as whites of the same sex to be treated with antihypertensive medication and nearly as likely to have their blood pressure controlled" (p. 110). Heckler also noted that from 1968 to 1982, stroke mortality in blacks declined 50 percent, and coronary heart disease also had decreased dramatically. Hypertension control has certainly been one of the factors responsible for this improvement; it is critical that efforts to treat hypertension in African American populations be continued. Unfortunately, appropriate care often has been complicated by limited access to care, discrimination, and poverty.

Tertiary prevention seeks to reduce disability and to prevent complications from developing. A major aim of nursing care when implementing tertiary activities is to help clients adjust to limitations in daily living, to increase coping skills, to control symptoms, and in general, to minimize the complications of disease by reducing the rate of residual damage in a given population. Cultural factors that should be considered in tertiary prevention programs for African Americans are shown Box 10-5.

Using Cultural Knowledge in Tertiary Prevention

Community nurses have demonstrated competence in the management of community hypertension programs. Although these programs are vital to the early diagnosis and management of hypertension, they also include a component that focuses on helping clients manage a chronic disease, an aspect of tertiary prevention. In addition, community health nurses are in the advantageous position of assessing clients and families in their own homes and neighborhoods. This provides an understanding of the daily life situation faced by clients that other health care professionals often lack. It is this understanding that community health nurses can bring to bear when helping clients with tertiary preventive activities.

Box 10-5 *Cultural Factors to Consider in Planning Tertiary Prevention for a Traditional African American Population*

Language:
African American communication concepts/patterns can be identified and used in community education programs.
Cultural health beliefs:
Good health comes from good luck.
Health is related to harmony in nature.
Illnesses are classified as "natural" or "unnatural."
Illness may be God's punishment.
Maintenance of health is associated with "reading the signs," i.e., the phase of the moon, seasons of the year, position of the planets.
Cultural health practices:
Use of herbs, oils, powders, roots, and other home remedies may be common.
Cultural healers:
Older woman ("old lady") in the community who has a knowledge of herbs and healing
Spiritualist who is called by God to heal disease or solve emotional or personal problems
Voodoo priest/priestess who is a powerful cultural healer who uses voodoo, bone reading, etc., to heal or bring about desired events
Root doctor who uses roots, herbs, oils, candles, and ointments in healing rituals
Time orientation:
May be present-time oriented, which makes preventive care more difficult to implement and maintain.
Nutritional practices:
Soul food takes it name from "a feeling of kinship" among African Americans and may be served at home, provided at church dinners, or served at homestyle restaurants.
Diets may reflect traditional rural southern foods such as greens, grits, corn bread, chick peas, etc.

(Continued)

Box 10-5. *(Continued)*

Economic status:
African Americans account for a large number of those persons in the lower socioeconomic strata in American society.

Educational status:
High aspirations for education, but socioeconomic status and other complex factors limit educational opportunities.

Family and social networks:
Often strong extended family networks with a sense of obligation to relatives.

Self-concept:
The importance of race has been a continual issue for the self-identity of African Americans.

Impact of racism:
Unfortunately, racism is still present, and a negative perception of the African American's skin color by health professionals will seriously interfere with efficacious health care.

Religion:
African American churches have tremendous influence on daily life of their members because they serve as a source of spiritual and social support.
The African American church acts as a caretaker for the cultural characteristics of African American culture (Roberson, 1985).

Biologic variations:
There is a high incidence of lactose intolerance and lactase deficiency; this has implications for diet planning if African American clients cannot tolerate milk or milk products.
There is a higher prevalence of hypertension among African Americans than among European Americans.
Sickle cell anemia is more common among African Americans.

Adapted from Bloch, B. (1983). Nursing care of black patients. In M. S. Orque, B. Bloch, & L. S. A. Monrroy (Eds.). *Ethnic Nursing Care: A Multicultural Approach,* pp. 81–113. St. Louis: C. V. Mosby; and Andrews, M. M., & Bolin, L. (1993). The African American community. In J. M. Swanson & M. Albrecht (Eds.). *Community Health Nursing: Promoting the Health of Aggregates,* pp. 443–458. Philadelphia: W. B. Saunders.

Summary

Cultural concepts related to community health nursing practice have been discussed. A framework for providing culturally sensitive nursing care has been introduced to help nurses and other health professionals provide care to individuals and groups with diverse cultural backgrounds. These frameworks help nurses use cultural knowledge in assessing, planning, and implementing nursing care. This chapter explored the role of the family in transmitting beliefs and practices of health and illness. Cultural diversity within communities was addressed, and various subcultures within the United States, including refugees and immigrants, were discussed.

Cultural concepts were explored as they relate to the community at large. A cultural assessment was described as an integral component of a community nursing assessment. A selected cultural assessment of Navajo (Native American) was presented as an example to provide cultural data to assist nurses in providing culturally sensitive nursing care to individuals and groups. Preventive care in the community is of particular importance to community health nursing. The use of cultural knowledge in primary, secondary and tertiary levels of prevention was introduced. Examples of cultural diversity and levels of prevention were described to illustrate how cultural knowledge can be used in community health nursing practice.

Review Questions

1. Describe four cultural concepts and discuss how they can be used to provide transcultural nursing care to families and aggregates.
2. Describe an example of how cultural factors influence the health of an aggregate group within the community. How do cultural factors influence illness levels in an aggregate group?
3. List major cultural considerations in implementing preventive programs for culturally diverse groups. How can cultural considerations be used to identify barriers and facilitators for preventive programs?
4. Identify special health considerations in immigrant groups within the community.
5. Describe an approach to primary preventive health care for several cultural groups, i.e., Hispanics, African Americans, Amish and Laotian.
6. Describe secondary and tertiary programs targeting hypertension for elderly Chinese Americans.
7. Describe similarities and differences between folk and scientific health care systems. Give an example of each.

Learning Activities to Promote Critical Thinking

1. Describe sociocultural factors and their impact on health care for a cultural group within your community. Evaluate access, availability and acceptability of various health care services. Is this cultural group at risk? Why?
2. Conduct a community cultural assessment of a group within your community. Critically analyze the cultural knowledge and/or information that should be considered when planning care for the group? Use the outline provided in Table 10-1 to identify and collect cultural assessment data, i.e., family and kinship, social life, political systems, language, world view, religious behaviors, health beliefs and practices and health concerns. Compare and contrast the assessment of other groups in your community.
3. Develop a program plan or intervention for a cultural group within your community that has components of primary, secondary, and tertiary prevention.
4. Attend religious services at a church, temple, synagogue, or place of worship to learn about a religion different from your own. Assess how each church meets the unique needs of its congregation.
5. Identify alternative health care practitioners within your community. Which subcultures do they serve? Describe the kinds of care that they offer to residents.

References

Anderson, E. T., & McFarlane, J. M. (1996). *Community as Partner: Theory and Practice in Nursing* (2nd ed.). Philadelphia, PA: J. B. Lippincott.

Andrews, M. M., & Bolin, L. (1993). The African-American community. In J. M. Swanson & M. Albrecht (Eds.). *Community Health Nursing: Promoting the Health of Aggregates,* pp. 433–458. Philadelphia: W. B. Saunders.

Aroian, K. J. (1993). Mental health risks and problems encountered by illegal immigrants. *Issues in Mental Health Nursing 14,* 379–397.

Bauwens, E., & Anderson, S. (1992). Social and cultural influences on health care. In M. Stanhope & J. Lancaster (Eds.). *Community Health Nursing: Process and Practice for Promoting Health* (3rd ed.). pp. 91–108. St. Louis, MO: C. V. Mosby.

Bell, R. (1994). Prominence of women in Navajo healing beliefs and values. *Nursing and Health Care 15,* 232–240.

Betrus, P. A., Elmore, S. K., & Hamilton, P. A. (1995). Women and somatization: Unrecognized depression. *Health Care for Women International 16,* 287–297.

Blendon, R. J., Aiken, L. H., Freeman, H. E., & Corey, C. R. (1989). Access to medical care for black and white Americans. *Journal of the American Medical Association 261*(2), 278–281.

Bloch, B. (1983). Nursing care of black patients. In M. S. Orque, B. Bloch, & L. A. Monrroy (Eds.). *Ethnic Nursing Care: A Multicultural Approach,* pp. 81–113. St. Louis, MO: C. V. Mosby.

Boyle, J. S., Ferrell, J., Hodnicki, D., & Muller, R. (1996). Going home: African American caregiving for adult children with human immunodeficiency virus disease. *Holistic Nursing Practice 11,* 27–35.

Boyle, J. S., Szymanski, M. T., & Szymanski, M. E. (1993). Improving home health care for the Navajo. *Nursing Connections 5*(4), 3–13.

Burk, M. E., Wieser, P. C., & Keegan, L. (1995). Cultural beliefs and health behaviors of pregnant Mexican American women: Implications for primary health care. *Advances in Nursing Science 17*(4), 37–52.

Clark, M. J. (1996). Care of the community or target group. In M. J. Clark (Ed.). *Nursing in the Community* (2nd ed.). pp. 389–421. Stamford, CT: Appleton & Lange.

Cookfair, J. M. (1991). *Nursing Process and Practices in the Community.* St. Louis, MO: C. V. Mosby.

Flynn, B. C. (1997). Are we ready to collaborate for community based health services? *Public Health Nursing 14*(3), 135–136.

Friedman, M. M., & Ferguson-Marshalleck, E. G. (1996). Sociocultural influences on family health. In S. M. Hanson & S. T. Boyd, *Family Health Care Nursing: Theory, Practice, and Research,* pp. 81–98. Philadelphia: F. A. Davis Company.

Goeppinger, J., & Schuster, G. F., III (1992). Community as client: Using the nursing process to promote health. In M. Stanhope & J. Lancaster (Eds.). *Community Health Nursing: Process and Practice for Promoting Health* (3rd ed.), pp. 253–276. St. Louis, MO: C. V. Mosby.

Healthy People 2000: National Health Promotion and Disease Prevention Objectives. (1991). Washington, DC: U.S. Department of Health and Human Services, Public Health Service.

Heckler, M. M. (1985a). *Report of the Secretary's Task Force on Black and Minority Health, Vol. I: Executive Summary.* Washington, DC: U.S. Department of Health and Human Services.

Heckler, M. M. (1985b). *Report to the Secretary's Task Force on Black and Minority Health, Vol.2: Crosscutting Issues in Minority Health.* Washington, DC: U.S. Department of Health and Human Services.

Huse, D. M., Osler, G., Kildeen, A. R., Lurey, M. T., & Coldez, G. A. (1989). The economic costs of non-insulin dependent diabetes mellitus. *Journal of the American Medical Association 8,* 391–406.

Huttlinger, K. W., & Tanner, D. (1994). The peyote way: Implications for culture care theory. *Journal of Transcultural Nursing 5,* 5–11.

Kluckhohn, C., & Leighton, D. (1974). *The Navaho.* Cambridge, MA: Harvard University Press.

Lancaster, J., Lowry, L. W., & Martin, K. S. (1996). Organizing frameworks applied to community health nursing. In M. Stanhope & J. Lancaster, *Community Health Nursing: Promoting Health of Aggregates, Families and Individuals* (4th ed.). pp. 179–205. St. Louis, MO: C. V. Mosby.

Leininger, M. (1978). *Transcultural Nursing: Concepts, Theories and Practices.* New York: John Wiley & Sons.

Leininger, M. (1991). Leininger's acculturation health care assessment tool for cultural patterns in traditional and nontraditional lifeways. *Journal of Transcultural Nursing 2*(2), 40–42.

Leininger, M. (1995). Teaching transcultural nursing in undergraduate and graduate programs. *Journal of Transcultural Nursing 6*(2), 10–26.

Meleis, A. I. (1997). Immigrant transitions and health care: An action plan. *Nursing Outlook 45,* 42.

National Institute of Nursing Research (1995). *Community-Based Health Care: Nursing Strategies.* Bethesda, MD: U.S. Department of Health and Human Services.

Neel, J. V. (1962). Diabetes mellitus: A "thrifty" genotype rendered detrimental by progress. *American Journal of Human Genetics 14,* 353–362.

Orque, M. S. (1983). Orque's ethnic/cultural system: A framework for nursing care. In M. S. Orque, B. Bloch, & L. A. Monrroy (Eds.). *Ethnic Nursing Care: A Multicultural Approach,* pp. 5–48. St. Louis, MO: C. V. Mosby.

Phillips, S., & Lobar, S. (1990). Literature summary of some Navaho child health beliefs and rearing practices within a transcultural nursing framework. *Journal of Transcultural Nursing 1,* 13–20.

Pender, N. J. (1987). Health and health promotion: Conceptual dilemmas. In M. E. Duffy & N. J. Pender (Eds.). *Proceedings of a Wingspread Conference: Conceptual Issues in Health Promotion,* pp. 7–23. Indianapolis: Sigma Theta Tau International, Honor Society of Nursing.

Rhodes, E. R., Hammond, J. M., Welty, T. K., Handler, A. O., & Amler, R. W. (1987). The Indian burden of illness and future health interventions. *Public Health Reports 102,* 361–368.

Roberson, M. H. B. (1985). The influence of religious beliefs on health choices of Afro-Americans. *Topics in Clinical Nursing 7*(3), 57–63.

Saunders, L. (1954). *Cultural Differences and Medical Care: The Case of the Spanish Speaking People of the Southwest.* New York: Russell Sage Foundation.

Scanlan, J. (1983). Who is a refugee? Procedures and burden of proof under the Refugee Act of 1980. *In Defense of the Alien 5,* 23.

Spector, R. E. (1996). *Cultural Diversity in Health and Illness* (4th ed.). New York: Appleton-Century-Crofts.

Stanhope, M., & Lancaster, J. (1996). *Community Health Nursing: Promoting Health of Aggregates, Families and Individuals* (4th ed.). St. Louis, MO: C. V. Mosby.

Weatherby, N. L., McCoy, H. V., Bletzer, K. V., McCoy, C. B., Inciardi, J. A., McBride, D. C., & Forney, M. A. (1997). Immigration and HIV among migrant workers in rural southern Florida. *Journal of Drug Issues* 27(1), 155–172.

West, K. (1978). *Diabetes in American Indians: Advances in Metabolic Disorders.* New York: Academic Press.

White, V. (1985). The Experience of Pregnancy among Hispanic Women. Unpublished master's thesis, University of Utah, Salt Lake City, Utah.

Young, S. A., & Kaufman, K. (1988). Promoting breastfeeding at a migrant health center. *Journal of the American Public Health Association 78,* 523–525.

U.S. Bureau of the Census (1992). *1990 Census of Population: General Population Characteristics.* Washington, DC: U.S. Government Printing Office.

U.S. Department of Health and Human Services. (1993). *Healthy People 2000 Review.* Washington, DC: U.S. Government Printing Office.

Four

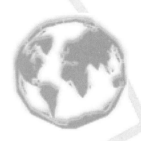

Contemporary Challenges in Transcultural Nursing

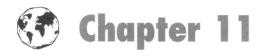

Chapter 11

Culture and Nutrition

Margaret M. Andrews

OBJECTIVES

1. Examine the cultural meanings of food for people from diverse backgrounds.
2. Identify guidelines for the nurse in assessing the nutritional status of clients from diverse cultures.
3. Explore health-related dietary beliefs and practices such as hot-cold and yin-yang theories as they relate to clients from diverse cultures.
4. Critically evaluate ways to adapt a menu for clients with special dietary needs in ways that are culturally congruent.
5. Examine cultural issues in nutrition in maternal and child health care.
6. Identify strategies that may be used to facilitate dietary change in culturally diverse clients.

As people of various cultural backgrounds and nationalities have settled in the U.S. and Canada, they have brought their food patterns with them, introducing a wide assortment of foods to their new homelands. New immigrants and their first-generation offspring usually adhere more closely to cultural food patterns than do subsequent generations. With increasing assimilation, subsequent generations may link to their past cultural food patterns only on holidays or at family gatherings. In some cases, they may give up cultural foods but retain traditional methods of preparation (Dudek, 1997). Even within a cultural group, food habits vary significantly among families and individuals.

Food patterns are generally developed during childhood and reflect the family's cultural heritage, lifestyle, socioeconomic status, religion, education, lifestyle, and individual factors such as nutritional requirements for age, gender and body size, health status, and taste physiology. The geographic region and urban/rural setting also exert an influence on food patterns for individuals, families, groups and communities. The literature abounds with studies reporting the observable food patterns of particular cultures and subcultures including food items consumed in different cultures, methods of production, preparation (e.g., seasonings, cooking techniques, cuisine, and culinary specialties), processing (e.g., canning, refrigerating, drying and fermenting), and kitchen tools (cooking and table utensils, dishes and recipes).

Perhaps one of the most important factors in promoting, maintaining, and restoring the client's health is your ability to encourage the intake of the right types and quantities of nutrients. The degree to which the nurse is successful may make the difference between a rapid return to health and a slow, prolonged recovery, or none at all. For centuries, diet has been used by many cultures in treating specific disease conditions, promoting health during pregnancy, fostering growth and development for infants and children, and instilling hope that the ingestion of certain foods could lead to the prolongation of one's earthly life. Recent research has linked nutritional components to many diseases, and diet is frequently considered in the prevention and/or treatment of many physical and emotional disorders.

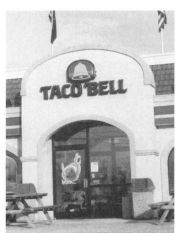 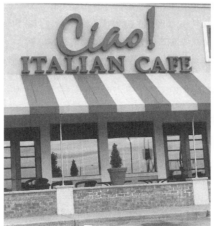 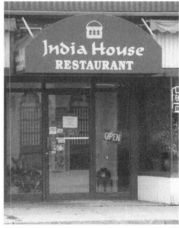

Restaurants featuring ethnic foods have proliferated across North America as people of different nationalities have introduced a wide assortment of cuisines to their new homeland.

Although food often makes people feel better both physically and psychologically, it also has many sociocultural functions. Transcultural nursing is concerned with different foods in diverse cultures, the food patterns of the cultures, and the ways foods help people stay healthy or cause them to become ill. In the following section, we will examine the cultural influences on dietary behaviors.

Cultural Influences on Dietary Behaviors

Most experts agree that the relationships between food-related behaviors and culture are complex and require a multidisciplinary approach to understand them. Nurses are primarily interested in the answer to the following questions: Which factors are the best predictors of the client's dietary behaviors? What culturally appropriate strategies can the nurse use to encourage the client to change unhealthy dietary behaviors into healthy ones? To answer these questions, various models and frameworks have been proposed. Figure 11-1 identifies the cultural influences on lifestyle and dietary behaviors.

Dietary behaviors are, in part, influenced by macro-level political, economic and social systems and by food production and distribution systems. Food production systems include commercially grown foods and those produced on a smaller scale such as foods grown in a backyard garden that are intended primarily for consumption by members of the household. In some agricultural countries or regions, a household is encouraged to produce sufficient food for its members. In Nigeria, for example, the federal government has launched a widespread campaign that encourages citizens to "Feed the nation, feed your family." Every family is urged to grow sufficient fruits and vegetables to feed its members. In the U.S. and Canada, most of the population resides in urban areas and relies on the distribution of food from rural to urban centers. A highly organized food distribution system includes rail, air and truck transportation and enables people to enjoy a variety of fresh meats, fruits and vegetables throughout the year, with some seasonal variation. These two systems in turn determine the locally available foods in restaurants and stores for people to purchase (or less frequently to barter or exchange for other goods or services).

As used in this discussion, the term *household* refers to individuals who reside in a common dwelling and share meals. Among the factors to be considered in understanding dietary behaviors is the *composition* of a household which includes the size, gender, and ages of household members. Economists have observed that given the same income, larger households spend more money on food than smaller ones, but the value of the food purchased per person decreases with increasing household size. Gender and age are physiological states that are influenced by culture and that in turn influence the individual's food consumption patterns. Across cultures, women consume, on average, less food than men. The more hours women spend employed outside the home, the fewer hours they spend in meal preparation, with estimates of 15–20 minutes per day for employed women compared to those who are not employed. They also tend to use more prepared convenience foods such as TV dinners and other frozen foods.

The *structure* of a household refers to members' relationship with one another and their household roles. Among the roles is that of *food gatekeeper*. In the now

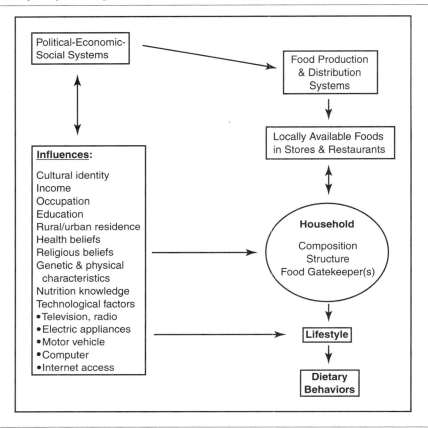

FIGURE 11-1. Cultural influences on dietary behavior.

classic *channel theory*, Lewin (1943) suggests that food moves through channels and the person who is primarily responsible for the food for a household is a *gatekeeper*. Nurses need to examine the social and psychological characteristics of the gatekeeper in order to understand his/her food acceptance. It should be noted that there may be more than one gatekeeper, especially in dual-income households. The theory states that once the food passes through the gate and onto the table, it will be eaten by household members. It should be noted that the theory does not account for households in which members eat out frequently or children are provided meals at school. Nonetheless, the theory still has considerable merit, and nurses should be sure to identify the food gatekeeper(s) when doing diet education.

Factors that influence the household dietary behaviors include cultural identity, income, occupation and education of household members, the rural/urban location of the residence, health and religious beliefs, genetic (e.g., lactose intolerance) and physical characteristics (e.g., gender, height, weight, percent body fat), knowledge of nutrition, level of activity and exercise (which may be interrelated with a sedentary or active occupation), and technological factors such as ownership of television, radio, computer and electric household appliances (stove, refrigerator, microwave oven, and various convenience items). In addition, dietary behaviors are influenced by people's access to transportation by privately owned motor vehicles, taxicabs, light rail, airplanes or other forms of public transportation. For the members of some cultures, travel by horse and buggy (Amish), dogsled (Native Alaskans), skis (Eskimos, Native Alaskans), canoes, kayaks and other watercraft (some Native Hawaiians, Eskimos, and American Indians), and/or walking may be used to reach food sources.

You should recognize that food itself is only one part of eating. In some cultures, social contacts during meals are restricted to members of the immediate or extended family. You should be aware of the individual's preference, particularly in situations fostering group dining, such as psychiatric/mental health institutions, extended-care facilities, and older adult or nursing homes, which sometimes encourage clients to eat in small groups. Traditional group nutrition education also may be inappropriate when it conflicts with cultural restrictions. In some Middle Eastern cultures, men and women eat meals separately, or women may be permitted to eat with their husbands but not with other males. Although certain practices may be unfamiliar to the U.S. or Canadian nurse, it is important that diversity related to meals be respected.

Cultural Meaning of Food

People often use food in building and maintaining human relationships. Food brings people together, promotes common interests, and stimulates the formation of bonds with other people and society. Sharing a meal frequently is a sign of affection and friendship, whereas refusal to eat with someone reflects anger, hostility, rejection, punishment, or mistrust. It is rare for enemies to share a meal. Box 11-1 presents some examples of the cultural meanings of food.

Cultural Functions and Uses of Food

Culture defines both the functions and uses of foods. According to Leininger (1995), there are seven *universal functions and uses of foods*, regardless of culture:

1. Although there is considerable debate concerning what constitutes the essential or basic nutritional needs of people in different settings, there is consensus that *food enables people to maintain body functions and produce energy.*
2. Food is used to *establish and maintain social and cultural relationships with relatives, friends, strangers, and others.* Rituals are frequently associated with food uses to bring people together. For example, in most of the U.S. and Canada, nurses expect a "coffee break," with *coffee* being a euphemism for whatever beverage or snack foods the individual prefers. Food may be used during particular life-cycle passages, sometimes referred to as *rites of passage.* Procuring and distributing foods are often interconnected with cultural status and prestige functions related to work, marriage, achievements, and other factors.
3. Food functions to *assess social relationships or interpersonal closeness or dis-*

Box 11-1 *Selected Examples of Cultural Meanings of Food*

Critical life force for survival
Relief of hunger
Peaceful coexistence
Promotion of health and healing
Prevention of disease or illness
Expression of caring for another
Interpersonal closeness or distance
Promotion of kinship and familial alliances
Solidification of social ties
Celebration of life events (e.g., birthday, marriage)
Expression of gratitude or appreciation
Recognition of achievement or accomplishment
Business negotiations
Information exchange
Validation of social, cultural, or religious ceremonial functions
Way to generate income
Expression of affluence, wealth, or social status

tance between people. The manner in which a culture is stratified, by castes, classes, or clans, determines who gets what foods.

4. A fourth universal function and symbolic use of food is to *cope with emotional stresses, conflicts and traumatic life events.* Compulsive eating and hoarding of food to relieve tensions are largely learned and patterned from cultural practices. Anorexia nervosa, bulimia, and compulsive overeating to relieve anxiety occurs more frequently in Western cultures where food is abundant.

5. Food is used to *reward, punish, and influence the behavior of others.* From early in childhood, food rewards such as candy, sugared cereals, cookies, cupcakes, and sweetened beverages are given to children to reinforce positive behaviors. In other cultures, children may be rewarded with non-refined foods such as fruits, vegetables, nuts, and meat.

6. Food *influences the political and economic status of an individual or group.* Food has been used to build and maintain harmonious relationships between politicians and their constituents, gain votes, and foster desired political alliances. Economically, the food is important in exchanges to maintain basic food supplies and provide diversity in people's diets. The production, accumulation, and distribution of food is of great concern worldwide. Periods of drought, floods, earthquakes, volcanic eruptions and other influences from the natural environment exert a significant influence on the production and distribution of foods in many countries.

7. Finally, food is used to *assess, treat, and prevent illnesses or disabilities* of people. For centuries, folk and professional healers have used diet to treat

specific disease conditions, promote health during pregnancy, foster child growth and development, and instill hope in people of all ages that the ingestion of certain foods could lead to the prolongation of their earthly life.

Body Image, Food and Culture

Definitions of the ideal body size and shape vary from one culture to another and change with time. Cultural images of ideal body size and methods used to achieve it have been the topic of lively discussion for many years, and the multi-million-dollar diet industry illustrates that much time, energy, and money is spent on people's efforts at achieving the culturally appropriate body build.

In addition to recognizing a group's definitions of ideal weight or size, nurses can benefit from an appreciation of the significance associated with thinness and fatness. Concern with ideal body size and shape begins in infancy. Research indicates that when asked to identify the ideal body size, most Puerto Ricans and Cubans selected a plumper body, whereas the majority of whites chose a thinner figure as ideal for infants.

Research has demonstrated that both excessively thin and excessively obese people have increased morbidity and mortality. Obesity, for example, has been shown to increase the risk of heart attack, stroke, hypertension, diabetes, musculoskeletal problems, and others. The hazards facing underweight people are not as well documented but include greater risks from infectious diseases. Research Application 11-1 summarizes a study of the determinants of body size perceptions and their relationship to dietary behavior in a multiethnic group of women.

Nutrition Assessment

You must consider cultural variation when assessing the client's nutritional state and food intake. Among the factors to consider are the frequency and number of meals eaten, form and content of ceremonial meals, snacking habits and the regularity of food consumption. Because potential inaccuracies may occur, the 24-hour dietary recalls or 3-day food records used traditionally for assessment may be inadequate when dealing with clients from diverse backgrounds. Another source of error may be reliance on dietary handbooks because information and exchange tables are generally based on European American diets.

Although it may seem self-evident, you may need to define what is meant by the term *food*. Each person classifies foods into five groups according to whether the food is considered *inedible, edible by animals (but not humans), edible by humans (but not my kind), edible by humans (but not by me),* and *edible by me*. Culture is a primary influence on how an individual decides which food belongs in which category. For example, certain Latin American groups do not consider vitamin-rich green vegetables to be food, and thus fail to list intake of these vegetables on daily records. Among Vietnamese Americans, dietary intake of calcium may appear inadequate, particularly with the low consumption of dairy products common among members of this group. However, you need to know that pork bones and shells are commonly consumed, thus providing adequate quantities of calcium to meet daily requirements. Clay is

Cultural Perspectives on the Perception of Body Size

Mossavar-Rahmani, Y., Pelto, G. H., Ferris, A. M., & Allen, L. H. (1996). Determinants of body size perceptions and dieting behavior in a multiethnic group of hospital women staff. *Journal of the American Dietetic Association, 96*(3), 252–256.

Using a convenience sample of N = 174 women from diverse cultural backgrounds working in an urban New York hospital, the investigators examined the factors that determine perceived body size and its relationship to dietary behavior. The findings revealed that height and weight-for-height were stronger predictors of accuracy of perceived body size than ethnicity. Tall, slight women were more likely to overestimate whereas short, heavy women were more likely to underestimate actual body size. European American women were more likely to perceive their body size as larger than actual compared with Afro-Caribbeans and African Americans. Women with a history of weight reduction dieting were more likely to overestimate their size and to view it as different from what is perceived as attractive to others.

Clinical Applications

Between 50 to 60 percent of women and adolescent girls in the United States are dissatisfied with the size of their body. Whether women perceive their bodies as too large or too small may reflect attitudes toward obesity and may be related to "dieting" behavior (i.e., the deliberate restriction of energy intake). Some women who feel the need to diet may correctly perceive their body size to be undesirably large in terms of health risks, whereas other women of similar body size may be less inclined to diet because they perceive their body size to be appropriate. Dieting may provide the behavioral link among perception of body image, body image preferences, and food intake, but there needs to be further research on these relationships.

Nurses must ensure that women acquire a realistic perception of their body size before undertaking a weight reduction diet. Nurses can play a positive role by encouraging healthy, realistic body image ideals. This study shows that helping patients achieve this goal requires attention to several factors, including ethnic background. For example, some Puerto Rican women have a view about body size that may, at first glance, appear to be similar to their European American counterparts. On closer examination, however, it becomes evident that they are experiencing inner conflict between wanting to be thin, which is valued by Anglo peers, and acquiescing to their family's preference for a larger body size. Although further study is needed, there may be intergenerational differences in body size perceptions, with older women preferring larger sizes than younger ones.

sold for consumption in parts of Africa but not in other parts of the world. In France, corn is considered animal feed not fit for human consumption, whereas corn is considered a sacred and essential diet staple by many Native Americans tribes. Due to religious beliefs, some Jewish, Muslim, and Seventh-Day Adventist clients consider pork inedible, whereas members of many other religions would eat it without hesitation. Eating dog, cat, or horse meat is unacceptable to most European Americans, yet these meats are enjoyed by some people having Asian or African heritage. Foods such as beef and chicken may be enjoyed by the majority of Americans and Canadians but not by those who follow a vegetarian diet.

You need to be aware that culture determines meal patterns. Asking a client what was eaten at breakfast, lunch, and supper reflects your ethnocentric bias that three meals are the norm. Among many Native American and Latin American groups, two meals a day are usually eaten. In Spain, four meals a day plus frequent snacks are customary. In some nomadic African tribes, one meal is consumed every other day. Furthermore, what foods constitute a meal may be a factor in diet analysis. For example, in India, a meal is only a meal if rice or another traditional grain food (such as flat bread) is served. Although other foods are eaten in large quantities, they may be considered snacks if no rice or bread is consumed. When a meal is eaten and the etiquette of eating also are culturally determined. Culture influences beliefs about what food should be eaten cooked or raw. For example, many Asian Americans eat significant quantities or cooked vegetables, but seldom consume them raw.

Among some African-American groups, particularly in rural southern areas, large quantities of rich foods may be consumed on weekends, whereas the intake of food on a weekday is typically much lighter. Many groups tend to feast, often in the company of family and friends, on selected holidays. For example, many Christians eat large dinners on Christmas and Easter and consume other traditional high-calorie, high-fat foods such as seasonal cookies, pastries, and candies. It should be noted that holy days may be celebrated at various times depending on the religious calendar followed. Many Jewish families celebrate Passover, Rosh Hashanah, Hanukkah, and other religious holy days with rich ethnic foods, often eaten in quantities that exceed consumption during the nonholiday period. Your need to be familiar with the religious and ethnic calendars of clients from various groups in order to be aware of the influence of religion and culture on diet. This information is especially significant for clients with diabetes, hypertension, gastric ulcers and other conditions in which diet plays a key role.

Stereotypically, in U.S. and Canadian white cultures, people eat bacon and eggs for breakfast in the morning, sandwiches for lunch around noon, and meat and potatoes or rice for supper in the evening. Some cultures make few distinctions between what is served at different meals, and others vary in what foods are considered appropriate. For example, soup is commonly eaten at every meal by Vietnamese, and beans are enjoyed at breakfast, lunch, and supper by many Mexicans. Cheese and olives are popular breakfast foods in the Middle East, and peanut butter is added to many dinner dishes in West Africa.

Religious and Civic Holidays

As discussed in Chapter 12, cultural food practices are often interconnected with religious dietary restrictions. In many religious traditions, foods are used symbolically in celebrations and rituals such as bread and wine (some groups substitute grape juice) served during many Christian communion services. The Hindu refrain from eating meat and show a high degree of reverence for cows. Many Jews and Muslims refrain from eating pork, and they ritually slaughter the animals whose meat is permitted to be eaten. Table 11-1 summarizes the food-related practices of selected religious groups.

TABLE 11-1
Food Restrictions for Selected Religions

Religious Group and Food Restrictions	Clinical Implications
Church of Jesus Christ of Latter-Day Saints (Mormonism)	
No alcoholic beverages	Avoid medicines containing alcohol such as some cough suppressants
No stimulants (caffeinated beverages such as coffee, tea, sodas)	For clients on liquid diets, substitute decaffeinated beverages for brewed and instant regular coffee, teas, cocoa, and carbonated beverages containing caffeine (e.g., colas). Avoid medicines containing caffeine such as the following OTCs *Analgesics* Anacin, Bromo-Seltzer, Cope, Empirin, Excedrin *Stimulants* No Doz Vivarin Caffedrine *Diet Pills* Dexatrim and similar generic brands Many cold preparations
Observant Mormons fast on the first Sunday of each month. Fasting means refraining from food and liquids.	Fasting is not required during illness nor by persons with diabetes, hypoglycemia, ulcers or other medical condition for which fasting is contraindicated.
Judaism	
Three major groups • Orthodox—strict observance • Conservative—nominal observance • Reform—less ceremonial emphasis and minimum observance of dietary laws	Kosher meals are available in hospitals and other health care settings. They usually are served on paper plates with plastic utensils that are sealed. Nurses should not unwrap the utensils or transfer food onto another dish.
The *laws of kashrut* dictate which foods are permissible under religious law:	Do not bring nonkosher foods into the home of a Jewish client who follows the laws of kashrut
1. Only meat from cloven-hoofed animals that chew cud (cattle, sheep, goat, ox, or deer) is allowed. These animals must be slaughtered ritually in a manner that results in minimal pain to the animal and maximal blood drainage. There are two methods used to prepare *kosher* (meaning "properly preserved" or "fit for eating") meats: a. The meat is soaked in cold water for 30 minutes, salted, and drained to deplete blood content. It is then washed under cold water and drained again before cooking. OR	

TABLE 11-1 (*Continued*)

Religious Group and Food Restrictions	Clinical Implications
b. The meat is first prepared by quickly searing or cooking over an open flame, which permits liver to be eaten.	Milk may not be used in coffee if served with a meat meal. Nondairy creamers can be substituted if they do not contain sodium caseinate, which is derived from milk.
2. Meat and dairy products cannot be served at the same meal, nor can they be cooked or served in the same set of dishes. Milk or milk products may be consumed just before a meal, but not until 6 hours after eating a meal in which meat has been consumed. Fish, eggs, vegetables, and fruits are considered *parve* or neutral and may be eaten with dairy products or meat meals.	When teaching clients about special diets, be sure that sample menus are congruent with dietary laws Be aware that keeping a kosher kitchen requires two sets of dishes, pots, & utensils.
3. Fish with fins and scales are allowed. No shellfish (crab, lobster, shrimp, clam, oyster) or scavenger fish (catfish, shark, porpoise) may be eaten. Crocodile, frog, snail, snake, and tortoise also are prohibited. Note: Kosher foods in stores are marked with one of two symbols: a. The letter "K" with a circle designating it is kosher, or b. The encircled letter "U" which is the seal of the Union of Orthodox Jewish Congregations of America	
Additional dietary laws are followed during the week of Passover. (No bread or product with yeast may be eaten; instead *matzah* or unleavened bread is eaten.) Products that are fermented or can cause fermenting or souring may not be eaten.	
There are a number of fast days in the Jewish calendar, with the holiest being Yom Kippur, or Day of Atonement, during which Jews abstain from food and drink from sunset the evening before the holy day until after sunset the following day.	The nurse should encourage Jewish clients to consult with a rabbi if their insistence on fasting may be detrimental to health (e.g., those with insulin-dependent diabetes, hypoglycemia, or ulcers). Maintaining one's health supercedes the laws of fasting.

Islam

Pork, pork products, animal shortening, and alcohol are strictly prohhibited.	Clients in hospitals and other health care settings may need assistance in identifying foods that have been prepared using animal shortenings or pork seasonings. They should avoid regular gelatin made with pork, marshmallow and other confections made with pork. Avoid medicines containing alcohol such as some cough suppressants. Avoid extracts such as vanilla or lemon that contain alcohol.
The slaughter of poultry, beef, and lamb must be done ritually by a Muslim to ensure that it is *halal*.	Although many hospitals and other health care settings do not routinely provide foods that are *halal*, these products are often available at specialty grocery stores, particularly in large urban areas.

TABLE 11-1 (*Continued*)

Religious Group and Food Restrictions	Clinical Implications
Fasting is common. During the month of Ramadan no foods or beverages are consumed until after sunset. Note: Recent immigrants from the Middle East may eat and pass food with the right hand. Because the left hand is used for toileting, it is considered extremely impolite to eat with the left hand.	Fasting is not required for persons who are ill.

Roman Catholicism

Abstinence from meat and meat products (gravy, soups) and fasting on Ash Wednesday and the Fridays during a 40-day period of religious observance called Lent. Rules of fasting apply to those between the ages of 12 and 65. Fasting refers to eating one regular meal and two smaller meals per day.	Fish, cheese, or other meat substitutes are offered on these days. Fasting is not required for children, the elderly, or anyone who is ill.

Seventh-Day Adventism

Fermented or alcoholic beverages are prohibited.	Avoid medicines containing alcohol such as some cough medicines. Avoid vanilla and lemon extract.
Optional vegetarianism may take three forms: (a) Strict vegetarians (syn. *vegans*)—people who include no animal-derived products in their diet; (b) ovolactovegetarians—people who use milk, milk products, and eggs but no meats in their diet; and (c) semivegetarians—Adventists who refrain from pork or pork products, shellfish, and blood.	Strict vegetarians may need assistance in selecting a balanced diet from the hospital menu.
Snacking between meals is discouraged.	Some clients with diabetes, hypoglycemia, or ulcers may require between-meal snacks.

Cultural foods are frequently served in the celebrations that follow religious rituals such as Catholic baptisms and confirmations, Jewish bar mitzvahs and bat mitzvahs, and similar religious ceremonies marking a *rite of passage*. In nearly every culture, food is an integral part of a wedding. Christian holidays such as Christmas and Easter, Jewish celebrations such as Passover, Rosh Hashana, and Hanukkah, and non-religious holidays such as Kwanzaa, government holidays in the U.S. and Canada and the Chinese New Year, are examples of events that are celebrated with special foods. See Figure 12-1 for selected religious and civic holidays in the U.S. and Canada. Knowing the client's religious beliefs about food enables the nurse to suggest improvements or modifications that will not conflict with religious dietary laws. Similarly, cultural dietary beliefs may be interconnected with yin/yang and hot/cold theories as they relate to health promotion across the life span, pregnancy, and the alleviation of the symptoms associated with disease and illness.

Understanding Cultural Influences on Dietary Change

Although North Americans have more extensive nutrition knowledge than ever before in history, many people are unable to apply it to their daily lives. As a consequence, obesity, heart disease, hypertension, and other diet-related disorders continue to afflict a significant proportion of the U.S. and Canadian populations, with those from diverse cultural backgrounds being at high risk. An understanding of culture change processes and intervention strategies form the foundation for the *directed change process*. There are three components in the directed change process that influence people's receptivity to change. These are the *client* and his/her significant others, the *nurse*, and the nature of the *recommended dietary change* itself.

Figure 11-2 provides a schematic representation of the interrelationships among the *client, nurse* and *recommended dietary change*.

Client Influences on Directed Dietary Change

Cultural attitudes, values, beliefs and practices concerning diet, exercise, and image of the ideal body affect the client's perceptions of recommended dietary change. The cultural value placed on change itself must also be considered. Although an attraction to novelty and modernity is widespread in some cultures, others embrace more traditional, time-proven values. The client who places a value on change is more receptive, overall, to diet-related changes.

Among the attitudes and values that play an especially important role in the adoption and rejection of dietary change are those concerning authority. In most societies, people rely on specialists for information and advice about religion, government, technology, health, and other aspects of life. The number and variety of specialists increases as society becomes more complex, and that society's dependence on authorities for solutions to problems also grows. The academic degrees and titles of nurses, dieticians, and other health care providers sometimes leads to their being perceived in an authority role, at least by some clients. Some people place a great deal of faith in the advice of these authorities and are readily influenced by professionals or recognized experts.

For example, some clients will consider dietary change only if it is recommended by an authority figure such as a nurse. An attitude closely associated with dependence on authority is the expectation of change. In some cultures, authorities provide people with new, effective solutions to their health-related problems and the public begins to expect authorities to produce changes that further improve their lives. Although openness to change has many positive aspects, it may also lead to problems. With this expectation, people grow increasingly receptive to change and willing to consider modifying their food patterns. Thus, the expectation of change in itself serves as a stimulus to the acceptance of change.

Not all change that is expected is also welcome. Clients may anticipate change but at the same time prefer the status quo. For example, a newly diagnosed diabetic client may realize from media publicity or contact with other diabetics that significant dietary change is needed but prefer to continue eating foods with high sugar content. Even if change is not desired, it is more likely to be accepted when it is anticipated than when it is not.

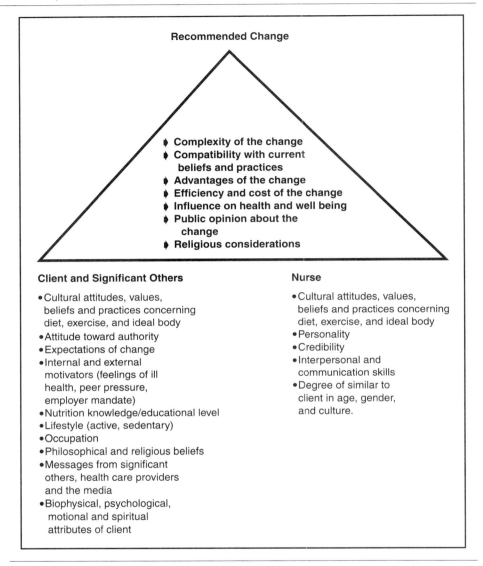

Recommended Change

- Complexity of the change
- Compatibility with current beliefs and practices
- Advantages of the change
- Efficiency and cost of the change
- Influence on health and well being
- Public opinion about the change
- Religious considerations

Client and Significant Others

- Cultural attitudes, values, beliefs and practices concerning diet, exercise, and ideal body
- Attitude toward authority
- Expectations of change
- Internal and external motivators (feelings of ill health, peer pressure, employer mandate)
- Nutrition knowledge/educational level
- Lifestyle (active, sedentary)
- Occupation
- Philosophical and religious beliefs
- Messages from significant others, health care providers and the media
- Biophysical, psychological, motional and spiritual attributes of client

Nurse

- Cultural attitudes, values, beliefs and practices concerning diet, exercise, and ideal body
- Personality
- Credibility
- Interpersonal and communication skills
- Degree of similar to client in age, gender, and culture.

FIGURE 11-2.   Cultural influences on dietary change.

In cultures that do not expect dietary changes to occur, nurses usually encounter resistance to new ideas or programs. Because nutrition change is not seen as natural or good, it proceeds more slowly than in situations where it is expected. In some cases, the client may be suspicious of your motives and skeptical of the benefits of the diet change.

The client's motivation for dietary change may have internal or external origins. Internal motivation may include the desire to feel more energetic, fit, or alert. In some instances, the client may be motivated by fear of undesirable consequences. For example, an African American with a family history of hypertension, stroke and premature death from cardiovascular disease may be highly motivated to follow the low-sodium diet recommended for hypertension out of fear for the devastating effects observed in others. External motivation may come from family members, peers, employers, nurses and other health care providers, members of the clergy, or folk healers. It also may be the result of media influence from television, radio, newspapers, or magazines. In more recent years, the internet, computer and video software, and other electronic sources may influence some clients.

The client's likelihood of making a dietary change is interrelated with knowledge of nutrition, educational level, occupation, income, and socioeconomic status which in turn determine whether the person has a relatively active or sedentary life style. Throughout the U.S. and Canada, adult education is widespread and nurses often use lecture-discussion groups, seminars and workshops to teach about dietary change. In some cultures, formal education is appropriate only for children, and adults may feel uncomfortable in the learner role. Even in cultures where adult education is widespread, some clients may find classroom programs unacceptable because such activities remind them of negative experiences they had in school. Philosophical and religious beliefs may influence the client's readiness to embrace dietary change. For example, some people follow a vegetarian diet because they believe philosophically that taking the life of an animal is immoral, whereas others cite religious scriptures for refraining from meat. Finally, unique characteristics related to the client's biophysical (age, gender, genetic makeup), psychological, emotional, and spiritual attributes must be considered as factors contributing to his or her willingness to embrace directed dietary change.

Directed Dietary Change

The directed change process, like many situations involving persuasion, relies heavily on the nurse advocating dietary change for its success. *Personality* is one of the inescapable attributes that contributes to your ability to direct dietary change in clients from diverse cultures. Engaging clients with likeable mannerisms will attract attentive consideration to both themselves and their recommendations about diet. People are more likely to listen, consider their opinions, and emulate the nurse with an outgoing, sociable personality. The client's perception of the nurse's *prestige* or *status* is also a factor to be considered.

Credibility refers to the nurse's expertness and trustworthiness as a change agent. Clients' beliefs about the nurse's knowledge of nutrition, education, and competence form their assessment of his/her credibility. Trustworthiness is based on clients' evaluation of the nurse's sincerity and personal motives for promoting dietary change. Related is the concept of prestige. A difficult concept to analyze, prestige encompasses a variety of interconnected traits such as competence, past accomplishments, reputation, wealth, and in many cases ascribed characteristics such as gender, age, or nationality. The nurse's prestige also varies according to the audience, the situation, and the subject. It should be noted that prestige alone is insufficient to influence others to alter their dietary behavior.

The nurse's interpersonal and communication skills will influence the client's decision to follow a recommended dietary change. The nurse-client relationship will affect the nurse's ability to persuade the client. In many communities people look primarily to professionals for leadership and direction in change, whereas others are more skeptical of change and unwilling to adopt new food patterns. People who are open to advice about dietary change from nurses and other health care providers from outside their community typically accept change first and are sometimes called *early adopters*. Those who are more resistant to change and follow community members rather than professionals are sometimes called *late adopters*.

Because nurses who come from outside a community are largely ineffective in persuading late adopters, it is often beneficial to recruit early adopters from within the group to support the dietary change. The effectiveness of using these in-group change agents is illustrated in research on infant feeding practices among Cubans, Puerto Ricans, and whites in Florida. Mothers did not adopt the advice of health care providers about controlling infant weight gain unless it also was advocated by a friend, relative or neighbor. For this reason, diet counseling is often more effective if a friend, neighbor, or relative attends the session and reinforces the advice given by the nurse. The nurse's cross-cultural communication skills and facility in the client's primary language also must be considered.

In some cultures (e.g., traditional Chinese, Mexican, and Arab groups), similarity in age, gender, ethnicity and other attributes of the nurse and client can promote effective cross-cultural communication and diet change. It is not, however, the position of this author that nurse and client must be from similar backgrounds in all cases. If the nurse has a solid grasp of transcultural nursing concepts, principles and theories, the differences in heritage should not be obstacles to promoting dietary change.

Nature of the Recommended Changes

Although the exact nature of the change varies according to the client's needs, nurses frequently encourage people to eat less sugar and fat and to exercise regularly. Certain characteristics of change are especially powerful influences on people's receptivity to change. They include *complexity, compatibility* with existing values and beliefs, relative *advantages* (efficiency, health, pleasure, economics, prestige), and *penalties* (illness, legal sanctions, public ridicule, religious censure).

Complexity refers to the degree to which the change is perceived as relatively difficult to understand and use. For example, a cooking technique that seems easy to master will be more readily adopted than one that appears difficult. Any dietary change makes certain performance demands on the person who adopts it. Some dietary recommendations require the client to calculate and tabulate the amount of nutrients daily, whereas others require the client to remember lists of foods that can and cannot be eaten. All require some relearning or reconditioning.

Compatibility with current beliefs refers to the degree to which the recommended change is perceived as consistent with the existing norms and practices of the client. In general, changes that do not conflict with existing traits are more readily accepted. Therapeutic diets, for example, may be incompatible with some cultural classifications of food. As discussed previously, in India, Latin America, the Near East and elsewhere, people classify foods, illness, and medicines as hot or cold. The exchange list diet would be incompatible with this belief system, though modification might be possible. Recommended dietary changes may be incompatible with existing norms pertaining to the preparation, storage, or appearance of foods.

The *relative advantage* of change refers to the degree to which a dietary modification is perceived as being better than the idea it supersedes. *Efficiency* refers to the effectiveness of a new idea, item, or practice and its ability to function well. Efficiency becomes more difficult to assess when the results require time before observable benefits are seen by the client. For example, the relative advantage of a weight reduction diet frequently requires many months, but it is still possible to monitor change by measuring the client's weight, blood pressure, hematocrit, serum cholesterol, blood glucose or other physiologic indicators at periodic intervals. These laboratory test results, if incorporated into the ongoing nursing care plan, provide systematic feedback of the diet's success or failure.

Next, let us examine the interconnection between diet and *health*. The extent to which people are willing to alter their diets for health reasons varies. In some individuals, certain foods cause gastrointestinal discomfort, allergic reactions or other acute symptoms of distress so severe that the client willingly avoids them, a situation that may lead to nutritional deficiencies. Feeling poorly when blood glucose levels rise after eating sugar serves as a powerful incentive for some people with diabetes to avoid sweets.

The *fear* of becoming sick, weak, or debilitated from eating something new is a deterrent to dietary change. For example, the recent pilot testing of snack foods containing olestra was met by public protest because some people experienced unpleasant gastrointestinal symptoms after eating foods with olestra. Pleasure derived from dietary change is another important consideration in people's receptivity to something new. Of course there is a high degree cultural relativity in the perception of taste pleasure. The literature abounds with examples of people rejecting dietary innovations because of dissatisfaction with the taste, texture, or other pleasure-giving qualities. New hybrid strains of corn in Mexico, wheat in India, and potatoes in Peru have been rejected despite superior yields, resistance to pests, and high nutritional qualities because they were not as pleasing to eat as traditional strains. Although *pleasure* is a powerful motive to acceptance of a new food or diet pattern, the long-term consequences of the new item may offset the immediate satisfaction. For example, people may avoid foods they like but suspect of containing carcinogens.

Financial considerations play a significant role in the decision to accept or reject a new food or dietary pattern. Often it is possible to replace expensive foodstuffs such as meat with less expensive items such as beans, rice, eggs, or peanut butter. Because cost is the major constraint for many clients, it is important that each dietary restriction recommended is necessary. When cost is not considered in formulating diet recommendations, adherence often declines. The *social advantages* of the diet change must be considered. Prestige is a major social attraction of many new practices and goods for some people.

Although the social advantages frequently outweigh the disadvantages, *penalties* commonly associated with dietary change include legal sanctions, public ridicule, and religious concerns. Many products never reach the consumer because they fail to meet government requirements or standards. Some products may be marketed with warnings designated to deter acceptance. For example, some low-calorie soft drinks warn that consumption by laboratory animals has been determined to cause cancer. In this way laws governing labelling sometimes deter acceptance by people who might otherwise consume the item. Adverse public opinion is another type of penalty that can impede change in food patterns. This may take the form of censure or ridicule.

Finally, fear of supernatural punishment prevents some people from accepting new foods and practices. In Chapter 12 the reader will find a discussion of the food-related beliefs and practices for selected religious groups.

Promoting Dietary Change

You should be aware that the degree to which clients from culturally diverse backgrounds adhere to advice concerning dietary change may be less than expected. If a client's values are inconsistent with the underlying rationale for recommended change, the probability of adherence is low. Clients may agree verbally to do something out of courtesy or fear but fail to act on your recommendations. Limited understanding of a health-related disorder may act as a disincentive for dietary change, particularly when there are no signs or symptoms to relieve. For example, clients with hypertension may perceive no need for a low-sodium diet because the clinical manifestations of disease are absent, hence the nickname "silent killer." You should explain the concept of blood pressure in a culturally meaningful manner and provide a rationale for the recommended dietary modification.

Knowledge that an eating practice is harmful does not necessarily promote change in that behavior, as is commonly seen in obese persons who continue to overeat, diabetics who persist in eating candy and other high-sugar foods, and so forth. This is true regardless of the client's cultural background, educational level, socioeconomic status, or religious affiliation. You must balance the clients' rights to determine their own future against your need to promote change. The goal should be to provide advice and recommendations in a positive and culturally appropriate manner, that encourages learning and promotes behavioral change in the desired direction. The decision to change behavior based on your advice is up to the client.

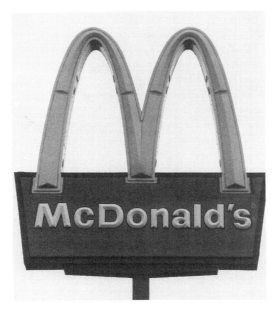

Some fast-food restaurants have expanded their menus to include salads and other foods aimed at meeting the needs of the growing number of health-conscious customers.

Although you will find advantages and disadvantages in each group's cultural food patterns, you should be mindful that these patterns have contributed to the group's survival over time. In some instances, this meant making significant adaptations in order to obtain a nutritious data from available food, especially in times of shortage. According to Davis and Sherer (1994), each food, food behavior, and tradition can be categorized as *beneficial, neutral,* or *potentially harmful.* Tofu, used in Asian cooking, is beneficial because it increases the protein and calcium content of the diet. Efforts should be made to alter only the patterns that affect the nutritional value in an undesirable manner. For example, given that many water-soluble vitamins are destroyed by heat, the practice of cooking foods for long periods should be discouraged unless the liquids are consumed and/or iron cookware is used (Davis & Sherer, 1994). An understanding of cultural food patterns can be used to encourage beneficial practices or incorporate them into the client's diet. Whether a food is categorized as *neutral* or *potentially harmful* depends on factors such as age, weight, genetics, and medical diagnosis. For example, candy is neutral for many people, but potentially harmful for diabetic clients.

Food patterns are generally deeply rooted, contribute to psychological stability, and are difficult to change. If it is necessary to change the client's diet for health-related reasons, you should suggest minimal modifications to traditional foods. Be sure the client and food gatekeepers in the family understand the meal plan and that the client has control over food choices. Although it is important to refrain from ageist judgments, cultural food patterns are likely to be used more consistently by older members of the household (Davis and Sherer, 1994).

Berlin and Fowkes (1983) have proposed a 5-step teaching framework for cross-cultural health care with the acronym LEARN—*l*isten, *e*xplain, *a*cknowledge, *r*ecommend and *n*egotiate.

In the LEARN model, the health care provider is first encouraged to *listen* to the client's perception of the problem. Strategies such as reflecting or restating the client's words and clarifying meanings should be used. For example, "I'm interested in knowing more about preparing Chinese vegetables. Please tell me again how the cooking

Food patterns are usually deeply rooted and difficult to change at any age. When health-related reasons necessitate dietary change, the nurse should assure that the client has control over food choices and that minimal modifications to traditional foods are suggested.

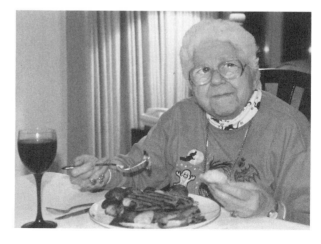

oil is used." or "I didn't quite understand what you just said." To promote effective communication, it is important for you to *explain* your understanding of the client's perception of the problem; for example, the nurse might say to a Chinese American client, "What I'm hearing you say is that you believe yin fruits and vegetables will be best for your diarrhea, which is a yang condition." You should then *acknowledge* the similarities and differences between the client and yourself. For example, the nurse might say to a Vietnamese American client, "You've indicated that bad wind has caused your chest pain. I believe that your high-cholesterol diet and obesity have contributed to your development of heart disease."

You should *recommend* dietary changes that are congruent with the client's culture and individual preferences. If recommendations are linked with the client's motivation for change, the probability of success is increased. When these recommendations are presented, household members who shop for and prepare the food should be included. Be sure to consider the timing of discussions about diet (e.g., proximity to discharge, signs of readiness by the client, calendar of religious or secular holidays). The nurse might plan to make recommendations when, for example, the spouse of a Mexican American client visits the hospital. By way of example, you might say, "I know that you want to continue working so you can support your family. To decrease your chance of having another heart attack, I would urge you to eat less fat and lose weight. When preparing tacos, use no-fat or low-fat cheese and sour cream. The entire family would reduce their risk of heart disease if they ate their tacos this way." Because of cultural differences in attitudes toward obesity and past experiences with food shortages, especially for immigrants from countries with famines, natural disasters or war, the client may be unwilling to follow recommendations about reducing caloric intake.

If you determine that the client is unlikely to follow the dietary recommendations, then alternatives such as increased activity or exercise should be suggested. In suggesting these alternatives, the nurse should identify the benefits of exercise in a manner that appeals to the client's motivation. For example, the known *benefits of exercise* include increased efficiency of the heart and lungs, increased energy and vitality, increased blood flow throughout the body, increased strength and coordination, improved elimination, enhanced self-image, improved appearance, decreased heart rate and blood pressure, and decreased anxiety, tension and depression. Finally, you should *negotiate* a plan of action that offers options congruent with the client's cultural beliefs. For example, after presenting several options, you might ask the client, "Which of the weight reduction plans would be easiest for you?" It is important to get clients and those significant to them to commit to a concrete plan of action that can subsequently be evaluated for its effectiveness and modified as needed. This plan of action sometimes takes the form of a health behavior *contract* that incorporates the principles of self-directed change by encouraging the client to assume responsibility for eating behaviors. The contract defines who will take what actions and when in an effort to obtain specific results over a reasonable period of time. Social support and reinforcement are motivating factors used in contracts. Because some clients are uncomfortable with written contracts, they may also be made verbally with the client, family member or friend.

A powerful strategy for teaching about change in dietary habits is the modeling of positive behavior by nurses and other health care providers. Be aware that credibility will be lost quickly if your behaviors are incongruent with recommendations given to clients. As a group, nurses tend to have poor eating habits, some of which relate to high job-related demands. For example, in many hospitals nurses skip meals or breaks because of the urgent, pressing and sometimes life-threatening situations involving their clients. Working nights or rotating shifts may disrupt their natural food patterns and habits. Many nurses are overweight, overstressed, dependent on alcohol, and often uncritical of their unhealthy work environments or lifestyles.

Although the value of a positive role model has merit, research demonstrates that clients are likely to experience a level of comfort when in the company of others who are like themselves. In studies of exercise and weight reduction among middle-aged sedentary, overweight women, it has been revealed that women generally prefer to exercise with others of similar age and body size (Gillett, et al., 1993, 1995). Many studies have demonstrated that time-limited programs of diet or exercise followed by a break have higher success rates, though optimal cardiovascular, aerobic power, and body composition changes may require periods in excess of 4 months. Rather than recommending a permanent, lifelong change, the nurse might suggest that the client commit to regular physical activity for more limited periods such as 16 weeks. The client may then take a brief break and commit to another time-limited program. Other factors that influence adherence to exercise include social networks, pleasurable feelings associated with increased energy and fitness, and an exercise leader with a health-related background (Gillett, et al., 1993). Unfortunately, some disease conditions do not permit temporary or short-term modifications in exercise or diet. For example, clients with diabetes, renal disease, food allergies and related conditions may need to sustain long-term or lifelong dietary change or face dire consequences.

Health-Related Dietary Beliefs and Practices

As discussed previously, foods are commonly used by many cultures in the prevention and treatment of illness. In the United States and Canada nutrition has become extremely important as a preventive measure for many physical and emotional disorders. Diabetes mellitus, hypertension, asthma, lactose intolerance and peptic ulcers are a few of the many disorders for which diet is a major component of the treatment regimen.

In many cultures of the world, people believe that the promotion of health and prevention of disease are dependent on the ability to maintain a state of *balance*, a concept not totally foreign to Western-educated nurses and other health care providers who recognize the need for *homeostasis*, achieved by balancing fluids and electrolytes within narrow margins. In many cultures, the nature and name of the balance differs. For example, some clients from Hispanic and Middle Eastern cultures may believe in the hot-cold theory whereas people of Asian descent are more likely to follow an ancient system of yin/yang balance. Let us examine the manner in which food is used to establish balance (and therefore, health) within the hot-cold and yin-yang theories.

Hot-Cold Theory

The beliefs and practices associated with the hot-cold theory originated in ancient Greece during the time of Hippocrates, who considered illness to be the result of humoral imbalance causing the body to become too hot or too cold. In this system, health is conceived as a state of *balance* among the body humors (blood, phlegm, black bile, and yellow bile) that manifests itself in a somewhat wet, warm body. Illness is believed to result from a humoral imbalance that causes the body to become excessively dry, cold, hot, wet, or a combination of these states. Food, herbs, and other medications, which are also classified as wet or dry, hot or cold, are used therapeutically to restore the body to its natural balance. Thus, according to this system, a cold disease such as arthritis, is cured by administering hot foods or medications.

The hot-cold theory describes intrinsic properties of a food, beverage, or medicine and its effect on the body. Although the terminology of the hot-cold system seems to suggest that it is based on the thermal state of the substance ingested, temperature or spiciness are *not* the qualities that determine the classification of specific substances. The classification of foods, beverages, and medicines as hot or cold varies within each cultural group. In general, warm or hot foods are believed to be easier to digest than cold or cool foods. In order to achieve balance, illnesses are treated with substances having the opposite property of the illness. Conditions thought to be caused by exposure to cold or chilling are cured by hot medicines as well as by ingesting hot foods and beverages. The opposite is true of illnesses believed to be caused by exposure to heat. For example, colds are commonly attributed to drafts, and arthritic pain in the hands is often said to come from exposing the hands to cold water after they have been immersed in hot. Similarly, an upset stomach may be attributed to eating too many foods that are classified as cold, thus chilling the stomach. Although there are considerable differences among cultural groups concerning the criteria used for classifying something into hot and cold categories, the hot-cold system functions in a similar way for each of them. Table 11-2 summarizes the hot-cold classification among Puerto Ricans, a group that has hot, cold, and cool categories of illnesses, bodily conditions, medicines, herbs, and foods. Iranians also classify foods into one of two categories, *garm* (hot), and *sard* (cold), which sometimes corresponds to high-calorie and low-calorie foods. If imbalance occurs, symptoms are treated by eating food from the opposite group. For example, conditions such as fever, diaphoresis, urticaria, and various rashes are thought to result from eating too many hot foods such as onions, garlic, spices, candy, walnuts, or honey. It is believed that the stomach may become chilled (e.g., symptoms of dizziness, weakness, nausea, and vomiting) by eating too many cold foods such as grapes, plums, cucumbers, or yogurt (Lipson & Hafizi, 1998).

New foods or medicines are incorporated into the hot-cold system according to the effect they have on the body. Penicillin, because it can cause hot symptoms such as a rash or diarrhea, is categorized by many groups as a hot substance, whereas a drug that might cause muscle spasms would be considered cold. The very fact that new items are still being incorporated into the hot-cold system attests to its vitality among certain cultural groups. You should be aware that some Hispanic clients may refuse foods or medications that violate their hot-cold beliefs. For example, some Mexican American clients will refuse hot medicines such as aspirin or penicillin when used to treat hot diseases such as sore throat or fever. Instead, the client is likely to seek treatments that will restore equilibrium such as cooling herbs brewed as teas, enemas (which are thought to remove heat), or by a change in the diet to include more cold foods.

TABLE 11-2
The Hot-Cold Classification Among Puerto Ricans

	Frío (Cold)	Fresco (Cool)	Caliente (Hot)
Illnesses or bodily conditions	Arthritis Colds *Frialdad del estómago** Menstrual period Pain in the joints *Pasmo†*		Constipation Diarrhea Rashes Tenesmus Ulcers
Medicine and herbs		Bicarbonate of soda Linden flowers Mannitol Mastic bark $MgCO_2$ Milk of magnesia Nightshade Orange flower water Sage	Anise Aspirin Castor oil Cinnamon Cod liver oil Iron tablets Penicillin Rue Vitamins
Foods	Avocado Bananas Coconut Lima beans Sugar cane White beans	Barley water Bottled milk Chicken Fruits Honey Raisins Salt cod Watercress	Alcoholic beverages Chili peppers Chocolate Coffee Corn meal Evaporated milk Garlic Kidney beans Onions Peas Tobacco

*Upset stomach due to ingestion of too many cold-classed foods.

†Tonic spasm of any voluntary muscle.

From Harwood, A. (1971). The hot-cold theory of disease: Implications for treatment for Puerto Rican patients. *Journal of the American Medical Association, 216*(7), 1155. Copyright © 1971 American Medical Association. Reprinted by Permission.

Yin-Yang Theory

For more than 3,000 years, the Chinese have used health foods and herb tonics to prevent and cure illness. These treatments originated in ancient legend and have been woven into philosophy, religion, and folklore. Diet therapy was an important part of Chinese traditional medicine, and was integrated with other forms of healing including meditation, acupuncture, and martial arts.

According to the ancient philosophy of *Tao* (pronounced "dow"), the balance of the two elements *yin* and *yang* maintains harmony in the universe. Yin represents female, cold, and darkness, whereas yang represents male, hot, and light. When foods are digested they turn into air which is either yin or yang. The terms yin and yang are often, though somewhat inadequately, translated into English as cold and hot. The balance of yin and yang components in the diet is considered essential to good health because excesses of either are believed to result in body imbalances recognized as diseases. Thus, yin conditions require yang foods or treatment. Some neutral foods (those that are neither yin nor yang) may be used to treat either type of condition. Table 11-3 summarizes some examples of yin, neutral, and yang foods.

TABLE 11-3
Yin, Neutral, and Yang Foods

Yin	Neutral	Yang
Bean curds	Noodles	Bamboo
Bean sprouts	Soft rice	Beef
Bland foods	Sugar	Broiled meat
Boiled foods	Sweets	Catfish
Broccoli		Chicken
Cabbage		Chicken soup
Carrots		Chinese dats
Cauliflower		Chiretta (an herb)
Celery		Eggplant
Cold (thermal) foods		Eggs
Congee		Fatty meats
Cucumber		Fried foods
Day lily		Garlic
Duck		Ginger root
Fish (some types)		Ginseng
Fruits (some types)		Glutinous rice
Ginko		Green peppers
Greens (most)		Hot (thermal) foods
Honey		Leeks
Melon		Liquor
Milk		Mushrooms
Pears		Onions
Pork		Peanuts
Potatoes		Persimmons
Seaweed		Pig's knuckle soup
Soybeans		Pork liver
Spinach		Red beans
Turnips		Red foods
Turtle (one type)		Red peppers
Water		Roasted peanuts
Watercress		Seasme oil
Watermelon soup		Shellfish
Winter melon		Sour foods
Winter pumpkin		Spicy foods
White foods		Tangerines
White turnips		Tomatoes
		Vinegar
		Wine

From Ludman, E. K., & Newman, J. M. (1984). Yin and yang in the health-related food practices of three Chinese groups. *Journal of Nutrition Education, 16,* 4. © Society for Nutrition Education. Reprinted with permission.

The Chinese culture, like many others, has folk beliefs linked to menstruation, pregnancy, and the postpartum period, all of which are yin conditions. Yang substances are considered necessary during these times to restore the balance needed for health and to build up the strength which is lost. Special yang foods are often used for "building blood" and are especially appropriate for the elderly who may already have "weak blood," and for pregnant women who are weakened by their condition.

Dietary Practices of Specific Cultural Groups

Asian and Pacific Americans

In general, people of Asian and Pacific Island descent have maintained strong ties to their native foods. Because there as so many different cultures and subcultures comprising the panethnic category referred to Asian/Pacific Islander, this discussion focuses on Asian food traditions, many of which are ancient and complex. Diet is intimately associated with health, and in a complex manner with the condition of the cosmos. The diets of Chinese, Hindus, and many other Asians are intimately linked philosophically to all other aspects of society and influence the individual's state of health.

Asian cookery is characterized by mixed dishes with the ingredients cut into small pieces. Although preparation is lengthy, the actual cooking time is usually brief, thus essential vitamins are generally retained. Characteristic foods include rice and wheat, pork, chicken, a variety of vegetables, eggs, various soy preparations, and tea. A favorite sauce combines sweet and sour flavors. Sodium intake is high, and fat consumption is typically very low. Although raw vegetables are rarely served, there are abundant vitamins in cooked vegetables and fresh fruits.

With adult *lactase deficiency* being virtually universal, milk use is rare. Overeating or obesity is not prevalent, perhaps because of the belief that one should leave the table only 70 percent full. The preference for fresh fruits and low-calorie bean dishes for dessert also fosters a low incidence of obesity. Nutritionally, the yin-yang system has been beneficial, creating variety in the diet and balancing the amounts of animal protein, grains, and vegetables. You should be aware that if a recommended diet isn't balanced in terms of yin and yang foods, it may not be followed.

African Americans

Although it is somewhat artificial to separate blacks from other Americans or Canadians in describing diet, several factors make it worthwhile to discuss African Americans' diet separately. First, there are more low-income blacks, and low incomes are associated with less nutritious diets. Second, many African Americans are lactose intolerant, and therefore, their consumption of dairy foods is lower. Designing a diet adequate in calcium requires special attention for nurses working with pregnant African American women or others requiring high-calcium diets. Third, *soul food,* a combination of dishes created with ingredients from Africa, the Caribbean, and the southern U.S., are popular among some African Americans. Well seasoned with salt and fat, soul foods provide an economical link between African Americans and their historic roots. A dish known as *chitlins* is made by scrubbing the skin of pig intestines, then boiling them with vinegar for hours. When tender, they are eaten with a spicy hot sauce. Soul food also includes many vegetables. Collard, turnip, and mustard greens contain

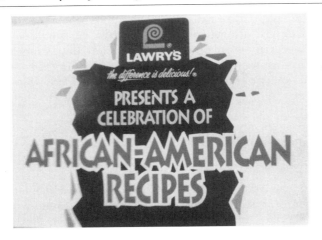

Although African Americans consume many of the same foods as others, their dietary patterns and food choices sometimes have distinctive characteristics. Recipes celebrating soul food and other African American specialty foods are featured in this pamphlet produced by a manufacturer of seasonings.

fiber, calcium, and large quantities of vitamin A. Beans and peas are excellent sources of low-fat plant protein. Sweet potatoes and other yellow vegetables are high in vitamin A. Unfortunately, the benefits can be lost if these foods are not prepared with nutrition in mind. For example, lima beans are not nearly as healthful when flavored with fatty ham hocks; the fiber in greens is broken down by overcooking; and most of the vitamins in greens are lost when cooking liquid (sometimes called *pot liquor*) is discarded.

Regional differences in food patterns should be noted. Southern diets are distinguishable because they contain more corn, rice, pork, lard, legumes, and greens than northern ones. Hot breads and fried foods are popular. An analysis of nutritional adequacy of 250 low-income black homes in Mississippi showed mean intakes of protein, vitamin A, thiamin, riboflavin, and ascorbic acid to be above the Recommended Dietary Allowances, whereas mean intakes of calories, calcium, iron, and preformed niacin were below recommended dietary allowances. Only calcium was determined to be inadequate. Adolescents had the least nutritious diets of the study subjects whereas adult women had superior intakes except for calcium and iron.

Important food beliefs that affect food selection among African Americans are shared by many groups. Foods may be classified as heavy (cornbread, greens, legumes) or light (fruit, white bread). A balanced meal consists of a mixture of heavy and light foods. Some foods are also identified as strength foods, such as vegetables, meat, and milk. For the middle-class American or Canadian, meat would be considered as more strengthening than vegetables, a factor that has socioeconomic and nutritional components.

Some African Americans believe that a healthy body displays a balance of hot and cold humors, with blood being categorized as hot. In this belief system *low blood*, a condition in which there is too little blood in the body, can be treated with diet. The dietary treatment consists of increased intake of liver, beets, rare meat, or milk. Note the emphasis on the color red and the bloodiness of the meat. The term low blood is sometimes confused with anemia, but biomedical and lay treatment may coincide so there are usually no adverse effects. *High blood* (excess blood in the body) can cause strokes and is believed to come from eating too much rich food or red meat, such as pork.

The treatment is believed to be dietary and involves use of astringent and acidic foods such as vinegar, lemons, pickles, or epsom salts to open the pores and let excessive sweat escape. Because pregnancy is classified as hot, the pregnant woman must control her diet to protect against high blood. This dietary control involves avoidance of meats and high-calorie foods or increasing the intake of sodium-rich foods. If the pregnant woman is told that she has *high blood pressure*, her assumption that this refers to high blood may lead her to decrease her already depleted protein intake and increase her consumption of foods thought to have cold properties, such as sodium-rich foods, thus increasing the probability that she will suffer from eclampsia. Nutrients that are often inadequate in African American women include calcium, magnesium, iron, zinc, vitamin B_6, vitamin E, and folacin. These nutrients plus vitamin A and riboflavin are frequently lacking in the diets of African American men (Davis & Sherer, 1994; Dudek, 1997).

Hispanic Americans

Although wide variations among the cultures and subcultures comprising the Hispanic panethnic group exist, some examples of dietary considerations will be examined. Although Mexican American and Puerto Rican diets differ, both groups base food selection on the hot-cold theory of health, and similarities exist in both subcultures. The staples of Mexican American diets feature beans and tortillas made from corn treated with lime (calcium carbonate). Other popular foods are eggs, chicken, lard, chili peppers, onions, tomatoes, squash, herb teas (especially mint and chamomile), sweetened packaged breakfast cereals, potatoes, bread, carbonated beverages, canned fruits, gelatin, ice cream, other sweets, and sugar. Milk is used primarily in hot beverages. Large breakfasts are common.

In the Southwest, chili, chili con carne, enchiladas, tamales, tostadas, chicken mole, and nopalitos are favored by many Hispanics. Among Mexican American migrant workers in California, favorite dishes include refried beans, tacos, tortillas, and, to a lesser extent, such middle-class American dishes as hamburgers, macaroni and cheese, and hot dogs. Compared with white counterparts, Mexican Americans use more carbonated beverages, beer, and sweetened beverage mixes, and less milk, coffee, and tea. Mexican American diets are generally adequate for protein and energy, but low for vitamins A and C, iron, and calcium largely because of overcooking. Obesity, diabetes mellitus and anemia are common.

Native Americans

In Native American cultures, food has religious, social, and cultural meaning. Health is believed to be a state in which the entire being is in *balance*, whereas illness indicates *disharmony* or *imbalance*. A complex set of tribe-specific rules are followed to maintain harmony, and herbs, chants, or healing ceremonies are used to treat the root cause of illnesses (versus symptoms only).

With more than 550 federally recognized tribes in the U.S., Native American dietary practices vary widely. There are, however, three staples that are considered sacred by most tribes—corn, squashes and beans. The contemporary American Indian diet usually combines indigenous natural foods with modern processed foods. In geographic areas providing game and fish, these items are important food sources. Fruits, berries, roots, and wild greens are highly valued foods, but scarce in many areas, particularly large urban centers. When indigenous foods are unavailable, the daily diet consists of commodity foods provided by the U.S. Department of Agriculture and foods purchased at stores. Access to fresh fruits and vegetables is frequently problematic due to unavailability or expense in areas in which these items are not locally grown.

Lack of refrigeration may greatly limit some Native Americans' consumption of fresh meat, milk, fruits, and vegetables. When relying on non-perishable foods for the bulk of the diet, there is often marginal or deficient states in key nutrients, whereas excessive amounts of refined sugar, cholesterol, fat, and calories are consumed.

Food acceptance is often tribe-specific. Among Navajo, meat and blue cornmeal are considered strong foods whereas milk is a weak food. Corn is a sacred food to many American Indian tribes and is used in ceremonies, such as weddings. Dietary taboos against many foods exist among different tribes. For example, some Plains Indians place a taboo on fish.

Although there is currently debate over the harmful affects of giving infants a bottle at nap and bedtime, an exceptionally high prevalence (50–80 percent) of tooth decay has been reported among Native American infants who are bottle-age. Some dental research has linked the so-called baby bottle decay to high bacteria levels in the mouth and bottles containing sweetened water (versus milk). Regardless of the cause, there has been a widespread effort to discourage parents and other providers of care from leaving a propped bottle in the infant's crib at bedtime with the hope that dental caries can be reduced in young Native American populations. Milk is seldom used after infancy.

Poor nutrition has been linked to several leading causes of death among Native Americans such as heart disease, stroke, diabetes mellitus, and cirrhosis of the liver. Perhaps the most serious risk-factor for more serious conditions is obesity. The high rate of alcoholism among American Indians contributes significantly to nutritional disorders and is interrelated with liver cirrhosis. The Pima Indians have the highest known rate of Non-insulin Dependent Diabetes Mellitus (NIDDM), with a prevalence of nearly 50 percent of those over 35 years of age. Diets on some reservations supply less than two-thirds of the recommended dietary allowance for calories, calcium, iron, iodine, riboflavin, and vitamins A and C. As a rule, diets are high in carbohydrate, saturated fat, sodium and sugar (Davis & Sherer, 1994; Dudek, 1997).

Maternal Health

Women from other cultures may refuse to seek early prenatal care because pregnancy is considered a normal state for women, not a medical abnormality. Fear, modesty, or cultural taboos may also keep some women from seeking health care during pregnancy as well as the desire to avoid examinations by members of the opposite sex, such as male obstetricians or nurses. Folk beliefs concerning diet and pregnancy are common among people from many cultures and subcultures. Contained among folk beliefs for various cultural groups is the belief that the fetus can be affected both positively and negatively by maternal experiences, emotions, exposures, and eating habits during pregnancy.

Certain foods are believed to promote a healthy delivery for mother and baby, whereas other foods are feared to result in a difficult delivery and a deformed, injured, or stillborn infant. For example, some women believe that failure to satisfy a food craving during pregnancy or overindulgence in a food can cause a birthmark resembling the craved food or an allergy to that food in the infant. Thus, an unsatisfied desire for strawberries or cherries is sometimes blamed for causing red birthmarks, whereas a chocolate craving is thought to cause brown marks. Aversions, usually to protein foods, alcohol, and caffeinated beverages, are believed by some to protect the mother and her developing fetus against harmful forces. Therefore, it becomes not only acceptable, but necessary for pregnant women adhering to such beliefs to satisfy their cravings.

Pica, the ingestion of non-food substances, such as laundry starch (*amylophagia*), clay or dirt (*geophagia*), ice, burnt matches, ashes, wall plaster, hair, and stones has been reported among certain cultural groups. Starch eating is more frequently reported among African American women, whereas clay eating is reported most commonly among Hispanic women. The reasons for pica are not well understood, but several theories have been suggested including the body's need to acquire certain missing nutrients, hunger, cultural tradition, prevention of nausea, and attention seeking. Regardless of the reason for pica, it is important for the nurse to determine if clients practice it and to what degree. Geophagia is harmful because the clay blocks absorption of iron, potassium and zinc, sometimes resulting in iron deficiency anemia and muscle weakness (from low potassium). Although it is most prevalent in pregnancy and early childhood, pica may also affect adult men.

When taking nutritional histories for pregnant women, you must include direct, non-judgmental questions such as, "Many women crave things to eat during pregnancy; are you having cravings for things that you don't usually eat such as laundry starch, dirt, or ice?" Although the ingestion of most non-food substances is harmless, some items such as wall plaster, laundry starch, toilet bowl freshener, and mothballs may have serious adverse effects. Large amounts of non-food items are likely to replace nutritious foods needed by a pregnant woman. When consumed in large quantities, clay can obstruct the gastrointestinal tract, so the nurse should inquire about signs and symptoms of obstruction. Fortunately, most women who practice pica during pregnancy do so on a limited basis and without adverse effects.

Although Western medicine recognizes the importance of adequate weight gain during pregnancy to produce larger and healthier infants, women from some cultures believe that weight gain must be restricted to produce a small infant and an easy delivery. This belief may have been founded in reality according to the level of obstetric care that was available to women in their native country.

Hot-cold theories of disease and health have an influence on practices in both the prenatal and postpartum periods. The third trimester of pregnancy is generally regarded by Hispanic women as hot. A client might prefer to avoid hot foods and medications, such as iron supplements, during this period. You should explain the reason for the extra iron and describe symptoms associated with iron deficiency anemia in an effort to gain the woman's cooperation in taking the medication. If this seriously violates the woman's belief system, then the nurse should discuss dietary sources of iron and encourage culturally-appropriate iron-rich foods.

Although cultural variation plays an important role in human nutrition, it has been difficult to determine the exact relationship between prenatal nutritional status and cultural influences, primarily because of the continuous process of environmental transition and acculturation that occurs in any cultural group. Most nurses, dieticians and other health care providers recommend a prenatal diet that is based on white, middle-class food preferences and scientifically derived nutrient levels. This diet recommends the intake of three to four servings per day of the basic four food groups, resulting in an emphasis on a high intake of animal protein (meat and eggs), dairy products (whole milk and cheese), citrus fruits, and fresh vegetables. Most health care providers routinely recommend a daily prenatal vitamin and iron supplement.

The concept of balance in this diet implies variety, which is expensive to provide both regionally and seasonally. In general, the risk of this diet is ethnocentricity. Economically disadvantaged families cannot afford such a diet, nor does the one quart of milk per day recommendation meet the needs of lactose intolerant women who are unable to digest the milk sugar. According to Overfield (1995), lactose intolerance affects approximately 94 percent of Asians, 79 percent of American Indians, 75 percent of African Americans, 50 percent of Mexican-Americans, and 17 percent of American Whites.

Calcium-rich alternatives to milk, such as aged cheese and sour milk products (e.g., yogurt) are safe to use for lactose intolerant persons because the lactose in these foods has been converted to lactic acid. Other excellent sources of calcium include beans, cabbage, collards, cauliflower, kale, rhubarb, egg yolk, and molasses. An import fact to remember in counseling women about calcium sources is that the high calcium content in green leafy vegetables, such as spinach, chard, and beet greens, cannot be utilized by the body as well as the calcium in other foods because it is bound to oxalic acid.

Although dietary knowledge and food intake patterns vary widely, the observance of various vegetarian and health food diets has some implications for nurses counseling pregnant women. The dietary beliefs and practices of vegetarians and health foodists are white, middle-class, educated Americans and Canadians who believe that food and health are interconnected. Health foodists usually choose foods such as whole grains and organically grown fruits and vegetables while avoiding red meat, chemical additives, tobacco, alcohol, caffeine, and drugs. Health foodists often take dietary supplements and sometimes very large doses of vitamins and minerals. Because vegetarian women, especially vegans, have lower protein and energy intake when compared with non-vegetarians, they have leaner bodies, experience later menarche, have lower pre-pregnancy weights, lower pregnancy weight gain, and altered milk composition during lactation.

Seventh-Day Adventists and other more traditional vegetarian groups seem to be at less nutritional risk when compared with vegan women, or those who follow strict macrobiotic diets and have little interaction with Westernized health care. Vegan diets, especially macrobiotic diets, are often deficient in nutrients deemed essential in pregnancy, such as proteins, calcium, vitamins (A, B_6, B_{12}, and riboflavin), iron, zinc, and copper. The importance of empathic, non-judgmental dialogue about food patterns and preferences cannot be overemphasized. Prenatal food guides are available that can be used to adapt nutrient requirements for pregnancy to individual beliefs and practices. In using print or media supplements for diet education, you should remember that the success of these materials is interrelated with the client's literacy level, language facility, educational background, religious beliefs, and health-related practices.

You may find that a woman of Hispanic background prefers to avoid cold foods for 1 to 2 months after delivery because cold foods are believed to slow the flow of blood and prevent the emptying of the uterus. Some Asian women may abstain from vegetables, fruits, and fruit juices for a month postpartum because these foods are considered too cold and could endanger their health. You should carefully assess the nutritional composition of the woman's overall diet while observing these and similar practices during pregnancy and the postpartum period. If specific deficiencies are identified, the nurse should discuss acceptable alternative foods that will provide sufficient amounts of the deficient nutrients. Emphasis should be placed on promotion of the mother's and the baby's optimum health while matter-of-factly discussing the consequences of prolonged deficiency of the nutrient(s) of concern.

Nurses counseling individuals for whom humoral practices and beliefs have special meaning should use principles of neutralization. Neutralization involves accommodating to beliefs by suggesting mixing of hot and cold foods. You must also accept food practices and preferences, and not try to change culturally established patterns. For example, a pregnant Puerto Rican woman who fails to take her prenatal vitamin and iron tablets, for iron deficiency anemia, may refuse to take the medicine because in her cultural meaning system, these medications are hot and therefore are to be avoided during pregnancy, a hot physical state. This woman may benefit from a suggestion to try taking vitamins and iron with fruit juice, a cold substance, thereby maintaining the proper balance of physical states.

Child Health

As discussed in Chapter 3, infant feeding practices are culturally determined. Although breastfeeding is the usual method in non-Western countries, women from those same cultures may elect to bottle feed when living in the U.S. or Canada. Middle- and upper-class Anglo women are more likely to breastfeed than other cultural groups. In contrast, African Americans have the lowest rate of breastfeeding. Members of the subcultures within each group , however, will vary in the extent to which they choose breast-feeding. For example, Puerto Rican women may choose breast-feeding more often than Cuban women. In general, cultural values influence women's perceptions about breast-feeding in terms of nutritional value, the father's beliefs, breast exposure, sexuality, and convenience. Breast-feeding may also be viewed by new immigrants as less modern and prestigious than bottle feeding. You should explain the advantages of breast-feeding versus bottle feeding and attempt to assist the woman in making an informed decision about the method of feeding her new infant.

Folk beliefs are sometimes instrumental in determining breast-feeding practices by women who elect this method of feeding. Among some Hispanic and Asian women, breastfeeding is delayed for several days after birth because colostrum is considered "dirty," and thus unacceptable for the baby. Some Hispanic women believe that stress

TABLE 11-4

*Growth Standards of Healthy Chinese Children and Adolescents (Urban)**

Age (Months or Years)	Boys				Girls			
	Weight (kg)	Height (cm)	Head Circumference (cm)	Chest Circumference (cm)	Weight (kg)	Height (cm)	Head Circumference (cm)	Chest Circumference (cm)
Birth	3.27	50.6	34.3	32.8	3.17	50.0	33.7	32.6
1 mo	4.97	56.5	38.1	37.9	4.64	55.5	37.3	36.9
2 mo	5.95	59.6	39.7	40.0	5.49	58.4	38.7	38.9
3 mo	6.73	62.3	41.0	41.3	6.23	60.9	40.0	40.3
4 mo	7.32	64.4	42.0	42.3	6.69	62.9	41.0	41.1
5 mo	7.70	65.9	42.9	42.9	7.19	64.5	41.9	41.9
6 mo	8.22	68.1	43.9	43.8	7.62	66.7	42.8	42.7
8 mo	8.71	70.6	44.9	44.7	8.14	69.0	43.7	43.4
10 mo	9.14	72.9	45.7	45.4	8.57	71.4	44.5	44.2
12 mo	9.66	75.6	46.3	46.1	9.04	74.1	45.2	45.0
15 mo	10.15	78.3	46.8	46.8	9.54	76.8	45.6	45.8
18 mo	10.67	80.7	47.3	47.6	10.08	78.4	46.2	46.6
21 mo	11.18	83.0	47.8	48.3	10.56	81.7	46.7	47.3
24 mo	11.95	86.5	48.2	49.2	11.37	85.3	47.1	48.2
2½ yr	12.84	90.4	48.8	50.2	12.28	89.3	47.7	49.0
3 yr	13.63	93.8	49.1	50.8	13.1	92.8	48.1	49.8

Age								
3½ yr	14.45	97.2	49.4	51.5	14.0	96.3	48.5	50.5
4 yr	15.26	100.8	49.7	52.2	14.89	100.1	48.8	51.2
4½ yr	16.07	103.9	50.0	53.0	15.63	103.1	49.1	51.8
5 yr	16.88	107.2	50.2	53.6	16.46	106.5	49.4	52.5
5½ yr	17.65	110.1	50.5	54.4	17.18	109.2	49.6	53.0
6 yr	19.25	114.7	50.8	55.6	18.67	113.9	50.0	54.2
7 yr	21.01	120.6	51.1	57.1	20.35	119.3	50.2	55.5
8 yr	23.08	125.3	51.4	58.8	22.43	124.6	50.6	57.1
9 yr	25.33	130.6	51.7	60.8	24.57	129.5	50.9	58.6
10 yr	27.15	134.4	51.9	62.0	27.05	134.8	51.3	60.7
11 yr	30.13	139.2	52.3	64.3	30.51	140.6	51.7	63.5
12 yr	33.05	144.2	52.7	66.5	34.82	146.6	52.3	67.2
13 yr	36.90	149.3	53.0	68.9	38.52	150.7	52.8	70.3
14 yr	42.03	156.5	53.5	72.4	42.26	153.7	53.1	73.3
15 yr	46.91	162.0	54.3	76.0	45.37	155.5	53.4	75.6
16 yr	50.90	165.6	54.9	78.8	47.43	156.8	53.8	76.6
17 yr	53.11	167.7	55.2	80.8	48.57	157.4	53.9	77.9

*Measurements of rural Chinese children are slightly lower.

NOTE: A comparison of the average growth of American and Chinese children demonstrates that on the standard NCHS growth charts the mean height and weight for Chinese children fall in the 10th percentile, as compared with the mean growth measurements for American children, which are in the 50th percentile.

From Whaley, L. F., & Wong, D. L. (1987). Nursing Care of Infants and Children (3rd ed.) St. Louis, MO: C. V. Mosby. Reproduced by permission.

and anger in the mother will produce "bad milk" and make the infant ill. Women with a tendency toward a bad temper may think that it is unwise for them to breast-feed. You should spend time with these women discussing the relative merits of breast-feeding but respect the individual's decision. If the mother perceives that her ill-tempered emotions will be transmitted to the infant during breast-feeding, then there is a strong possibility that her beliefs will become self-fulfilling prophecies.

According to most pediatricians and pediatric nurse practitioners, the introduction of solid foods is frequently associated with some aspects of infant development, such as ability to hold up the head, swallow, and sit with support. In other cultures, introduction of solid foods may relate to the eruption of the first tooth, the reaching out for adult foods, or the cessation of breast-feeding. In many cultures, the mother is judged by how much her infant eats and how quickly the infant gains weight. Thus, an obese infant may be desired because it is perceived to reflect positively on the mothering skills of the woman. On the other hand, in some Asian cultures it is common for a 16-month old child to be fed entirely on milk without any solid foods. Sometimes rice water, which is low in calories and iron, is added at 6–8 months of age.

You should discuss the infant's nutritional needs with the mother and with key significant others in the family. Because these culturally-based infant feeding practices may result in failure-to-thrive syndrome, a serious condition characterized by poor weight gain, slow development, and in extreme cases, diminished intellectual function-

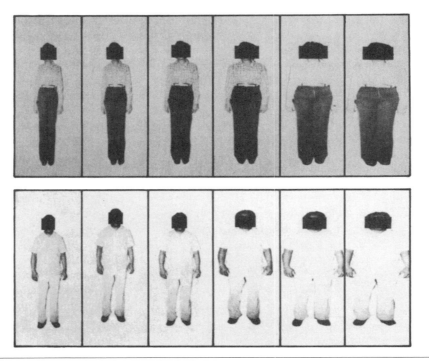

Body imagery. (From Emily B. Massara and Albert J. Stunkard, International Journal of Obesity 1979 [3], pp. 149–52.)

ing, you should share your concerns in earnest and urge the parents to bring the child to a health care provider for frequent monitoring of growth and development. You should take the time to explain a standard growth chart to the parents and to teach them how to weigh the baby, watch for developmental milestones, and observe for symptoms of nutritional deficiency. Table 11-4 illustrates a growth chart developed specifically for Asian children. Hot-cold classifications also apply to the health of infants and children. Rashes, diarrhea, fever, and many other childhood diseases are classified as hot, and therefore, require cold or cool foods.

Summary

You must conduct a complete nutritional assessment on each client and must make an effort to understand health-related dietary beliefs and practices that may impact on dietary intake for culturally diverse clients. Such beliefs as hot-cold and yin-yang theories may influence nursing care significantly and may make the difference between a rapid recovery and a slow one, for persons of all ages. Special attention to maternal and child nutritional practices has been presented because cultural food prescriptions surrounding pregnancy and childhood are common. Although it is impossible to suggest food preferences based on stereotypical generalizations about Asian, African American, Hispanic or Native American foods, several types of cultural food preferences were presented. In addition to identifying some typical foods for selected cultural groups, the strengths and potential dietary deficiencies of the typical diet were examined. Finally, the influence of cultural food patterns during pregnancy and early childhood were discussed.

Review Questions

1. Critically examine the cultural influences on food patterns and dietary behaviors.
2. Discuss the common or universal cultural functions and uses of food by people from different cultural backgrounds.
3. Critically explore the interrelationship between food patterns and religion.
   a. Compare and contrast the dietary practices of Islam, Judaism, and Seventh-day Adventism.
   b. Identify the nursing implications in caring for clients with special religious dietary needs.
4. Compare and contrast the hot-cold and yin-yang theories as they relate to cultural food patterns.
   a. Which cultural groups are most likely to embrace hot-cold and yin-yang theories?
   b. What is the function of *balance* in the hot-cold and yin-yang theories?
   c. What are the nursing implications of these two theories in caring for clients from diverse cultures?
5. Choose one of the panethnic minority groups (African American, Hispanic, Asian/Pacific Islander or Native American) and identify the major strengths and limitations of the cultural food patterns for that group. Criti-

cally examine the limitations of stereotyping diverse cultures and subcultures into a single panethnic grouping?

6. Critically examine strategies you might use in promoting dietary change in clients from diverse cultural backgrounds.

Learning Activities to Promote Critical Thinking

1. When working with bulimic, anorexic or obese clients, you should avoid reinforcing negative media messages concerning body size by assuring clients that health can be maintained within a range of weights and a variety of sizes and shapes. Using the photographs below, answer the following questions about body size and compare your responses with those of your classmates or coworkers.
   a. Which body size would you prefer to have?
   b. Which body size do you think is most healthy?
   c. Which body size do you think is most attractive?
   d. Which body size do you prefer in people of the opposite gender?
   e. Which body size do you prefer in people of the same gender?
2. Visit an ethnic restaurant in your community and answer the following questions.
   a. Which menu items have become integrated into the food patterns of the larger society, i.e., are available as packaged or frozen food selections in grocery stores?
   b. Besides the food that is served, what other evidence of the culture is apparent in this restaurant (e.g., cultural serving dishes or eating utensils, pictures, statues, shrines, incense, music, and so forth)?
   c. In what way is the language of the country integrated into the dining experience?
   d. Critically evaluate the authenticity of the restaurant and its menu. How *anglicized* has the menu and dining atmosphere become? What cultural diversity is apparent among the restaurant staff and patrons?
   e. If possible, interview the restaurant owner to learn more about the food patterns of the culture. If more than one type of cuisine is served (e.g., Mandarin Chinese and Thai foods), ask the owner why the combinations were chosen.
3. Keep a food diary for 1 week. What cultural foods or beverages have you consumed during this period?
4. Make an appointment with a dietician in a hospital or other health care facility. Ask about the types of diets available to accommodate the cultural needs of clients from diverse groups. What are the most common requests by clients? How are the religious dietary needs of clients met? Ask to see trays prepared to meet the cultural and religious needs of clients.
5. There are more than 200,000 internet sites concerning nutrition. Visit five of these sites and critique the information in terms of accuracy, credibility, reliability, and cultural appropriateness for diverse clients. The Nutrition

Navigator helps sort out credible sources from those selling products. Summarize your findings in written or electronic format for future reference.

References

Berlin, E. A., & Fowkes, W. C. (1983). A teaching framework for cross-cultural health care: Application in family practice. *Western Journal of Medicine 139*, 934–938.

Davis, J. R., & Sherer, K. (1994). *Applied Nutrition and Diet Therapy for Nurses*. Philadelphia: W. B. Saunders.

Dudek, S. G. (1997). *Nutrition Handbook for Nursing Practice*. Philadelphia: J. B. Lippincott.

Gillett, P. A., Caserta, M. S., White, A. T., & Martinson, L. (1995). Response of 49- to 59-year-old sedentary, overweight women to four months of exercise conditioning and/or fitness education. *Activities, Adaptation and Aging 19*(4), 13–22.

Gillett, P. A., Johnson, M., Juretich, M., Richardson, N., Slagle, L., & Farikoff, K. (1993). The nurse as exercise leader. *Geriatric Nursing: American Journal of Care for the Aging 14*(3), 133–137.

Leininger, M. M. (1995). *Transcultural Nursing: Concepts, Theories, Research and Practices*. New York: McGraw Hill, Inc.

Lewin, K. (1943). Forces behind food habits and methods of change. In *The Problem of Changing Food Habits: Report of the Committee on Food Habits, 108*, pp. 35–36. Washington, DC: National Academy of Science.

Lipson, J. G., & Hafizi, H. (1998). Iranians. In L. D. Purnell & B. J. Paulanka (Eds.). *Transcultural Health Care: A Culturally Competent Approach*, pp. 323–351. Philadelphia: F. A. Davis Company.

Lipson, J. G., & Steiger, N. J. (1996). *Self-Care Nursing in a Multicultural Context*. Thousand Oaks, CA: Sage Publications.

Overfield, T. (1995). *Biologic Variation in Health and Illness: Race, Age and Sex Differences*. New York: CRC Press.

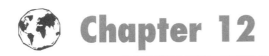

Chapter 12

Religion, Culture, and Nursing

Margaret M. Andrews
Patricia A. Hanson

OBJECTIVES

1. Explore the meaning of spirituality and religion in the lives of clients across the life span.
2. Identify the components of a spiritual needs assessment for clients from diverse cultural backgrounds.
3. Examine the ways in which spiritual and religious beliefs can be incorporated into the nursing care of clients from diverse cultures.
4. Discuss cultural considerations in the nursing care of dying or bereaved clients and families.
5. Describe the health-related beliefs and practices of selected religious groups in North America.

As an integral component of culture, religious beliefs may influence a client's explanation of the cause(s) of illness, perception of its severity, and choice of healer(s). In times of crisis, such as serious illness and impending death, religion may be a source of consolation for the client and family and may influence the course of action believed to be appropriate.

Dimensions of Religion

Religion is complex and multifaceted in both form and function. Religious faith and the institutions derived from that faith become a central focus in meeting the human needs of those who believe. "Not a single faith fails to address the issues of illness and wellness, of disease and healing, of caring and curing. Stated more positively, most faiths were born as, at least in part, efforts to heal" (Marty, 1990, p.14). Consequently, the influence of religion on health-related matters requires a few preliminary remarks.

First, it is necessary to identify specific religious factors that may influence human behavior. No single religious factor operates in isolation but rather exists in combination with other religious factors. Faulkner and DeJong (1966) have proposed five major dimensions of religion: experiential, ritualistic, ideological, intellectual, and consequential.

The *experiential* dimension recognizes that all religions have expectations of members and that the religious person will at some point in life achieve direct knowledge of ultimate reality or will experience religious emotion. Every religion recognizes this subjective religious experience as a sign of religiosity.

The *ritualistic* dimension pertains to religious practices expected of the followers and may include worship, prayer, participation in sacraments, and fasting.

The *ideological* dimension refers to the set of beliefs to which its followers must adhere in order to call themselves members. Commitment to the group or movement as a social process results, and members experience a sense of belonging or affiliation.

The *intellectual* dimension refers to specific sets of beliefs or explanations or to the cognitive structuring of meaning. Members are expected to be informed about the basic tenets of the religion as well as to be familiar with sacred writings or scriptures. The intellectual and the ideological are closely related because acceptance of a dimension presupposes knowledge of it.

The *consequential* dimension refers to religiously defined standards of conduct and includes religiously defined standards of conduct and proscriptions that specify what followers' attitudes and behaviors should be as a consequence of their religion. The consequential dimension governs people's relationships with others.

Obviously, each religious dimension has a different significance when related to matters of health and illness. Different religious cultures may emphasize one of the five dimensions to the relative exclusion of the others. Similarly, individuals may develop their own priorities related to the dimension of religion. This affects the nurse providing care to clients with different religious beliefs in several ways. First, it is the nurse's role to determine from the client, or from significant others, the dimension or combinations of dimensions that are important so that the client and nurse can have mutual goals and priorities. Second, it is important to determine what a given member of a specific religious affiliation believes to be important. The only way to do this is to ask either the client or, if the client is unable to communicate this information personally, a close family member.

Third, the nurse's information must be accurate. Making assumptions about clients' religious belief systems on the basis of there cultural, or even religious, affiliation is imprudent and may lead to erroneous inferences. The following case example illustrates the importance of verifying assumptions with the client.

Observing that a patient was wearing a star of David on a chain around his neck and had been accompanied by a rabbi upon admission, a nurse inquired whether he would like to order a kosher diet. The patient replied, "Oh, no. I'm a Christian. My father is a rabbi, and I know it would upset him to find out that I have converted. Even though I'm 40 years old, I hide it from him. This has been going on for 15 years now."

The key point in this anecdote is that the nurse validated an assumption with the patient before acting. Furthermore, it should be noted that not all Jewish persons follow a kosher diet or wear a star of David.

Fourth, even when individuals identify with a particular religion, they may accept the "official" beliefs and practices in varying degrees. It is not the nurse's role to judge the religious virtues of clients but rather to understand those aspects related to religion that are important to the client and family members. When religious beliefs are translated into practice, they may be manipulated by individuals in certain situations to serve particular ends, that is, traditional beliefs and practices are altered. Thus, it is possible for a Jewish person to eat pork or for a Catholic to take contraceptives to prevent pregnancy.

Although some find it necessary to label this as an exceptional or accidental occurrence, such a point of view tends to ignore the fact that change can and does occur within individuals and within groups. Homogeneity among members of any religion cannot be assumed. Perhaps the individual once embraced the beliefs and practices of the religion but has since changed his/her views, or perhaps the individual never accepted the religious beliefs completely in the first place. It is important for nurse to be open to variations in religious beliefs and practices and to allow for the possibility of change. Individual choices frequently arise from new situations, changing values and mores, and exposure to new ideas and beliefs. Few people live in total social isolation, surrounded by only those with similar religious backgrounds.

Fifth, ideal norms of conduct and actual behavior are not necessarily the same. The nurse is frequently faced with the challenge of understanding and helping clients cope with conflicting norms. Sometimes conflicting norms are manifested by guilt or by efforts to minimize or rationalize inconsistencies.

Sometimes norms are vaguely formulated and filled with discrepancies that allow for a variety of interpretation. In religions having a lay organization and structure, moral decision-making may be left to the individual without the assistance of members of church hierarchy. In religions having a clerical hierarchy, moral positions may be more clearly formulated and articulated for members. Individuals retain their right to choose regardless of official church-relate guidelines, suggestions, or even religious laws; however, the individual who chooses to violate the norms may experience the consequences of that violation, including social ostracism, public removal from membership rolls, or other forms of censure.

Religion and Nursing Care

For many years nursing has emphasized a holistic approach to care in which the needs of the total person are recognized. Most nursing textbooks emphasize the physical and psychosocial needs of clients rather than ways to address spiritual needs. Guidelines for providing spiritual care to culturally diverse clients is a subject about which little has been written. As you provide holistic health care, addressing spiritual needs becomes essential.

Religious concerns evolve from and respond to the mysteries of life and death, good and evil, and pain and suffering. Although the religions of the world offer various interpretations of these phenomena, most people seek a personal understanding and interpretation at some time in their lives. Ultimately, this personal search becomes a pursuit to discover a God, or some unifying truth, that will give meaning, purpose, and integrity to existence (Ebersole & Hess, 1994).

Before spiritual care for culturally diverse clients is discussed, an important distinction needs to be made between religion and spirituality. *Religion* refers to an organized system of beliefs concerning the cause, nature, and purpose of the universe, especially belief in or the worship of God or gods; *spirituality* is born out of each person's unique life experience and his or her personal effort to find purpose and meaning in life.

The goal of spiritual nursing care is to assist clients in discovering their own God or unifying truth, the ultimate reality that gives meaning to their lives in relationship to the health care crisis that has precipitated the need for nursing care. Spiritual nursing care promotes clients' physical and emotional health as well as their spiritual well-being. When providing care, you must remember that the goal of spiritual intervention is not, and should not be, to impose your religious beliefs and convictions.

Although spiritual needs are recognized by many nurses, spiritual care is often neglected. Among the reasons that nurses fail to provide spiritual care are the following: (1) they view religious and spiritual needs as a private matter concerning only an individual and his/her Creator; (2) they are uncomfortable about their own religious beliefs or deny having spiritual needs; (3) they lack knowledge about spirituality and the religious beliefs of others; (4) they mistake spiritual needs for psychosocial needs; and (5) they view meeting the spiritual needs of clients as a family or pastoral responsibility, not a nursing responsibility.

Spiritual intervention is appropriate if you care about clients' spiritual well-being as much as their biologic, physical and psychosocial health and if you recognize that the balance of physical, psychosocial, and spiritual is essential to overall good health. Nursing is an intimate profession, and nurses routinely inquire without hesitation about very personal matters such as hygiene and sexual habits. The spiritual realm also requires a personal, intimate type of nursing intervention.

In 1971 the White House Conference on Aging defined the spiritual dimension as pertaining to people's inner resources, especially their ultimate concern, the basic value around which all other values are focused, the central philosophy of life, which guides their conduct, the supernatural and non-material dimensions of human nature. The spiritual dimension encompasses the person's need to find satisfactory answers to questions about the meaning of life, illness, or death (Ebersole & Hess, 1994; Moberg, 1971).

In 1978 the Third National Conference on the Classification of Nursing Diagnoses recognized the importance of spirituality by including "spiritual concerns," "spiritual distress" and "spiritual despair" in the list of approved diagnoses. Because of practical difficulties, these three categories were combined at the 1980 National Conference into one category, "spiritual distress," which is defined as disruption in the life principle which pervades a person's entire being and which integrates and transcends one's biological and psychosocial nature. Moberg (1981) acknowledges the multidimensional nature of spiritual concerns and defines these as the human need to deal with sociocultural deprivations, anxieties and fears, death and dying, personality integration, self-image, personal dignity, social alienation, and philosophy of life.

Spiritual Care and the Phenomenon of Nursing

As discussed in Chapter 2, cultural assessment includes assessment of the relationship among religious and spiritual issues as they relate to the health care status of the client. In the case of integration of health care and religious/spiritual beliefs, the focus of the nursing plan is to help the client maintain his/her own beliefs in the face of the health care crisis and to use those beliefs to strengthen their individual coping patterns. In the event that the religious beliefs are contributing to the overall health problem (i.e. guilt, remorse, expectations etc.) you can be therapeutic by asking questions that clarify the problem and non-judgmentally supporting the client's problem solving.

Summarized in Box 12-1 are guidelines for assessing spiritual needs in clients from diverse cultural backgrounds.

Religion and Childhood Illnesses

Religion is especially important to clients during periods of crisis. In a broad sense, any hospitalization or serious illness can be viewed as stressful and therefore has the potential to develop into a crisis situation. You may find that religion plays as especially significant role in situations involving the serious illness of a child and in circumstances that include dying, death, or bereavement.

Illness during childhood may be an especially difficult clinical situation. Children as well as adults have spiritual needs that vary according to their developmental level and the religious climate that exists in the family. Parental perceptions about the illness of their child may be partially influenced by religious beliefs. For example, some parents may believe that a transgression against a religious law has caused a congenital anomaly in their offspring. Other parents may delay seeking medical care because they believe that prayer should be tried first.

You should be respectful of parents' preferences regarding the care of their child. When parental beliefs or practices threaten the child's well-being and health, you are

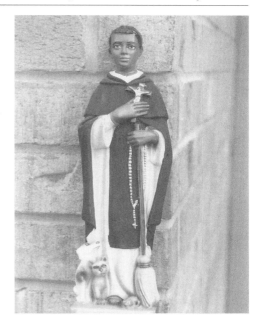

This statue commemorates the Catholic saint Martin De Porres. Born in Peru during the 16th century to a Spanish father and Negro mother, Martin De Porres studied medicine, which he later, as a member of the Dominican Order, put to use in helping the poor. He is honored by some Catholics as the patron saint of African Americans. When assessing the needs of clients from diverse religious backgrounds, nurses can observe for the presence of religious objects in the client's home or yard.

obligated to discuss the matter with the parents. It may be possible to reach a compromise on which parental beliefs are respected and necessary care is provided. On rare occasions, it may become a legal matter. Religion may be a source of consolation and support to parents, especially those facing the unanswerable questions associated with life-threatening illness in their children.

Nursing Care for the Dying or Bereaved Client and Family

"All Americans do not mourn alike. Mourning is cultural behavior and we live in a multicultural society. But the way we are raised dictates patterns we regard as proper or natural. Just as we celebrate holidays or marriages differently, we also mourn differently. The mourning customs of others may seem unusual when compared to your tradition, but like yours, they help people cope with death."

Memory and Mourning American Expressions of Grief
Strong Museum, 1994, Rochester, NY.

Nurses inevitably focus on restoring health, or fostering environments in which the client returns to a previous state of health or adapts to physical, psychological, or emotional changes. However, one aspect of *care* that is often avoided or ignored, though it is every bit as crucial to clients and their families, is death and the accompanying dying and grieving processes.

Death is indeed a universal experience, but one that is highly individual and personal. Although each person must ultimately face death alone, rarely does one person's death fail to affect others. There are many rituals, serving many purposes, that people use to help them cope with death. These rituals are usually determined

Box 12-1 *Assessing Spiritual Needs in Culturally Diverse Clients*

Environment:

- Does the client have religious objects, such as a bible, prayer book, devotional literature, religious medals, rosary or other type of beads, photographs of historic religious persons or contemporary church leaders (e.g., pope, church president), paintings of religious events or persons, religious sculptures, crucifixes, objects of religious significance at entrances to rooms (e.g., holy water founts, a *mezuzah,* or small parchment scroll inscribed with an excerpt from the Bible), candles of religious significance (e.g., Pascal candle, menorah), shrine, or other?
- Does the client wear clothing that has religious significance (e.g., head covering, undergarment, uniform)?
- Are get-well greeting cards religious in nature or from a representative of the client's church?
- Does the client receive flowers or bulletins from his or her church?

Behavior:

- Does the client appear to pray at certain times of the day or before meals?
- Does the client make special dietary requests (e.g., kosher diet, vegetarian diet, or diet free from caffeine, pork, shellfish, or other specific food items)?
- Does the client read religious magazines or books?

Verbalization:

- Does the client mention God (Allah, Buddha, Yahweh), prayer, faith, church, or religious topics?
- Does the client ask for a visit by a clergy member or other religious representative?
- Does the client express anxiety or fear about pain, suffering, or death?

Interpersonal relationships:

- Who visits? How does the client respond to visitors?
- Does a priest, rabbi, minister, elder, or other church representative visit?
- How does the client relate to the nursing staff? To his or her roommate(s)?
- Does the client prefer to interact with others or to remain alone?

Spiritual Care: The Nurse's Role, 3d Ed., by Judith Allen Shelly and Sharon Fish. © 1988 by InterVarsity Press, Christian Fellowship of the USA. Used by permission of InterVarsity Press, P.O. Box 1400, Downers Grove, IL 60515.

by cultural and religious orientation. Situational factors, competing demands, and individual differences are also important in determining the dying, bereavement, and grieving behaviors that are considered socially acceptable.

The role of the nurse in dealing with dying clients and their families varies according to the needs and preferences of both the nurse and client, as well as the clinical setting in which the interaction occurs. By understanding some of the cultural and religious variations related to death, dying and bereavement, you can individualize the care given to clients and their families.

Nurses are often with the client through various stages of the dying process and at the actual moment of death. particularly when death occurs in a hospital, nursing

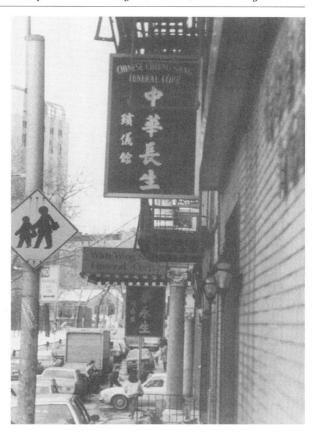

In order to preserve traditions associated with death and burial practices, some Chinese Americans prefer to use Chinese funeral directors, such as this one located in New York City's Chinatown.

home, extended care facility or hospice. You often determine when and whom to call as the impending death draws near. Knowing the religious, cultural and familial heritage of a particular client as well as his/her devotion to the associated traditions and practices may help you determine whom to call when the need arises.

Religious Beliefs Associated with Dying

Universally people want to die with dignity. Historically this was not a problem when individuals died at home in the presence of their friends and families. Now, when more and more people are dying in institutions (hospitals, nursing homes and extended care facilities) ensuring dignity throughout the dying process is a more complex task. Once death is seen as a problem for professional management, the hospital displaces the home, and specialists with different kinds and degrees of expertise take over for the family.

The way in which people commemorate death tells us much about their attitude and philosophy of life and death. Although it is beyond the scope of this book to explore the philosophical and psychological aspects of death in detail, some points will be made that relate to nursing care.

A nurse may or may not actually participate in the rituals associated with death. When people die in the United States, and Canada, they are usually transported to a mortuary, where the preparation for burial occurs.

In many cultural groups, preparation of the body has traditionally been very important. Whereas many cultural groups have now adopted the practice of letting the mortician prepare the body, there are some, particularly new immigrants, who want to retain their native and/or religious customs. For example, for certain Asian immigrants it is customary for family and friends of the same sex to wash and prepare the body for burial or cremation.

If a person dies in an institution, it is common for the nursing staff to "prepare" the body according to standard procedure. Depending on the ethno-religious practices of the family, this may be objectionable—the family may view this washing as an infringement on a special task that belongs to them alone. If the family is present, you should ask family members about their preference. If ritual washings will eventually take place at the mortuary, you may carry out the routine procedures and reassure the family that the mortician will comply with their requests, if that has in fact been verified.

North American funeral customs have been the topic of study in lively discussion. The initial preparation of the body has been described in the following way (Kalish & Reynolds, 1981, p. 65):

> After delivery to the undertaker, the corpse is in short order sprayed, sliced, pierced, pickled, trussed, trimmed, creamed, waxed, painted, rouged and neatly dressed...transformed from a common corpse into a beautiful memory picture. This process is known in the trades as embalming and restorative art, and is so universally employed in the U.S. and Canada that the funeral director does it routinely without consulting the corpse's family. He regards as eccentric those few who are hardy enough to suggest it might be dispensed with. Yet no law requires it, no religious doctrine commends it, nor is it dictated by considerations of health, sanitation or even personal daintiness. In no part of the world but in North America is it widely used. The purpose of embalming is to make the corpse presentable for viewing in a suitably costly container, and here too the funeral director routinely without first consulting the family prepares the body for public display.

This extensive preparation and attempt to make the body look "alive," "just as he used to" or "just as if she/he were asleep" may reflect the fact that Anglo Americans have been less in contact with death and dying than other cultural groups. The Anglo American group is a culturally bound ethnic group, and the avoidance of death may reflect cultural and religious differences. For example, if a patient died and a family member does not want to see the body until the mortician has "fixed it up" this request needs to be respected, regardless of your personal beliefs.

Funeral Practices

By their very nature, people are social beings who need to develop social attachments. When these social attachments are broken by death, people have a need to bring closure to the relationships. The funeral is an appropriate and socially acceptable time for the expression of sorrow and grief. Although there are some mores that dictate acceptable behaviors associated with the expression of grief, such as crying and sobbing, the wake and funeral are generally viewed as times when members of the living social network can observe and comfort the grieving survivors in their mourning, and say a last goodbye to the dead person.

Customs for disposal of the body after death vary widely. Muslims have specific rituals for washing, dressing, and positioning the body. In traditional Judaism, cosmetic restoration is discouraged, as is any attempt to hasten or retard decomposition by artificial means. As part of their lifelong preparation for death, Amish women sew white burial garments for themselves and for their family members (Wenger, 1991). For the viewing and burial, faithful Mormons are dressed in white temple garments. Burial clothes and other religious or cultural symbols may be important items for the funeral ritual. If such items are present, you should ensure they are taken by the family or sent to the funeral home.

Believing that the spirit or ghost of the deceased person is contaminated, some Navaho are afraid to touch the body after death. In preparation for burial, the body is dressed in fine apparel, adorned with expensive jewelry and money, and wrapped in new blankets. After death, some Navaho believe that the structure in which the person died must be burned.

Funeral arrangements vary from short, simple rituals to long, elaborate displays. Among the Amish, family members, neighbors and friends are relied upon for a short, quiet ceremony. Many Jewish families use unadorned coffins and stress simplicity in burial services. Some Jews fly the body to Jerusalem for burial in ground considered to be holy. Regardless of economic considerations, some groups believe in lavish and costly funerals.

Attitudes Toward Death

In some cultures, people believe that particular omens such as the appearance of an owl or a message in a dream warn of approaching death. Breaking a taboo may be believed to cause death, and the nurse may be seen as the responsible agent! The literature contains numerous reports of incidents in which nurses have removed objects of religious and spiritual significance that are believed to have healing powers from clients/patients of all ages—rosaries from the cribs of infants, necklaces worn by elderly Native Americans, and so forth. In some cases the intention of the nurse was benevolent as in the instance in which the nurse indicated that the item was removed in order to keep it in a safe place with other valuables.

Voodoo beliefs and practices are known to exist in North America. Incidents of sudden death or minor injuries following hexing have been attributed to the power of suggestion and to total social isolation, which have been thought to trigger fatal physiologic responses and sensitization of the autonomic nervous system.

Acceptance of sudden, violent death is difficult for family members in most societies. For example, suicide is strictly forbidden under Islamic law. In the Filipino culture, suicide brings shame to the individual and to the entire family. Many Christian religions prohibit suicide and may impose sanctions even after death for the "sin." For example, a Catholic who commits suicide may be denied burial in blessed ground or in a Catholic cemetery. In some religions a "church funeral" is not permitted for a suicide victim, requiring the family to make alternative arrangements. This imposition of religious law can further add to the grief of surviving family members and friends.

The Northern Cheyenne believe that suicide, or any death resulting from a violent accident, disturbs the individual's spiritual balance. This disharmony is termed *bad death* and is believed to render the spirit earthbound in its wanderings, thus preventing it from entering the spirit world. A bad death, by contrast, occurs unexpectedly and violently, leaving the victim without a chance to settle affairs or to say good-bye.

> A "bad death" is "bad" because evil caused it, which leaves the soul of the dead unrestful, unfulfilled, and desirous of returning to the living out of a longing for what has been taken away. The soul returns to the living, although not out of malevolence, to visit loved ones. It is on these visits, that the dead can bring a form of *ka:cim mum-kidag* (staying—Indian—sickness), to the living—hence their dangerousness (Kozak, 1991, p. 214).

In addition to exploring Tohono O'odham (Papago) categories of death, Kozak looks at the larger causes of the increase in violent deaths, arguing "that shifting mortality trends indicate shifts in other aspects of society" (Kozak, 1991, p. 211). Increased deaths are tied to declining economic conditions on the reservation, where jobs have disappeared.

> ...the O'odham's economic transition has meant either migrating away from family and friends to find work or remaining on the reservation at home usually to confront extreme unemployment and welfare dependency. Neither option is considered satisfactory or desirable. The social-psychological side-effects of these economic transformations are highlighted, in an inverse relationship in alcohol and drug abuse, violence, and a general increase in dependency (Kozak, 1991, p. 213).

Death-memorials provide a place for the dead to go without bringing harm to the living, and a place for the living to go to help the dead to a proper afterlife. Among the Tohono O'odham, there has been a notable increase in violent deaths, particularly for young males, since 1955. The majority of these violent deaths are the result of motor vehicle accidents, and are marked by the Tohono O'odham people with roadside death-memorials or shrines. Suicides and homicides are also sometimes commemorated with death-memorials. A good death among the Tohono O'odham comes at the end of a full life, when a person is prepared for death.

Deaths from non-violent but untimely causes can be equally difficult for the patient, family and friends. Cancers and chronic diseases may give the patient and family time to "prepare" for the death, but the death still occurs and must receive attention.

The Tohono O'odham's categories of "good" and "bad" deaths have implications for research on excess deaths. Accidents, homicide and suicide produce bad deaths; in Tohono O'odham eyes, these are deaths that should not occur, deaths that should be avoided if possible. "Bad" deaths are excess deaths. If the medical community's concern is with eliminating excess deaths, it must also be concerned with the larger cultural, social, and economic context in which these deaths occur. Other causes of death, while still important, may impact a people to a much lesser degree. Diabetes mellitus, for example, most often affects people of more advanced years, and because of its slow progress, allows them to prepare for death. This is still an excess death by Western medical standards, but it is not a "bad" death (cf., Hickey & Hall, 1993; Huttlinger et al., 1992).

Buddhism has a holistic approach to death. To the Buddhist way of thinking, illness is inevitable and is a consequence of events and actions taken. These may not be necessarily in this life but can also be in previous lives. The belief is in the cause and effect of events in this life as well as in previous lives. There is an acceptance of death, which means that the choice has been made to anticipate the grief and accept the inevitability of death. This does not mean resignation or the denial of conventional medicine. It does mean moving peacefully into the next existence from the presence of loving family and friends.

The Death of a Child

Although there is a great deal written about children's conceptions of death, cross-cultural studies have not yet been reported. Children develop a concept of death through innate cognitive development, which has significant cultural variations, and through acquired notions conveyed by the family, which vary according to the family's cultural beliefs. Thus, it is unsafe to assume that all children, regardless of their family's culture, will develop parallel concepts of and reactions to death.

Most children's initial experience with death occurs with the loss of a pet rather than a person. Due to reduced childhood mortality and delayed adult mortality, Western children are much less exposed to family death than they used to be and tend to be sheltered from the experience. The current lack of direct exposure of children to death is both a class and cultural phenomenon.

In many societies of the Western world, children are considered precious, valued, and vulnerable; they are protected and often the first to be saved in emergencies. In less developed societies, by contrast, parents are less likely to see most of their children grow into adulthood because of a very high infant mortality rate. As a result, a child's life may be viewed as less valued and precious than an adult's, but is still viewed as valuable to the parents and other loved ones. Regardless of the sociocultural situation, each society has a special view of the significance of children and their death as it affects the bereaved family.

Awareness of Dying

The issue of whether individuals should be made aware of their impending death has been debated extensively by physicians, nurses, and others. In the Kalish and Reynolds (1981) study, 71 percent of Anglos, 60 percent of African Americans, 49 percent of Japanese Americans, and 37 percent of Mexican Americans favored telling clients that they were dying. Each cultural group believed the physician was the most appropriate person to communicate the information, whereas a family member was the second most appropriate choice. However, individual preferences should be respected. In some cultures, not telling the dying individual of their empending death is a way for them to be allowed to "save face."

Bereavement, Grief, and Mourning

Bereavement is a sociological term indicating the status and role of the survivors of a death. *Grief* is an affective response to a loss, while *mourning* is the culturally patterned behavioral response to a death. What differs between races and cultural groups is not so much the feelings of grief but their forms of expression or mourning.

Different family systems may alleviate or intensify the pain experienced by bereaved persons. In the typical nuclear Anglo or European-American family, the death of a member leaves a great void because the same few individuals fill most of the roles. By contrast, cultural groups in which several generations and extended family members commonly reside within a household may find that the acute trauma of bereavement is softened by the fact that the familial role of the deceased is easily filled by other relatives. It should be noted, however, that the loss is experienced and mourned irrespective of the person's cultural background.

Although nurses frequently encourage clients and their families to express their grief openly, many people are reluctant to do so in the institutional setting. The nurse often sees the family at a time when members are still in shock over the death and are responding to the situation as a crisis, rather than expressing their grief. Three fourths of the African American, Japanese, and Anglos stated they would try hard to maintain control of their emotions in public, while less than two thirds of Mexican Americans were concerned with the public expression of grief. When asked about crying, either publicly or privately, 88 percent of Mexican American, 71 percent of Japanese, 70 percent of Anglos, and 60 percent of African Americans indicated that this was acceptable, particularly in private (Kalish & Reynolds, 1981)

When asked who would be sought for comfort and support in time of bereavement, these groups most frequently named a family member or a member of the clergy. In an institutional setting, a nurse who has been with the patient and family throughout the dying process may be surprised at the time of death when the grieving persons turn to other family, and the nurse is "left out."

Although the experience of grief is a universal phenomenon, a nurse should recognize that the expression of grief is strongly influenced by cultural factors. For example, mourning may vary according to the lines of emotional attachment. With matrilineal societies a woman may be expected to grieve for male members of her maternal family, such as fathers and brothers, but not for her spouse.

It is not uncommon for a surviving spouse to have a serious illness within a year or two following the death. Although the exact reasons for this are unknown, the stress of losing a spouse seems to render the surviving partner more vulnerable to illness. Caring for a person who is seriously ill, but also mourning a recent death requires added sensitivity by the nurse to the patient's emotional needs.

Some mourning rituals are highly structured and lengthy, while others are relatively simple and short. In the Jewish tradition, there are five successive stages of mourning which extend for a year and include practices that influence virtually every aspect of life. The examination of the following four ethnic groups is intended to provide the nurse with insight into specific cross-cultural bereavement behaviors.

Spanish Speaking Groups

With 17.4 million members, the Spanish-speaking represent the second largest cultural group in the United States (U.S. Bureau of the Census, 1990). Of these, 59 percent are of Mexican origin, 15 percent Puerto Rican, 6 percent Cuban, and 20 percent of other Hispanic origin. Although little is known about specific bereavement patterns of each group, the Puerto Ricans have been studied, and the resulting information may help the nurse to empathize with the client from this cultural group. However the nurse should not generalize for all members of the group, nor assume that mourning will be the same for other Hispanic groups.

Many Puerto Ricans believe that a person's spirit will not be free to enter the next life if that person has left something unsaid before death. For this reason, it is important for friends and family to complete their relationships with a dying person. With sudden death such closure is obviously impossible, but in the case of chronic illness, those close to the dying client should be given the privacy necessary to accomplish this task. Atypical grief may arise when grieving Puerto Ricans feel that the relationship has not been properly completed (Eisenbruch, 1984b).

Following the death, the family meets together to comfort one another and to pray for the dead. Called a "wake," this event offers a mechanism for mobilizing community support and for the expression of grief. With the predominant religion being Roman Catholic, religious rituals such as masses, rosaries, and novenas are observed to benefit both the deceased and the surviving family members. In North America time restrictions for wakes are often imposed by funeral directors, but traditionally, last for several days.

Grief is sometimes expressed in a syndrome called *el ataque*, which is characterized by seizure-like behavior, hyperkinetic episodes, a display of aggression, and sometimes stupor. Such behavior is acceptable and socially sanctioned within the Puerto Rican culture as a way for bereaved persons to discharge anger. Anglo American nurses, however, may view this behavior as aberrant. In keeping with beliefs about **machismo**, in which males in general are raised to keep all feeling of suffering inside, bereaved Hispanic men are often unreceptive to grief counseling and may resent being told by the nurse that "it's okay to cry." Economic stress may add a burden to the bereaved. Many Puerto Rican families wish to accompany the body of the deceased to Puerto Rico for burial. The family, community, and church may provide financial assistance; the traditional leave with pay given in the United States. Still, the economic necessity of returning to work after only 3 days of mourning (the traditional leave with pay given by employers in the United States) may interfere with the ability to grieve.

Kalish and Reynolds (1981) found that for Mexican Americans the family protective network is prominent. Of all groups studied, the Mexican Americans were the most likely to want to protect both the dying and the bereaved, such as small children who might have difficulty with the death. Mexican Americans often rally around the hospitalized client and take turns in shifts of vigil. They tend to encourage the open expression of feeling of anguish and grief (Eisenbruch, 1984b).

Urban African-Americans

The way people handle the problems surrounding death indicates the way in which they deal with life. There are very few new resources available to an individual who faces critical illness or death. The decision-making process used to cope with life-threatening illness is likely to be similar to the process used during other times in the individual's life.

With the help of the media, the belief has been perpetuated that African Americans have more contact with death than Whites, particularly violent deaths and accidents. Bereaved African Americans (and Anglo Americans) are likely to rely on friends, church members, neighbors, and other non-relatives when faced with the death of a loved one. African Americans are less likely to express their grief overtly and publicly. Patterns of coping with death will vary widely among urban Blacks depending upon the educational and socioeconomic background of the bereaved, more than in many other ethnic groups.

One stereotype is that when faced with a crisis African Americans, because of a closely knit supportive family network, can look after themselves. However, the extended family does not predominate among either rural or urban Blacks. With a preponderance of female-headed, single-parent family units, it is unrealistic to expect the bereaved to rely solely on the family for the needed support.

Besides the cultural idiom of bereavement, Blacks may experience different modes of death. Fewer whites die violently than do African Americans. Those who survive violence often need to rely on the biomedical system for help over an extended period of time (Kalish & Reynolds, 1981).

Ethnic Chinese and Related Groups

Included in this group are not only people from China but also ethnic Chinese from all of southeast Asia. Even though many Chinese Americans have been assimilated into Western society, the attitudes toward death in classical Chinese society have pervaded. In general Chinese Americans tend to be stoic and fatalistic when faced with terminal illness and death. This outward stoicism, however, does not negate the inner feelings of sorrow and loss that accompany the loss of a loved one.

Traditional Chinese society recognized that the family was the basic social unit, and codified the concept in laws of degrees of kinship. *Wu-fu*, meaning "the five kinds of clothing," defines degrees of relationships and determines the severity of mourning in terms of closeness of the deceased to the mourner.

The Chinese traditionally follow a system of double burial. The initial burial in a coffin lasts for seven years, after which time the remains are exhumed and stored in an urn for years or decades more. Reburial in an elaborate tomb marks the second burial, after which time the deceased is able to have a beneficial effect on descendants. Many Chinese Americans are unaware of these traditional customs (Eisenbruch, 1984b). They have adopted an American Christian religion while maintaining non-Christian cultural beliefs related to death, dying and burial. In such cases it is especially critical to know whom to call in the event of an emergency and particularly at the time of death.

Southeast Asian Refugees

During recent years Southeast Asian refugees have developed into an important cultural group in the United States and Canada. Included in the group are at least five distinct categories: Vietnamese, Kampucheans, Hmong, Laotian, and Lao-Theung.

Refugees are particularly vulnerable to the stress of bereavement; many have already suffered the loss of close family members as a result of war in Southeast Asia, and the refugee experience is itself a stressful event. Furthermore, traditional mourning practices must be modified in the United States due to cultural differences. Major differences in mourning among the subgroups of Southeast Asians exist and include the following: the color of mourning clothes and the duration for which they are worn, the commemorative celebration on the anniversary of the death, and marriages of the deceased person's spouse and children.

When the bereaved are unable to carry out meaningful traditional rituals, their stress may be amplified when the cultural mechanisms for support are impeded. Some traditional Vietnamese practices include preparation of the body by family members, including placement of a coin in the deceased person's mouth to help the spirit at various stages of its journey, and use of special divination when choosing the grave site. American morticians are usually unwilling or unable to comply with request of this nature because, for example, rigor mortis has set in by the time the body reaches the funeral home, making opening the mouth difficult. Furthermore, cemeteries have specific regulations about grave sites, some of which are governed by zoning, health, and sanitation laws. Thus, bereavement codes of the immigrant may violate laws of the host country.

Social and religious practices among the refugees from Southeast Asia vary markedly. The Vietnamese and ethnic Chinese may be Mahayana or Theravada Buddhist, and the Hmong and other hill tribes are usually animist in their beliefs (Eisenbruch, 1984b), Each group has its own ritual prescriptions and proscriptions. The nurse should become aware of differences and avoid stereotyping all Southeast Asian in order to prevent embarrassing errors that could lead to further distress for the client and family.

Summary of Beliefs Related to Death and Dying

The contemporary bereavement practices of various cultural groups discussed here demonstrate the wide range of expressions of bereavement. Each group reflects practices that best meet its members' needs. Once you understand this, you can better appreciate their role in promoting a culturally appropriate grieving process. Conversely, hindering or interfering with practices that the client and family find meaningful can disrupt the grieving process. Bereaved people can develop physical and psychological symptoms, and may succumb to serious physical illnesses, leading even to death. Although bereavement is regarded as a "universal" stressor, the magnitude of the stress and its meaning to the individual varies significantly cross-culturally. For example, one Western misconception is that it is more stressful to mourn the death of a child than the death of an older or more distant relative. Yet cross-cultural studies show that emotional attachments to relatives vary significantly and are not based on Western concepts of kinship (Eisenbruch, 1984b).

Although traditional funeral and post-funeral rituals have benefitted both bereaved persons and their social groups in their original settings, the influence of the contemporary Western urban setting is unknown. It is likely that in North America, most individuals have assimilated United States and Canadian practices in varying degrees. You should obtain information from individual clients in a caring manner, explaining that they wish to provide culturally appropriate nursing care.

Religious Trends in the United States and Canada

The United States and Canada are cosmopolitan nations to which all of the major and many of the minor faiths of Europe and other parts of the globe have been transplanted. With an influx of refugees from Southeast Asia, many Eastern religions have become increasingly prevalent. With such a complex mosaic of religions, no one has succeeded in enumerating all of the denominations. According to the 1990 Yearbook of American and Canadian churches, there are 358,194 congregations representing over 1,200 different religious denominations. Religious bodies with 60,000 or more members in the United States and Canada are identified in Table 12-1.

As discussed, a wide range of beliefs frequently exist within religions, a factor that adds complexity. Some religions have a designated spokesperson or leader who articulates, interprets, and applies theological tenets to daily life experiences, including those of health and illness. These include a Jewish rabbi, a Catholic priest, and a Lutheran minister. Some churches rely more heavily on individual conscience, whereas others entrust decisions to a group of individuals, or to a single person vested with ultimate authority within their church.

Although it is impossible to address the health related beliefs and practices of any religion adequately, this chapter offers a brief overview of some groups. Some of the world's religions fall into major branches or divisions such as Vaishnavite and Shaivite Hinduism, Theravada and Mahayana Buddhism, Orthodox, Reform and Conservative Judaism, Catholic, Orthodox and Protestant Christianity, and Sunnite and Shi'ite Islam. There also are subdivisions into what are often called denominations, sects or schools of thought and practice.

Contributions of Religious Groups to the Health Care Delivery System

Many denominations own and operate health care institutions and make significant fiscal contributions that help control health care costs. For example, the Catholic Church, the largest single denomination in the U.S., is also a major stakeholder in the health care field. According to the *Catholic Almanac* (1997), the nation's 600 Catholic hospitals treat 15.3 million patients annually and account for approximately 10 percent of all hospital beds. In addition, the Catholic church is responsible for treating 3.9 million patients at its 556 health centers and 143,000 individuals at its 1,018 day care and extended day care centers. Moreover, there are under direct Catholic auspices 94 nonresidential schools for the handicapped, 1,531 specialized homes, 14 facilities for the deaf and hearing impaired, 4 centers for the blind and visually impaired, 517 facilities for the aged, 72 facilities for abused, abandoned, neglected, and emotionally disturbed children, 116 centers for those with developmental disabilities, 2 residences for the orthopedically/physically handicapped, 8 cancer hospitals, and 11 substance abuse centers. Catholic Charities U.S.A., an umbrella agency that oversees the non-hospital work, reports that its agencies serve more than 12 million people each year, often functioning as a centralized referral source for clients ultimately treated in non-Catholic agencies (Angrosino, 1996; Foy & Avato, 1997).

Similarly, there are many Jewish hospitals, day care centers, extended care facili-

TABLE 12-1
Membership for Selected Religious Bodies in the United States and Canada

Religious Body	Membership
African Methodist Episcopal Church	3,500,000
African Methodist Episcopal Zion Church	1,231,000
American Baptist Association	250,000
American Baptist Churches in the U.S.A.	1,508,000
Antiochian Orthodox Christian Archdiocese of North America	300,000
Armenia Apostolic Church of America	150,000
Assemblies of God	2,325,000
Baha'i International Community	363,000
Baptist Bible Fellowship International	1,500,000
Baptist General Conference	135,000
Baptist Missionary Association of America	230,000
Buddhist	401,000
Christian and Missionary Alliance	302,000
Christian Brethren (a.k.a. Plymouth Brethren)	98,000
Christian Church (Disciples of Christ)	938,000
Christian Churches and Churches of Christ	1,071,000
Christian Congregations, Inc.	112,000
Christian Methodist Episcopal Church	719,000
Christian Reformed Church in North America	211,000
Church of God (Anderson, IN)	216,000
Church of God (Cleveland, TN)	723,000
Church of God in Christ	5,500,000
Church of God of Prophecy	71,000
Church of Jesus Christ of Latter-Day Saints	4,613,000
Church of the Brethren	144,000
Church of the Nazarene	598,000
Churches of Christ	1,651,000
Conservative Baptist Association of America	200,000
Coptic Orthodox Church	180,000
Cumberland Presbyterian Church	772,000
Diocese of the Armenian Church of America	414,000
Episcopal Church	2,505,000
Evangelical Covenant Church	90,000
Evangelical Free Church of America	227,000
Evangelical Lutheran Church of America	5,199,000
Free Methodist Church of North America	75,000
Church of Friends (Quakers)	130,000
General Association of Regular Baptist Churches	136,000
General Baptists (General Association of)	74,000
Grace Gospel Fellowship	60,000
Greek Orthodox Diocese of North & South America	1,950,000
Hindu	227,000

TABLE 12-1 (Continued)

Religious Body	Membership
Independent Fundamental Churches of America	70,000
International Church of the Foursquare Gospel	223,000
International Council of Community Churches	500,000
International Pentecostal Holiness Church	150,000
Jehovah's Witnesses	946,000
Jewish	3,137,000
Lutheran Church—Missouri Synod	2,597,000
Mennonite Church	96,000
Muslim/Islamic	527,000
National Association of Congregational Christian Churches	70,000
National Association of Free Will Baptists	200,000
National Baptist Convention of America, Inc.	3,500,000
National Baptist Convention, U.S.A., Inc.	8,200,000
National Missionary Baptist Convention, U.S.A., Inc.	2,500,000
Old Order Amish Church	81,000
Orthodox Church in America	2,000,000
Pentecostal Assemblies of the World	1,000,000
Pentecostal Church of God, Inc.	113,000
Polish National Catholic Church of North America	282,000
Presbyterian Church in America	258,000
Presbyterian Church (U.S.A.)	3,698,000
Progressive National Baptist Convention, Inc.	2,500,000
Reformed Church in North America	309,000
Reorganized Church of Jesus Christ of Latter-Day Saints	150,000
Roman Catholic Church	60,191,000
Romanian Orthodox Episcopate of America	65,000
Salvation Army	443,000
Serbian Orthodox Church in the U.S.A. and Canada	67,000
Seventh-day Adventist Church	4,303,000
Southern Baptist Convention	15,614,000
Unitarian Universalist	502,000
United Church of Christ	1,501,000
United Methodist Church	8,584,000
United Pentecostal Church International	550,000
Wesleyan Church (USA)	177,000
Wisconsin Evangelical Lutheran Synod	415,000

Data from U.S. Bureau of the Census (1996). *Statistical Abstracts of the United States: 1996,* (116th ed.). Washington, DC: U.S. Government Printing Office.

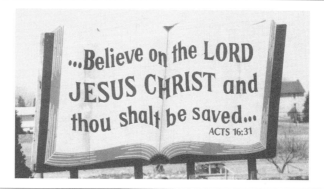

Eighty-five percent of North Americans report religious affiliation with a Christian church. Of the 60 percent affiliated with Protestant groups in the United States, Baptists account for 21 percent; Methodists, 9 percent; Lutherans, 7 percent; Presbyterians, 5 percent; and Episcopalians, 2 percent. Catholics comprise 26 percent. Those belonging to non-Christian religions total 6 percent of the population whereas those reporting no religious affiliation account for 9 percent.

ties, and organizations to meet the health care needs of Jewish and non-Jewish persons in need. For example, the National Jewish Center for Immunology and Respiratory Medicine is a research and treatment center for respiratory, immunologic, allergic and infectious diseases, whereas the Council for Jewish Elderly provides a full range of social and health care services for seniors including adult day care, care/case management, counseling, transportation and advocacy.

Many other denominations such as Lutheran, Mennonite, Methodist, Muslim and Seventh-day Adventist groups own and operate hospitals and health-care organizations similar to those described previously.

The remainder of this chapter will examine in alphabetical order the health-related beliefs and practices of selected North American denominations.

Listing of Selected Religions

Amish

The term *Amish* refers to members of several ethno-religious groups who choose to live separately from the modern world through manner of dress, language, family life, and selective use of technology. There are four major *orders* or affiliating groups of Amish: (1) *Old Order Amish*, the largest group which is often used synonymously with "the Amish"; (2) the ultraconservative *Swartzentruber* and *Andy Weaver Amish*, both more conservative than the Old Order Amish in their restrictive use of technology and *shunning* of members who have dropped out or committed serious violations of the faith; (3) the less conservative *New Order Amish* which emerged in the 1960s with more liberal views of technology but emphasizing high moral standards in restricting alcohol and tobacco use and in courtship practices; and (4) the *Liberal Beachy Amish*.

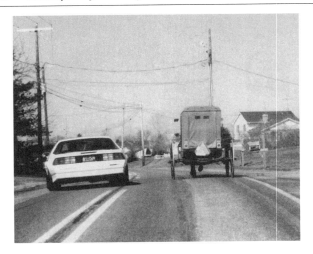

Although Amish restrict their use of technology for reasons that are, in part, health-related, they ironically find themselves at high risk for accidents that frequently result from the careless use of technological developments by non-Amish neighbors.

The total population of Amish is estimated at 160,000 spread throughout 220 plus settlements in 21 states and one Canadian province (about 1/20th of 1 percent of the total U.S. and Canadian populations). In 1900, there were approximately 5000 Amish, which represented the number who immigrated to the U.S. during the 18th and 19th centuries. During the 20th century, however, the population grew as the Amish became less frequent targets for conversion and growing numbers of children (80–85 percent) chose, as adults, to be baptized Amish. As a result, the population grew to 85,000 by 1979 and has nearly doubled that number today. More than half are younger than age 18 (Donnermeyer, 1997).

Beliefs and Religious Practices

The imperative to remain separate is the common theme of the nearly 500-year history of the Amish and is based on the following scripture passage:

> "Be not conformed to this world, but be ye transformed by the renewing of
> your mind...."
>> Romans (12:2)
> "Be ye not unequally yoked together with unbelievers; for what fellowship
> hath righteousness with unrighteousness? and what communion hath light
> with darkness?"
>> Corinthians II (6:14)

The Amish are direct descendants of a branch of *Anabaptists* (which means to be re-baptized) that emerged during the Protestant Reformation and resided in Switzerland, The Netherlands, Austria, France and Germany. Anabaptists stressed adult baptism, separation from and non-assimilation with the dominant culture, conformity in dress and appearance, marriage to others within the group, non-proselytization, non-participation in military service, and a disciplined lifestyle with an emphasis on simple living, basic tenets that remain today.

A former Catholic priest from The Netherlands named Menno Simmons (1496–1561) wrote down the beliefs and practices of the Anabaptists, who became known as *Mennonites.* In 1693 under the leadership of a church elder named Jacob Ammann (1656–1730), a more conservative group broke away forming the group currently known as the Amish.

According to Donnermeyer (1997) there are five core characteristics of the Amish. First, the Amish are a *subculture,* a group that has distinctive beliefs, values and behaviors from the greater culture of which the group is a part. The Amish maintain their separateness and distinctiveness from U.S. and Canadian societies in a variety of ways. Geographically, the Amish live close together in areas referred to as *settlements* and rely primarily on the horse and buggy for transportation.

The Amish continue to practice their faith in the tradition of Anabaptism, which includes small church districts of a few dozen families led by a bishop; church services that rotate from house to house of each family (no church building); the practice of adult baptism, communion twice a year, and shunning. Church leaders are chosen through a process of nomination and drawing by lot, and they serve for life. All but a few Amish marry, extended family remains important, and divorce is rare. The Amish dress in distinctive clothing (plain colors and mostly without buttons and zippers). They speak a form of German among themselves known as Pennsylvania Dutch or High German, and they sometimes refer to non-Amish as the "English."

The second core feature of the Amish is the *ordung* which is used for passing on religious values and way of life from one generation to the next. Parts of the *ordung* are based on specific biblical passages, but much of it consists of rules for living the Amish way.

The third characteristic of the Amish is called *meidung* or the practice of *shunning.* After all members of the church district have discussed the case and agreed to impose *meidung,* the individual is separated from the rest of his/her community. It is the church's method of enforcing the ordung. *Meidung* is an important way of maintaining both a sense of community among Amish and a sense of separation from the rest of the world. Sanctions for violations against important values, beliefs and behaviors that define distinctiveness from the majority culture enable the Amish to retain their religious and cultural identity. In most cases when *meidung* is applied, it is for a limited time. *Meidung* applies only to Amish adults who have been baptized, not to their unbaptized children. Children of Amish who choose not to be baptized often become members of neighboring Mennonite congregations and maintain contact with their Amish relatives.

With less serious violations of the *ordung,* a member is visited privately by the deacon and a minister and the matter is resolved quietly. For more serious offenses, the punishment is carried out publicly during a church service. A few offenses, such as adultery and divorce, are automatically conditions of *excommunication.* By displaying deep sorrow and repentance for an offense, excommunicated members can be allowed back but this is not easily accomplished.

The fourth core characteristic is the *selective use of technology.* The Amish selectively use many modern technologies, but only if they do not threaten their ability to maintain a community of believers. Technologically, the Amish restrict the use of electricity in their homes and farms and they limit their use of telephones. Although they ride in automobiles, trains, and airplanes, they do not operate them. Tractors for farm field work might reduce the opportunity for sons and daughters to help parents with farm chores, and the farm would become larger, reducing the number available for future generations. Thus, technology is not inherently bad, but when its consequences result in destruction of family and community life, it is avoided.

The fifth and final core characteristic of the Amish is *gelassenheit*. This term means "submission" or yielding to a higher authority and represents a general guide for behavior among Amish members. *Gelassenheit* represents the high value that the Amish place on maintaining a sense of community which is accomplished by not drawing too much attention to one's self. Amish cite gelassenheit as the reason they avoid having their photographs taken and prohibit mirrors in their homes.

HOLY DAYS. Amish hold church services every other Sunday on a rotating basis in the homes or barns of church district members. The church services last several hours with hymns, scriptures and services in High German or Penn Dutch. The family hosting the services is expected to provide a meal for all in attendance. Christmas celebrations include family dinners and gift exchange. Weddings last all day and include eating and singing. An important part of Amish life is informal visiting. Families often visit one another without advance notice, and it is common for unexpected visitors to stay for a meal.

SACRAMENTS. Adult baptism. Communion twice a year.

RELIGION AND HEALING. Illness is seen as the inability to perform daily chores with physical and mental illness being accepted equally. Health care practices within the Amish culture are varied and include folk, herbal, homeopathic and Western biomedicine. Unlike the use of episodic biomedicine, however, preventative medicine may be seen as against God's will. The use of the Western biomedical health care system is largely episodic and crisis-oriented. If Western biomedicine fails, there is no hesitancy in visiting an herb doctor, pow-wow doctor (those who practice a folk healing art known as *brauche* in which touch is used to heal) or a chiropractor. Folk, professional, and alternative care are often used simultaneously. Cost, access, transportation, and advice from family and friends are the major factors influencing healing choices (Wenger, 1990).

DIET, MEDICATIONS, AND PROCEDURES. The use of alcoholic beverages, tobacco and narcotic drugs is prohibited. There are no restrictions against the use of blood, blood products or vaccines if advised by health care providers.

Controversial Issues Related to Health Care

BIRTH CONTROL. The Amish believe that the fundamental purpose of marriage is the procreation of children, and couples are encouraged to have large families. Children are an economic asset to the family as they assist their parents with housework, farm chores, gardening and family business. Women are expected to have children until menopause. If situations arise that justify sterilization (e.g., removal of cancerous reproductive organs), those called upon to make the decisions would rely on the best medical advice available and the council of the church leaders. Although the Amish family structure is patriarchal, the grandmother is often a key decision maker concerning reproductive and other health-related issues.

ABORTION. Inconsistent with Amish values and beliefs.

ARTIFICIAL INSEMINATION, GENETICS, AND EUGENICS. Inconsistent with Amish values and beliefs.

SOCIAL ACTIVITIES (DATING, DANCING). The Amish strive for high standards of conduct in both their private and public lives; this includes chastity before marriage and humility in dress, language, and behavior. The function of dating is to afford individuals an opportunity to become acquainted with each other's character. Couples contemplating marriage may engage in a practice called *bundling* in which the fully clothed couple lies next to each other in bed without having sexual contact.

SUBSTANCE USE. Alcoholic beverages and drugs are forbidden unless prescribed by a physician. Tobacco use is prohibited.

Religious Support System for the Sick
VISITORS. Individual members of local and surrounding communities assist and support each other in time of need. From cradle to grave each person knows he/she will be cared for by those in their community. *Friendscraft* is a unique three-generational extended family support network inherent in the Amish community that provides informal support, emotional and financial assistance and advice. The extended family consists of aunts, uncles, cousins and grandparents who usually live only a few miles away and can be counted on to assist in times of illness.

TITLE OF RELIGIOUS REPRESENTATIVE. Religious titles are not used. There are approximately 1,100 Amish church districts in the U.S. and Canada, each representing about 20–35 families and a minimal hierarchy of church leaders (a bishop, deacon and two ministers). The bishop is the spiritual head; the deacon assists the bishop and is responsible for donations to help members with medical bills and other expenses; and the ministers help the bishop with preaching at church services and providing spiritual direction for the church district and its members. Although bishops meet periodically, there is no church hierarchy above the level of the church district. Because the Amish are surrounded by American and Canadian societies which continuously exert strong economic and cultural pressures that are incompatible with Amish values, the Amish represent a subculture that is among the most "self-consciously engineered of all societies" (Donnermeyer, 1997, p. 9).

CHURCH ORGANIZATIONS TO ASSIST THE SICK. Individual members of local church districts look after the needs of the sick person and his/her family.

Issues Related to Death and Dying
PROLONGATION OF LIFE (RIGHT TO DIE). A personal matter that may be discussed with the bishop, ministers, and/or family members.

EUTHANASIA. A personal matter that may be discussed with the bishop, ministers, and/or family members.

AUTOPSY.   Acceptable in the case of medical necessity or legal requirement but seldom performed on the Amish.

DONATION OF BODY.   Although there is no specific prohibition, the Amish usually prefer to bury the intact body and generally do not donate body parts for medical research.

DISPOSAL OF BODY AND BURIAL.   Bodies are buried in small cemeteries located in Amish communities on private property.

ADDENDUM: MEETING HEALTH EXPENSES.   The Amish beliefs in self-sufficiency, separation from the world, and mutual aid have resulted in their rejection of formal assistance that comes from outside the Amish community. For example, they obtained exemption for self-employed workers from Social Security, including Medicare, in 1965 on religious grounds and received exemption for all Amish workers from these programs in 1988. Amish seldom purchase commercial health insurance; rather, than commercial health insurance, the Amish have traditionally relied on personal savings and various methods of mutual assistance within the immediate and larger Amish community to meet their medical expenses. It is expected that each family has planned for future health care needs (e.g., birth of a child and minor illness), but it is recognized that catastrophic illnesses resulting in extensive medical expenses do sometimes occur. In these instances, the Amish community provides assistance, usually through participation in one of the Amish Hospital Aid plans.

As indicated in Research Application 12-1, changing occupational patterns among the Amish have resulted in shifting views toward commercial health insurance. According to Donnermeyer (1997), in Holmes County, Ohio only 32.9 percent of Amish breadwinners earn their living as farmers—24.5 percent are active farmers, 4% are retired farmers and 3.4 percent hold dual occupations (both farm and non-farm). Similar trends have been reported among other Amish settlements, where 30–80 percent of adult males work in non-farm wage labor jobs in construction, factories, and home-based shops (e.g., cabinet making , harness making, black smithing, and so forth). The underlying reasons for the change are attributed to two factors: (1) population growth, and (2) difficulty finding sufficient farmland for the growing numbers of Amish.

Baha'i International Community

The Baha'i Faith is an independent world religion. It has members in approximately 340 countries and localities and represents 1900 ethnic groups and tribes.

MEMBERSHIP.   North America, 363,000; worldwide, 5.4 million

Beliefs and Religious Practices

The writings that guide the life of the Baha'i International Community comprise numerous works by Baha'u'llah, prophet-founder of the Baha'i Faith. Central teachings are the oneness of God, the oneness of religion, and the oneness of humanity. Baha'u'llah proclaimed that religious truth is not absolute but relative; that Divine Revelation is a continuous and progressive process; that all the great religions of the world are divine in origin; and that their missions represent successive stages in the spiritual evolution of human society.

For Baha'is, the basic purpose of human life is to know and worship God, and to carry forward an ever-advancing civilization. To achieve these goals, they strive to fulfill certain principles:

1. Fostering of good character and the development of spiritual qualities, such as honesty, trustworthiness, compassion, and justice.
2. Eradication of prejudices of race, creed, class, nationality, and sex.
3. Elimination of all forms of superstition hampering human progress, and achievement of a balance between material and spiritual aspects of life. An unfettered search for truth and belief in the essential harmony of science and religion are two aspects of this principle.
4. Development of the unique talents and abilities of every individual through the pursuit of knowledge and the acquisition of skills for the practice of a trade or profession.
5. Full participation of both sexes in all aspects of community life, including the elective, administrative, and decision-making processes, along with equality of opportunities, rights, and privileges of men and women.
6. Fostering of the principle of universal compulsory education.

Baha'is may not be members of any political party but may accept nonpartisan government posts and appointments. They are enjoined to obey the government in their respective countries and, without political affiliation, may vote in general elections and participate in the civic life of their community.

The Baha'i administrative order has neither priesthood nor ritual; it relies on a pattern of local, national, and international governance, created by Baha'u'llah. Institutions and programs are supported exclusively by voluntary contributions from members.

The Baha'i International Community has consultative status with the United Nations Economic and Social Council and with the United Nations Children's Fund. It is also affiliated with the United Nations Environment Program and with the United Nations Office of Public Information.

The World Center of the Baha'i Faith is in Israel, established in the two cities of Haifa and 'Akka. The affairs of the Baha'i world community are administered by the Universal House of Justice, the supreme elected council, situated in Haifa.

HOLY DAYS.   Extending from sunset to sunset are Baha'i holy days, feast days, and days of fasting. These holy days are not contraindications to medical care or surgery.

SACRAMENTS.   Although the Baha'i Faith does not have sacraments in the same sense that Christian Churches do, it does have practices that have similar meanings to members. These practices include the recitation of obligatory prayers, and participation in observance of holy days and the Nineteen-Day Fast, which is mandatory for all Baha'is between the ages of 15 and 70 years. Exceptions are made for illness, travel away from home, and pregnancy. Fasting occurs from sunrise to sunset for an entire Baha'i month, which consists of 19 days.

RELIGION AND HEALING.   With an attitude of harmony between religion and science, Baha'is are encouraged to seek out competent medical care, to follow the advice of those in whom they have confidence, and to pray.

DIET, MEDICATIONS, AND PROCEDURES.   The use of alcoholic beverages and narcotic drugs is prohibited except by prescription. There are no restrictions against the use of blood, blood products, or vaccines if advised by health care providers.

SURGICAL PROCEDURES.   Amputations, organ transplantation, biopsies, circumcision, and amniocentesis are permitted if advised by health care providers.

Controversial Issues Related to Health Care

BIRTH CONTROL.   Baha'is believe that the fundamental purpose of marriage is the procreation of children. Individuals are encouraged to exercise their discretion in choosing a method of family planning.

Baha'u'llah taught that to beget children is the highest physical fruit of man's existence. The Baha'i teachings imply that birth control constitutes a real danger to the foundations of social life. It is against the spirit of Baha'i law, which defines the primary purpose of marriage to be the rearing of children and their spiritual training. It is left to each husband and wife to decide how many children they will have. Baha'i teachings state that the soul appears at conception. Therefore, it is improper to use a method that produces an abortion after conception has taken place (e.g., intrauterine device). Methods that result in permanent sterility are not permissible under normal circumstances. If situations arise that justify sterilization (e.g., removal of cancerous reproductive organs), those called upon to make the decision would rely on the best medical advice available and their own consciences.

ABORTION.   Members are discouraged from using methods of contraception that produce an abortion after conception has taken place (e.g., intrauterine device). A surgical operation for the purpose of preventing the birth of an unwanted child is strictly forbidden.

Baha'i teachings state that the soul of man comes into being at conception. Abortion and surgical operations for the purpose of preventing the birth of unwanted children are forbidden unless circumstances justify such actions on medical grounds. In this case, the decision is left to the consciences of those concerned, who must carefully weigh the medical advice they receive in the light of the general guidance given in the Baha'i writings.

ARTIFICIAL INSEMINATION.   Although there are no specific Baha'i writings on artificial insemination, Baha'is are guided by the understanding that marriage is the proper spiritual and physical context in which the bearing of children must occur. Couples who are unable to bear children are not excluded from marriage, since marriage has other purposes besides the bearing of children. The adoption of children is encouraged.

EUGENICS AND GENETICS. The Baha'is view scientific advancement as a noble and praiseworthy endeavor of humankind. Baha'i writings do not specifically address these two branches of science.

SOCIAL ACTIVITIES (DATING, DANCING). Baha'is strive for high standards of conduct in both their private and public lives; this includes chastity before marriage, moderation in dress, language, and amusements, and complete freedom from prejudice in their dealings with peoples of different races, classes, creeds and orders.

The Baha'i Faith forbids monastic celibacy, noting that marriage is fundamental to the growth and continuation of civilization. The function of dating is to afford individuals an opportunity to become acquainted with each other's character. Those contemplating marriage are encouraged to engage in some form of work and service together, a practice intended to promote assessment of their own maturity and readiness for marriage as well as to improving their knowledge of the character and values of the prospective marriage partner.

SUBSTANCE USE. Alcoholic beverages and drugs are forbidden unless prescribed by a physician. Tobacco use is strongly discouraged.

Religious Support System for the Sick

VISITORS. Individual members of local and surrounding communities assist and support each other in time of need.

TITLE OF RELIGIOUS REPRESENTATIVE. Religious titles are not used.

CHURCH ORGANAIZATIONS TO ASSIST THE SICK. Individual members of local communities look after needs.

Issues Related to Death and Dying

PROLONGATION OF LIFE (RIGHT TO DIE). Since human life is the vehicle for the development of the soul, Baha'is believe that life is unique and precious. The destruction of a human life at any stage, from conception to natural death, is rarely permissible. The question of when natural death has occurred is considered in light of current medical science and legal rulings on the matter.

EUTHANASIA. Same as above.

AUTOPSY. Acceptable in the case of medical necessity or legal requirement.

DONATION OF BODY. Baha'is are permitted to donate their bodies for medical research and for restorative purposes.

DISPOSAL OF BODY. Local burial laws are followed. Cremation is prohibited.

BURIAL. Unless required by state law, Baha'i law states that the body is not to be embalmed. Cremation is forbidden. The place of burial must be within 1 hour's travel from the place of death. This regulation is always carried out in consultation with the family, and exceptions are possible.

Buddhist Churches of America

Buddhism is a general term that indicates a belief in Buddha and encompasses many individual churches. In 1993 there were 554,000 Buddhists in North America. World-wide membership is 309 million.

The Buddhist Churches of America is the largest Buddhist organization in mainland United States. This group belongs to the largest subsect of Jodo Shinshu Buddhism (Shin Buddhism), Honpa Hongwanji, which is the largest traditional sect of Buddhism in Japan. The Jodo Shinshu sect was started by Shinran (1173–1263) in Japan. The headquarters of Jodo Shinshu Buddhism are in Kyoto, Japan. The group of churches in Hawaii is a different organization of Shin Buddhism, called Honpa Hongwanji Mission of Hawaii. There are numerous Buddhist sects in the United States, including Indian, Sri Lankan, Vietnamese, Thai, Chinese, Japanese, Tibetan, and so on.

Buddhism was founded in the sixth century B.C. in northern India by Gautama Buddha. In the third century B.C., Buddhism became the state religion of India and spread from there to most of the other Eastern nations. The term Buddha means *enlightened one.*

At the beginning of the Christian era, Buddhism split into two main groups: Hinayana, or southern Buddhism, and Mahayana, or northern Buddhism. Hinayana retained more of the original teachings of Buddha and survived in Sri Lanka (formerly

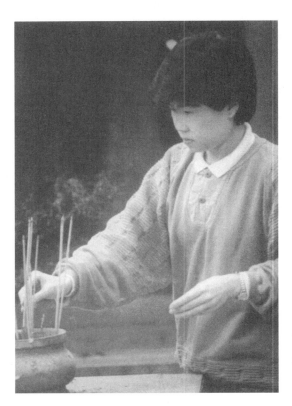

Buddhist woman lights incense in remembrance of deceased ancestors during the Chinese New Year celebration.

Ceylon) and southern Asia. Mahayana, a more social and polytheistic Buddhism, is strong in the Himalayas, Tibet, Mongolia, China, Korea, and Japan.

Beliefs and Religious Practices

Buddha's original teachings included Four Noble Truths and Noble Eightfold Way, the philosophies of which affect Buddhist response to health and illness. Four Noble Truths expounds on suffering and is the foundation of Buddhism. The truths consist of (1) the truth of suffering, (2) the truth of the origin of suffering, (3) the truth that suffering can be destroyed, and (4) the way that leads to the cessation of pain.

Noble Eightfold Way gives the rule of practical Buddhism, which consists of (1) right views, (2) right intention, (3) right speech, (4) right action, (5) right livelihood, (6) right effort, (7) right mindfulness, and (8) right concentration. Nirvana, a state of greater inner freedom and spontaneity, is the goal of all existence. When one achieves Nirvana, the mind has supreme tranquility, purity, and stability (Hinnell, 1984).

Although the ultimate goals of Buddhism are clear, the means of obtaining those goals are not religiously prescribed. Buddhism is not a dogmatic religion, nor does it dictate any specific practices. Individual differences are expected, acknowledged, and respected. Each individual is responsible for finding his/her own answers through awareness of the total situation.

HOLY DAYS.   Special holy days occur on January 1 and 16, February 15, March 21, April 8, May 21, July 15, September 1 and 23, and December 8 and 31. Although there is no religious restriction for therapy on those days, they can be highly emotional, and a Buddhist patient should be consulted about his or her desires for medical or surgical intervention.

SACRAMENTS.   Buddhism does not have any sacraments. A ritual that symbolizes one's entry into the Buddhist faith is the expression of faith in the Three Treasures (Buddha, Dharma, and Sangha).

RELIGION AND HEALING.   Buddhists do not believe in healing through a faith or through faith itself. However, Buddhists do believe that spiritual peace, and liberation from anxiety by adherence to and achievement of awakening to Buddha's wisdom, can be important factors in promoting healing and the recovery process.

DIET, MEDICATIONS, AND PROCEDURES.   There are no prescriptions in Buddhism for any of these things. Buddha's teaching on the middle path may apply here; he taught that extremes should be avoided. What may be medicine to one may be poison to another, so generalizations are to be avoided. Medications should be used in accordance with the nature of the illness and the capacity of the individual. Whatever will contribute to the attainment of Enlightenment is encouraged.

SURGICAL PROCEDURES.   Treatments such as amputations, organ transplants, biopsies, amniocentesis, and other procedures that may prolong life and allow the individual to attain Enlightenment are encouraged.

Research Application 12-1

Old Order Amish and Commercial Health Insurance

Greksa, L. P., & Korbin, J. E. (1997). Influence of changing occupational patterns on the use of commercial health insurance by the Old Order Amish. *Journal of Multicultural Nursing & Health, 3*(2), 13–18.

Although Old Order Amish families have in the past been prohibited from using commercial health insurance on religious grounds, the increasing cost of hospitalization combined with changing occupational patterns by the Amish has resulted in a change in health care utilization patterns. The data for the study were obtained through participant observation and informal open-ended interviews with Old Order Amish families residing in Geauga County, Ohio. The findings indicate that there is an increasing tendency for Old Order Amish families in this county to utilize health insurance provided by non-Amish employers. The pattern is associated with an increased utilization of biomedical health services, which is related to the availability of extensive health services and facilities in neighboring Cleveland.

Clinical Application

The Old Order Amish are a dynamic group that has managed to survive at least partially because they have selectively incorporated new components into their cultural system. One important change over the last few generations involves the transition from an agrarian way of life to one based on wage labor and the accompanying increased use of employer-provided commercial health insurance. The researchers also noted that an additional cost for the Amish seeking biomedical health care is transportation, a sum that may equal or exceed that paid to the health care provider. Perhaps the most important consideration for nurses is to understand is that Old Order Amish society is dynamic and that there is greater heterogeneity between and within congregations than might be expected by outward manifestations of conformity in dress and selective use of technology.

Controversial Issues Related to Health Care

The immediate emphasis is on the person living now and the attainment of Enlightenment. If practicing birth control or having sterility testing will help the individual attain Enlightenment, it is acceptable.

Buddhism does not condone the taking of a life. The first of Buddha's Five Precepts is abstention from taking lives. Life in all forms is to be respected. Existence by itself often contradicts this principle (e.g., drugs that kill bacteria are given to spare a patient's life). With this in mind, it is the conditions and circumstances surrounding the patient that determine whether abortion, therapeutic or on demand, may be undertaken.

Religious Support System for the Sick

TITLE OF RELIGIOUS REPRESENTATIVE.   Priest.

Issues Related to Death and Dying

PROLONGATION OF LIFE (RIGHT TO DIE).   If there is hope for recovery and continuation of the pursuit of Enlightenment, all available means of support are encouraged.

EUTHANASIA. If life cannot be prolonged so that the person can continue to search for Enlightenment, conditions may permit euthanasia.

DONATION OF BODY OR PARTS. If the donation of a body part will help another continue the quest for Enlightenment, it may be an act of mercy and is encouraged.

AUTOPSY AND DISPOSAL OF BODY. The body is considered but a shell; therefore, autopsy and disposal of the body are matters of individual practice rather than of religious prescription.

BURIAL. Burials are usually a brief grave side service after a funeral at the temple. Cremations are common.

ADDENDUM. The headquarters of the Buddhist Churches of America are located at 1710 Octavia Street, San Francisco, California 94109 (Telephone: [415] 776–5600). Additional material is available at the Buddhist Bookstore of the Buddhist Churches of America Headquarters.

Catholicism (According to the Roman Rite)

With a North American membership of approximately 96 million and a worldwide membership of more than 1 billion, some 32 rites exist within Catholicism. Of these, the Roman Rite is the major body.

Beliefs and Religious Practices

HOLY DAYS. Catholics are expected to observe all Sundays as holy days. Sunday or holy day worship services may be conducted anytime from 4:00 PM on Saturday to Sunday evening. In addition, there are 7 days set aside for special liturgical observance: Christmas (December 25th), Solemnity of Mary, Mother of God (January 1st), Ascension Thursday (The Lord's Ascension Bodily into Heaven—observed 40 days after Easter), Feast of the Assumption (August 15th), All Saints Day (November 1st), and the Feast of the Immaculate Conception (December 8th).

SACRAMENTS. The Roman Catholic Church recognizes seven sacraments. These are Baptism, Reconciliation (formerly Penance or Confession), Holy Communion or Eucharist, Confirmation, Matrimony, Holy Orders, and Anointing of the Sick (formerly Extreme Unction).

RELIGION AND HEALING. In time of illness, the basic rite is the Sacrament of the Sick, which includes anointing of the sick, communion, if possible, and a blessing by a priest. Prayers are frequently offered for the sick person and for members of the family. The Eucharist (a small unleavened wafer made of flour and water) is often given to the sick as the food of healing and health. Other family members may participate if they wish to do so.

Diet, Medications, and Procedures

DIET (FOODS AND BEVERAGES). The goods of the world have been given for use and benefit. The primary obligation people have toward foods and beverages is to

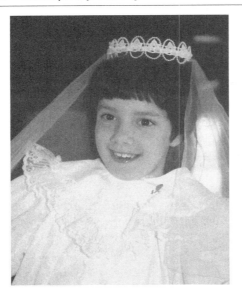

In the Roman Catholic tradition, when children reach the age of reason (about 7 years) they continue the ongoing initiation into their religion by making their First Communion. In addition to the religious ritual, there are sometimes cultural traditions surrounding this event, many of which involve a family celebration after the religious services have concluded.

use them in moderation and in such a way that they are not injurious to health. Fasting in moderation is recommended as a valued discipline. There are a few days of the year when Catholics have an obligation to fast or to abstain from meat and meat products. Catholics fast and abstain on Ash Wednesday and Good Friday, and abstinence is required on all of the Fridays of Lent. The sick are never bound by this prescription of the law. Healthy persons between the ages of 18 and 62 are encouraged to engage in fasting and abstinence as described.

MEDICATIONS.   As long as the benefits outweigh the risk to the individuals, judicious use of medications is permissible and morally acceptable. A major concern is the risk of mutilation. The Church has traditionally cited the "principle of totality," which states that use of medications is allowed as long as the medications are used for the good of the whole person.

BLOOD AND BLOOD PRODUCTS.   As above.

AMPUTATIONS.   Acceptable if consistent with the "principle of totality."

ORGAN TRANSPLANTS.   The transplantation of organs from living donors is morally permissible when the anticipated benefit to the recipient is proportionate to the harm done to the donor, provided that the loss of such an organ does not deprive the donor of life itself nor of the functional integrity of his body.

BIOPSIES.   Permissible.

CIRCUMCISION.   Permissible.

AMNIOCENTESIS.   The procedure in and of itself is not objectionable. However, it is morally objectionable if the findings of the amniocentesis are used to lead the couple to decide on termination of the pregnancy or if the procedure injures the fetus.

Controversial Issues Related to Health Care

BIRTH CONTROL. The basic principle is that the conjugal act should be one that is love-giving and potentially life-giving. Only natural means of contraception, such as abstinence, the temperature method, and the ovulation method, are acceptable. Ordinarily, artificial aids and procedures for permanent sterilization are forbidden. Birth control (anovulents) may be used therapeutically to assist in regulating the menstrual cycle.

ABORTION. Direct abortion is always morally wrong. Indirect abortion may be morally justified by some circumstances (e.g., treatment of a cancerous uterus in a pregnant woman). Abortion on demand is prohibited. The Roman Catholic Church teaches the sanctity of all human life, even the unborn, from the time of conception.

STERILITY TESTS. Use of such tests for the purpose of promoting conception, not misusing sexuality, is permitted.

ARTIFICIAL INSEMINATION. Although debated heavily, traditionally this has been looked on as illicit, even between husband and wife.

EUGENICS AND GENETICS. Objectionable. This violates the moral right of the individual to be free from experimentation. It also interferes with God's right as master of life and man's stewardship of his life. Some genetic investigations to help determine genetic diseases may be used, depending upon their ends and means.

SOCIAL ACTIVITIES (DATING, DANCING). The major principle is that Sunday is a day of rest; therefore, only unnecessary servile work is prohibited. The 6 holy days are also considered days of rest, although many persons must engage in routine work-related activities on some of these days.

SUBSTANCE USE. Alcohol and tobacco are not evil per se. They are to be used in moderation and not in a way that would be injurious to one's health or that of another party. The misuse of any substance is not only harmful to the body but also sinful.

Religious Support System for the Sick

VISITORS. Although a priest, deacon, or lay minister usually visits a sick person alone, he may invite the family or other significant people to join in prayer. In fact, that is most desirable, since they, too, need support.

The priest, deacon, or lay minister will usually bring the necessary supplies for administration of the Eucharist or administration of the Sacrament of the Sick (in the case of a priest). The nursing staff can facilitate these rites by ensuring an atmosphere of prayer and quiet and by having a glass of water on hand (in case the patient is unable to swallow the small wafer-like host). Consecrated wine can be made available but is usually not given in the hospital or home. The nurse may wish to join in the prayer. Candles may be used, although not if the patient is on oxygen. The priest, deacon, or lay minister will usually appreciate any information pertaining to the patient's ability to swallow. Any other information the nurse believes might help the priest or deacon respond to the patient with more care and effectiveness would be appreciated.

Catholic lay persons of either sex may visit hospitalized or homebound elderly or sick persons. Although they may not administer the Sacrament of the Sick or the Sacrament of Reconciliation, they may bring Holy Communion (the Eucharist).

TITLE OF RELIGIOUS REPRESENTATIVE.   Father (priest); Mr. or Deacon (deacon); Sister (Catholic woman who has taken religious vows); Brother (Catholic man who has taken religious vows).

ENVIRONMENT DURING VISIT BY RELIGIOUS REPRESENTATIVE.   Privacy is most conducive to prayer and to the administration of the sacraments. In emergency cases, such as cardiac or respiratory arrest, medical personnel will need to be present. The priest will use an abbreviated form of the rite and will not interfere with the activities of the health care team.

CHURCH ORGANIZATIONS TO ASSIST THE SICK.   Most major cities have outreach programs for the sick, handicapped, and elderly. More serious needs are usually handled by Catholic Charities and other agencies in the community or on the local parish level. Organizations such as the St. Vincent DePaul Society may provide material support for the poor and needy as well as some counseling services, depending on the location. The Catholic Church owns and operates hospitals, extended care facilities, orphanages, maternity homes, hospices, and other health care facilities. It is usually best to consult the pastor or chaplain in specific cases for local resources.

Issues Related to Death and Dying

PROLONGATION OF LIFE (RIGHT TO DIE).   Members are obligated to take ordinary means of preserving life (e.g., intravenous medication) but are not obligated to take extraordinary means. What constitutes extraordinary means may vary with biomedical and technological advances and with the availability of these advances to the average citizen. Other factors that must be considered include the degree of pain associated with the procedure, the potential outcome, the condition of the patient, economic factors, and the patient's or family's preferences.

EUTHANASIA.   Direct action to end the life of patients is not permitted. Extraordinary means may be withheld, allowing the patient to die of natural causes.

AUTOPSY.   This is permissible as long as the corpse is shown proper respect and there is sufficient reason for doing the autopsy.

DONATION OF BODY.   The principle of totality suggests that this is justifiable, being for the betterment of the person doing the giving.

DISPOSAL OF BODY.   Ordinarily, bodies are buried. Cremation is acceptable in certain circumstances, such as to avoid spreading a contagious disease.

BURIAL.   Since life is considered sacred, the body should be treated with respect. Any disposal of the body should be done in a respectful and honorable way.

Christian Science (Church of Christ, Scientist)

Christian Science accepts physical and moral healing as a natural part of the Christian experience. Members believe that God acts through universal, immutable, spiritual law. They hold that genuine spiritual or Christian healing through prayer differs radically from the use of suggestion, willpower, and all forms of psychotherapy, which are based on use of the human mind as a curative agent. In emphasizing the practical importance of a fuller understanding of Jesus' works and teachings, Christian Science believes healing to be a natural result of drawing closer to God in one's thinking and living.

MEMBERSHIP.   The church does not keep membership data; there are 3,000 congregations worldwide.

Beliefs and Religious Practices
HOLY DAYS.   Besides the usual weekly day of worship (Sunday), other traditional Christian holidays are observed on an individual basis. Wednesday evenings are observed worldwide as times for members to gather for testimony meetings.

SACRAMENTS.   Although sacraments in a strictly spiritual sense have deep meaning for Christian Scientists, there are no outward observances or ceremonies. Baptism and holy communion are not outward observances but deeply meaningful inner experiences. Baptism is the daily purification and spiritualization of thought, while communion refers to finding one's conscious unity with God through prayer (Christian Science Publishing Society, 1994).

RELIGION AND HEALING.   Viewed as a byproduct of drawing closer to God, healing is considered proof of God's care and one element in the full salvation at which Christianity aims. Christian Science teaches that faith must rest not on blind belief, but on an understanding of the present perfection of God's spiritual creation. This is one of the crucial differences between Christian Science and "faith healing" (Christian Science Publishing Society, 1994).

The practice of Christian Science healing starts from the Biblical basis that God created the universe and man "and made them perfect." Christian Science holds that human imperfection, including physical illness and sin, reflects a fundamental misunderstanding of creation and is therefore subject to healing through prayer and spiritual regeneration.

An individual who is seeking healing may turn to Christian Science practitioners, members of the denomination who devote their full time to the healing ministry in the broadest sense. In cases requiring continued care, nurses grounded in the Christian Science faith provide care in facilities accredited by the mother church, the First Church of Christ, Scientist, in Boston, Massachusetts. Individuals may also receive such care in their own homes. Christian Science nurses are trained to perform the practical duties a patient may need, while also providing an atmosphere of warmth and love that supports the healing process. No medication is given, and physical application is limited to the normal measures associated with hygiene. The Christian Science Journal, a monthly publication, contains a directory of qualified Christian Science practitioners and nurses throughout the world.

Before they can be recognized and advertised in The Christian Science Journal, practitioners must have instruction from an authorized teacher of Christian Science and provide substantial evidence of their experience in healing. There are some 4,000

Christian Science practitioners throughout the world. Practitioners who speak other languages may also be listed in appropriate editions of The Herald of Christian Science, which is published in 12 languages.

The denomination has no clergy. Practitioners are thus lay members of the Church of Christ, Scientist, and do not conduct public worship services or rituals. Their ministry is not an office within the church structure but is carried out on an individual basis with those who seek their help through prayer. Both members and nonmembers are welcome to contact practitioners by telephone, by letter, or in person for help or for information.

Christian Science practitioners are supported not by the church but by payments from their patients. Their ministry is not restricted to local congregations but world-wide. Many insurance companies include coverage of payments to practitioners and Christian Science nursing facilities in their policies. In spite of such superficial resemblances with the health professions, the work of Christian Science practitioners involves a deeply religious vocation, not simply alternative health care. Practitioners do not employ medical or psychological techniques.

The term healing applies to the entire spectrum of human fears, griefs, wants, and sin, as well as to physical ills. Practitioners are called upon to give Christian Science treatment not only in cases of physical disease and emotional disturbance but also in family and financial difficulties, business problems, questions of employment, schooling problems, theological confusion, and so forth. The purpose of prayer, or Christian Science treatment, is to deal with these interrelated and complex problems of establishing God's law of harmony in every aspect of life. When healings are accomplished through perception and living of spiritual truth, they are effective and permanent. Physical healing is often the manifestation of a moral and spiritual change (Christian Science Publishing Society, 1978, 1994).

Ordinarily, a Christian Science practitioner and a physician are not employed on the same case, since the two approaches to healing differ so radically. During childbirth, however, an obstetrician or qualified midwife is involved. Since bone-setting may be accomplished without the use of medication, a physician is also employed for repair of fractures, if the patient requests this medical intervention. In the case of a contagious or infectious disease, Christian Scientists observe the legal requirements for reporting and quarantining affected individuals. The denomination recognizes public health concerns and has a long history of responsible cooperation with public health officials.

Christian Scientists are not arbitrarily opposed to doctors. They are always free to make their own decisions regarding treatment in any given situation. They generally choose to rely on spiritual healing because they have seen its effectiveness in the experience of their own families and fellow church members, experience that goes back over 100 years and in many families for three or four generations. Where medical treatment for minor children is required by law, Christian Scientists strictly adhere to the requirement. At the same time, they maintain that their substantial healing record needs to be seriously considered in determining the rights of Christian Scientists to rely on spiritual healing for themselves and their children. They do not ignore or neglect disease, but they seek to heal it by the means they believe to be most efficacious.

Diet, Medications, and Procedures
DIET.   No restrictions.

MEDICATIONS. Christian Scientists ordinarily do not use drugs. Immunizations/vaccines are acceptable only when required by law.

BLOOD AND BLOOD PRODUCTS. Ordinarily not used by members.

AMPUTATIONS. A Christian Scientist who has lost a limb might seek to have it replaced with a prosthesis.

ORGAN TRANSPLANTS. Christian Scientists are unlikely to seek transplants and are unlikely to act as donors.

BIOPSIES. Christian Scientists do not normally seek biopsies or any sort of physical examination.

CIRCUMCISION. This is considered an individual matter.

AMNIOCENTESIS. Christian Scientists are unlikely to seek this type of procedure.

Controversial Issues Related to Health Care

BIRTH CONTROL. Matters of family planning are left to individual judgment.

ABORTION. Since abortion involves medication and surgical intervention, it is normally considered incompatible with Christian Science.

ARTIFICIAL INSEMINATION. This is unusual among Christian Scientists.

EUGENICS AND GENETICS. Christian Scientists are opposed to compulsory programs in this field.

SOCIAL ACTIVITIES (DATING, DANCING). Members are encouraged to be honest, truthful, and moral in their behavior. Although every effort is made to preserve marriages, divorce is recognized. The Christian Science Sunday School teaches young people how to make their religion practical in daily life as related to school studies, social life, sports, and family relationships.

SUBSTANCE USE. Members abstain from alcohol and tobacco; some abstain from tea and coffee.

Religious Support System for the Sick

Christian Scientists have their own nurses and practitioners (see section on Religion and Healing).

TITLE OF RELIGIOUS REPRESENTATIVE. No special religious titles are used Although each branch church elects two Readers for Sunday and Wednesday services. Christian Scientists are a church of laymen and laywomen.

CHURCH ORGANIZATIONS TO ASSIST THE SICK. Benevolent Homes staffed by Christian Science nurses; visiting home nurse service.

Issues Related to Death and Dying

PROLONGATION OF LIFE (RIGHT TO DIE). A Christian Science family is unlikely to seek medical means to prolong life indefinitely. Family members pray earnestly for recovery of a person as long as the person remains alive.

EUTHANASIA.   This is contrary to the teachings of Christian Science.

DONATION OF BODY.   Most Christian Scientists believe that they can make their particular contribution to the health of society and of their loved ones in ways other than this.

DISPOSAL OF BODY.   This is left to the individual family to decide.

BURIAL.   The form of burial and burial service is decided by the individual family.

ADDENDUM.   A wide variety of books and journals are published by the Christian Science Publishing Society, Boston, Massachusetts. Most major cities have Christian Science Reading Rooms, which carry these publications and which are staffed by church members, who are available to provide additional information.

The Church of Jesus Christ of Latter-Day Saints (Mormonism)

The Church of Jesus Christ of Latter-Day Saints, commonly known as Mormonism, is a Christian religion established in the United States in the early 1800s. It now has a North American membership of 7 million, and a worldwide membership approaching 10 million (1997).

Beliefs and Religious Practices

HOLY DAYS/SPECIAL DAYS.   Sunday is the day observed as the Sabbath in the United States. In other parts of the world the Sabbath may be observed on a different day; in Israel, for example, Mormons observe the Sabbath on Saturday.

Sacraments (commonly called ordinances)

Ordinances of Salvation
1. Baptism at the age of accountability (8 years or after); never performed in infancy or at death; always by immersion.
2. Confirmation at the time of baptism to receive the gift of the Holy Ghost.
3. Partaking of the sacrament of the Lord's Supper at Sunday sacrament meetings.
4. Endowments.*
5. Celestial Marriage.*
6. Vicarious ordinances*

Ordinances of Comfort, Consolation, and Encouragement
1. Blessing of babies.
2. Blessing of the sick.
3. Consecration of oil for use in blessing of the sick.
4. Patriarchal blessings.
5. Dedication of graves.

---

*These ordinances occur in temples. Temples are sacred places of worship that are accessible only to observant Mormons, who are "worthy" to enter them as deemed by their local religious leaders.

After being deemed worthy to go to a temple, a Mormon will wear a special type of underclothing, called a garment. While in a health care setting the garment may be removed to facilitate care. As soon as the individual is well, he or she is likely to want to wear the garment again. The elderly may not wish to part with the garment in the hospital. The garment has special significance to the person, symbolizing covenants or promises the person has made to God.

RELIGION AND HEALING. Mormons believe that the power of God can be exercised in their behalf to bring about healing at a time of illness. The ritual of blessing the sick consists of one member (Elder) of the priesthood (male) anointing the ill person with oil and a second Elder "sealing the anointing with a prayer and a blessing." Commonly both Elders place their hands on the individual's head. Faith in Jesus Christ and in the power of the priesthood to heal, requisite to the healing use of priesthood, does not preclude medical intervention but is seen as adjunct to it. Mormons believe that medical intervention is one of God's ways of using humans in the healing process.

Diet, Medications, and Procedures

DIET. Mormons have a strict dietary code called the Word of Wisdom. This code prohibits all alcoholic beverages (including beer and wine), hot drinks (i.e., tea and coffee, although not herbal tea), and tobacco in any form.

Fasting to a Mormon means no food or drink (including water), usually for a 24-hour period. Fasting is required once a month on the designated fast Sunday. Pregnant women, the very young, the very old, and the ill are not required to fast. The purpose of fasting is to bring oneself closer to God by controlling physical needs. The person is expected to donate the price of what has not been eaten to the church to be used to care for the poor.

MEDICATIONS. There is no restriction on the use of medications or vaccines in Mormon Church doctrine. It is not uncommon to find many members of the Mormon Church using herbal folk remedies, and it is wise to explore in detail what an individual may have done or taken to help themselves.

BLOOD AND BLOOD PRODUCTS. There is no restriction on the use of blood or blood components.

SURGERIES/PROCEDURES. Surgical intervention is a matter of individual decision in cases of amputations, transplants, and organ donations (both of donor and recipient). Biopsies and resultant surgery are also a matter of individual choice.

Circumcision of infants is viewed as a medical health promotion measure and is not a religious ritual. Amniocentesis is a matter of individual choice. However, even if the fetus is found to be deformed, abortion is not an option unless the mother's life is in danger.

Controversial Issues Related to Health Care

BIRTH CONTROL. According to Mormon belief, one of the major purposes of life is procreation; therefore, any form of prevention of the birth of children is contrary to church teachings. Exceptions to this policy include ill health of mother or father and genetic defects that could be passed on to offspring.

ABORTION.   Abortion is forbidden in all cases except when the mother's life is in danger. Even in these circumstances abortion would be looked upon favorably only if the local priesthood authorities, after fasting and prayer, received divine confirmation that the abortion is acceptable.

In the event of pregnancy resulting from rape, the church position is that the child should be born and put up for adoption if necessary, rather than be aborted. The final decision rests with the mother. No official church sanction would be employed if she chose to abort the child.

Abortion on demand is strictly forbidden.

STERILITY/FERTILITY TESTING.   Since bearing children is so important, all measures that can be taken to promote having children are acceptable.

ARTIFICIAL INSEMINATION.   Acceptable if the semen is from the husband.

SOCIAL ACTIVITIES (DATING, DANCING).   The Mormon Church has a wide variety of activities for its youth and encourages group activities until young people are at least 16.

Young men are highly encouraged to perform "missions" for the church for 2 years at their own expense. The earliest age one can elect to do this is 19 years. Women may go on missions when they are 21, but marriage is more strongly emphasized for them.

SUBSTANCE USE.   Alcohol, caffeinated beverages (such as tea, coffee and soda pop), and tobacco are forbidden. In recent years "recreational drugs," and non-medically indicated use of sedative and narcotics have also been considered forbidden substances.

Religious Support System for the Sick

VISITORS.   Mormonism has a highly organized network, and many church representatives are likely to visit a hospitalized member, including the bishop and two counselors (leaders of the local congregation), home teachers (two men assigned to visit the family each month), and visiting teachers (two women assigned to visit the female head of household each month). Friends within the local congregation can also be expected to visit.

TITLE OF RELIGIOUS REPRESENTATIVE.   A variety of titles are used for members of the Mormon hierarchy. The term Elder is generally acceptable regardless of a man's position, and the term Sister is acceptable for women.

ENVIRONMENT NEEDED FOR HEALTH-RELATED RITUALS.   To perform a blessing of the sick, the Elders performing the blessing need privacy and, if possible, quiet. They generally bring a vial of consecrated oil with which to anoint the person. If they want to perform a Sacrament of the Lord's Supper, they usually bring what they need with them. Bread and water are used for this ordinance.

CHURCH ORGANIZATIONS TO ASSIST THE SICK.   The Relief Society is the Mormon organization for helping members. It is organized by the women of the church, who work closely with priesthood leaders to determine general needs of members, including use of the church-run welfare organization. Church members who are in need may receive local help, such as child care for children when parents are ill or hospitalized and money for medical expenses.

Issues Related to Death and Dying

PROLONGATION OF LIFE (RIGHT TO DIE). Whenever possible, medical science and faith healing are used to reverse conditions that threaten life. When death is inevitable, the effort is to promote a peaceful and dignified death. Mormons firmly believe that life continues beyond death and that the dead are reunited with loved ones; therefore, the belief is that death is another step in eternal progression (Green, 1992a; 1992b).

EUTHANASIA. Life and death are in the hands of God, and humans must not interfere in any way.

AUTOPSY. Permitted with the consent of the next of kin and within local laws.

DISPOSAL OF BODY PARTS. Organ donation is permitted; it is an individual decision.

BURIAL. Cremation is discouraged but not forbidden; burial is customary. Graves are dedicated by a local priesthood member.

Hinduism

The Hindu religion may be the oldest religion in the world. There are over 719 million Hindus in worldwide, with a North American following of approximately 1.3 million members.

Beliefs and Religious Practices

No common creed or doctrine binds Hindus together. There is complete freedom of belief. One may be monotheistic, polytheistic, or atheistic. The major distinguishing characteristic is the social caste system.

The religion of Hinduism is founded on sacred, written scripture called the Vedas. Brahman is the principle and source of the universe and the center from which all things proceed and to which all things return. Reincarnation is a central belief in Hinduism.

Life is determined by the law of karma. According to karma, rebirth is dependent on moral behavior in a previous stage of existence. Life on earth is transient and a burden. The goal of existence is liberation from the cycle of rebirth and re-death and entrance into what in Buddhism is called nirvana (a state of extinction of passion).

The practice of Hinduism consists of roles and ceremonies performed within the framework of the caste system. These rituals focus on the main socioreligious events of birth, marriage, and death. Hindu temples are dwelling places for deities to which people bring offerings. There are numerous places for religious pilgrimage.

Holy Days (based on a lunar calendar)

1. Purnima (day of full moon)
2. Janamasthtmi (birthday of Lord Krishna)
3. Ramnavmi (birthday of Rama)
4. Shivratri (birth of Lord Shiva)
5. Naurate (nine holy days occurring twice a year; in about April and October)
6. Dussehra
7. Diwali
8. Holi

RELIGION AND HEALING.   Some Hindus believe in faith healing; others believe illness is God's way of punishing people for their sins.

Diet, Medications, and Procedures

DIET.   The eating of meat is forbidden because it involves harming a living creature.

MEDICATIONS.   Acceptable.

BLOOD AND BLOOD PRODUCTS.   Acceptable.

AMPUTATIONS.   Persons who lose a limb are not outcasts from society. Loss of a limb is considered due to "sins of a previous life."

ORGAN TRANSPLANTS.   Donation and receipt of organs are both acceptable.

AMNIOCENTESIS.   Acceptable, although not often available.

Controversial Issues Related to Health Care

BIRTH CONTROL.   All types are acceptable.

ABORTION.   No Hindu policy exists on abortion, either therapeutic or on demand.

ARTIFICIAL INSEMINATION.   No religious restriction exists; not often practiced owing to lack of availability.

SOCIAL ACTIVITIES (DATING, DANCING).   Strictly limited by caste system.

SUBSTANCE USE.   No Restrictions

Religious Support System for the Sick

TITLE OF RELIGIOUS REPRESENTATIVE.   Priest.

CHURCH ORGANIZATIONS TO ASSIST THE SICK.   None; help is provided by family and friends within the caste.

Issues Related to Death and Dying

PROLONGATION OF LIFE (RIGHT TO DIE).   There is no religious custom or restriction. Life is seen as a perpetual cycle, with death considered just one more step toward nirvana.

EUTHANASIA. Not practiced.

AUTOPSY. Acceptable.

DONATION OF BODY OR PARTS. Acceptable.

DISPOSAL OF BODY. Cremation is most common. Ashes are collected and disposed of in holy rivers.

BURIAL. As described above under "Disposal of Body." Fetus or newborn is sometimes buried.

Islam

Islam is a monotheistic religion founded between 610 and 632 A.D. by the prophet Muhammad. Derived from an Arabic word meaning submission, Islam literally translated means "submission to the will of God." A followers of Islam is called Moslem or *Muslim* which means "one who submits." Current U.S. membership is 2.6 million with worldwide membership of 950 million.

Muhammad, revered as the prophet of Allah (God), is seen as succeeding and completing both Judaism and Christianity. Good deeds will be rewarded at the last Judgment, whereas evil deeds will be punished in hell.

Beliefs and Religious Practices

Islam has five essential practices, or *Pillars of Faith*. These are (1) the *profession of faith (shahada)*, which requires bearing witness to one true God and acknowledging Muhammad as his messenger; (2) *ritual prayer* five times daily; dawn, noon, afternoon, sunset, and night, facing Mecca, Saudi Arabia, Islam's holiest city (salat); (3) *alms giving (zakat)* to the needy reflects the Koran's admonition to share what one has with those less fortunate, including widows, orphans, homeless persons and the poor; (4) *fasting* from dawn until sunset throughout Ramadan during the ninth month of the Islamic lunar calendar; and (5) *making a pilgrimage to Mecca* (located in Saudi Arabia) at least once during one's lifetime (*hajj*).

The sources of the Islamic faith are the Qur'an (Koran), which is regarded as the uncreated and eternal Word of God, and Hadith (tradition), regarded as sayings and deeds of the prophet Muhammad. All Muslims recognize the existence of the *sharia* and the five categories into which it divides human conduct: required, encouraged, permissible, discouraged and prohibited.

Various sects of Islam have developed. When Muhammad died, a dispute arose over the leadership of the Muslim community. One faction, the Sunni, derived from the Arabic word for "tradition," felt that the caliph, or successor of Muhammad, should be chosen, as Arab chiefs customarily are, by election. Therefore, they supported the succession of the first four, or the rightly guided caliphs who had been Muhammad's companions. The other group maintained that Muhammad chose his cousin and son-in-law, Ali, as his spiritual and secular heir and that succession should be through his bloodline. In 680 A.D., one of Ali's sons, Hussein, led a band of rebels against the ruling caliph. In the course of the battle Hussein was killed and with his death began the Shi'a, sometimes called the Shi'ite movement, whose name comes from the word meaning "partisans of Ali." The Shi'a and Sunni are the two major branches of Muslims, with the Sunni constituting about 85 percent of the total. The Sunni are found in Lebanon, the West Bank, Jordan, and throughout Africa whereas the Shi'a, are located in Iran, Iraq, Yemen, Afghanistan, and Pakistan. The Shi'a and the Sunni also have different rituals, practices, structural and political orientations.

HOLIDAYS AND SPECIAL OBSERVANCES.   Days of observance in Islam are not "holy" days but days of celebration or observance. The Muslims follow a lunar calendar, so the days of observance change yearly.

Each Muslim observance has its own significance. They are listed here in the same order in which they occur in the Muslim lunar calendar, and their standard Arabic names are used. However, the Arabic spellings for the names of the holidays may vary, or local names may be used.

Muharam 1 Rasal-Sana (or New Year): The first day of the first month, celebrated much the same as the first day of the year is celebrated throughout the world.

Muharam 10 Ashura (the 10th of the first month): A religious holiday through which pious Muslims may fast from dawn to sunset. For Shi'ite Muslims, this is a special day of sorrow commemorating the assassination of the prophet's grandson, Hussein.

Rabi'i 12 Maulid al-Nabi: The birthday of the prophet Muhammad. In some regions this holiday goes on for many days, a time of festivities and exchange of gifts.

Rajab 27 Lailat al-Isra wa al Miraj (literally, "The Night of the Journey and Ascent"): Commemorates Muhammad's night journey from Mecca to the al-Aqsa mosque in Jerusalem and his ascent to heaven and return on the same night.

Sh'ban 14: This is the 14th night of the eighth month of Sh'ban. It is widely celebrated by pious Muslims, sometimes called the Night of Repentance. It is treated in many parts of the Muslim world as a New Year's celebration.

Ramadan (the ninth month of the Muslim year): This entire month is devoted to meditation and spiritual purification through self-discipline. It is a period of abstinence from eating, drinking, smoking and sexual relations. The fast is an obligation practiced by Muslims throughout the world unless they are old, infirm, traveling, or pregnant. The fast is from sunup to sundown, at which time a meal (*iftar*) is taken.

Ramadan 27 Lailat al-Qadir (next to the last night of the fasting month): This is simply called the Night of Power and Greatness, and it is by custom a very special holy time. It is the night that commemorates when revelation was first given to Muhammad.

Shawwal 1 "Id ad-Fitr": This is called the Lesser Feast because it begins immediately after the month-long Ramadan feast. It is perhaps Islam's most joyous festival, marking as it does the month of abstinence and the cleansing of the believer. It usually lasts for 2 or 3 days. Families and friends visit each others' homes, new clothes and presents are exchanged, and sweet pastries are a favorite treat.

Dhu al-Hijjah 1–10: Muslims, if they are able, are obliged to undertake a pilgrimage to Mecca at least once in their lifetime. This journey, called the Hajj, is performed during the last month of the Muslim calendar, Dhu al-Hijjah.

Dhu al-Hijjah 10: All Muslims, whether they are on the pilgrimage or at home, participate in the feast of the sacrifice, Id al-Adha, which marks the end of the Hajj on the tenth of Dhu al-Hijjah. The feast is the "Feast of the Sacrifice," called the Greater Feast, and is observed by the slaughtering of animals and distribution of the meat. In some places this is done individually. The meat is shared equally among the family and the poor. Sometimes the slaughtering takes place in public areas, and the meat is then distributed.

SACRAMENTS. None.

RELIGION AND HEALING. Faith healing is not acceptable unless the psychological health and morale of the patient is deteriorating. At that time, faith healing may be employed to supplement the physician's efforts.

Diet, Medications, and Procedures

DIET. Eating pork and drinking intoxicating beverages are strictly prohibited. In all cases moderation in one's life is expected. Some Muslims consume meat that has been ritually slaughtered by the process called *halal,* which means "the lawful or that which is permitted by Allah".

Fasting during the month of Ramadan is one of the pillars of Islam. Children (boys, 7 years old; girls, 9 years old) and adults are required to fast. Pregnant women, nursing mothers, and the elderly, as well as anyone whose physical condition is so fragile that a physician recommends that they not fast, are exempt from fasting but expected to fast later in the year or to feed a poor person to make up for the unfasted Ramadan days.

MEDICATIONS. There are no restrictions as far as medications are concerned. Even items normally forbidden (e.g., pork derivatives) are permitted if prescribed as medicine.

BLOOD AND BLOOD PRODUCTS. No restrictions.

AMPUTATIONS. Acceptable; no restrictions.

ORGAN TRANSPLANTS. Acceptable for both donor and recipient.

BIOPSIES. Acceptable; no restrictions.

CIRCUMCISION. No age limit is fixed, but circumcision is practiced on male children at an early age. For adult converts it is not obligatory, although it is sometimes practiced.

AMNIOCENTESIS. Available in many Islamic countries, used by "progressive" doctors and expectant parents only. Used only to determine the status of the fetus, not the sex of the child; this is left in the hands of God.

Controversial Issues Related to Health Care

BIRTH CONTROL.   All types of birth control are generally acceptable in accordance with the law of "what is harmful to the body is prohibited." Family physician's advice on method of contraception is required. Husband and wife should agree on the method.

ABORTION.   No official policy on abortion, either therapeutic or on demand. There is a strong religious objection to abortion, which is based on Muhammad's condemnation of the ancient Arabian practice of burying alive unwanted newborn females.

ARTIFICIAL INSEMINATION.   Permitted only if from husband to his own wife.

EUGENICS AND GENETICS.   No official policy exists. Different Islamic schools of thought accept differing opinions.

SUBSTANCE USE.   Alcohol is strictly forbidden.

Religious Support System for the Sick

CHURCH ORGANIZATIONS TO ASSIST THE SICK.   None; family and friends provide emotional and financial support.

Issues Related to Death and Dying

PROLONGATION OF LIFE (RIGHT TO DIE).   The right to die is not recognized in Islam. Any attempt to shorten one's life or terminate it (suicide or otherwise) is prohibited.

EUTHANASIA.   Not acceptable.

AUTOPSY.   Permitted only for medical and legal purposes.

DONATION OF BODY PARTS OR BODY.   Acceptable; no restrictions.

DISPOSAL OF BODY.   It is important in Islam to follow prescribed burial procedure. Under conditions that cause fragmentation of the body, sections of the burial ritual may be omitted.

BURIAL.   Burial of the dead, including fetuses, is compulsory. The five steps of the burial procedure consist of:

1. Ghasl El Mayyet: Rinsing and washing of the dead body according to Muslim tradition. Muslim women cleanse a woman's body; Muslim men, a man's body.
2. Muslin: After being washed three times, the body is wrapped in three pieces of clean white cloth. The Muslim word for "coffin" is the same as that for "muslin."
3. Salat El Mayyet: Special prayers for the dead are required.
4. The body should be processed and buried as soon as possible. The body should always be buried so that the head faces towards Mecca.
5. Burial of a fetus: Prior to a gestational age of 130 days, a fetus is treated like any other discarded tissue. After 130 days the fetus is considered a fully developed human being and must be treated as such.

Jehovah's Witnesses

MEMBERSHIP. North American, 1,485,426; worldwide, 4,709,889

Beliefs and Religious Practices

Many Americans have at one time or another encountered ministers of the Watch Tower Bible and Tract Society, known as Jehovah's Witnesses. The name Jehovah's Witnesses, the name that members prefer, is derived from the Hebrew name for "God" (Jehovah) according to the King James Bible. Thus, Jehovah's Witnesses is a descriptive name, indicating that members profess to bear witness concerning Jehovah, his God-ship, and his purposes. Every Bible student devotes approximately 10 hours or more each month to proselytizing activities.

HOLY DAYS. Although Witnesses do not celebrate Christmas, Easter, or other traditional Christian holy days, a special observance of the Lord's Supper is held. Witnesses and others may attend this important meeting, but only those numbered among the 144,000 chosen members (Revelations 7:4) may partake of the bread and wine as a symbol of the death of Christ and the dedication to God. This memorial of Christ's death should take place on the day corresponding to Nisa 14 of the Jewish calendar, which occurs sometime in March or April. These elite members will be raised with spiritual bodies (without flesh, bones, or blood) and will assist Christ in ruling the universe. Others who benefit from Christ's ransom will be resurrected with healthy, perfected physical bodies (bodies of flesh, bones, and blood) and will inhabit this earth after the world has been restored to a paradisiacal state.

SACRAMENTS. No sacraments are observed.

RELIGION AND HEALING. The practice of faith healing is forbidden. However, it is believed that reading the scriptures can comfort the individual and lead to mental and spiritual healing.

Diet, Medications, and Procedures

MEDICATIONS. To the extent that they are necessary, medications are acceptable.

BLOOD AND BLOOD PRODUCTS. Blood in any form, and agents in which blood is an ingredient, are not acceptable. Blood volume expanders are acceptable if they are not derivatives of blood. Mechanical devices for circulating the blood are acceptable as long as they are not primed with blood initially. In some cases children have been made wards of the court so they could receive blood when a medical condition mandating blood transfusion was life-threatening. This can threaten the standing of the child in the community and must be approached with great care.

The determination of Jehovah's Witnesses to abstain from blood is based on scriptural references and precedents in the history of Christianity. Courts of Justice have often upheld the principle that each individual has a right to bodily integrity, yet some physicians and hospital administrators have turned to the courts for legal authorization to force blood to be used as a medical treatment for an individual whose religious convictions prohibit the use of blood (Sugarman, et al., 1991).

SURGICAL PROCEDURES. Although surgical procedures are not in and of themselves opposed, administration of blood during surgery is strictly prohibited (Smith, 1986).

AMPUTATIONS.   There is no church rule pertaining to the loss of limbs or the amputation of body parts.

ORGAN TRANSPLANTS (DONOR AND RECIPIENT).   If they are a violation of the principle of bodily mutilation, transplants are forbidden. However, this is usually an individual decision. Blood may not be used in this, or any, surgery.

BIOPSIES.   Acceptable.

CIRCUMCISION.   Individual decision.

AMNIOCENTESIS.   Acceptable.

Controversial Issues Related to Health Care
BIRTH CONTROL.   Sterilization is prohibited because it is viewed as a form of bodily mutilation. Other forms of birth control are left up to the individual.

ABORTION.   Both therapeutic and on-demand abortions are forbidden.

STERILITY TESTS.   This is an individual decision.

ARTIFICIAL INSEMINATION.   This is forbidden both for donors and for recipients.

EUGENICS AND GENETICS.   Jehovah's Witnesses do not condone any activities in these areas; they are considered to interfere with nature and therefore are unacceptable.

SOCIAL ACTIVITIES (DATING, DANCING).   Youth are encouraged to socialize with members with their own religious background.

SUBSTANCE USE.   Members abstain from the use of tobacco and hold that drunkenness is a serious sin. Alcohol used in moderation, however, is acceptable.

Religious Support System for the Sick
VISITORS.   Individual members of congregation, including elders. Visitors pray with the sick person and read scriptures. Since members do not smoke, it is preferred that patients be placed in rooms with nonsmokers.

TITLE OF RELIGIOUS REPRESENTATIVE.   If male, Mr. or Elder; if female, Ms. or Mrs. Religious titles are not generally used.

CHURCH ORGANIZATIONS TO ASSIST THE SICK.   Individual; members of congregation look after needs.

Issues Related to Death and Dying
PROLONGATION OF LIFE (RIGHT TO DIE).   The right to die or the use of extraordinary methods to prolong life is a matter of individual conscience.

EUTHANASIA.   This practice is forbidden.

AUTOPSY.   An autopsy is acceptable only if it is required by law. No parts are to be removed from the body. Man's spirit and body are never separated.

DONATION OF BODY.   This practice is forbidden.

DISPOSAL OF BODY.   This is a matter of individual preference.

BURIAL. Burial practices are determined by local custom. Cremation is permitted if the individual chooses it.

ADDENDUM. Jehovah's Witnesses are opposed to saluting the flag, serving in the armed forces, voting in civil elections, and holding public office. These prohibitions are related to belief in a theocracy that is in harmony with New Testament Christianity. Governed by a body of individuals, members united with the theocracy are to dissociate themselves from all activities of the political state and give full allegiance to "Jehovah's organization." This practice is related to the belief that Jesus Christ is King and Priest and that there is no need to hold citizenship in more than one kingdom. Members also refrain from gambling.

A pamphlet entitled Jehovah's Witnesses and the Question of Blood may be obtained free of charge by contacting the World Headquarters for the Jehovah's Witnesses at 117 Adams Street, Brooklyn, NY, 11201.

Judaism

Judaism is an Old Testament religion that dates back to the time of the prophet Abraham. Worldwide there are approximately 18 million Jews. U.S. membership consists of approximately 7 million members.

Beliefs and Religious Practices

Judaism is a monotheistic religion. Jewish life historically was based on interpretation of the laws of God as contained in the Torah and explained in the Talmud and in oral tradition.

Ancient Jewish law prescribed most of the daily actions of the people. Diet, clothing, activities, occupation, and ceremonial activities throughout the life cycle are all part of Jewish daily life.

JEWISH CULTURE AND TRADITIONS. Today there are at least three schools of theological thought and social practice in Judaism. The three main divisions include Orthodox, Conservative, and Reform. There is also a fundamentalist sect, called Hasidism. Hasidic Jews cluster in metropolitan areas and live and work only within their Jewish communities.

Any person born of a Jewish mother or anyone converted to Judaism is considered a Jew. All Jews are united by the core theme of Judaism, which is expressed in the Shema, a prayer that professes a single God.

HOLY DAYS. The Sabbath is the holiest of all holy days. The Sabbath begins each Friday 18 minutes before sunset and ends on Saturday, 42 minutes after sunset, or when three stars can be seen in the sky with the naked eye.

Other Holy Days are:

1. Rosh Hashanah (Jewish New Year)
2. Yom Kippur (Day of Atonement, a fast day)
3. Succot (Feast of Tabernacles)
4. Shmini Atzeret (8th Day of Assembly)
5. Simchat Torah
6. Chanukah (Festival of Lights, or Rededication of the Temple in Jerusalem)

7. Asara B'Tevet (Fast of the loth of Tevet)*
8. Fast of Esther
9. Purim
10. Passover
11. Shavuot (Festival of the Giving of the Torah)
12. Fast of the 17th of Tammuz
13. Fast of the 9th of Ave (Commemoration of the Destruction of the Temple)

Holy days are very special to practicing Jews. If a condition is not life-threatening, medical and surgical procedures should not be performed on the Sabbath or on holy days.

Preservation of life is of greatest priority and is the major criterion for determining activity on holy days and the Sabbath. If a Jewish patient is hesitant to receive urgent and necessary treatment because of religious restrictions, a rabbi should be consulted.

SACRAMENTS/RITUALS. Brit milah, the covenant of *circumcision,* is performed on all Jewish male children on the eighth day following birth. Although circumcision is a surgical procedure, for Jews it is a fundamental religious obligation. Circumcision is usually performed by a *mohil,* a pious Jew with special training, or by the child's father. Since the severing of the foreskin constitutes the essence of the ritual, the practice of having a non-Jewish or non-observant physician perform the circumcision in the presence of a rabbi or other person who pronounces the blessing is not acceptable according to Jewish law.

Circumcision may be delayed if medically contraindicated. For example, if the child has *hypospadias,* a congenital defect of the urethral wall for which surgical repair usually occurs at age 3 years and requires the use of the foreskin in reconstructive plastic surgery, the circumcision may be delayed. At times, Jewish law requires postponement of circumcision though contemporary medical science recongnizes no potential threat to the health of the baby, e.g., for physiologic jaundice. As soon as the jaundice disappears, the *milah* may be performed. In Reform and Conservative traditions, girls mark the eighth day of life with a *dedication* ceremony in which prayers and blessings are invoked on her behalf.

The *bar mitzvah* (meaning "son of the commandment") is a confirmation ceremony for boys at age 13 that has been preceded by extensive religious study including mastery of key Torah passages in Hebrew. In Reform and Conservative traditions, the *bas (or bat) mitzvah* (meaning "daughter of the commandment") is the equivalent ceremony for girls.

RELIGION AND HEALING. Medical care from a physician in the case of illness is expected according to Jewish law. There are many prayers for the sick in Jewish liturgy. Such prayers and hope for recovery are encouraged.

Diet, Medications, and Procedures

DIET. The dietary laws of Judaism are very strict; the degree to which they are observed varies according to the individual. Strictly observant Jews never eat pork,

---

*Not observed by liberal/Reform Jews.

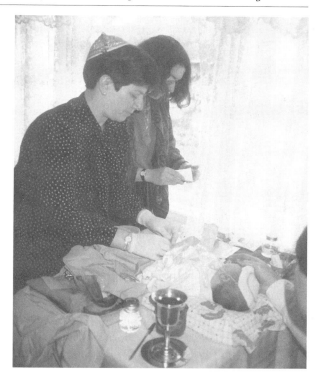

The *brit milah* or covenant of circumcision is being performed in the home of this 8-day-old Jewish infant by 2 *mohils*, one of whom is a Jewish pediatrician.

never eat predatory fowl, and never mix milk dishes and meat dishes. Only fish with fins and scales are permissible; shellfish and other water creatures are prohibited.

Kosher is a Jewish word that means "properly preserved." All animals must be ritually slaughtered to be kosher. This means that the animal is to be killed by a sochet, quickly, with the least possible pain. More colloquially, many people think kosher refers to a type of food. If a patient asks for kosher food, it is important to determine what he means.

MEDICATIONS.   There are no restrictions when medications are used as a part of therapeutic process.

BLOOD AND BLOOD PRODUCTS.   There is a prohibition in Judaism against ingesting blood (e.g., blood sausage, raw meat). However, this does not apply to receiving blood transfusions.

Controversial Issues Related to Health Care
BIRTH CONTROL.   It is said in the Torah that Jews should be fruitful and multiply; therefore, it is a "mitzvah" to have at least two children. Since the Holocaust of World War II, it has been increasingly acceptable to have more children to replace those that were lost. It is permissible to practice birth control in traditional and liberal homes (Forsythe, 1991).

In the past, contraception was limited to the female; vasectomy was prohibited.

Currently, Judaism permits contraception by either partner, although Hasidic and Orthodox Jews rarely employ vasectomy.

ABORTION.   Although therapeutic abortion is always permitted if the health of the mother is jeopardized, traditional Judaism regards the killing of an unborn child to be a serious moral offense, whereas liberal Judaism permits it with strong moral admonition (i.e., it is not to be used as a means of birth control). The fetus, although not imbued with the full sanctity of life, is a potential human being and is acknowledged as such.

STERILITY TESTING.   Permissible when the goal is to enable the couple to have children.

ARTIFICIAL INSEMINATION.   Permitted under certain circumstances. A rabbi should be consulted in each individual case.

EUGENICS AND GENETICS.   Jews have an understandable aversion to genetic engineering because of the experimentation carried on during the Nazi era. At the same time, eugenics are permitted under a limited range of circumstances. The Jewish belief in the sanctity of life is a guiding factor in rabbinical counseling.

SOCIAL ACTIVITIES (DATING, DANCING).   Like all ethnic groups, Jews tend toward endogamy. Social activities that might lead to marriage outside the faith are discouraged. However, it is recognized that a significant number of individuals in Jewish society will seek partners outside. When this occurs, every effort is made to bring the non-Jewish partner into Judaism and to keep the Jewish partner a member and part of Jewish society.

SUBSTANCE USE.   The guideline is moderation. Wine is a part of religious observance and used as such. Drunkenness is not a sign of a good Jew. Historically, Jews well connected with their faith have had a low incidence of alcoholism.

Religious Support System for the Sick

VISITORS.   The most likely visitors will be family and friends from the synagogue. To visit the sick is a "mitzvah" of service (an obligation, a responsibility, and a blessing). There are often many Jewish social service agencies to help those in need. The Jewish Federation and Jewish Community Service are two large organizations that provide services to fulfill a variety of needs.

TITLE OF RELIGIOUS REPRESENTATIVE.   The formal religious representative from a synagogue is the *rabbi*. A visit from the rabbi may be spent talking, or the rabbi may pray with the person alone or in a minyan, a group of 10 adults 13 years or older. If the patient is male and strictly observant, he may wish to have a prayer shawl (tallit), a cap (kippa), and tefillin (special symbols tied onto the arms and forehead). If the patient's own materials are not at the hospital, it may be necessary to ask that they be brought. Prayers are often chanted. If possible, privacy should be provided.

Issues Related to Death and Dying

PROLONGATION OF LIFE (RIGHT TO DIE).   A person has the right to die with dignity. If a physician sees that death is inevitable, no new therapeutic measures that would artificially extend life need to be initiated. It is important to know the precise time of death for the purpose of honoring the deceased after the first year has passed.

EUTHANASIA. Prohibited under any circumstances. It is regarded as murder. However, in the administration of palliative medications that carry the calculated risk of overdose, the amelioration of pain is paramount.

AUTOPSY. Any *unjustified* alteration in a corpse is considered a desecration of the dead to be avoided in normal circumstances. When postmortem examinations are justified, they must be limited to essential organs or systems. Needle biopsy is preferred. All body parts must be returned for burial. Jewish family members may ask to consult with a rabbinical authority before signing an autopsy consent form.

DONATION OF BODY PARTS. This is a complex matter according to Jewish law. If it seems necessary, consultation with a rabbi should be encouraged.

BURIAL. The body is ritually washed at a funeral home following death, if possible by members of the *Chevra Kadisha* (Ritual Burial Society). The body is then clothed in a simple white burial shroud. Embalming, a process wherein the blood of the deceased is replaced by an embalming fluid, and cosmetic treatment of the body are forbidden. Public viewing of the body is considered a humiliation of the dead. Relatives are forbidden to touch or embrace the deceased, except when involved in preparation for interment. The exact time of burial is significant for sitting *shiva*, the mourning period. Following death in an institution, a nurse may wash the body for transport to the funeral home. Ritual washing then occurs later. Human remains, including a fetus at any stage of gestation, are to be buried as soon as possible. Cremation is not in keeping with Jewish law.

ADDENDUM. Additional information can be obtained from: Synagogue Council of America, 432 Park Avenue South, New York, NY 10016. (212) 686-8670.

Mennonite Church

MEMBERSHIP. United States, 260,000.

Beliefs and Religious Practices

HOLY DAYS. The Mennonites observe the religious days of the traditional Christian churches. Observance places no restrictions on health-related procedures on these days.

SACRAMENTS. Mennonites observe Baptism and Holy Communion as official church sacraments. Patients will request sacraments as necessary. Neither sacrament is believed necessary for salvation.

RELIGION AND HEALING. Healing is believed to be a part of God's work in the human body through whatever means he chooses to use, whether medical science or healing that comes in answer to specific prayer. There is no religious ritual to be applied unless the patient asks for one in whatever way is personally meaningful. Sometimes anointing of oil is practiced.

Diet, Medications, and Procedures

No specific guidelines or restrictions.

BLOOD AND BLOOD PRODUCTS.   Acceptable; no restrictions.

SURGICAL PROCEDURES.   No restrictions.

Controversial Issues Related to Health Care

BIRTH CONTROL.   All types of contraception are acceptable. The choice is left to the individual.

ABORTION.   Therapeutic abortions are acceptable. Mennonites generally believe that on-demand abortion must be decided according to the specifics of individual cases. The church has chosen to avoid making a ruling that must be followed unquestionably. The individual must follow her own conscience and learn to live with the consequences. Some parts of the Mennonite Church have adopted statements opposing abortion on demand.

ARTIFICIAL INSEMINATION.   The church does not have regulations regarding artificial insemination. The individual conscience and point of view of the patient needs to be respected. Usually, artificial insemination is sought only if husband and wife are donor and recipient, respectively.

EUGENICS AND GENETICS.   The church accepts scientific endeavor as a valid activity that needs to respect all of God's creation. The concerns of eugenics and genetics in its future potential have not been fully confronted. Mennonites believe that God and man work together in caring for and improving the world.

SOCIAL ACTIVITIES (DATING, DANCING).   No restrictions.

Issues Related to Death and Dying

PROLONGATION OF LIFE (RIGHT TO DIE).   The church does not believe that life must be continued at all cost. Health care professionals should decide whether to take heroic measures on the basis of the patient's individual circumstances and the emotional condition of the family. When life has lost its purpose and meaning beyond hope of meaningful recovery, most Mennonites feel that relatives should not be censured for allowing life-sustaining measures to be withheld.

EUTHANASIA.   Euthanasia as the termination of life by an overt act of the physician is not condoned.

AUTOPSY.   Acceptable; no restrictions.

DONATION OF BODY.   Acceptable; no restrictions.

DISPOSAL OF BODY.   Per local law and custom.

BURIAL.   Burial practices follow local customs and legal requirements.

ADDENDUM.   Mennonites believe that each person is responsible before God to make decisions based on his or her understanding of the Bible. For this reason, there are a minimum of official statements or regulations. Even when these are to be found, they are perceived by members as guidelines rather than proclamations to supplant individual responsibility. It should also be noted that the Mennonite faith encompasses a wide spectrum of cultural circumstances, which are more responsible for variations among individual Mennonites than is the basic theology, which is relatively uniform.

It is therefore necessary to ascertain individual preferences and to work with patients on a one-to-one basis rather than stereotyping according to religious affiliation.

Native American Churches

Differentiating Native American health care practices from their religious and cultural beliefs is much more difficult than with the other religions presented in this chapter. Native Americans represent 2 million people and more than 300 tribal units within North America. Each group has individual beliefs and practices, yet they maintain a similar nonprescriptive attitude toward health care.

There is in the United States today a specific religion called the Native American Church or Peyote Religion. Encompassing members of many tribes, its focus is on the revival of Native American culture and beliefs.

When trying to support a Native American in physical or psychological crisis, the nurse needs to remember a number of seemingly unrelated facts. First, the non-Westernized Native American belief about disease is not necessarily based on symptoms. Disease may be attributed to intrusive objects, soul loss, spirit intrusion, breach of taboo, or sorcery. Disease may also be attributed to natural or supernatural causes (Vogel, 1970). Second, the Native American may embrace an organized, usually Christian religion, as well as be a member of a particular Native American tribe. Native Americans also balance "modern theories of disease" with long-standing tribal beliefs or customs. Therefore, during illness and particularly hospitalization, Native Americans may ask to see a priest or minister as well as a tribal "medicine man" or curandero. Visits from these persons will likely be spiritually supportive in nature, although the form of the support may vary greatly.

The spiritual basis for much of Native American belief and action is symbolized by the number four. This number, which pervades much American Indian thought, is seen in the extended hand, which means life, unity, equality, and eternity. The clasped hand symbolizes unity, the spiritual law that binds the universe.

It is this unity upon which decisions should be made. Questions about abortion, use of drugs, giving and receiving blood, right to life, euthanasia, and so on do not have dogmatic "yes" or "no" answers; rather, answers are based on the situation and the ultimate unity/disunity that a decision would produce.

To the Native American, everything is cyclical. Communication is the key to learning and understanding; understanding brings peace of mind; peace of mind leads to happiness; and happiness is communicating. Other guidelines also function in groups of four (Steiger, 1975).

Four guidelines toward self-development are:

1. Am I happy with what I am doing?
2. What am I doing to add to the confusion?
3. What am I doing to bring about peace and contentment?
4. How will I be remembered when I am gone, in absence and in death?

The four requirements of good health are:

1. Food
2. Sleep

3. Cleanliness
4. Good thoughts

The four divisions of nature are:

1. Spirit
2. Mind
3. Body
4. Life

The four divisions of goals are:

1. Faith
2. Love
3. Work
4. Pleasure

The four ages of development are the:

1. Learning age
2. Age of adoption
3. Age of improvement
4. Age of wisdom

The four expressions of sharing are:

1. Making others feel you care
2. An expression of interest
3. An expression of friendship
4. An expression of belonging

Unity, the great spiritual law, also can be expressed in four parts:

1. Going into the silence in spirit, mind, and body
2. The union through which all spirituality flows
3. A goal toward communicating with all things in nature
4. Recognized through sense, emotions and impressions.

In concert with the belief in the interconnectedness of all things natural remedies in the form of herbal medicine are often used. (It is interesting to note that Native American folk medicine and herbal remedies provided the forerunners of many of today's pharmaceutical remedies.) Herbal treatments are still used today and may be requested by Native American patients in a Western medical setting.

A nurse caring for a Native American client should be careful to obtain a careful and complete history, including a list of whatever native remedies have been tried. The patient may not know the names of herbs used in treatment, and the tribal medicine man or woman may need to be consulted.

Respecting the concept that religion, medicine, and healing are inseparable to the Native American, one must be sensitive to the fact that asking for names of native medicines or descriptions of healing practices tried in an attempt to cure the person before his entrance into the Western medical system is not just simply obtaining a history, but also entering into the realm of what might be not only private but also very sacred. The nurse must use care and sensitivity and show deep respect for the information received.

Seventh-Day Adventists

MEMBERSHIP.   Worldwide, 7.5 million; North American, 783,000

Beliefs and Religious Practices

Seventh-Day Adventists believe that because the body is the temple of God, it is appropriate to abstain from any food or beverage that could prove harmful to the body. Since man's first diet consisted of fruits and grains, the Church encourages a vegetarian diet. However, not all members follow such a diet.

HOLY DAYS.   The seventh day (Saturday) is observed as the Sabbath, from Friday sundown to Saturday sundown. The Sabbath is the day that God blessed and sanctified. It is a sacred day of worship and rest. Saturday worship services are held, as are weekly evening prayer meetings (usually midweek).

SACRAMENTS.   There are three church ordinances: (1) baptism by immersion, (2) the Ordinance of Humility, and (3) the Lord's Supper or Communion. There is no requirement for a final sacrament at death.

RITUALS AT TIME OF BIRTH.   None.

RITUALS AT TIME OF DEATH.   Anointing, if requested by individual or family member.

RELIGION AND HEALING.   The church believes in divine healing and practices anointing with oil and prayer. This is in addition to healing brought about by medical intervention. Since 1865 the church has maintained chaplains and physicians as inseparable in its institutions.

Diet, Medications, and Procedures

DIET.   Although the church encourages a vegetarian diet, some members prefer to eat meat and poultry. Based on a passage in Leviticus Chapter 11, Verse 3, non-vegetarian members refrain from eating foods derived from any animal having a cloven hoof that chews its cud (e.g., meat derived from pigs, rabbits, or similar animals). Although fish with fins and scales are acceptable (e.g., salmon), shellfish are prohibited. Consumption of some birds is prohibited, but common poultry such as chicken and turkey are acceptable. Fermented beverages are prohibited.

Fasting is practiced, but only when members of a specific church elect to do so. Practiced in degrees, fasting may involve abstention from food or liquids. Fasting is not encouraged if it is likely to have adverse effects on the individual.

MEDICATIONS.   Adventists operate one of the world's largest religiously operated health systems, including a medical school. Physical medicine and rehabilitation are emphasized and recommended, along with therapeutic diets. There are no restrictions on the use of vaccines.

BLOOD AND BLOOD PRODUCTS.   No restrictions.

AMPUTATIONS.   No restrictions.

ORGAN TRANSPLANTS AND DONATION OF ORGANS.   No restrictions.

BIOPSIES.   No restrictions.

CIRCUMCISION.   No restrictions.

AMNIOCENTESIS.   No restrictions.

Controversial Issues Related to Health Care

BIRTH CONTROL.   This is an individual decision; the church prohibits cohabitation except between husband and wife.

ABORTION.   Therapeutic abortion is acceptable if the mother's life is in danger and in cases of rape and incest. On demand, abortion is unacceptable, since Adventists believe in the sanctity of life.

ARTIFICIAL INSEMINATION.   If between husband and wife, there is no objection.

EUGENICS AND GENETICS.   Although the church views this as an individual decision, it upholds the principle of responsibility in dealing with children.

SOCIAL ACTIVITIES (DATING, DANCING).   Dancing is not encouraged as a form of recreation or social activity. Members are encouraged to date other members or persons holding similar beliefs and values.

SUBSTANCE USE.   Abstinence from the use of fermented beverages and tobacco products.

Religious Support System for the Sick

VISITORS.   At the request of the sick person or the family, the pastor and elders of the church will come together to pray and anoint the sick person with oil.

TITLE OF RELIGIOUS REPRESENTATIVE.   Doctor, Pastor, Elder.

CHURCH ORGANIZATIONS TO ASSIST THE SICK.   There is a worldwide Seventh Day Adventists health system, which includes hospitals and clinics.

Issues Related to Death and Dying

PROLONGATION OF LIFE (RIGHT TO DIE).   Although there is no official position, the church has traditionally followed the medical ethics of prolonging life.

EUTHANASIA.   As above.

AUTOPSY.   Acceptable.

DONATION OF ENTIRE BODY OR PARTS.   Acceptable.

DISPOSAL OF BODY.   No directives or recommendations.

BURIAL.   No specific directives concerning burial; this is an individual decision.

ADDENDUM.   The Seventh-Day Adventists church is opposed to the use of hypnotism in the practice of medicine or under any other circumstance.

Unitarian/Universalist Church

MEMBERSHIP.   Worldwide Unitarian Universalist membership is 200,599, with a North American membership of 199,472.

Beliefs and Religious Practices

Unitarianism was officially organized in 1774 in England. This organization occurred after a long history of debate and dissension regarding the nature of God, particularly regarding the Trinitarian concept, which existed in various forms in the Catholic and Protestant religions.

HOLY DAYS.   No religious holy days are celebrated. Members come from various cultural and religious backgrounds and observe special days according to their own heritage and desire.

SACRAMENTS.   Normal milestones of life (birth, marriage, death) may be celebrated religiously. Although it is uncommon, puberty and divorce may include religious observances.

Unitarian Universalism does not believe in a need for sacraments. Baptism of infants and occasionally of adults is sometimes performed as a symbolic act of dedication. The Lord's Supper is administered in some congregations.

RELIGION AND HEALING.   Faith healing is considered largely superstitious and wishful thinking. Members believe in use of the empirical method reason, and science to facilitate healing.

Diet, Medications, and Procedures

DIET.   No restrictions.

MEDICATIONS.   No restrictions.

BLOOD AND BLOOD PRODUCTS.   No restrictions.

AMPUTATIONS.   No restrictions.

ORGAN TRANSPLANTS.   No restrictions.

BIOPSIES.   No restrictions.

CIRCUMCISION.   Viewed as a health practice, not a religious one.

AMNIOCENTESIS.   No restrictions; encouraged if medical evaluation deems it necessary.

Controversial Issues Related to Health Care

BIRTH CONTROL.   Strongly favor all types as a human right.

ABORTION.   Both therapeutic and on-demand abortion are acceptable. Strongly favor the right of the mother to decide.

STERILITY TESTING.   Acceptable; more research is encouraged.

ARTIFICIAL INSEMINATION.   Both donation and receipt are acceptable. Strongly favor this as a human right.

SUBSTANCE USE.   No restrictions. Use according to reason.

Issues Related to Death and Dying

PROLONGATION OF LIFE (RIGHT TO DIE).   Favor the right to die with dignity. "Personhood" is sacred, not the spark of life.

EUTHANASIA.   Members tend to favor nonaction, including withdrawal of technical aids when death is imminent or when the patient has made a written request in advance.

AUTOPSY.   Recommended.

DONATION OF BODY.   Acceptable.

DISPOSAL OF BODY/BURIAL.   Cremation is most common. Donation to a medical school for study is not uncommon. Burial of a fetus is rare.

FUNERAL.   Memorial service in the church or at home without the body present is customary.

Research Application 12-2 provides information regarding other research done on this topic, and Box 12-2 summarizes some of the religious and nonreligious holidays covered in this chapter.

Review Questions

1. When assessing the spiritual needs of clients from diverse cultural backgrounds, what are the key components that you should consider?
2. In providing nursing care for the dying or bereaved client and family, what cultural considerations should the nurse include in the plan?
3. Compare and contrast the religious beliefs and practices concerning diet, medications, and procedures for five of the religious groups discussed in the section of the chapter called Listing of Selected Religions.
4. Analyze the contributions of religious bodies to the U.S. (or Canadian) health care delivery system.
5. What affect do health care facilities that are owned and operated by religious groups have on the overall cost and quality of health care in the U.S. and Canada?
6. What religious rituals mark significant developmental milestones for children and adolescents? Identify the ritual/ceremony, approximate age at which the child or adolescent participates in it, and the name of the religion(s) associated with it.

Research Application 12-2

A question that may be asked in relationship to religious beliefs and health is Do the religious beliefs have a positive effect on the health of practicing members? There is a body of research, mostly experimental or quasiexperimental in design, that seems to document a salutary effect of some force, energy, or field considerably more subtle than Western biomedicine is able to demonstrate within three-dimensional physical reality. This effect has been demonstrated in more than 150 published empirical studies of these types of healing in human beings. Included in this section is a review of selected studies that examine the health-promoting and healing aspects of religious beliefs and practices, including prayer.

Burkhardt, M. A. (1993). Characteristics of spirituality in the lives of women in a rural Appalachian community. *Journal of Transcultural Nursing, 4*(2), 12–18.

This qualitative study reports the results of research investigating how women in rural Appalachia experience and describe spirituality in their daily lives. Characteristics described by the five subjects in this study included belief in God or Greater Source, prayer/meditation, and a sense of relationship or connectedness with others, nature, and oneself. The dominant theme that emerged relative to these relationships was that of self-reliance or inner strength. Spirituality for these women relates to the whole of life and is relational.

Mills, P. K., Beeson, W. L., Phillips, R. L., & Fraser, G. E. (1994). Cancer incidence among California Seventh-day Adventists, 1976–1982. *American Journal of Clinical Nutrition, 59* (supplement), 1136S–42S.

In this longitudinal study cancer incidence was monitored in a population of 34,000 Seventh-day Adventists in California. By religious belief, Adventists do not consume tobacco, alcohol, or pork and approximately one half adhere to a lactovegetarian lifestyle. Comparisons of cancer incidence rates in this population with an external reference population were calculated using standardized morbidity ratios (SMRs) for all cancer sites. Relative risks were calculated by using data obtained from a detailed lifestyle questionnaire that members of the study population completed. For all cancer sites (except prostate), the SMR was lower in the male Adventists. For females, the all-cancer SMR was lower (except for endometrial cancer) but not reduced enough to be considered statistically significant.

The researchers conclude that the unique lifestyle of Adventists may afford greater protection for males than females. Whereas males traditionally are exposed to cigarette smoke, alcohol, and a high-fat diet more than are females, the lack of exposure to these substances may enhance the health of males more than females. When examining specific cancer sites, both males and females have substantially lower SMRs for respiratory cancer, an expected finding given the almost complete lack of reported cigarette smoking by Adventists. For discussion of other cancer sites, the reader is encouraged to review the research results reported in the article.

Luna, L. (1994). Care and cultural context of Lebanese Muslim immigrants: Using Leininger's theory. *Journal of Transcultural Nursing, 5*(2), 12–20.

In this ethnonursing study, the meanings and experiences of care for Lebanese Muslims as influenced by cultural context in selected natural and community settings were examined. Using Leininger's Theory of Cultural Care Diversity and Universality, the researcher posed questions aimed at discovering the meanings and experiences of care as influenced by world view, social structure, and cultural context in the hospital, clinic, and home. Ethnonursing research methods were used with 13 key and 30 general informants in an urban U.S. community. The majority of informants were new immigrants living fewer than 10 years in the United States. Universal themes of care that were similar in the three contexts reflected care as a religious obligation in Islam, care as equal but different gender responsibilities, and care as individual and collective meanings of honor. The researcher concludes by applying Leininger's three modes of decision and action—cultural care preservation/maintenance, cultural care accommodation/negotiation, and cultural care repatterning/restructuring—in the provision of culturally congruent care for Lebanese Muslim clients.

Clinical Applications

Knowledge of the positive influence of religious and spiritual beliefs in health promotion, disease prevention, and healing enables nurses to provide culturally competent care. In some cases, religious dietary practices have been demonstrated to prevent serious diseases such as cancer and cardiovascular conditions. Whenever possible, the nurse should reinforce healthy religious behaviors and discuss with clients the research-based data supporting the health benefits of their religious practices.

Box 12-2 *Religious and Nonreligious Holidays in the United States and Canada*

This calendar is a guide to religious and nonreligious holidays that are celebrated in the United States and Canada. The list is not exhaustive, but is given to encourage the reader to be aware of the many holidays and festivals that are reflective of the great mixture of religious and ethnic groups that exist in North America.

B = Buddhist	J = Jewish	O = Eastern Orthodox Christian
Ba = Baha'i	Ci = Civic Holiday	P = Protestant
C = Christian (general)	Ja = Jain	RC = Roman Catholic
H = Hindu	M = Mormon	S = Sikh
I = Islam		

JANUARY

1 New Year's Day Ci	6 Epiphany C	3rd Monday Martin Luther King, Jr.
Feast of St. Basil O	7 Nativity of Jesus Christ O	Birthday Observance Ci

FEBRUARY

Black History Month (U.S.)   14 Valentine's Day Ci   Mid-month President's Day (U.S.) Ci
8 Scout Day Ci

Other holidays that often fall in February according to the lunar calendar

Chinese New Year	Nehan-e (Death of Buddha) B	Ash Wednesday C
Ramadan (30 days) I	Vasant Panchami (Advent of Spring) H, Ja	Purim J

MARCH

Women's History Month (U.S.)   17 St. Patrick's Day C   25 Annunciation C

Other holidays that often occur in March according to the lunar calendar

Eastern Orthodox Lent begins O	Palm Sunday RC, P	Good Friday RC, P
Higan-e (First Day of Spring) B	First Day of Passover (8 days) J	Easter C, RC, P, M
Naw-Ruz (Baha'i and Iranian	Holi (Spring Festival) H, Ja	Mahavir Jayanti
New Year)	Maunday Thursday RC, P	(Birth of Mahavir) Ja

APRIL

16 Yom Ha'atzmaut (Israel Independence Day) J

Holidays that often occur in April according to the lunar calendar

Hanamatsuri (Birth of Buddha) B	Baisakhi (Brotherhood) S	Palm Sunday O
Yom Hashoah	Huguenot Day P	Holy Friday O
(Holocaust Remembrance Day) J, Ci	Ramavani (Birth of Rama) H	Easter O

Box 12-2. *(Continued)*

MAY

5   Cinco de Mayo   Ci
13   Ascension Day   RC, P

23   Victoria Day (Canada)

30   Memorial Day   Ci

Holidays that often occur in May according to the lunar calendar
Shavuot   J

Idul-Adha (Day of Sacrifice)   I

Pentecost   RC, P

JUNE

9   Ascension Day   O
12   Anne Frank Day

14   Flag Day (U.S.)   Ci

24   Nativity of St. John the Baptist   RC, P

Holidays that often occur in June according to the lunar calendar
Muharram
Ratha-yatra

Islamic New Year

Hindu New Year

JULY

1   Canada Day (Canada)   Ci

4   Independence Day (U.S.)   Ci

24   Pioneer Day   M

Holidays that often occur in kJuly according to the lunar calendar
Obon-e   B

AUGUST

6   Transfiguration   C
      Hiroshima Day   Ci

15   Feast of the Blessed Virgin Mary   RC, O

SEPTEMBER

1st Monday   Labor Day (U.S.)   Ci
15   National Hispanic Heritage
        Month (30 days)   Ci

17   Citizenship (U.S. Constitution)   Ci
19   San Gennaro Day   RC

25   Native American Day   Ci

Holidays that often occur in September according to the lunar calendar
Higan-e (First Day of Fall)   B

Rosh Hashanah (Jewish New York: 2 days)   J

OCTOBER

12   Columbus Day (U.S.)   Ci
      Thanksgiving Day (Canada)   Ci

24   United Nations Day   Ci

31   Reformation Day   P
      Halloween   RC, Ci

Holidays that often occur in October according to the lunar calendar
Dusserah (good over Evil)   H, JA
Yom Kippur (Atonement)   J

Sukkot (Tabernacles)   J
Shemini 'Azeret (end of Sukkot)

Diwali, or Dipavali
   Festival of Lights)   H, Ja

NOVEMBER

1   All Saints Day   RC, P
11   Veterans Day   Ci

25   Religious Liberty Day   Ci
1st Tuesday   Election Day (U.S.)   Ci

4th Thursday   Thanksgiving Day
   (U.S.)   Ci

Holidays that often occur in November according to the lunar calendar
Baha'u'llah Birthday   Ba

Guru Nanak Birthday   S

Box 12-2. *(Continued)*

DECEMBER

6   St. Nicholas Day   C
8   Feast of the Immaculate
      Conception   RC
10 Human Rights Day   Ci

12 Festival of Our Lady of Guadalupe
      (Mexico-Hispanic)

25 Christmas   C, RC, P, M, Ci

Holidays that often occur in December according to the lunar calendar
Bodhi Day (Enlightenment)   B   Hanukkah (Jewish Festival of Lights: 8 days)   J   Kwanzaa (7 days)

Learning Activities to Promote Critical Thinking

1. Visit a church not of your own belief system and interview a member of the clergy or an official church representative about the health-related beliefs of that religion. Discuss with him/her the implications of those beliefs for someone hospitalized for an acute illness or a chronic illness. Inquire about the ways in which nurses can be of most help to hospitalized members of this religion.

2. Interview members of various religions about their beliefs about health and illness. Compare these interviews with the published beliefs or official statements from these religions. Discuss the implications of the differences (if any) that you found.

3. Interview fellow students, classmates, or coworkers (if you are employed) about what they know about health beliefs of various religions, especially those religions most often encountered among the patients you work with most often. Make a poster, or prepare a presentation comparing the results of your interviews with the official beliefs of those religions. Share this information with your classmates.

4. Interview 4 or more members of the same religious group but that are of various ages themselves (i.e. children, teenagers, young adults, middle aged and elderly). Ask them about their religious beliefs and how they effect their health. Compare the results, commenting on similarities and differences.

5. If you have thought about the above exercises in terms of physical health, consider each of the questions from the perspective of mental health and spiritual health.

References

Angrosino, M. V. (1996). The Roman Catholic church and U.S. health care reform. *Medical Anthropology Quarterly* 10(1), 3–19.

Backman, M. (1983). *Christian Churches of America.* New York: Charles Scribner & Sons.

Chapman, A. (1991). The Buddhist way of dying. *Nursing Praxis in New Zealand* 6(2), 23–26.

Christian Science Publishing Society (1978). *What is a Christian Science Practitioner?* Boston: Christian Science Publishing Society.

Christian Science Publishing Society (1994). *Science and Health.* Boston: Christian Science Publishing Society.

Donnermeyer, J. F. (1997). Amish society: An overview. *The Journal of Multicultural Nursing & Health* 3(2), 6–12.

Ebersole, P., & Hess, P. (1994) *Toward Healthy Aging.* St. Louis, MO: C. V. Mosby.

Eisenbruch, M. (1984a). Cross-cultural aspects of bereavement. I. A conceptual framework for comparative analysis. *Culture, Medicine, and Psychiatry* 8, 283–309.

Eisenbruch, M. (1984b). Cross-cultural aspects of bereavement. II. Ethnic and cultural variations in the development of bereavement practices. *Culture, Medicine, and Psychiatry* 8, 315–347.

Faulkner, J. E., & DeJong, C. F. (1966). Religiosity in 5 D: An empirical analysis. *Social Forces* 45, 246–254.

Forsythe, E. (1991). Religious and cultural aspects of family planning. *Journal of the Royal Society of Medicine* 84(3), 177–178.

Foy, F. A., & Avato, R. M. (1997). *Catholic Almanac 1997.* Huntington, IN: Our Sunday Visitor Publishing Division.

Glock, C. Y., & Stark, R. (1965). *Religion and society in tension.* Chicago: Rand McNally.

Green, J. (1992a). Death with dignity: Christianity. *Nursing Times* 88(3), 25–29.

Green, J. (1992b). Death with dignity: Jehovah's Witnesses. *Nursing Times* 88(5), 36–37.

Greksa, L. P., & Korbin, J. E. (1997). Influence of changing occupational patterns on the use of commercial health insurance by the Old Order Amish. *The Journal of Multicultural Nursing & Health* 3(2), 13–18.

Hickey, M. E., & Hall, T. R. (1993). Insulin therapy and weight change in Native American NIDDM patients. *Diabetes Care* 16(1), 364–368.

Hinnell, J. R. (1984). *The Penguin Dictionary of Religions.* New York: Penguin Books.

Hostetler, J. A. (1993). *Amish Society.* Baltimore: Johns Hopkins University Press.

Huttlinger, K., Krefting, L., Drevdahl, D., Tree, P., Bacca, E., &

Benally, A. (1992). Doing battle: A metaphorical analysis of diabetes mellitus among Navajo people. *American Journal of Occupational Therapy* 46(8), 706–712.

Kalish, R. A., & Reynolds, D. K. (1981). *Death and Ethnicity: A Psychocultural Study.* New York: Baywood.

Marty, M. M. (1990). Health, medicine, and the faith traditions. *Healthy People 2000: A Role for America's Religious Communities.* Emory University: The Carter Center and the Park Ridge Center.

Moberg, D. (1971). *Spiritual Well-Being.* Washington, DC: White House Conference on Aging.

Moberg, D. (1981). Religion and the aging family. In P. Ebersole and P. Hess (Eds.). *Toward Healthy Aging,* pp. 349–351. St. Louis, MO: C.V. Mosby.

Smith, E. B. (1986). Surgery in Jehovah's Witnesses. *Journal of National Medical Association* 78(7), 668–669.

Steiger, B. (1975). *Medicine Talk.* New York: Doubleday & Co.

Sugarman, J., Churchill, L. R., Moore, J. K., & Waugh, R. A. (1991). Medical, ethical, and legal issues regarding thrombolytic therapy in the Jehovah's Witnesses. *American Journal of Cardiology* 68(15), 1525–1529.

Vogel, V. J. (1970). *American Indian Medicine.* Norman, OK: University of Oklahoma Press.

Weiss, D. W. (1988). Organ transplantation, medical ethics and Jewish law. *Transplantation Proceedings* 20(1), 1071–1075.

Wenger, A. F. (1990). The culture care theory and the Old Order Amish. In M. M. Leininger (Ed.). *Culture Care Diversity and Universality: A Theory of Nursing.* New York: National League for Nursing Press, 147–178.

Wenger, A. F. (1991). Culture specific care and the Old Order Amish. *IMPRINT,* April–May, 80–85.

Yearbook of American and Canadian Churches, Annual. (1990). New York: National Council of the Churches of Christ in the United States of America.

1990 Census of the Population and Housing Data Paper Listing (CPH-L-133). Washington, DC: U.S. Government Printing Office.

Chapter 13

Ethics and Culture: Contemporary Challenges

Mary E. Norton

KEY TERMS

Bioethics
Common Morality
Customary Morality
Eastern Ethical Perspectives

Ethics
Ethical Principles
Moral

Moral Anthropology
Theory
Value

OBJECTIVES

1. Evaluate a personal value system.
2. Compare Eastern and Western ethical perspectives.
3. Discuss ethical theories that can be used transculturally.
4. Apply ethical principles and theories in transcultural health care settings.
5. Use reflection, dialogue and critical thinking strategies in applying the Transcultural Ethical Decision Making Model.

Western Ethical Perspectives

> The nurse ... promotes an environment in which the values, customs, and spiritual beliefs of the individual are respected."
> International Council of Nurses, 1973

Providing culturally relevant health care within an ethical framework is a challenge for health care professionals throughout the world. This responsibility is further complicated when clients coming from one country or culture are introduced to a health care system in another part of the world, a system that has different cultural and moral traditions. The magnitude and complexity of the problem is reflected in the number of immigrants throughout the world. Currently, there are 85 million immigrants worldwide; 17 million are living on the North American continent (Bolini & Siemm, 1995). As a result, in the United States and Canada transcultural encounters are becoming more frequent in the delivery of health care.

While the populations of the United States and Canada are becoming more culturally diverse, the largest group of health care providers remains homogeneous. The nursing work force is composed primarily of European American women, most of whom are from working- and middle-class backgrounds. Consequently, the graduates of nursing programs must be prepared to care for clients from diverse cultural backgrounds who may have value and ethical systems different from their own. Chapter 14 discusses some of the problems and challenges inherent in a multicultural workforce.

The purposes of this chapter are to describe how health care providers can engage clients of health care in a dialogue that fosters mutual understanding through the sharing of values and beliefs. The second purpose is to provide a framework within which nurses can discuss and systematically resolve transcultural ethical issues. This framework encourages the health care provider and client to analyze traditional health care practices from an ethical perspective and then challenge their moral acceptability. Lastly, the third purpose is to provide the reader with a culturally relevant ethical decision-making model.

To achieve these purposes, the chapter begins by stressing the importance of values clarification for the professional and for clients. Personal values underlie the perspectives about the worth of any person, object or behavior. It is essential for nurses and clients to examine and understand their own value systems before they can respect those of others, or collaborate in ethical decision making. A values clarification tool for professionals and a transcultural values clarification tool for clients will be introduced and described. This discussion will be followed by definitions of ethics and bioethics, a discussion of various transcultural ethical perspectives, and a summary of the international and transcultural progress of bioethics during the last decade. Ethical theories and principles that provide a basic foundation to identify and analyze contemporary transcultural ethical issues will be explored.

Traditional cultural practices are discussed in the context in which they occur and ethical acceptability of several of the practices are challenged. An intervention strategy will be introduced to help readers analyze ethical problems arising from traditional cultural practices that might be commonly encountered by the nurse. The cultural examples used in this chapter are *not intended* to stereotype any particular cultural group. Rather, they are used to heighten the reader's awareness to different health beliefs and behaviors. The examples also illustrate the influence of personal values and culture on the identification of ethical issues and on the ethical approach used to resolve them. The use of ethical principles in transcultural nursing practice as well as challenges to ethical theories are discussed. Influences on transcultural health care delivery as a result of cultural differences are described, and examples are provided. Lastly, a culturally sensitive transcultural ethical decision making model is introduced. Critical thinking skills of the reader are strengthened by completing selected learning activities and analyzing case studies.

Transcultural Values Clarification

Values are a freely chosen set of personal beliefs or attitudes about truth, the worth of any thought, object, person or behavior (Kozier, Erb & Blais, 1997). Values give direction and meaning to one's life and play a significant role in making choices.

Health care providers and clients cannot take for granted common value systems or common understanding of disease or illness. In addition, misunderstandings can arise about causation, treatment and adherence to medical regimens (Gerteis, Daley & Delbanco, 1993; Dugger, 1997; Knight, 1997). Nor can providers and/or clients assume similar perspectives exist toward accidents, illness, health, or the traditions surrounding transitional life events, such as birth and death (Mydan, 1995). In addition, value differences also exist among different groups within the same culture. These value differences are based on age, caste, class, education, gender, geographic location, political and religious beliefs, and traditions (Nasr, 1981). Value differences within a culture are less noticeable when the members share a common language. The nurse cannot assume that people who share the same culture and language also share the same values. However, it is true that transcultural differences between health care providers and clients are more conspicuous when they are deeply rooted and based on different ways of everyday living, different systems of meaning, and different ways of social understanding (Jecker, Carrese & Pearlman, 1995).

Personal values also underlie the perspectives from which health care providers and clients attempt to resolve ethical issues. Therefore, it is important for health professionals and clients to have a clear understanding of their personal values and beliefs before engaging in any kind of ethical decision-making in crises conditions.

The Nurse

It is expected that the nurse, while providing care, will promote an environment in which the values, customs and spiritual beliefs of clients will be respected (International Council of Nurses, 1973). Nurses must understand their own values and beliefs before they can respect those of clients. The process of values clarification provides the nurse with an opportunity for deeper self-understanding as well as the discovery of those values that are prized and cherished. Values clarification also enables the nurse to identify and understand which values are fixed or those that are changing or emerging (Steele & Harmon, 1983; Eliason, 1993; Spector, 1996). These personal values provide a foundation for the development of professional values. As a professional nurse continues to grow and change, his/her values and beliefs may also change. Many changes often occur during the educational process as the student is exposed to new ideas, new people and different life situations. Changes in values continue throughout life. The process of self-examination should be an ongoing practice to enable nurses to continually clarify and reevaluate their value systems. There are several values clarification strategies by which health care providers can come to know themselves (Spradley & Allender, 1996). Box 13-1 contains a learning activity that is helpful for nurses and others to use to clarify and understand their own values.

The Client

In a transcultural health care setting, sometimes the clients' value and beliefs systems are ignored or greatly misunderstood. It is essential for health care professionals to understand the values and beliefs that guide the lives of the clients in their care. Helping clients clarify their beliefs and values will also aid nurses in better understanding *each particular client,* fostering an understanding between themselves and clients, and

Box 13-1. *Understanding Own Values*

After answering the following questions you will understand some of own unique values.

Step 1   Please take an index card and proceed as follows:

1. In the center of the card write your name.
2. Underneath your name write a word or statement that best describes you.
3. In one corner write the title of the best book you ever read. Why?
4. In another corner name one thing you do well.
5. In the third corner name one thing you would like to do better.
6. In the fourth corner write two values from you childhood.
   a. Write the name of the person who taught you that value.
   b. Do these values influence you today? How?
   c. If not, why not?

Step 2   Now examine the values you have just described.

1. Have your values changed from childhood?
2. Which values have changed? Why?
3. Which values have not changed? Why?
4. Prioritize your values. Which values will guide your behavior in ethical situations?
5. What one word or phrase would you now use to describe yourself?

Step 3   Now exchange your value sheet with a classmate—preferably someone from another culture or geographic area—and discuss the following questions.

1. Are your values similar? Why?
2. Are your values different? Why?
3. Will the differences in values lead to ethical conflicts? Why? Why not?
4. Dialogue with this person regarding your feelings about working with people who have values different from yours. And also share your views of the values of people from other cultures.

(Spradley B. W. & Allender J. A., 1996; Chitty K. K., 1997; Clark M. J., 1996)

delivering culturally relevant care. Understanding each client's values will prevent the nurse from assuming that clients share the values of the nurse's cultural group. Indeed, the client may not adhere to cultural values that are shared by others of the same culture. Some clients may be questioning their traditional values or may have rejected them.

The assessment and clarification of values requires clients to thoughtfully reflect on serious and often intimate subjects that may be difficult to think about and discuss. One way to approach this assessment is to share questions about health care decisions with a particular client and ask him or her to think about the questions and write down the answers. Of course, this approach assumes that the nurse has already assessed the client's literacy and writing ability. Some clients are not comfortable writing down answers to questions, or they may find this approach a bit patronizing. Another technique would be to ask clients to discuss the questions and their responses with their family members or other significant others. This method would foster communication among all "key" persons in the client's life. It may also help the family

Box 13-2 *Transcultural Assessment and Clarification of Values and Beliefs*

To the client—The health care professionals assigned to care for you want to understand your *values and beliefs* so they can deliver culturally relevant health care. Please assist them in better understanding you by completing this form.

Background Information

1. Where were you born?
2. How long have you lived in the United States?
3. Did you receive any formal education in the United States? How much?
4. Where were your family members born?

Relationships

5. Who are the decision makers in your family?
6. Who do you consider "family?"
7. Who do you want to make health care decisions for you?
8. In the event you cannot make health care decisions for yourself, who would you appoint to make these decisions for you?

Communication

9. What language do you consider your "mother" tongue?
10. Do you read and write in your "mother" tongue?
11. In which language do you prefer to receive health information?

Cultural Bonds

12. What cultural traditions do you observe in your home?

Religious Affiliation

13. Do you have a religious affiliation? If so, what is the affiliation?
14. Do your cultural or religious beliefs influence your attitude toward health care?
    a. Do these beliefs influence your attitude toward prevention of illness? If so, how?
    b. Do these beliefs influence your attitude toward treatment of illness? If so, how?
15. How would you describe your health status?
16. Do you have *any* symptoms that require "healing?"
17. How long have you had these symptoms?
18. What "healing" strategies do you use to relieve these symptoms?
19. Do these symptoms affect your ability to work or fulfill other obligations?
20. During your course of treatment what cultural/religious beliefs would you like us to consider?

Other

21. Is there anything else you would like to share with us that would help us care for you in a more sensitive way?

If clinically related to the diagnosis or chief complaint, it may be useful to collect data about transplantation, organ donation, autopsy, blood transfusions, drugs containing alcohol or caffeine, or foods that are taboo or prohibited.

Box developed using data from Spector, R. E. (1996). *Cultural Diversity in Health and Illness* (4th ed.). Stamford, CT: Appleton & Lange.

to know and understand the feelings of the client on topics they would not usually discuss because they might believe that they implicitly know the answers. After the task has been completed, the health care professional, the client, the family and/or significant others could discuss the responses. This kind of discussion will help health care professionals better understand the cultural and ethical issues of health care delivery from the client's perspective. Box 13-2 contains an assessment form; however, a word of caution is in order as it is not meant to be an exhaustive inventory of clients' beliefs and values. Rather, it is a starting point in the dialogue to foster mutual understanding among providers and recipients of health care.

Transcultural Assessment and Clarification of Values and Beliefs

Ethics and Bioethics

Ethics is a systematic philosophical method of inquiry that assists people in under-standing the morality (rightness or wrongness) of human behavior and social policies. Ethics also refers to the standards of behavior expected of members of professional groups. These standards are described in codes of professional conduct (Fry, 1994). It is important for nurses to have a knowledge of ethics in order to develop an ethical framework to guide their professional practice and to cope with ethical uncertainties stemming from work with clients, families, and colleagues. Ethical uncertainties will become more challenging during the next century with the increased use of health care technology (Leininger, 1997). Ethical knowledge also prepares nurses to fully participate in multidisciplinary ethical discussions as members of bioethics com-mittees.

Bioethics is the utilization of ethical inquiry to generate moral responses while analyzing difficult questions arising in health care delivery and social policies. The principal historic starting point of the field of bioethics as a discipline was in 1970 (Reich, 1996). The word *bioethics* was first introduced in 1971 by the American oncologist Van Rensselaer Potter in his book *Bioethics: Bridge to the Future*. He stated, "A science of survival must be more than a science alone, and I therefore propose the term *Bioethics* in order to emphasize the two most important ingredients in achieving the new wisdom that is so desperately needed: biological knowledge and human values" (p. 2).

The distinctive feature of bioethics is that it widens the field of medical ethics to include all issues of life, health, health care and the ethical problems and issues that arise in all health professions. Moreover, it extends to biomedical and behavioral research and includes a broad range of social and political issues such as the allocation of health care nationally and internationally, problems in public and occupational health, and population control (Reich, 1996). Therefore, bioethics fosters awareness that general health is dependent upon factors that are not inherently "medical" such as nutrition, hygiene, housing, work conditions and lifestyle. Bioethics is society's attempt to manage the new and far-reaching powers over life, powers coming from developments in the scientific community. Attempting to bridge the gap that separates the worlds of scientific facts and ethical values has been one of the most important accomplishments of bioethical reflection in the last 20 years.

Bioethics: An International and Transcultural View

Bioethics is a distinctive creation of North American culture. It is widely accepted that the field of bioethics originated in the United States, where it has gained an impressive position in academia, public policy and public education (Reich, 1996). Bioethics has also emerged and advanced in other countries and languages to an extraordinary degree, especially during the last decade (Dell'oro & Viafora, 1996). International developments in bioethics address a different range of issues, present different models of ethical analysis and provide new insights into the discipline. Moreover, bioethics as developed in countries with distinctively different moral mentalities and intellectual approaches has promoted international, intercultural and cross cultural dialogue (Norton, Walami & Hashim, 1995).

In the Mediterranean basin, for example, the multitude of cultural traditions have created a strong association with virtue, character and moral anthropology as the method of ethical analysis. Anthropology usually refers to one particular aspect of a group such as culture, sociology or psychology, whereas moral anthropology or philosophical anthropology considers the human being in its totality (Viafora,1996). An anthropological model illustrates a particular image of what a human being *is*. Within this perspective the human being is considered to be more than a quantitative and functional boundary. Ethical values are seen as a requirement for personhood. In addition, there is a constant search for the values upon which the human dimension of existence is grounded. Ethical issues are not reduced to questions of maximizing happiness but embrace issues of meaning and value. The anthropological model also helps develop a system of values that shapes the meaning of life, suffering and death. Finally, it determines patterns of behavior, criteria of evaluation and motivation for action. It also influences the understanding of other concepts such as health, therapy, and healing (Viafora,1996).

In contrast, in the North American continent during the 1960s and 1970s, a process of patients' emancipation gave rise to the patients' rights movement. The movement promoted a respect for patient autonomy and the principle of informed consent. During this time physicians were persuaded not only to share information with patients about their illnesses, but also to ensure that patients had sufficient understanding of the information to give an informed consent for treatments, procedures and participation in research. Thus, the role of the patient evolved from one of dependence on the physician to make clinical decisions to one of mutual participation in designing treatment plans (Szasz & Hollender, 1956). The process found expression in the language of rights; such as the right of informed consent. It was a language quite familiar in the Western cultural context that arose from the various rights movement of the decade; for example; the civil rights and/or women's rights movement. In addition, the human rights movement supported the patient's rights movement and the bioethical movement in general (Viafora, 1996). As a result, it was the language of rights that influenced the development of bioethics in the West in contrast to the language of virtues and duties, which characterized ethical traditions in other parts of the world.

Currently, bioethics occupies an increasingly important place in public discussions in a number of different countries on all continents (Suborne, 1992; McDonald, Machizawa & Satoh, 1992; Tong & Spicer, 1994; Al-Awadi, 1996; Dell'oro & Viafora,

1996). The First International Congress on Bioethics was held in Mexico City in 1994 (Fluss, 1995). Because of the differences in value systems and approaches to ethics across cultures, it is extraordinary difficult to write ethical texts for world populations. The Convention on Human Rights and Biomedicine is a document that exemplifies the difficulty of the task. It took a decade and a half of discussions and debates before the Committee of Ministers of the Council of Europe approved the document for adoption by its 39 members in November of 1996 (de Wachter, 1997). Two international organizations have taken a leading role in global ethics. The first is the Council for International Organizations of Medical Sciences. The second is the World Health Organization. During 1997 meetings in Switzerland, both organizations addressed and linked the issues of ethics and equity with human rights considerations. Such international developments in bioethics illustrate a marked change from 15 years ago, when there was very little activity in the discipline outside of the United States. The recent developments also have illustrated the complexity of ethical discussion across national boundaries (Lie, 1995).

Survey of Ethical Theories

Ethical theory provides a framework within which professionals can reflect on the moral nature (rightness or wrongness) of actions and can evaluate moral judgments and moral character as well as proposed policies (Beauchamp & Childress, 1994). Some knowledge of these theories is essential for reflective ethical decision making. The term *theory* is used to refer to systematic reflection and argument and to an integrated body of principles. Moral reality is very complex and any one theory may give only a partial insight to moral truth. It would be best to consider each theory as a partial contribution to a comprehensive moral vision (Arras, 1995). It is important for nurses to be aware of the various ethical frameworks to help in structuring and resolving the ethical uncertainties in contemporary professional practice. Furthermore, nurses care for clients from various cultural backgrounds and traditions and should be aware of ethical models that will enable them to deliver ethical health care within a transcultural nursing framework.

There are several ways to classify ethical theories. Since it is predicted that diverse spiritual and ethical issues will be emphasized in the next century and principles of transcultural nursing care require a respect for cultural diversity, consideration will be given to both the *Eastern* and *Western* classifications of ethical perspectives and theories (Leininger, 1991, 1997).

Eastern ethical theories are based on Asian or Indian philosophies and may also be influenced by religious systems of belief. Confucianism is an example of an Eastern ethical theory. All the teachings of this theory involve human relations and it emphasizes the virtues of righteousness (*yi*) and benevolence (*yen*) that combine all virtues and can be considered the perfect virtue. This theory views man as an essentially social creature bound to his fellow man by *jen,* that is sympathy, human-heartedness or loving others. Jen is expressed through the five relations: sovereign and subject, parent and child, elder and younger brother, husband and wife, and friend and friend. An important aspect of benevolence is the concept of mutuality or reciprocal benevolence (*shu*) that stresses treating others as we would want to be treated. Ritual and etiquette help these relations function smoothly. Correct conduct proceeds through a sense of virtue developed by observing appropriate models of ethical conduct (Fry, 1994). In Eastern theories, the standard for conduct or measuring square comes from within the person. If after thoughtful consideration a person finds an action morally acceptable, they should act upon it without any hesitation (Chao, 1991).

Taoism was another philosophical school developed in China during the sixth century B.C. Taoism is concerned with the origin and meaning of life. This school believes that human happiness is achieved in following the natural order. It also emphasizes trusting in one's intuitive knowledge (Parry, 1995). Taoism focuses on the observation of nature in order to discover the characteristic of the Tao, or the way of life. This is in contrast to Confucianism, which focuses on man and values social conventions and rituals.

Western ethical theories are based on European or American philosophies and are influenced by Judeo-Christian belief systems. The western ethical theories that are briefly explored here are those believed to be the primary theories; for example, consequentialist and nonconsequentialist. *Consequential* theories are those that only examine the consequences of actions: Underlying these theories is a firm believe that the consequences of actions are the only relevant considerations in any assessment of behavior. Consequentialists claim that an action is right according to the balance of good consequences it produces. The action is wrong according to the balance of bad consequences it produces. The best known consequence-based theory is *utilitarianism*. The major principle of this theory is that of utility (Beauchamp & Childress, 1994). John Stuart Mill is the one individual who had the most significant influence on this theory as we know it today. The core of the theory is the greatest happiness principle. Actions are right in proportion that they tend to promote happiness and wrong as they tend to produce unhappiness (Arras, 1995). The theory provides the rationale for resource allocation and raises questions concerning the greatest net benefit from the allocation for a population. The theory is also closely related to cost effectiveness. For example, how much benefit is possible from health care expenditures (Bryant, Khan & Hyder, 1997).

An advantage of utilitarianism is that it requires us to consider the outcome of actions. The theory is sometimes referred to as the *calculus morality* because it requires us to calculate the probable consequences of every action, both long and short term to determine the amount of happiness or unhappiness the action will produce. For example: What are the long- and short-term consequences of genetic engineering and gene therapy? A disadvantage of utilitarianism is that money and resources will be given to projects that will serve the largest segment of the population even if these practices conflict with the principle of justice. Utilitarians do not believe that suffering and sacrifice have any intrinsic moral worth as the right action is the one that promotes the most happiness or the greatest pleasure (Arras, 1995).

A nonconsequentialist perspective is that in which ethical decisions are *not* based on the outcomes of an action, rather on the *rightness or wrongness of the action itself* (Childress, 1989).

Such a theory is known as *duty-based ethics*. Professional codes of ethics are based on ideas of duty and stem from nonconsequentialist perspectives. A major proponent of nonconsequentialist perspectives was Immanuel Kant. In Kant's work or theory, an action was considered moral if it originated from good will or good intention (Chitty, 1997). Kant also believed an *action could bring about happiness and might still be wrong and that consequences can never make an wrong action right.* For example: six terminally ill patients are in need of transplants. It is permissible to hasten another patient's death in order to distribute the organs and save these six lives? Utilitarians would say this is the maximum benefit—saving six lives at the expense or sacrifice of only one. Kant would say the act of murder is *intrinsically wrong* and cannot make the action right, regardless of the number of lives that could be saved.

The emphasis of Kant's theory is on the ability of a person to think and plan; that is, to reason. This ability gives humans a special moral status that leads to a respect for persons, their plans and goals. Showing respect for other individuals is demonstrated by telling them the truth and insisting on informed consent for clients and research subjects (Arras, 1995). Consequentialist and nonconsequentialist theories shape moral issues into frameworks structured by a single dominant principle. The principle is expressed in the context of Western language as rights and obligations. A limited comparison of Eastern and Western ethical perspectives is presented in Box 13-3.

Other ethical theories pertaining to nursing and transcultural delivery of health care are character ethics, community-based ethics, the ethics of care, and common morality. *Character ethics,* or virtue ethics, emphasizes the *people who perform actions and make choices* (Beauchamp & Childress, 1994) and originally was introduced by Aristotle (Arras, 1995). Character ethics suggests that moral issues in health care should be discussed in the framework of virtues; the belief is that character is more important than mere conformity to rules (Beauchamp & Childress, 1994). The essence of this model and moral life is reliable character, moral good sense, and emotional responsiveness. A person who has these characteristics will possess the *focal virtues* of integrity, discernment, compassion, and trustworthiness (Beauchamp & Childress, 1994). One may experience conflicting motivation arising from different virtues, and questions occur as to which one is the most appropriate to use; therefore, principles are essential to guide conduct. The implementation of the principles requires judgment, which flows from character, moral discernment and a person's sense of responsibility and accountability.

Virtues in character ethics can be inculcated through education, interactions, and role models. This theory has implications for health science faculties not only to teach these virtues in their educational programs but also to demonstrate them as role models in their human interactions. Faculties should also create a climate that motivates learners in the health care professions to desire the best for their clients rather than just imposing rules (Beauchamp & Childress, 1994). Virtues are also important in Confucianism, which emphasizes that proper behavior proceeds through a sense of virtue developed by observing suitable models of ethical behavior (Fry, 1994). From Confucius to Aristotle to Mill, most philosophers agree that *the most important ingredient in a person's moral life is a developed character that provides the inner motivation and strength to do what is right and good.*

Community-based theory (communitarianism) views ethical theory from communal values, the common good, social goals and traditional practices (Beauchamp & Childress, 1994). The proponents of this theory ask which rules, acts, and policies

Box 13-3 *Comparison of Eastern and Western Ethical Perspectives*

Eastern Ethical Theories

During the sixth century BC two philosophical systems developed in China—Confucianism and Taoism. The theories developed in these systems are based on Asian/Indian philosophies and may also be influenced by religious beliefs. The theories serve as ethical guidelines for living.

Confucianism

A. All teachings of this theory emphasize human relations.
B. Emphasizes the virtues of:
   1. Righteousness (yi)
   2. Benevolence (yen)
This virtue combines all virtues and is considered "perfect virtue."
Another aspect of benevolence is Shu, which stresses treating others as we would want to be treated.
C. This theory views humans as essentially social creatures.
   1. Humans are bound together by jen, that is, sympathy, human-heartedness, or loving others.
   2. Jen is expressed through five relations;
      —Sovereign and Subject
      —Parent and Child
      —Elder/Younger/Brother
      —Husband and Wife
      —Friend and Friend
      Ritual and etiquette help these relations function smoothly.
D. Correct conduct proceeds through a sense of virtue developed by observing appropriate models of ethical conduct (Fry, 1994).
E. The standard of conduct comes from within a person.
F. If after thoughtful consideration a person finds an action morally acceptable, that person should act without any hesitation (Chao, 1991).

Western Ethical Theories

Theories are based on European or American philosophies and are influenced by Judeo-Christian beliefs.

Consequentialism

A. John Stuart Mill had the greatest influence on the theory as we know it today.
B. The theory only examines consequences of action.
C. An action is right if it produces good consequences.
D. An action is wrong if it produces bad consequences.
E. Best known consequence-based theory is utilitarianism.
   1. The only principle is utility (Beauchamp & Childress, 1994).
   2. The core of the theory is "the greatest happiness principle."
   3. Actions are right if they tend to promote happiness and wrong if they tend to promote unhappiness (Arras, 1995)
F. The theory provides the rationale for resource allocation.
   1. It is concerned with getting the greatest net benefit from resource allocation and health care expenditures to a population, a project, or the development of a new drug (Bryant, Khan, & Hyder, 1997).
G. Advantages of this theory
   1. It requires consideration of the outcomes of actions.
   2. It requires calculating of the probable consequences of every action, both long and short term.
H. Disadvantages of this theory
   1. There are many disadvantages of this theory. In principle it permits the interests of the majority to override the rights of the minority (Beauchamp & Childress, 1994).
   2. Another is the possibility of conflicts with other moral principles such as justice, truth telling, and keeping promises in order to achieve maximal good consequences (Arras, 1995).

Box 13-3. *(Continued)*

Eastern Ethical Theories

Taoism

Taoism is the other philosophical system developed in China during the sixth century BC

A. Taoism is concerned with the origin and meaning of life.

B. This system believes that human happiness is achieved in following the natural order.

C. It emphasizes trusting in one's intuitive knowledge.

D. Taoism focuses on the observation of nature in order to discover the "characteristic of the Tao," or the way of life.

 Taoism focuses on the observation of nature to discover the way of life, whereas Confucianism focuses on man and values, social conventions and rituals.

Western Ethical Theories

Nonconsequentialism

Theories are those in which ethical decisions are not based on the outcome of an action but on the *rightness or wrongness of the action itself* (Childress, 1989).

A. The major proponent of this theory was Immanuel Kant.

B. The theory is commonly known as *duty-based ethics.*

 1. Professional codes of ethics are based on this theory (Clark, 1996).

C. The theory also proposes that an action could bring about happiness and might still be wrong, *and consequences could never make a wrong action right.*

D. Humans have the ability to think, and this ability confers a special moral status.

 1. The special moral status of humans requires us to respect people and their goals.

 2. Respect for persons is demonstrated by telling them the truth and by insisting on informed consent for clients and research subjects (Arras, 1995).

Consequentialism and nonconsequentialism shape moral issues into frameworks structured by a single dominant principle. This principle is expressed in the Western language context in terms of rights and obligations.

best reinforce and promote communal values including family values. The question to be asked is, What is most conducive to a good society? Not, Is it harmful or does it violate autonomy? (Callahan, 1990). The theory accepts the pluralistic conceptions of the *good life* and its recognition of some individual rights. It depends on democratic initiatives to fashion a community conception of the *good life* into policies and laws. One vision of the implementation of the theory is found in community health planning when citizen members deliberate their conception of the *good life* and debate policies and allocation of health care resources in their community (Emmanuel, 1991). Communitarians emphasize the need to foster neighborhood associations, create communal ties and promote public health. This empowers the community to assert control over factors that affect their health (Airhihenbuwa, 1995). Moreover, this theory supports the general transcultural principles of respect for the cultural diversity of clients so that appropriate health and nursing care can be provided (Leininger, 1991)

The *ethic of care* originated in feminist writings. These writings explored how women display an ethic of care, in contrast to men who predominantly exhibit an ethic of rights and obligations. Carol Gilligan, a psychologist, has played a prominent role in the development of this theory (Beauchamp & Childress, 1994). The theory is applicable to nursing because care is a concept that is of interest to nursing and nursing theorists. In fact, the way in which professionals should care is an ethical question (Ray, 1994). Ray (1994) suggested that in a culturally diverse society, ethical questions expand to include how people ought to live with members of communities who share the same world but hold different views of human virtues, ethical principles, cultural values and religious beliefs.

The ethics of care theory emphasizes traits valued in intimate personal relationships, for example: sympathy, compassion, fidelity, and discernment. Caring refers to care for, emotional commitment to, and a willingness to act on behalf of persons with whom we have a significant relationship. Although care and its action derivative caring have numerous and diverse meanings, Ray (1994) emphasized that caring is a relational discipline. A common theme in nursing is interrelatedness, or the way in which one stands with or is connected to the other. In the ethics of care theory, Kantian universal rules, impartial utilitarian calculations and individual rights are de-emphasized. *The ethics of care theory emphasizes that actions are important, as well as the promotion of positive relationships* (Beauchamp & Childress, 1994). This principle is found also in Eastern ethical theories.

The ethics of care theory maintains that the clients in the health care system are vulnerable, and the appropriate moral response from the health care provider is attentiveness to their needs, more than just a respect for their rights. The ethics of care also has a strong cognitive dimension since it involves an insight into and understanding of another's circumstances, needs, and feelings. In contrast to the rights-based theories, then, the ethics of care gives emotions a moral role.

A common morality theory takes its basic assumptions from the morality shared in common by the members of society such as common sense and tradition (Beauchamp & Childress, 1994). Common morality theories are pluralistic although they emphasize principles of obligation as consequence and non consequence-based theories, they do not advocate one principle to support all actions in the model. In addition, common morality ethics stresses ordinary shared moral beliefs for their content rather than depending on pure reason. *Common morality* is *not* synonymous with *customary morality* that is based on local customs and attitudes. *Common morality* is a pretheoretic moral point of view that transcends local customs and attitudes and is based on principles universally accepted by other ethical theories. An important function of the principles of the common morality theory is to challenge local customs and attitudes that fail to acknowledge *common moral* viewpoints and *basic moral principles* such as autonomy and justice (Beauchamp & Childress, 1994). The principles of the common morality theory that apply to nursing are autonomy, beneficence, justice, veracity, and fidelity and are defined in Box 13-4 (Fry, 1994). The principles primarily order, classify and group moral norms. Nurses, in thinking about ethical issues, should link together the strands of more general rules, rights and virtues that are the highest importance to health care ethics with the more particular feelings and perceptions.

Box 13-4 *Ethical Principles*

Autonomy is the ethical principle that states individuals ought to be permitted to determine their own actions according to plans they have chosen (Fry, 1994). To respect individuals as autonomous persons is to accept their choices, which stem from personal beliefs and values. When applying this principle cross culturally, one should remember that the way patients exercise their autonomy will be shaped by their sociocultural context, including religion and other beliefs. Autonomous patients may choose to delegate decision making to others, as frequently occurs among many ethnic groups (Beauchamp & Childress, 1994).

Beneficence is the obligation to do good and avoid doing harm. Nurses are obliged to implement actions that benefit clients (Kozier, Erb, & Blais, 1997). The first duty of this principle is not to inflict harm on the patient.

Fidelity is defined as the obligation to remain faithful to one's commitments (Fry, 1994). These commitments are obligations implicit in a trusting relationship between patient and health care provider, such as keeping promises and maintaining confidentiality. Contemporary nursing roles sharpen obligations of fidelity to patients such as being a patient advocate. Fidelity is supported by the code of nursing ethics. When acting as a patient advocate, the nurse may create conflict with other members of the health care team who may not agree with this viewpoint (Beauchamp & Childress, 1994). Nurses may be negotiating with members of the health care team who may be members of subcultures of the dominant society, and their values and perceptions of the principles may differ from the dominant society. For example, a nurse may be advocating for patients who want their advance directives honored when they are unable to speak for themselves. Other members of the team, who are not members of the dominant society, may not want to honor these directives because they believe it is their duty to always preserve life.

Justice is a principle that requires equals to be treated equally, and those with unequal needs to be treated differently (Fry, 1994). This statement means when people have equal health needs they should be treated the same, but if their needs are greater, they should receive additional help or resources.

Veracity is the obligation to tell the truth and not deceive others (Fry, 1994). Truthfulness is regarded as essential to the existence of trust in many cultures. Based on this tradition, truthfulness has a special significance in health care relationships in many parts of the world. It is expected as part of the respect owed persons. However, some cultures regard truthfulness in health care relationships differently from other cultures. Truthfulness is required but may be carried out differently. Instead of telling the truth to the patient, the health care provider may be obliged to first tell the other members of the family. The family may then decide not to tell the patient. This method is considered in some cultures to be supportive to family relationships (Fry, 1994; Norton, Walani, & Hashim, 1995).

Discussion of Ethical Principles Transculturally

Although the principles of ethics are fairly clear, they may conflict with each other when one applies them transculturally. Generalizations about clients and their families without careful attention to their cultural background, their values and norms could lead to considerable difficulties in the patient/provider relationship. Issues surrounding informed consent, disclosure of diagnosis and prognosis and discussions of termination of treatment often are reflections of Western cultural values. These particular issues represent respect for the individual and autonomy of clients as well as a respect for openness in communication (Meleis & Jonsen, 1983). A good example of how individualism is reflected in cultural values and norms can be see in the manner in which clients exercise autonomy, which is prototypically expressed in the language of rights.

Let us discuss a situation where this may occur. A client could come from a variety of cultures such as Italian Pakistani or Japanese where the family would expect that the health care provider would share bad news with them first before talking with the individual client (Surbone, 1992; Norton, Walani & Hashim, 1995; Kristof, 1995). The family, in turn, will decide what information should be given to the client. Traditionally in these cultures, the emphasis is on beneficence, that is, on trying to shield clients from distressing information that may cause them increased anxiety. The pronounced emphasis on autonomy that prevails in the United States does not exist in numerous other cultures. In Japan the custom has been to share information regarding a poor prognosis only if adequate treatment is available (Kristof, 1995). In some societies or groups, it is culturally implicit to delegate decision making to others. Pellegrino (1992) suggests that some clients expect to be buffered from negative information about their prognosis and to provide them with details about their condition may be a harmful interpretation of respect for autonomy. In this situation *the obligation to respect the patient's autonomy remains,* although the pull of another principle—beneficence—may be stronger.

Thus, it is *very important* to remember that clients may vary in their views of wanting to know information about their illnesses. These differences may be due to variations of education, socioeconomic class, religious beliefs, degree of acculturation, as well as differences among cultural groups (Lane & Rubenstein, 1996). A study conducted of one group for whom dominant Western bioethical principles are not applicable is found in the accompanying Research Application 13-1 entitled Responses to Sharing of Information About a Serious Illness in Karachi.

Research Application 13-1   *Responses to Sharing of Information About a Serious Illness in Karachi*

Norton, M. E., Walani, S., & Hashim, F. (1995). Individuals' responses to sharing information about a serious illness: A survey in Karachi. In J. Wang (Ed.). *Health Care and Culture.* Morgantown, WV: University of West Virginia Press.

Health care professionals in Pakistan usually do not share health status information with seriously ill patients. The practice is to share information with the family who usually withholds the information from the patient. Therefore, patients cannot make informed decisions related to their treatment. Currently, there is no literature related to Pakistan on truth telling, patient autonomy or informed consent. This exploratory study describes individuals' responses to receiving essential information concerning their health status if they are seriously ill and the rationale for withholding or sharing information with a family member regarding the seriousness of a client's illness. A convenience sample consisted of 50 Pakistani adults, with a mean age of 37.4 years, from diverse educational and occupational backgrounds. Data were collected using a semi-structured interview guide. Ninety-three percent of the sample wanted essential information if they were seriously ill. However, only 35 percent would inform a family member of the seriousness of their illness, 40 percent would not inform them, 23 percent said it depends on the characteristics of the patient and nature of the disease. The study considers the cultural implications of data collection, and provides preliminary, culturally based data on disclosure of health status information to the seriously ill in Pakistan.

Clinical Application

• Ask family members (usually the eldest son, the father or oldest male) if it is appropriate to share information about the diagnosis or seriousness of the patients condition.

Carrese and Rhodes (1995) studied traditional values in a Navajo population and found that members of their sample did not share the values and moral perspectives of the white dominant society. In particular, values surrounding such things as negative information, disclosure of risk or bad news were markedly different in this study group. For example, in traditional Navajo culture, thought and language have the power to shape reality and control events. It is extremely important that health care professionals, as well as others, think and speak in a positive way and avoid negative thinking and speaking. Advance care planning, such as advanced directives and end-of-life treatment decisions may be a dangerous violation of traditional Navajo values and ways of thinking.

In many Eastern cultures, the debate continues about the use of Western ethical decision-making models in trying to resolve ethical questions. However, the theory of common morality and ethical principles can be utilized across cultures by various health care professionals in concert with the caring and communitarian theories. The health care professional, utilizing the virtues of integrity, compassion, trustworthiness and discernment in a caring and sensitive manner, can share with the family and client information about an illness and its treatment. It can be done within different cultural frameworks and should be based on the values and beliefs of the individual client and family.

Ethics and Culture—Challenges to Ethical Theories

Ethical relativism occurs when the rightness or wrongness of an action or practice cannot be resolved apart from the cultural or social context in which it occurs (Arras, 1995). Relativism views morality as relative to the community within which an individual lives and the manner in which the individual was raised. For example, freedom of speech would only be a moral value for cultures that believe in it, or for cultural groups for whom it is a cultural value. Therefore, moral values are *only right* in sociocultural contexts *that think they are right*. This type of thinking does not allow for criticism of intolerant practices of others, now or in the past (Arras, 1995). However, the belief that morality occurs in a cultural context can be incorporated into a nonrelativist approach called *multiculturalism*.

Multiculturalism encourages us to try to understand other cultures and traditional practices within the sociocultural context in which they occur. This method fosters the understanding that there is a range of ways to live and solve problems. However, *it is not,* and *should not be,* an uncritical acceptance of the values and customs of others, or even one's own for that matter. Some examples of uncritical examples of other customs include slavery in the United States and traditional female genital surgeries conducted on African and some Middle Eastern and Asian women (Kluge, 1993; James, 1994; Lane & Rubenstein, 1996).

Now, of course, we are all aware of the dehumanizing aspects of slavery during the early development of the United States. Even when it was a fairly common practice, it was criticized and finally, legal procedures were initiated which demanded the practice be abolished. However, the female genital surgeries, broadly known as female circumcision and practiced since the 2nd Century B.C., have been a source of international debate only since the 1970s (Lane & Rubenstein, 1996). These various surgical procedures, done during childhood and performed without anesthesia or sterile surgical instruments, remove part or all of the external genitalia of women. The wound edges are sutured together and when healed, the scar tissue covers the urinary meatus and most of the vagina.

The procedure is performed on 80–114 million women in 27 different countries (Lane & Rubenstein, 1996). The immediate health effects of the procedure are hemorrhage, shock, infection, pain, and urinary retention. The long term health effects include urinary tract infections, obstructed labor, and chronic pelvic infections, all of which may contribute to infertility, and in some parts of the world, high rates of maternal mortality (Lane & Rubenstein, 1996). Concerns with virginity, marriageability and the husband's sexual pleasure are some of the commonly stated reasons for performing the procedure. Women from some of the countries where the surgeries are commonplace have requested political asylum in the United States to avoid forced circumcision for themselves or their daughters. Arab and African feminists condemn the medicalization of these surgeries because they believe that this would promote the continuance of this procedure, rather than its abandonment.

On the other hand, many members of societies that practice female genital surgeries do not view the result as mutilation. Women who are not circumcised are viewed as unclean and are not considered marriageable as "no man would want them." In a study conducted in 1996, when circumcised women were asked if they planned to circumcise their daughters, an overwhelming majority were in favor of the procedure (Lane & Rubenstein, 1996). In fact, these women questioned how a mother could neglect such an important part of her daughter's preparation for womanhood. Female genital surgeries are only one practice in an extremely complex array of issues that include, among others, East–West relations, gender issues, and the status of women. The practice also illustrates that not all members of a society adhere to a single set of norms. With increased numbers of immigrants and refugees now living in the United States, it is possible that nurses working in multicultural clinical settings may encounter parents who want these procedures for their daughters. Therefore, it is essential that the nurse be familiar with an intervention strategy for resolving ethical conflicts of traditional cultural practices. A suggestion for one such strategy is shown in Box 13-5.

> **Box 13-5** *Intervention Strategy for Ethical Problems of Traditional Cultural Practices*
>
> 1. A culturally responsive effort to address problematic practices should be honest and *respectful.*
> 2. It also involves *listening to* and *valuing* the perspective of the other person.
> 3. The intervention should be in a *"voice"* that engages the *"other"* as an equal partner.
> 4. The language, while expressing a respect of the practices of all cultures, *also recognizes that traditional practices, in some cases, must be viewed in a new light* (Lane, 1996). This can be done by collaborating with the client to:
>   A. Identify the current values.
>   B. Prioritize the values.
>   C. Identify the goal of the value.
>   D. Identify alternative methods to achieve the same goal.

Influences on Transcultural Health Care Delivery

In a culturally diverse environment, the nurse must be aware that all cultures have their own "ideal" health practices, lifestyles and values (Leininger, 1991). It is important to consider, and *appreciate,* the differences between the provider and recipient of health care. Differences in values can create ethical dilemmas. Differences in behaviors can create barriers to the delivery of culturally competent health care. Although, it would be impossible to develop a complete list of all possible variations, health care providers must be aware of some basic cultural and religious differences that may result in a delay in seeking health care, use of traditional cultural methods of healing, or even refusal of some medical procedures such as blood transfusions or immunizations.

Health Customs and Behaviors

Clients from diverse cultural backgrounds may delay seeking health care advice when they become ill. This behavior may be due to factors such as lack of health insurance or financial inability to take time off from work to visit a clinic. Often clients that come from other cultural groups or are recent immigrants may be poor and are not employed in positions that offer benefits such as health insurance. Sometimes, clients perceive that as long as they can work, they are not ill even though they may not feel well. As a result, symptoms of an illness may be ignored if they do not interfere too much with work responsibilities. Moreover, some clients may first seek the help of a traditional healer. Others may use traditional home remedies or herbal mixture before they seek the help of a Western trained physician (Huang, 1996).

Eastern health care practices emphasize the mobilization of the individual's innate capacity for self-healing. This self-healing mechanism also is used to enhance the quality of life. In addition, Western health care practices are believed to be limited and reductionist and may only concentrate on one aspect of health such as an elevated cholesterol level. This is in contrast to Eastern health care practices, which call for

Box 13-6 *Transcultural Health Behaviors Vignette*

In some Middle Eastern cultures, the usual custom is to first serve food to the husband and children, and then to women. As a result women get the leftovers, and this may be a small quantity. This practice results in a poor nutritional status for women, particularly for those of childbearing age. This practice, coupled with women having multiple pregnancies, puts their health in great jeopardy.

1. Is there an ethical issue in this vignette?
2. If there is an ethical issue, what theory would you use to resolve the issue? Why would you use this theory?
3. What whould you do about this practice if you were the community health nurse in this area?

a more holistic approach. Eastern healers believe that the mind, body and spirit form an integral whole, and generally speaking, healers concentrate more on the person than the disease (Sheikh & Sheikh, 1989; Presswalla, 1994). Some groups of the Indian subcontinent focus on quality of life in the treatment of imperiled newborns rather than sanctity of life because of the strong belief in rebirth (Lie, 1995). Some Arab clients believe words have power to control life events, so they may minimize symptoms and refrain from discussing negative incident, such as previous illnesses (Meleis, Lipson, Solomon & Omidian 1989; Via, Callahan, Barry, Jackson & Gerber, 1997). These health beliefs and behaviors are significantly different from the Western scientific orientation to disease and treatment with the emphasis on medical diagnosis. An example of different beliefs and practices that influence health is shown in Box 13-6.

Preventative Health Behaviors

Preventative health measures are not considered important in some cultures, and some may even may be forbidden in some groups. Therefore, by time the client seeks health care, the illness may have progressed to an advanced stage and death may be a possible outcome. Usually this behavior causes health care providers to feel frustrated, since they believe the illness could have been prevented. An example is the polio outbreak that occurred in the Netherlands in 1992. See the vignette described in Box 13-7.

Communication

Communication is another important consideration in delivering culturally competent health and nursing care. The fact that English is not the primary language of many Americans may create communication difficulties for health care providers. Because of the language diversity in health care institutions, the American Hospital Association Bill of Rights for Patients contains a provision for ensuring that *patient rights* include being able to meet their communication needs (Guido, 1997). This provision is particularly important for patients who speak English poorly, are unable to express themselves clearly, or misunderstand what is said to them.

To prevent these occurrences many hospitals now have "language banks" or lists

Box 13-7 *Transcultural Health Prevention Vignette*

In this situation, members of a religious group considered immunizations as an act against the will of God. Therefore, the group members refused the polio immunization. When a group member developed polio, it sparked an outbreak of the disease and posed a serious health threat to the community. As a result, 71 people developed the disease and 2 died. Even after the outbreak, compliance within the high-risk group was scattered and their immunity remains uncertain (Oostvagel, 1995).

1. What is the ethical issue in this vignette?
2. How would you frame this ethical issue for discussion?
   a. What theory would you use to resolve the issue?
   b. Why would you use this theory?
3. What would you do in the situation described in this vignette if you were the community health nurse in this community?

of bilingual staff to assist in communicating with culturally diverse clients. However, sometimes the interpreter is a nonmedical staff member and does not understand the medical information that is to be communicated; this can be very problematic (Turner, 1997). To ensure accuracy, it is important that the person translating have an understanding of the material to be communicated. When an interpreter is used, the preference is for a person of the same gender and relative age as the client. In addition, it is important that interpreters translate the information exactly as it is stated. If interpreters simply summarize the information to be conveyed, it can contribute to confusion and lack of understanding by the client.

Cultural courtesy in communications also requires that health care providers refrain from calling clients by their first names since this practice may be considered rude in some cultures, particularly if the client is older than the health care provider. An important consideration in Western communication is direct eye contact, as well as a direct approach to problems. On the other hand, Muslim cultures strongly discourage direct eye contact between genders, and in Asian cultures, direct eye contact is considered impolite. Members of Asian cultures prefer subtlety and indirectness over a direct approach to solving problems. In addition, nearly all cultures have well-developed systems of nonverbal communication. For example, for individuals from Pakistan, a clicking sound made by the tongue along with a tilting of the head, indicates a negative response. Another consideration is the volume of the message to be delivered. Arab clients will perceive the importance of the message based on how loud, forceful and emphatic it is delivered (Via et al., 1997; Nydell, 1987). See the accompanying vignette in Box 13-8.

Ethnicity of Health Provider and Recipients

Clients may feel culturally distant from health care providers. Clients may come from one of the federally defined minority groups and the health professional from the dominant society. The reverse may also be true, with the professionals coming from a minority group. Both scenarios can cause difficulty in communication. See the vignette described in Box 13-9.

Box 13-8 *Transcultural Communications Vignette*

An older Muslim man from Nepal comes to a clinic in the United States complaining of back pain. Since he speaks little English, he is accompanied by his young adult grand-daughter who will serve as his translator. At the end of the visit, the client is asked to have several diagnostic tests done before a treatment plan is developed.

When the client returns the next week, the nurse learns he has not completed the diag-nostic tests. Again his granddaughter accompanies him and she tells the nurse he wants a massage. The nurse reiterates that the diagnostic tests must be completed be-fore anything else is done. After repeating this same scenario for two or more visits, the client is labeled "noncompliant."

1. Is there a problem in cross-cultural communication in this vignette? If so, describe the cross-cultural communication problems.
2. What could be done to improve the communication?
3. Is the patient "noncompliant?"

Box 13-9 *Transcultural Ethnicity of Health Provider Vignette*

The following scenario occurred during a case presentation in a large, inner-city metro-politan Health Sciences Center. The clients were an American family, and the physi-cian was Asian. In the Asian culture "losing face" and politeness are very important cultural considerations. The family had accused the physician of being lazy and negli-gent in caring for their child. It was obvious during the case presentation that the phy-sician felt she was "losing face" and she mentioned several times how hurt she was by the accusations. The physician then went on to emphasize how polite and courte-ous the father had been in the past, and now he was acting so arrogant. The physi-cian continued to reiterate how hurt she was by the family's accusations. When asked about reports from the family's previous health care providers, the physician reported she did not have them. The physician, fearing that the family would think she was checking up on them and that this would jeopardize their relationship, did not contact previous health providers. The participants in the case presentation respected the phy-sician's feelings and the physician was asked, "If the father apologized would you con-sider continuing to treat the family?" The physician agreed to continue to treat the family without an apology but again stated that she was very hurt by the accusations.

1. Even though the family members and the health provider spoke English, do you think they had a communication problem?
2. What are the cultural implications in this communication?
3. Do you think the physician has a clear understanding of *her own values* and how they impact patient care?
4. What are the ethical implications of the case?
5. What suggestions would you give to this physician for understanding clients from other cultures?

Educational Variations

Another consideration is the educational variation between the recipient and provider of health care. The client may not have a high educational level and may not understand the health care instructions. He or she may be embarrassed or ashamed to admit his/her lack of understanding of the information or instructions that the physician or nurse provide. As a result, clients may not follow the instructions, show minimal improvement and be labeled as *non-compliant.*

Time Perceptions

Clients from other cultures frequently have a different conception of time from the health care provider. The health care provider may measure time by appointments and punctuality, whereas the client measures it in terms of activities. So, if clients are involved in an another activity, they may fail to keep a clinic appointment. The health care provider may be future oriented and make appointments for follow-up visits, whereas clients, particularly Middle Eastern clients, may believe that life follows a preordained course and they should not interfere with it by making appointments for the future.

A Culturally Sensitive Ethical Decision-Making Model

Ethical decision-making models provide a framework in which ethical issues can be analyzed in an orderly manner. Most often the literature that is read by health care professionals in the United States frames the principles of ethics in health care within Western ethical traditions. Therefore, it is easy to neglect discussing potentially conflicting values held by clients from non-Western cultures. However, diverse transcultural ethical perspectives, such as the work of Dell'oro and Viafora (1996) and others are beginning to appear in the literature and will add to the transcultural analysis of ethical issues. A suggested Transcultural Ethical Decision Making Model is presented in the accompanying Box 13-10.

Box 13-10 *Transcultural Ethical Decision-Making Model*

Assumptions

1. Health professional and clients are persons of integrity.
   a. Integrity is a disposition to act in accordance with one's own moral beliefs and character (Gabriele and Gaita, 1981).
   b. With dialogue, people of integrity may develop alternative resolutions for problems (Thomasana, 1984).
2. The health professional and client are regarded as having equally important ethical concerns.

Gather Information

1. Health professionals critically examine their own values. What values and goals do they bring to the ethical encounter?

Box 13-10. *(Continued)*

2. Health professionals and clients humanly engage.
   a. Health care professionals learn about the clients' cultural orientation, ethical values, and health goals.
   b. This information is gathered from the client and significant other people in the client's life.
3. Identify the roles and responsibilities of the health professionals and the clients.
4. Identify the role and responsibility of other significant people involved in the situation.
5. Identify information about the clinical parameters of the case.

Identify the Ethical Problem

1. Involve all the decision makers in the discussions.
2. Ask all the people involved in the ethical issue to explain their view of the problem.
3. Identify the significance of the ethical problem.
4. Identify the significance of the values involved. Identify whose values are most significantly involved.

Identify Strategies

1. Identify the timeline for making the decision.
2. Identify each possible course of action.
   a. Identify how each option *adheres to the clients'* culture, value, and belief system.
   b. Identify any options that *violate the health professionals'* value or belief system.
   c. Identify positive and negative outcomes of each option.
   d. Identify the risks and benefits of each option.
3. Identify alternative choices of action. Prioritize alternatives based on clients' values.
4. Which option does the health professional recommend?
   a. Why?
   b. Does this option coincide with the clients' culture, value, and belief systems?
5. Sometimes even people of integrity will not agree on a resolution; one or the other considers the values involved wrong or offensive. Cross-cultural disagreement should be publicly negotiated. For example, in an ethics committee meeting, avoid imposing your own values on either health professionals or clients (Jecker, Carrese, & Pearlman, 1995).
6. Are there any other resources to help you in your decision-making process?

Make the Decision

1. Key decision makers choose a course of action based on their *best* judgment.

Evaluation of the Decision-Making Process

1. Were all significant participants included in the decision-making process?
2. Were all the significant participants satisfied with the decision-making process?
3. Were the outcomes as anticipated?
4. What could have been done differently?
5. Future recommendations?

Developed using data from Curtin, L. (1978). A proposed model for critical ethical analysis. *Nursing Forum (17),* 12–17; Fry, S. T. (1994). *Ethics in Nursing Practice: A guide to Ethical Decision Making.* Geneva: International Council of Nurses; Jecker, N. D., Carrese, J. A., & Pearlman, R. A. (1995, January-February). Caring for patients in cross-cultural settings. *Hastings Center Report,* 6–14.

Summary

This chapter stressed the importance of health professionals and clients being aware of their personal values. Values clarification tools were developed and presented. Ethics and bioethics were defined. The historical development of bioethics in the United States and selected European countries were discussed, and basic ethical principles were explored. The ethical theories pertaining to nursing and transcultural delivery of health care were explored. Character ethics, which stresses the importance of the character of individuals who perform actions and make choices, was explored, as was *caring,* which stresses the traits of sympathy, compassion and discernment. Differences between *customary morality*—that is, the importance of local customs, and *common morality,* a view that transcends local customs and attitudes, were compared and contrasted.

Intervention strategies were developed and presented for dealing with ethical problems of traditional cultural practices. The challenges to ethical theories of ethical relativism and multiculturalism were differentiated and explored in relation to delivery of culturally and ethically sensitive health care. Transcultural influences on health care were discussed in detail. Vignettes were included throughout the chapter to help the reader understand and apply the content. Lastly, a Transcultural Ethical Decision Making Model was introduced.

Review Questions

1. Identify and explain at least four causes of value differences *within* a culture.
2. Define bioethics and explain how the term is used to describe current standards of professional conduct.
3. Critically analyze the differences in European and American approaches to ethical decision making.
4. Identify one Eastern and one Western ethical theory. Critically analyze the differences and similarities in the two approaches?
5. Critically evaluate which of the Western ethical theories you think is most appropriate to use transculturally.
6. Critically examine the reasons for cross cultural misunderstandings in the resolution of ethical dilemmas.

Learning Activities to Promote Critical Thinking

1. Attend a Bioethics Committee meeting or Ethical Rounds and write about your experiences. Address the following issues:
   a. State the type of Bioethics Committee meeting. Which specialty area?
   b. Who are the members (disciplines and number of members)?
   c. What was the topic or case presentation for discussion?
      1. Was the client or their family present?
      2. Who represented them?
   d. How were ethical issues framed?

   e. Were there any transcultural issues?
      1. If the answer was yes—who spoke for the client?
      2. Was any type of transcultural values assessment conducted?
      3. Were any transcultural issues missed?
   f. Briefly explain how you would address the transcultural issues.
   g. Briefly describe the discussion that occurred.
   h. What would be your recommendations?
   i. Briefly discuss what you learned from the experience? Could you have this information in another way ?

2. Identify one new fact that you learned about your own value system from the Identification Seal learning activity? Critically analyze how this new knowledge will influence your thinking and behavior?

3. Select one Eastern (Confucianism or Taoism) and one Western (consequentialism or non-consequentialism) theory that is presented in Box 13-3. Analyze the following case study based on each of the selected theories.

CASE STUDY 13.1

In an intensive care unit, six patients are in need of organ transplants. Patient A is a microbiologist researcher on the brink of discovering a cure for AIDS and needs a heart transplant. Patient B is an economist who is an essential member of the task force developing a national health policy and needs a liver transplant. Patient C is a missionary who has spend forty years working with the poor in India and needs a kidney transplant. Patient D is the mother of ten children and needs a lung transplant. Patient E is a prominent political leader who is pivotal in the negotiations for peace in the Middle East and Central Europe and needs a lung transplant. Patient F is a former President of the United States who is currently involved in humanitrian work with the United Nations and is need of a kidney transplant.

Another patient in the intensive care unit is near death. This elderly patient is a prisoner serving a life sentence for murder. Is it permissible to hasten the death of the prisoner in order to procure organs and save the lives of six people who have made outstanding contributions to humanity.

4. Analyze the following case study using the Intervention Strategy for Ethical Problems of Traditional Cultural Practices shown in Box 13-5.

CASE STUDY 13.2

A woman comes into the clinic accompanied by her 14-year-old daughter requesting that the daughter be circumcised. List the steps of the process you would use to *humanly engage* the identified client in a voice that regards the clients as equal partners? What cultural considerations regarding value differences within subgroups of a culture should you keep in mind? List the specific steps you would take to explore the client's personal and cultural values regarding this traditional cultural practice. Would you ask the daughter to participate in the discussion? Why?

Ethics Resources

....

The Hastings Center
255 Elm Road
Briarcliff Manor
New York, NY

The Center for Medical Ethics and Health Policy
Baylor College of Medicine
Houston, TX

Pope John Center for the Study of Ethics in Health Care
186 Forbes Road
Braintree, MA

The Kennedy Center for the Study of Ethics
Georgetown University
Washington, DC
1-800-MED-ETHX

MacLean Center for Clinical Medical Ethics
University of Chicago
Chicago, IL

Center for Bioethics
University of Pennsylvania Medical Center
Philadelphia, PA

Medical College of Wisconsin
Bioethics Online Service

References

Airhihenbuwa, C. O. (1995). *Health and Culture: Beyond the Western Paradigm*. London: Sage Publications.

Al-Awadi, A. R. (1996). Medical ethics at the crossroads. *The Journal of Kuwait Medical Association 28,* 395–396.

Arras, J. D. (1995). *Ethical Issues in Modern Medicine* (4th ed.). London: Mayfield Publishing Co.

Beauchamp, T. L., & Childress, J. F. (1994). *Principles of Biomedical Ethics* (3rd ed.). New York: Oxford University Press.

Bolini, P., & Siemm, H. (1995). Health needs of migrants. *World Health 48*(6), 20–21.

Bryant, J. H., Khan, K. S., & Hyder, A. (1997). Ethics, equity and renewal of WHO's health-for-all strategy. *World Health Forum 18,* 2.

Callahan, D. (1990). *What Kind of Life*. New York: Simon and Schuster.

Carrese, J., & Rhodes, L. (1995). Western bioethics on the Navajo reservation. *Journal of the American Medical Association 274,* 826–829.

Chao, Y. M. (1991). *Moral Values in Nursing from Confucian Perspective*. Unpublished manuscript.

Childress, J. F. (1989). *The normative Principles of Medical Ethics*. In R. M. Veatch (Ed.). *Medical Ethics*, pp. 27–48. Boston: Jones and Bartlett.

Chitty, K. K. (1997). *Professional Nursing: Concepts and Challenges* (2nd ed.). Philadelphia: W. B.Saunders.

Clark, M. J. (1997). *Nursing in the Community* (2nd ed.). Stamford, CT: Appleton & Lange.

Curtin, L. (1978). A proposed model for critical ethical analysis. *Nursing Forum 17,* 12–17.

Dell'oro, R., & Viafora, C. (Eds.). (1996). *History of Bioethics: International Perspectives*. San Francisco: International Scholars Publications.

de Wachter, M. (1997). The European Convention on Bioethics. *Hastings Center Report 27,* 13–23.

Dugger, C. W. (1997, January 7). City of immigrants becoming more so in 90's. *New York Times*, p. 1.

Eliason, M. J. (1993). Ethics and transcultural nursing care. *Nursing Outlook 41,* 225–228.

Emmanuel, E. J. (1991). *The Ends of Human Life: Medical Ethics in a Liberal Policy*. Cambridge, MA: Harvard University Press.

Fluss, S. S. (1995, March/April). Ethics in health: Some current perspectives. *World Health 2,* 13–17.

Fry, S. T. (1994). *Ethics in Nursing Practice: A Guide to Ethical Decision Making*. Geneva: International Council of Nurses.

Gabriele, T., & Gaita, R. (1981). Integrity. *Proceedings of the Aristotelian Society Supplement 55,* 143–159.

Gerteis, E. S., Daley, J., & Delbanco, T. L. (Eds.). (1991). *Through the Patient's Eyes.* San Francisco: Jossey-Bass Publishers.

Guido, G. W. (1997). *Legal Issues in Nursing* (2nd ed.). Stamford, CT: Appleton & Lange.

Huang, L. H. (1996). Will they take their pills? *Reflections* 22(4), 15–16.

International Council of Nurses (1973). *International Council of Nurses Code for Nurses.* Geneva, Switzerland.

James, S. A. (1994). Reconciling international human rights and cultural relativism: The case of female circumcision. *Bioethics* 8(1), 1–26.

Jecker, N. D., Carrese, J. A., & Pearlman, R. A. (1995). Caring for patients in cross-cultural settings. *Hastings Center Report,* Vol. 25, No. 1, p. 6–14.

Kluge, E. (1993). Female circumcision: When medical ethics confronts cultural values. *Canadian Medical Journal* 149(2), 288–289.

Knight, H. (1997, April 9). Census report: 1 out of 10 in U.S. Are foreign born. *The Star-Ledger,* p. 9.

Kozier, B., Erb, G., & Blais, K. (1997). *Professional Nursing Practice: Concepts and Perspectives* (3rd ed.). New York: Addison-Wesley.

Kristof, N. D. (1995, February). When the doctor won't tell cancer patient the truth. *New York Times International,* p. 4.

Laffrey, S. C., Meleis, A. I., Lipson, J. G., Solomon, M., & Omidian, P. A. (1989). Assessing Arab-American health care needs. *Social Science & Medicine* 29, 877–883.

Lane, S. D., & Rubinstein, R. A. (1996). Judging the other: Responding to traditional female genital surgeries. *Hastings Center Report* 26(3), 31–40.

Leininger, M. (1991). Transcultural care principles, human rights, and ethical considerations. *Journal of Transcultural Nursing* 3(1), 21–23.

Leininger, M. (1997). Transcultural nursing in the 21st century. *International Nursing Review* 44, 19–23.

Levine, R. J. (1991). Informed consent: Some challenges to the universal validity of the Western model. *Law, Medicine and Health Care* 19(3), 207–213.

Lie, R. K. (1995). Cross-cultural medical ethics. http// www.well.com/user/reidar/pittsburgh.html.

McDonald, S. P., Machizawa, S., & Satoh, H. (1992). Diagnostic disclosure: A tale of two cultures. *Psychological Medicine* 22(1), 147–157.

Meleis, A. F., & Jonsen, A. R. (1983). Ethical crises and cultural differences. *Western Journal of Medicine* 138(6), 889–893.

Mydan, S. (1995). Many immigrant's views on death are out of U.S. mainstream. *New York Times News Service.* http:/ www.latino.com/heal/912html.

Nasr, S. H. (1981). *Islamic Life and Thought.* London: George Allen and Uwin.

Norton, M. E., Walani, S., & Hashim, F. (1995). Individuals' responses to sharing information about a serious illness: A survey in Karachi. In Janet Wong (Ed.). *Health Care and Culture.* Morgantown, WV: University of West Virginia Press.

Nydell, M. K. (1987). *Understanding Arabs: A Guide for Westerners.* Yarmouth, ME: Intercultural Press.

Oostvagel, P. (1995). Paying the price for one's beliefs. *World Health* 48(1), 22–23.

Pellegrino, E. D. (1992). Is truth telling to the patient a cultural artifact? *Journal of the American Medical Association* 268, 1734–1735.

Potter, V. R. (1971). *Bioethics: Bridge to the Future.* Englewood Cliffs, NJ: Prentice Hall.

Presswalla, J. L. (1994). Insights into Eastern health care: Some transcultural nursing perspectives. *Journal of Transcultural Nursing* 5(1), 21–24.

Ray, M. A. (1994). A framework and model for transcultural ethical analysis. *Journal of Holistic Nursing* 12(3), 251–264.

Reich, W. (1996). Bioethics in the United States. In R. Dell'oro & C. Viafora (Eds.). *History of Bioethics: International Perspectives,* pp. 83–118. San Francisco: International Scholars Publication.

Seelye, K. Q. (1997, March 27). The new U.S.: Grayer and more Hispanic. *New York Times,* p. 16.

Sheikh, A., & Sheikh, K. (1989). *Eastern and Western Approaches to Healing: Ancient Wisdom and Modern Knowledge.* New York: John Wiley.

Spector, R. E. (1996). *Cultural Diversity in Health and Illness* (4th ed.). Stamford, CT: Appleton & Lange.

Spradley, B. W., & Allender, J. A. (1996). *Community Health Nursing: Concepts and Practice* (4th ed.). Philadelphia: Lippincott.

Steele, S. M., & Harmon, V. M. (1983). *Values Clarification in Nursing* (2nd ed.). Norwalk, CT: Appleton-Century-Crofts.

Surbone, A. (1992). Letter from Italy: Truth telling to the patient. *Journal of the American Medical Association* 258(13), 1661–1662.

Szasz, T. S., & Hollender, M. H. (1956). A contribution to the philosophy of medicine: The basic models of the doctor-patient relationship. *Archives of Internal Medicine* 97, 585–592.

Thomasana, D. C. (1984). The context as a moral rule in medicine. *Journal of Bioethics* 5(1), 63–79.

Tong, K. L., & Spicer, B. J. (1994). The Chinese palliative patient and family in North America: A cultural perspective. *Journal of Palliative Care* 10(1), 26–28.

Turner, P. C. (1997, July 27). Hospital speaks the language of service. *The Sunday Star-Ledger,* p. 9.

Via, T., Callahan, S., Barry, K., Jackson, C., & Gerber, D. E. (1997). Middle East meets midwest: The new health care challenge. *The Journal of Multicultural Nursing & Health* 3, 1.

Viafora, C. (1996). Ethics today: An historic and systematic account. In R. Dell'oro & C. Viafora (Eds.). *History of Bioethics: International Perspectives.* p. 11. San Francisco: International Scholars Publication.

WHO Regional Office for Europe (1994). *A Declaration on the Promotion of Patients' Rights in Europe.* Copenhagen: WHO Regional Office for Europe.

Chapter 14

Cultural Diversity in the Health Care Workforce

Margaret M. Andrews

KEY TERMS

Multicultural Workplace
Multicultural Workforce
Cultural Diversity
Transcultural Nursing
   Administration
Corporate Culture
Organizational Climate
Ethos
Hatred

Prejudice
Bigotry
Racism
Race Relations
Social Amnesia
Discrimination
Ethnoviolence
Attitude Change

Cultural Values
Conflict
Dress Code
Hygiene
Family Obligations
Cross-Cultural Communication
Cultural Self-Assessment
   (individual and organizational)

OBJECTIVES

1. Analyze past, present, and future trends in the racial and ethnic composition of the health care workforce.
2. Identify the cultural meaning of work and its influence on the corporate culture and organizational climate of health care organizations.
3. Critically examine the manner in which hatred, prejudice, racism, discrimination and ethnoviolence manifest themselves in the health care workplace.
4. Critically analyze the cultural origins of conflict in the health care workforce.
5. Evaluate strategies for promoting effective cross-cultural communication and preventing conflict in the multicultural workplace.
6. Examine the process and content of cultural self-assessment for nurses and for health care organizations, institutions and agencies.

According to the U.S. Department of Health and Human Services (1993), 9 percent, or 207,000 of the 2.24 million registered nurses in the U.S., come from racial/ ethnic minority backgrounds. Estimates for each group are indicated in Table 14-1. Although fewer than 4 percent of licensed nurses in the U.S. are foreign educated, this represents 73,423 nurses. They tend to be clustered on the East and West coasts,

TABLE 14-1
Racial/Ethnic Diversity Among Registered Nurses in the United States

Black (non-Hispanic)	Hispanic	Asian/Pacific Islander	American Indian Alaska Native	Graduates of Foreign Program
90,600	30,400	76,000	10,000	73,000

Source: U.S. Department of Health and Human Services, Bureau of Health Professions (1993). *Fact Sheet. Selected Facts About Minority Registered Nurses.* Washington, DC: U.S. Government Printing Office.

and in the so-called sunbelt, so the numbers are large in some hospitals—usually those with more than 500 beds and those serving inner-city, low income populations. These figures do not reflect other types of cultural diversity nor the variation that exists within each of federally defined population categories.

As we enter the 21st century, there will continue to be an increasingly diverse workforce. According to the Bureau of Labor Statistics, the net rate of growth between 1986 and 2000 in the U.S. labor force of Hispanic females (85 percent), Asian females (83 percent), Hispanic males (68 percent), Asian males (61 percent), African American females (33 percent), and African American males (24 percent) will outpace the net rate of growth of white females (22 percent) and white males (−9 percent) (Schwartz & Sullivan, 1993).

The emerging American workforce is dramatically different from the former one. In many health care settings there is diversity in race, ethnicity, religion, age, sexual orientation, and national origin. Recent strides in the women's movement have called attention to important gender differences and the manner in which changing societal roles of both men and women influence relationships in the multicultural workplace. The interrelationship between culture and the physical, mental and emotional handicaps and disabilities of some health care workers also must be considered in the complex web called the multicultural workforce.

Women have historically comprised the majority of personnel in nursing and in many allied health disciplines. For the past two decades, women and members of racially and ethnically diverse groups have made significant inroads into health professions once overwhelmingly the province of white men. Table 14-2 summarizes the numbers of first professional degrees conferred to women by health field of study and race/ethnicity. The largest gains for most culturally diverse groups, however, occurred during the mid- to late-1970s. Since that time, with the exception of Asians and Hispanics, cultural diversity in the health fields has been relatively stable.

For most racial and ethnic groups, increases in the numbers of new health care professionals during the 1980s reflect increases in the number of degrees awarded in various fields. For African Americans in medicine and dentistry, the gains have been largely the result of an increase in the numbers of African American women. The number of first professional degrees awarded to black men in these fields declined between 1980 and 1990. Increasing numbers of underrepresented minority health professionals requires continued, systematic, and substantial gains. The loss of black male professionals in some fields and their failure to make the same gains as women

TABLE 14-2

Percent Change in the Numbers of First Professional Degrees Conferred to Women by Health Field of Study and Race/Ethnicity, 1981–1990

Health Professionals	All Women	White	Black	Hispanic	American Indian	Asian/Pacific
Allopathic medicine	34	20.1	42.9	117.8	83.3	313.7
Osteopathic medicine	135.5	130.6	−20	600	400	216.7
Dentistry	60.3	26.9	24.6	264.7	500	326.7
Pharmacy	150.5	146.7	108.3	200	−100	176.9
Optometry	105.8	99.4	133.3	233.3	−100	142.1
Podiatry	163.8	133.3	257.1	250	0	550

Source: Ninth Report to Congress (1993). *Health Personnel in the United States.* Washington, DC: U.S. Government Printing Office.

in others has resulted in critical setbacks. The declines have been attributed to the disproportionate participation of members of diverse groups in a number of trends in education. Among these trends are declining numbers of racial and ethnic minority male applicants to health professions schools, the declining popularity of undergraduate pre-medical majors and declining college participation rates for African Americans and their higher high school drop-out rates. Factors underlying these trends include a high rate of poverty and lack of economic security.

Population Changes and Implications for Health Care Needs

A significant number of the national health goals for the year 2000 involve specific objectives for improving the health status of the panethnic minority groups identified by the U.S. federal government, particularly those with low incomes. Meanwhile, culturally diverse cohorts of children, women of childbearing age, and the elderly are expected to grow, exacerbating the need for culturally and gender-sensitive providers of health care. Since 1972 there has been an explosion in the numbers of people migrating to the U.S., both with and without legal documentation. Although data concerning the number of recent immigrants working in health care settings are unavailable, overall 8 percent or 19.8 million people in the U.S. are foreign-born residents from other North American nations (41 percent), Asia (25 percent), Europe (29 percent), South America (5 percent), Africa (2 percent), the former Soviet Union (2 percent), and Oceana (1 percent) (U.S. Bureau of the Census, 1993).

The Challenges and Opportunities of Diversity

Before the current health care reform movement, foreign-born physicians, nurses, and others with health-related skills were actively recruited by U.S. hospitals, especially during the 1970s and 1980s. Because the health care workplace is a microcosm of the changing demographic patterns in society at large, the growing diversity among nurses and other members of the health care team frequently poses challenges and opportunities in the multicultural work setting. Consider the following cases.

CASE STUDY 14.1

When an African American patient was admitted to a small rural hospital with predominantly white staff and patients, nurses from one shift would include "black male" in their report to the oncoming shift. When one of the few African American nurses began using "white male" or "white female" in her report, she was accused of "having an attitude" and "trying to instigate racial trouble."

CASE STUDY 14.2

When informed that a patient was requesting medication for pain, a Lutheran nurse of German heritage responded to a fellow nurse, "She's just a Jewish princess who complains about pain all the time." A Jewish laboratory technician overheard the remark and demanded to know what the nursing supervisor was going to do about "the blatant anti-Semitism" on the unit.

CASE STUDY 14.3

A slightly built African American male nurse asks to meet with the operating room nurse manager about a surgeon who has recently immigrated from Russia. The nurse complains, "Dr. Ivanovich keeps asking me why I became a nurse. He asks very personal questions about my sexual orientation and wants to know if I'm 'queer.' I consider this a hostile work environment and refuse to scrub for his surgical cases anymore."

CASE STUDY 14.4

After receiving report on a critically ill victim of a motor vehicle accident, Dr. Juan Valdez-Rodriguez, the physician on call, asked for the patient's name. The reporting nurse said, "I don't know. Martinez, Hernandez, something like that. You'll recognize him when you see him—just another drunk Mexican who ran his pickup truck into a tree." Upon entering the exam room, the physician immediately recognized the victim as his cousin.

CASE STUDY 14.5

A nurse enters into a conversation with a Chinese American food service worker. Ms. Chin remarks that for the past 4 days she has been asked to be the interpreter for an elderly Chinese man on one of the units where she delivers food. "I don't want to offend the nurse manager who asked me to translate but it is not right for a younger woman to speak for an older man. It is not our custom. Besides, my supervisor scolded me for being so slow to do my work. She thinks I have become lazy. Would you talk to the nurse manager for me?"

CASE STUDY 14.6

Mrs. Patel, a native of India, is a nurse manager in a small rural hospital that has difficulty attracting qualified professional staff. Mrs. Patel tells her supervisor that she must "take some time off" due to a family emergency in her homeland. When the supervisor inquires about the details, he learns that Mrs. Patel already has purchased a non-refundable airline ticket with a return flight in 6 weeks. Mrs. Patel's husband is the chief executive officer for the town's major industry and chairman of the hospital's Board of Directors.

Transcultural Nursing Administration

According to Leininger (1996) *transcultural nursing administration* refers to "a creative and knowledgeable process of assessing, planning, and making decisions and policies that will facilitate the provision of educational and clinical services that take into account the cultural caring values, beliefs, symbols, references, and lifeways of people of diverse and similar cultures for beneficial or satisfying outcomes." (p. 30). Transcultural nursing administrative perspectives are essential for survival, growth, satisfaction, and achievement of goals in the multicultural workplace.

In the contemporary health care industry, nurse administrators necessarily focus their time and energy on issues such as cost–benefit outcomes, downsizing, territorial struggles with members of other disciplines, appropriate use of technology, and other important topics. With increasing frequency, nurse administrators are realizing the critical importance of transculturally based administrative practices that positively influence cost benefits and quality outcomes. With the increasing diversity among members of the health care workforce, nurses are challenged to develop and practice a new kind of administration known as *transcultural nursing administration*.

Cultural Perspectives on the Meaning of Work

The earliest recorded ideas about work refer to it as a curse, punishment or necessary evil needed to sustain life. People of high status did not work, whereas slaves, indentured servants and peasants worked. In contemporary society, the concept of work must be considered in its historical and cultural context. Cultural views about caring for the sick also must be considered because it may be perceived as a divine calling for those with supernatural powers (some African tribes), a religious vocation (some ethnic Catholic groups), or an undignified occupation for lower class workers (some Arab groups such as Kuwaitis and Saudi Arabians).

Cultural norms influence a staff member's consideration of group interest as opposed to individual interests in the multicultural workplace. Scholars have identified two major orientations embraced by people, *individualism and collectivism*. With *individualism,* importance is placed on individual inputs, rights, and rewards. Individualists emphasize values such as autonomy, competitiveness, achievement and self-sufficiency. Most English-speaking and European countries have individualist cultures.

Collectivism entails the need to maintain group harmony above the partisan interests of subgroups and individuals. In collectivist cultures values such as interpersonal harmony and group solidarity prevail. Staff whose ethnic heritage is Asian or South American are likely to be influenced by collectivism. Amish and Mennonite groups also are considered collectivist cultures.

One of the most notable distinctions between people from individualist and collectivist cultures is the meaning of work. Individualists work to earn a living. People are expected to work and need not enjoy it. Leisure or recreational activities frequently are pursued to alleviate the monotony of work. People from individualist cultures tend to dichotomize work and leisure. Individualist concepts of work reflect an orientation toward the future.

It also is useful to understand cultural differences about appropriate and desired behavior in the workplace. People from most individualist cultures are typically achievement oriented. Stereotypically, they want to do better, accomplish more, and take responsibility for their actions. They tend to develop personality traits such as assertiveness and competitiveness that facilitate this. In many collectivist cultures, however, qualities such as commitment to relationships, gentleness, cooperativeness, and indirectness are valued.

Some researchers have suggested that the motivation strategies of Japanese managers must appeal to the Japanese worker's sense of loyalty, commitment and group orientation, whereas motivation strategies of North American managers must appeal to the worker's sense of contract, rules, and individuality. Although some individuals exhibit a combination of the two, most staff members will display either an individualistic or collectivistic orientation in the workplace. Nurses in leadership positions need to recognize the fundamental value system embraced by their staff order to understand why they behave as they do at work.

Corporate Cultures and Subcultures

Health care organizations are mini-societies that have their own distinctive patterns of culture and subculture. One organization may have a high degree of cohesiveness with staff working together like members of a single family toward achievement of common goals. Another may be highly fragmented, divided into groups that think about the world in very different ways or that have different aspirations as to what their organization should be. Just as individuals in a culture can have different personalities while sharing much in common, such is the case with groups and organizations. It is this phenomenon that is referred to as *corporate culture. Corporate culture* refers to a process of reality construction that allows staff to see and understand particular events, actions, objects, communications or situations in distinctive ways. These patterns of understanding help people cope with the situations encountered and provide a basis for making behavior sensible and meaningful.

Shared values, beliefs, meaning, and understanding are components of the corporate culture. The corporate culture is established and maintained through an ongoing, proactive process of reality construction. It is an active, living phenomenon through which staff members jointly create and recreate their work place and world. One of the easiest ways to appreciate the nature of corporate culture and subculture is to observe the day-to-day functioning of the organization. Observe the patterns of interaction among individuals, the language that is used, the images and themes explored in conversation, and the various rituals of daily routine. Historical explanations for the ways things are done will emerge in discussions of the rationale for certain aspects of the culture.

The corporate culture metaphor is useful because it directs attention to the symbolic significance of almost every aspect of organizational life. Structures, hierarchies, rules and organizational routines reveal underlying meanings that are crucial for understanding how organizations function. For example, meetings carry important aspects of organizational culture which may convey a sense of conformity and order or causal informality. The environment in which the meetings are held reflects the formality or informality of the organization.

It is useful to pose the following questions when determining the corporate culture of a health care organization, institution or agency. Does the person presiding over the group stand or sit? Does the presider encourage discussion among group members or engage in a monologue? Are group members encouraged to express opinions freely or is there pressure to silence those who express opposing points of view? How do group leaders and members dress? What message does the institutional dress code convey about the acceptance of cultural diversity ? Do policies allow for cultural expressions in clothing, accessories, hair style and related areas? Although most institutions require employees to wear identification badges or name tags, what flexibility does the individual have for self-expression and expression of cultural identity and affiliation? The answers to the previous questions will provide a beginning understanding of the corporate culture of the organization.

Health care work environments are social settings that encompass many elements of a social system. It is useful to distinguish between the *organizational climate* of the work environment and the *corporate culture.* According to Flarey (1993), the organizational climate usually measures perceptions or feelings about the organization or work environment. The corporate or organizational culture, on the other hand, is what its members share—beliefs, values, assumptions, rituals—often unconsciously. Culture provides the community, the sameness, and the consensus that makes those people unique and special.

Hatred, Prejudice, Bigotry, Racism and Discrimination in the Multicultural Workplace

In some organizations, the use of racial, ethnic, sexual, and other derogatory remarks signals a disturbing underlying problem in the workplace. Why does hatred exist in the workplace? Although the reasons are complex and interconnected, some of the contributing factors include the early socialization of children to cultural and gender stereotypes, personal experiences (or lack of them) with people from diverse backgrounds, and exposure to negative societal attitudes.

According to Henderson (1994), *hatred* in the workplace is exacerbated during times of rapid immigration, periods of economic recession or depression, and high unemployment. Competition for sexual partners also is cited as a cause for hatred. Hatred can be the cause of tremendous hostility in the workplace. In some organizations, technology is being used to transmit derogatory remarks electronically to individuals or targeted groups by e-mail or fax. There is a proliferation of sites on the internet that allow free expression of hatred, using First Amendment rights to guarantee their right to freedom of expression.

The term *prejudice* refers to inaccurate perceptions of others and results in conclusions that are drawn without adequate knowledge or evidence. All people are prejudiced for or against other people. Prejudices found in the community at large are acted out in the workplace. *Bigotry* connotes narrowmindedness and refers to the obstinate or blind attachment to a particular opinion or viewpoint. The bigot blames members of out-groups for various misfortunes. In their efforts to make expedient decisions, bigots react to concepts rather than people. Whereas prejudice and bigotry refer to attitudes, *discrimination* refers to behaviors and is defined as the act of setting one individual or group apart from another, showing a difference or favoritism. Discriminatory behaviors, not attitudes, comprise the majority of intergroup problems. Although there are many laws against discriminatory behaviors, especially in the workplace, there are none against prejudice or bigotry (Henderson, 1994).

The nurse in Case 14.1, who pointed out in report that the patient was black, may not have any conscious discriminatory intent. By departing from the usual practice of not mentioning race, however, she made a statement that race was a variable that needed to be mentioned, which in turn, gave opportunity for prejudices in the minds of the other nurses to surface. Keeping people of color exploitable is a foundation of racial inequality.

Contrary to popular writings, prejudices in the workplace are not limited to black–white conflicts and confrontations. There is prejudice against various members of the workforce including women, older workers, individuals with disabilities, foreign-born workers, and white workers.

In Case 14.2, the nurse's characterization of the patient experiencing pain as "a Jewish princess" is a transparently anti-Semitic remark. The ability to control the lives of people is a psychological aspect of nursing that is often unconsciously manifest. The nurse in the case study may be exercising a certain degree of power over the patient, knowing that she was at the nurse's mercy for the relief of her pain. It also may reflect an underlying *scientific racism*, i.e., that there are biologic differences between certain groups. The nurse may believe that there are different pain thresholds among persons of diverse backgrounds and that Jewish patients tend to have a relatively low pain tolerance.

As discussed in Chapter 8 (Transcultural Aspects of Pain), the nurse's own ethnic background, religious affiliation and personal experience with pain may contribute to her perceptions of the patient's need for pain relief. Although the nurse may use scientific racism to rationalize her belief that the patient is requesting more pain relief than the average person, there is no excuse for the racist reference to her patient as "a Jewish princess." The nurse's racism adversely affected not only the patient, but a fellow nurse and a laboratory technician. The racial slur is an example of an implicit cue passed on to others, in which the nurse perpetuated both prejudice against and stereotypes about Jewish people. The laboratory technician is likely to view the nurse, and perhaps by extension the entire multicultural workplace, as hostile to Jews.

There also is prejudice based on sexual orientation as illustrated in Case 14.3. The African American nurse has expressed his concern with the hostile work environment created by the imposing Russian surgeon who asked inappropriate questions about his sexual orientation. Because the offender is a recent immigrant, he may be unaware of cultural differences concerning appropriate topics for discussion in the workplace—though it is doubtful that his behavior would be widely accepted in a Russia operating room setting either. Furthermore, the surgeon may have a limited English vocabulary and/or be unaware of the negative connotation of the slang term "queer." These explanations for the surgeon's inappropriate behavior in the workplace do not excuse him, but rather are offered as factors worthy of the nurse manager's consideration when attempting to address the problem.

Racism implies that superior or inferior traits and behavior are determined by race. Racism connotes prejudice and discrimination. To understand racism in the workplace, distinctions need to be made among (1) institutional structures and personal behavior, and the relationship between the two; (2) the variation in both degree and form of expression of individual prejudice; and (3) the fact that racism is merely one form of a larger and more inclusive pattern of ethnocentrism that may be based on various factors—racial and non-racial in nature (Henderson, 1994).

Racism is caused by a complex web of factors including ignorance, apathy, poverty, historic patterns of discrimination against particular groups, and social stratification. According to Brown (1973), society "is racially divided and its whole organization...promotes racial distinctions" (p. 8). With this frame of reference, racial bias and discrimination have been built into most U.S. and Canadian institutions and every citizen is a product of institutional racism. According to Henderson (1994), "What is commonly called racism is part of the larger problem of ethnic identification, of power and powerlessness, and of the exploitation of the weak by the strong....What most writers commonly call *race relations* should be properly understood in the larger context of *human relations*" (p. 21).

In the multicultural workplace, the expression of negative attitudes and behaviors by people toward others according to their identification as members of a particular group is of particular concern. The expression of these attitudes and behavioral patterns is learned as part of the cultural process. Negative group attitudes and destructive group conflicts are less likely to arise when employees treat each other as individuals and respond to each other on the basis of individual characteristics and behaviors.

In Case 14.4, the nurse's remark "just another drunk Mexican" is an example of a stereotype that may have an element of truth in it but is inaccurate. Although it is true that the majority of motor vehicle accidents are alcohol related, and that in this hospital a large proportion of those are Mexican Americans, it is untrue that all Mexican-American men are alcoholics. By overgeneralizing in this way, the nurse has failed to assess important information about the individual person and has depersonalized him through the stereotype. The nurse's apparent insensitivity to Dr. Valdez-Rodriguez' ethnic heritage is appalling. The pathos of the situation is further realized when the physician learns that "just another drunk Mexican" accident victim turns out to be his cousin.

According to Schwartz and Sullivan (1993), selective mistreatment, often in the absence of adequate social support, undermines the work experiences of individuals who are identified with groups that are the targets of discriminatory behavior. The career potential of staff from diverse backgrounds frequently is undermined by the relative lack of access to informal networks and mentors and by the expectation that they will assimilate into organizational cultures that are often intolerant of the cultures with which these staff identify. These manifestations of discrimination can be expected to undermine the functioning of the health care organization. Paradoxically, the victims of mistreatment are often the perpetrators as well. The victim of mistreatment may, in turn, mistreat others. One explanation for this phenomenon is that people are likely to exhibit a form of internalized oppression as a result of low self-esteem.

According to Holmes (1994), black, Hispanic, and Asian Americans resent one another almost as much as they do whites. This raises doubt about the strategy of merely hiring more minorities. Unless there is systematic training to help all staff to accept each other, conflicts of racial and ethnic origin will increase (Henderson, 1994).

Formation of Attitudes

Attitudes are learned, not innate. Researchers have found that as children grow older, they tend to forget that they were instructed in attitudes by their parents and significant other people. Around the age of 10, most children regard their attitudes toward people from different cultural backgrounds as being innate. Seldom do they recall being coached. *Social amnesia* develops, and elaborate rationalizations are presented to account for learned attitudes (Henderson, 1994).

The superiority or inferiority of a group (versus an individual) is usually less obvious than an individual's behavior. Most staff bring their cultural baggage to work with them, and they are molded and shaped by peer pressure. The values, behaviors, and customs those in the out-group are labeled as strange or unusual. As children, many staff learned to reject culturally different people and to view different synonymously with "inferior." In the insightful words of Carl Jung (1968):

> We still attribute to the other fellow all the evil and inferior qualities that we do not like to recognize in ourselves, and therefore have to criticize and attack him, when all that has happened is that an inferior soul has emigrated from one person to another. The world is still full of *betes noir* and scapegoats, just as it formerly teemed with witches and werewolves." (p. 65).

Violence in the Workplace

Although not all hatred leads to violence, there is a significant increase in the number of attacks on gays, anti-Semitic incidents, and reported cases of *ethnoviolence*. According to Henderson (1994), African Americans, Hispanics, homosexual males, and Jews are the primary targets of hate crimes, many of which occur in the workplace. Although it is impossible to protect all employees and patients from violence in health care settings, reasonable steps must be taken to protect those believed to be at risk. Verbal threats and/or assaults by or against staff members should not be tolerated.

Health care administrators have a moral imperative to take reasonable steps in assuring the physical safety of staff, patients/clients, and visitors. The institution's security officers and/or local police should be notified whenever violence is threatened. Some institutions require staff and visitors to pass through a metal detector when entering the premises, whereas others have posted security officers at entrances to ensure that only authorized persons are admitted. In extreme cases, it may be necessary to obtain a court order to prohibit an individual or group from the premises or to establish a safe perimeter so patients and staff may safely access the facility.

In recent years attorneys representing health care institutions have sometimes found it necessary to obtain a court order to ensure a safe work environment during times of racial, ethnic, religious and social discord. Unfortunately, some demonstrators with strong convictions have violated others' civil liberties and engaged in violent acts against those who disagree with their point of view. The shooting of staff at clinics where abortions are performed is an extreme example of hatred that has resulted in violence. This violence is caused by a complex web of interconnected factors including religious, moral, ethical, social, political and cultural differences.

Changing Attitudes

Although some argue that the focus should be on behavior rather than attitudes, others maintain that hatred, prejudice, bigotry, racism, discrimination and ethnoviolence begin with an individual's attitudes toward certain groups. There are several ways in which staff attitudes can be changed, but they require commitment by all levels of management within an organization. They also require an certain degree of openness and receptivity by the individual.

Efforts to change staff attitudes about people from culturally diverse groups should center on communication. Several approaches have been used by organizations. The first is called the *formal attitude change approach* is based on learning theories. This approach is based on the assumption that people are rational, information-processing beings who can be motivated to listen to a message, hear its content and incorporate what they have learned when it is advantageous to do so. There is an actual or expected reward for embracing diversity.

The second is known as the *group dynamics approach* assumes that staff are social beings who need culturally diverse co-workers as they adjust to environmental changes. The amount of change depends on people's attitudes toward diversity, their attention to the message and to the communicator, their understanding of the message and their acceptance of the message. Acceptance of diversity is likely to be enhanced by activities that provide tangible rewards for staff. It is seldom enough for the top management staff to urge staff to embrace diversity as a moral imperative.

Cultural Values in the Multicultural Workplace

Cultural values frequently lie at the root of cross-cultural differences in the multicultural workplace. Values form the core of a culture. Time orientation, family obligations, communication patterns (including etiquette, space/distance, touch), interpersonal relationships (including long-standing historic rivalries), gender/sexual orientation, education, socioeconomic status, moral/religious beliefs, hygiene, clothing, meaning of work, and personal traits exert influences on individuals within multicultural health care setting.

What is the importance of learning about the values of people from diverse cultural groups?

Values exert a powerful influence on how each person behaves, reacts, and feels. In the multicultural workplace, values affect people's lives in four major ways. Values underlie *perceived needs, what is defined as a problem, how conflict is resolved,* and *expectations of behavior.* When cultural values of individual staff members conflict with the organizational values or those held by co-workers, challenges, misunderstandings and difficulties in the workplace become inevitable. You must use these inevitable conflicts as opportunities to foster cross-cultural understanding among staff from diverse backgrounds and to enhance cross-cultural communication.

Cultural Perspectives on Conflict

The term *conflict* is derived from Latin roots [*confligere,* to strike against] and refers to actions that range from intellectual disagreement to physical violence. Frequently, the action that precipitates the conflict is based on different cultural perceptions of the situation. According to some social scientists, when participants in a conflict are from the same culture, they are more likely to perceive the situation in the same way and organize their perceptions in similar ways.

By examining proverbs used by members of various cultural groups, it is possible to better understand differences in the way conflict is viewed. Table 14-3 summarizes selected proverbs that relate to conflict and its resolution. The dominant culture's proverbs emphasize that people should behave assertively and deal with conflict through direct confrontation. Other cultures—particularly collectivist groups—may promote avoidance of confrontation and emphasize harmony (e.g., Native Americans, Alaska Natives, Amish, and Asians). The culture-based choices that lead people in these opposite directions are a major source of conflict in the workplace.

Many people from individualist cultures view conflict as a healthy, natural, and inevitable component of all relationships. People from many collectivist cultures, on the other hand, have learned to internalize conflict and value harmonious relationships above winning arguments and "being right." To many people of Native American and Asian descent conflict is not healthy, desirable, or constructive. In the Arab world,

TABLE 14-3
Cross-Cultural Perspectives on Proverbs and Conflict

Proverb	Value
Dominant Culture:	
The squeaky wheel gets the grease	Aggressiveness
	Direct confrontation
Tell it like it is	Direct confrontation
	Honesty even if it hurts the other
Take the bull by the horns	Direct confrontation
Shoot first, ask questions later	Aggressiveness
	Direct confrontation
	Protection of individual rights (versus good of the group)
Might makes right	Aggressiveness
	Dominance
Japanese:	
The nail that sticks out gets hammered.	Not calling attention to oneself
	Going along with the group
	Harmony and balance
Senegalese:	
Misunderstandings do not exist; only the failure to communicate does.	Strive to understand the other's point of view
	Harmony and balance is normal state, not conflict and confrontation
Zen:	
He who knows does not speak and he who speaks does not know	Listen to the other's side during conflict
	Silence
Arab:	
The hand of Allah is with the group	Primacy of group good (versus individual)
Haste comes from the devil	Patience
	Conflict resolution takes time

mediation is critical in resolving disputes, and confrontation seldom works. Mediation allows for saving face and is rooted in the realization that all conflicts do not have simple solutions.

The assertive, confrontational, direct style of communicating is characteristic of people from individualistic cultures, whereas the cooperative, conciliatory style is a more collectivist or Eastern mode of managing conflict. When attempting to influence others during a disagreement, for example, nurses from China, Japan and other collectivist cultures may employ covert conflict prevention strategies in order to minimize interpersonal conflicts. Nurses from individualistic cultures are more likely to rely on the overt confrontation of ideas and argumentation by reason.

In Case 14.5, the Chinese American food service worker has demonstrated the cultural value for harmonious relationships, indirect communication, and non-confrontational resolution of conflict. The nurse manager inadvertently placed Mrs. Chin in an awkward position by violating Chinese norms concerning gender and age. In traditional Chinese culture, it is inappropriate for a younger person to speak for an older one and for a female to speak for a male. Serving as an interpreter for the elderly Chinese man has been uncomfortable for her and the patient. Mrs. Chin's value for harmonious relationships in the workplace prevent her from speaking directly to the nurse manager and food service supervisor about the problem. By involving the staff nurse as an intermediary with the nurse manager, she is attempting to convey her dissatisfaction with the situation in a non-confrontational, indirect, and polite manner. She also is attempting to avoid appearing like a complaining, disgruntled employee who is unwilling to cooperate with other workers. For these reasons, she is reluctant to bring the problem to her food service supervisor's attention. She believes that she must please those in authority, foster harmonious relationships and avoid direct confrontation if she is to be a valuable employee of the hospital.

Cultural Origins of Conflict

Let's examine some cultural values and the manner in which they may result in conflict in the multicultural workplace. The origins of cultural conflict result from influences on the organization and on individuals. As indicated in Figure 14-1, political, economic, technological, and legal factors influence the corporate culture and organizational climate of both organizations and their employees. For organizations owned and operated by religious groups, religious influences must be considered. For example, in a hospital owned and operated by a Catholic religious order, abortions, tubal ligations, and other gynecologic procedures may be prohibited. Factors such as educational background, socioeconomic status, culture, moral and religious beliefs and personal traits of employees. Staff contribute to the perception that values are in conflict. Although there are many conflicting values that underlie problems, the following areas will be explored in the remainder of this chapter: Cultural perspectives on time orientation, interpersonal relationships (including historic rivalries between groups), cross-cultural communication (including etiquette and touch), family obligations, gender/sexual orientation, moral and religious beliefs (including dietary practices), personal hygiene, and clothing.

Cultural Perspectives on Family Obligations

Although family is important in all cultures, the constellation (nuclear, single-parent, extended, same-sex, etc.), emotional closeness among members, social and economic commitments among members, and other factors vary cross-culturally. Both staff nurses and those in administrative positions frequently report difficulty with requests from nurses of diverse cultural backgrounds that pertain to family obligations.

Some nurses from different cultures have been labeled as uncommitted to their

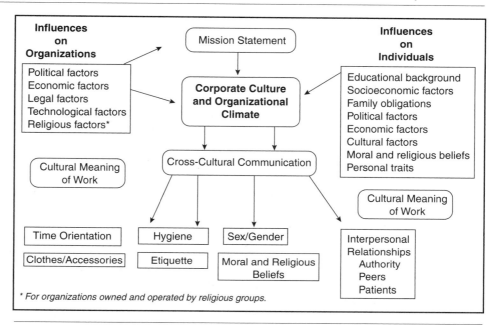

FIGURE 14-1.   Origins of conflict in the multicultural health care setting.

work and/or disinterested in their nursing careers because family is a higher priority than job or career. It should be noted that the so-called appliance nurse has long been recognized among members of the dominant culture as well. Given that it is highly unlikely (and undesirable) that the nurse manager would be successful at changing fundamental family-related values, the most useful approach is to focus on the problematic behavior. For example, if excessive absenteeism is the undesirable behavior, the nurse manager should arrange for a face-to-face meeting in which the problematic behavior is discussed. In addition, the use of peer pressure by coworkers also can be helpful in changing the undesirable behavior as fellow workers communicate to the individual why his/her behavior is troublesome. It is generally useful to identify the reason(s) for the excessive absenteeism and to explore culturally appropriate strategies for resolving the problem, such as utilization of the natural social support that is culturally expected of extended family members. The solution is seldom simple, as the following case analysis illustrates.

In Case 14.6, Mrs. Patel, the nurse manager from India, reflects the high value placed on family relationships and obligations when she tells her supervisor that she plans to absent herself from work for 6 weeks in order to help with a family emergency in India. Although she has a large extended family in India, she believes that it is her duty to be present during this family crisis. By purchasing a nonrefundable airline ticket, she has demonstrated her resolve.

The significant community influence exerted by Mrs. Patel's husband in this small rural community and his position in the hospital hierarchy further complicate the situation. The nursing supervisor is posed with an awkward dilemma because Mrs.

Patel is not entitled to 6 weeks' vacation, nor has she adequately planned to cover her unit's needs during her absence. The 6 weeks that she has requested exceeds the leave time permitted by hospital policy. Although it has been nearly impossible for this small rural hospital to recruit qualified professional staff, the nursing supervisor must consider dismissing Mrs. Patel. By allowing Mrs. Patel to be gone for 6 weeks, the supervisor would need to shift the burden to other nursing staff who will need to adjust their workloads. Granting authorized leave would set a precedent that may leave the hospital vulnerable if other staff decide to make similar requests for extended time off. Because of Mr. Patel's powerful influence in the both the hospital and community arenas, the nursing supervisor is cognizant of the external pressures that are likely to be exerted on him from multiple sources both inside and outside of the hospital. In his decision-making process, the supervisor must consider the cultural, ethical, legal, social and economic dimensions the situation from the perspectives of both the institution and the employee.

The value of independence from the family, for example, is highly valued by many from the dominant cultural groups in the U.S. and Canada but ranks very low in the hierarchy of people from most Middle Eastern and Asian cultures. In the latter groups, the family is highly valued, and the individual's life-long duties toward the family are explicit. Thus, absence from work for family-related reasons may be considered legitimate and important by workers from some cultures but may be perceived as an unnecessary inconvenience to the supervisor. For example, a Mexican American staff member may submit a last-minute request for vacation time in order to visit with a distant cousin who unexpectedly arrived in town after traveling a great distance. The Mexican American staff member thinks, "What a great opportunity to develop a stronger relationship with a distant member of my mother's family. How nice that cousin Juan has travelled so far to see me. I've been thinking about making a trip to Mexico next year, so perhaps I can stay with Juan during my visit. Surely my nurse manager understands how important family relationships are to Mexican Americans and will be able to rearrange the unit schedule to accommodate my request." The nurse manager may think, "What's wrong with these Mexican American staff ? Don't they want to work? This vacation request means that I'll have to re-do the schedule for the entire unit. If I permitted everyone to submit last-minute vacation requests, I'd go crazy. What's the big deal about a distant cousin coming to visit, anyway?"

Ideas about the importance of anticipating and controlling the future vary significantly from culture to culture. Whereas some staff place a high priority on planning for retirement, accumulating sick days, and purchasing insurance, other staff, particularly recent immigrants with family obligations in their homeland, might be more concerned with current obligations and living in the present. Similarly, some workers in high-risk jobs will participate actively in preventive immunization programs aimed at hepatitis and influenza, whereas others bewilder managers by saying, "What will be, will be. I can't spend time worrying about something that may or may not happen in the future."

Cultural Perspectives on Personal Hygiene

Another value that influences behavior is found in the proverb, "cleanliness is next to godliness." This proverb highlights the value for cleanliness, including an obsession

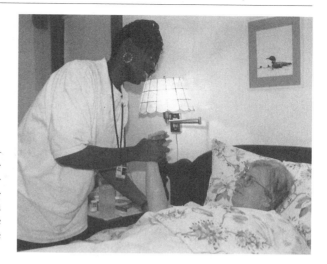

Effective cross-cultural communication is necessary for optimum patient healing. This African American home health care provider teaches a white patient how to perform range of motion exercises.

with eliminating or minimizing natural bodily odors—as evidenced by the plethora of deodorants, douches, body lotions, mouthwashes and the like with hundreds of different fragrances. Members of the dominant culture sometimes have difficulty staff from other cultures who are not unduly bothered by body odors and refrain from masking nature's original smells. In some cases, the staff member may come from a country in which water is scarce and bathing is restricted. Other times the staff member may be following religious or cultural practices that prohibit bathing during certain phases of the menstrual cycle, after delivery of a baby, and other times. Nurse managers and other supervisors frequently find the sensitive topic of hygiene difficult to discuss with staff from diverse cultural backgrounds.

Cross-Cultural Communication

Underlying the majority of conflict in the multicultural health care setting are issues related to effective cross-cultural communication, verbal and/or non-verbal. Even when dealing with staff from the same cultural background, it requires administrative skill to decide whether to speak with someone face-to-face, send an electronic or paper memorandum, contact by telephone or opt not to communicate about a particular matter at all. The nurse must exercise considerable judgment when making decisions about effective methods for effectively communicating with staff and patients/clients from diverse cultural backgrounds including a sense of timing, tone and pitch of voice, choice of location for face-to-face interactions, and related considerations. It should be noted that communication difficulties caused by language/accent issues become compounded on the telephone. It is sometimes necessary to counsel recent immigrants from non–English-speaking countries) to refrain from giving or receiving medical orders by telephone until their English language skills have developed.

Approximately 32 million people (14 percent of the total U.S. population) speak languages other than English. In rank order the most frequently spoken languages are Spanish, 54 percent; French, 6 percent; German, 5 percent; Italian, 4 percent;

and Chinese, 4 percent. As the 21st Century draws near it is estimated that the United States will continue to attract about two thirds of the world's immigration and 85 percent of the immigrants will come from Central and South America (U.S. Bureau of the Census, 1993). Box 14-1 suggests strategies for promoting effective cross-cultural communication in the multicultural workplace.

Cultural Perspectives on Touch

Differences in behavioral norms in the multicultural workforce are often inaccurately perceived. Typically, people from Asian cultures are not as overtly demonstrative of affection as Anglo Americans or African Americans. Generally they refrain from public embraces, kissing, and loud talking or laughter. Affection is expressed in a more reserved manner. Anglo and African Americans may be perceived as boisterous, loud, ill-mannered, or rude by comparison. In some cases, staff from different cultures may send messages through their use of touch that are not intended. Special attention is warranted for male–female relationships in the multicultural workplace. In general, it is best to refrain from touching staff of either sex unless warranted for accomplishment of a job-related task such as the provision of safe patient care. For nurses who tend to be more tactile, it is important to consciously refrain from placing one's hand on another's arm or shoulder, as frequently happens during ordinary conversation. For further discussion of this topic see Chapter 2.

Cultural Perspectives on Clothing and Accessories

Most health care institutions have a dress code or policy statement about clothing and accessories worn by staff in various parts of the facility (e.g., delivery room, operating room, specialty units, and so forth). It is important to review these documents periodically from a cultural perspective. For example, modification of the dress code might be necessary to accommodate Hindu women dressed in the *sari*, Sikh men who wear a turban, Amish and Mennonite women who wear bonnets and men who wear straw or black felt hats, Muslim women and Catholic nuns who cover their heads with veils, and Arab men who wear a *khafia*. Special consideration may need to be given to some African Americans and others who wear jewelry and other accessories in their hair, particularly when the hair is braided.

Cultural Perspectives on Time Orientation

In some cases cultural differences in time orientation create difficulty in the workplace. This may manifest itself when staff from diverse cultures are tardy, take excessive time for breaks and fail to complete assignments within the expected time frame. These differences may be interrelated with the cultural meaning of work, religious practices, and cross-cultural communication issues. It is important to be explicit in the job-related expectations about punctuality, schedule for breaks, and time allotted for assignments.

If a staff member develops a pattern of tardiness, the reason(s) should be explored. Although there needs to be a uniform standard applied to all staff concerning punctual-

Box 14-1 *Strategies to Promote Effective Cross-Cultural Communication in the Multicultural Workplace*

- Pronouce names correctly. When in doubt, ask the person for the correct pronunciation.
- Use proper titles of respect: "Doctor," "Reverend," "Mister." Be sure to ask for the person's permission to use his or her first name or wait until you are given permission to do so.
- Be aware of gender sensitivities. If uncertain about the marital status of a woman or her preferred title, it is best to refer to her as Ms. (pronounced mizz) initially, then ask how she prefers to be called at the first opportunity.
- Be aware of subtle linguistic messages that may convey bias or inequality. For example, referring to a white male as Mister while addressing an African American female by her first name.
- Refrain from Anglicizing or shortening a person's given name without his or her permission. For example, calling a Russian American "Mike" instead of Mikhael, or shortening the Italian American Maria Rosaria to Maria. The same principle applies to the last or surname.
- Call people by their proper name. Avoid slang such as "girl," "boy," "honey," "dear," "guy," "fella," "babe," "chief," "mama," "sweetheart" or similar terms. When in doubt, ask people if they are offended by the use of a particular term.
- Refrain from using slang, pejorative, or derogatory terms when referring to persons from ethnic, racial, or religious groups and convey to all staff that this is a work environment in which there is zero tolerance for the use of such language. Violators should be counseled immediately.
- Identify people by race, color, gender, and ethnic origin only when necessary and appropriate.
- Avoid using words and phrases that may be offensive to others. For example, "culturally deprived" or "culturally disadvantaged" imply inferiority and "nonwhite" implies that white is the normative standard.
- Avoid cliches and platitudes such as "Some of my best friends are Mexicans" or "I went to school with African Americans."
- Use language in communications that includes *all* staff rather than excludes some of them.
- Do not expect a staff member to know all the other employees of his or her background or to speak for them. They share ethnicity, not necessarily the same experiences, friendships, or beliefs.
- Communications describing staff should pertain to their job skills, not their color, age, race, sex, or national origin.
- Refrain from telling stories or jokes demeaning to certain ethnic, racial, age, or religious groups. Also avoid those pertaining to gender-related issues or persons with physical or mental disabilities. Convey to all staff that there will be zero tolerance for this inappropriate behavior. Violators should be counseled immediately.
- Avoid remarks that suggest to staff from diverse backgrounds that they should consider themselves fortunate to be in the organization. Do not compare their employment opportunities and conditions with those people in their country of origin.
- Remember that communication problems multiply in telephone communications because important nonverbal cues are lost and accents may be difficult to interpret.
- Provide staff with opportunities to explore diversity issues in their workplace and constructively resolve differences.

ity, it may be useful to listen to the staff member's explanation and ask what he/she thinks will rectify the problem. Reasons for punctuality problems may range from child care to car repair needs. Solutions may include the mobilization of cultural resources such as using extended family members to look after dependents or net-working with coworkers who might be able to recommend a reliable auto mechanic. It is important to listen attentively without rendering judgment or dictating solutions that the person has not agreed to.

It is sometimes useful to divide an assignment into sub-tasks with specific time lines for each activity. If the staff member has difficulty completing the assignment within the allotted time, it is important to follow-up with a discussion of the reasons why there were problems. This follow-up should be conducted in a positive, pro-active manner and viewed as an opportunity to promote cross-cultural communication, not as a punitive or disciplinary measure.

Cultural Perspectives on Interpersonal Relationships

As indicated in Figure 14-2, there are cultural differences in interpersonal relationships involving authority figures, peers, subordinates, and patients/clients. To examine, these cultural differences, consider the following example. Dr. Kelly, an Irish American physician, gave an order for vital signs to Kim Li, a Chinese-American nurse. The nurse perceived the order as unnecessary (but not harmful) to the patient, i.e., she thought the physician was requesting vital signs more frequently than warranted by the patient's condition. Nurse Li refrained from questioning the physician or negotiat-ing with him out of respect for his position of authority and the value she places on maintaining harmony in the relationship. Nurse Li said nothing and carried out the physician's order.

At the change of shift, the charge nurse became angry because she concurred with the assessment that Dr. Kelly had ordered vital signs too frequently and thought Nurse Li should have confronted the physician about the order. Nurse Li intentionally chose to avoid questioning Dr. Kelly's order because she perceived him as an authority

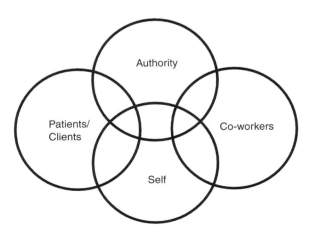

FIGURE 14-2. Cultural per-spectives on interpersonal rela-tionships.

figure and wanted to foster harmony and balance. In her cultural value system, causing conflict through direct confrontation would be perceived negatively. She would have experienced lowered self-esteem and "loss of face" if she had been responsible for causing disharmony in the nurse–physician relationship. The charge nurse, on the other hand, perceives the physician as a colleague whose respect will be earned by assertive, direct communication with him.

Long-standing Historic Rivalries

Some historians refer to the 1900s as the Century of War. At any given moment, there is armed conflict between two or more nations or factions within them. On occasion, the multicultural workplace becomes a battleground where long-standing historic rivalries and more recent geopolitical differences are reenacted in the form of interpersonal conflict between two or more staff members. After ruling out other potential sources of conflict, it may be worth examining the ethnic heritage and national origins of staff for possible reasons. For example, the nurse manager may observe a pattern of strained relationships between an Israeli physician and Palestinian physicians, nurses, laboratory technicians, physical therapists and other health care providers. Similar observations may be made concerning staff from known rival countries such as North and South Koreans, Russians and Armenians, Iranians and Iraqis, Indians and Pakistanis, and so forth.

Cues that may signal underlying historic rivalries include (1) the expression of high levels of emotional energy when interacting with a person from a rival group when the topic does not seem to warrant it; (2) sudden, uncharacteristic behavior changes when in the presence of a person from the rival group, e.g., an ordinarily cordial staff member unexpectedly becomes acrimonious for no apparent reason; (3) the repeated expression of strong opinions about historical, political and current events involving rival nations or factions; and (4) inappropriate attempts to persuade others to adopt his/her partisan views about the rivalry.

Cultural Perspectives on Etiquette

Values frequently underlie cultural expectations of behavior including matters of *etiquette,* the conventional code of good manners that governs behavior. For example, some people from Hispanic, Middle Eastern and African cultures expect the nurse manger to engage in social conversation and establish personal/social rapport before giving assignments or orders for the day's work. In developing interpersonal relationships, there is a high value placed on getting to know about a person's family, personal concerns, and interests before discussing job-related business. The nurse manger's reluctance to engage in self-disclosure about personal matters may leave the impression that he/she is uncaring and disinterested in the staff member. These behaviors by the manager are not conducive to building productive, harmonious relationships and may be misunderstood by staff from diverse backgrounds. Similarly, some cultures value formal greetings at the start of the day or whenever the first encounter of the day occurs, a practice found even among close family members. For example, it is important to

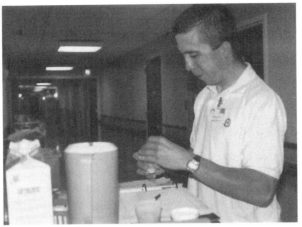

Although women historically have comprised the majority in nursing, men make significant professional contributions. In considering diversity in the multicultural workplace, the role of men in nursing must be included along with an examination of racial, ethnic, religious, and other types of differences.

say, "Good Morning, Mr. Okoro. There has been a change in your patient's insulin orders" rather than immediately "getting to the point" without recognizing by name the person to whom you are speaking.

Cultural Perspectives on Gender and Sexual Orientation

Women historically have comprised the majority of personnel in nursing and in many allied health disciplines. Currently, women comprise 97 percent of the nursing profession. Although Chapter 2 provides information about gender and sexual orientation, a few remarks about issues in the multicultural workplace will be made.

The complex interrelationship between gender and culture has been studied extensively. In the health care setting, nurses of both genders may face the biases and preconceptions of physicians, fellow nurses and other health care providers. The issue is further complicated by cultural beliefs about relationships with authority figures and cross-national perspectives on the status of various health care disciplines. For example, in many less developed nations nursing is a low status occupation. In some oil-rich Arab countries (e.g., Saudi Arabia, Kuwait) care for the sick is carried out by health care providers who are hired from abroad for the purpose of caring for the bodily needs of the sick—an activity that is considered unacceptable in its cultural context.

Males in nursing and other female-dominated health care disciplines continue to struggle as minority members of their professions. In the multicultural health care workplace, both men and women face the gender biases that exist in society. These issues frequently emerge in verbal and nonverbal communication and in interpersonal relationships. Our language also belies covert gender biases and preconceptions. For example, the expression *male nurse* is sometimes used but seldom does one hear about the *female nurse* because it is considered redundant and unnecessary. Beyond the scope of this text is an extensive analysis of workplace issues concerning gay, lesbian and bisexual staff, but these types of diversity must be considered in the multicultural workplace.

Cultural Perspectives on Moral and Religious Beliefs

In some circumstances, *moral and religious beliefs* may underlie conflicts in the multicultural workplace. Consider the following dilemmas:

- A nurse who believes that it is morally wrong to drink alcohol refuses to carry out a physician's order for the therapeutic administration of alcohol as a sedative/hypnotic or to administer medicines with an alcohol base (e.g., cough syrup).
- A nurse who believes that humankind should not unleash the power of nuclear energy refuses to care for irradiated cancer patients.
- A Roman Catholic nurse working in the operating room refuses to scrub for abortions, tubal ligations, vasectomies and similar procedures due to religious prohibitions.
- A Jehovah's Witnesses nurse refuses to hang blood or counsel patients concerning blood or blood products.
- A Seventh-Day Adventist nurse who cites biblical reasons for following a vegetarian diet is unwilling to conduct patient education involving diets that contain meat.
- Muslim and Jewish staff express concern that the hospital cafeteria fails to serve foods that meet their religious requirements.

The moral and religious issues mentioned are reflections of the diversity that characterizes staff in the health care workplace. The challenge is to balance the health care needs and rights of patients with the moral and religious beliefs of health care providers. In some instances, it may be impossible to provide the services demanded by the organization's mission statement if all nurses refused to engage in a particular activity. There may be legal implications for refusing to provide patients with certain services, e.g., those related to reproductive health. In the clinical world, the options available to accommodate the diverse moral and religious beliefs of staff frequently depend on the size of the organization, moral and religious proclivities of coworkers, attitudes and beliefs of managers, organizational climate, fiscal constraints and other factors. The challenge facing nurse managers is to balance the conflicting moral and religious beliefs of diverse groups with achievement of organizational goals. This must be accomplished in a manner that is respectful of the moral and religious beliefs of staff.

Conflicting Role Expectations: Staff Educated Abroad

According to the Commission on Graduates of Foreign Nursing Schools (Personal Correspondence, 1997), as of December 1993, there were 64,844 graduates of foreign nursing programs who are currently practicing as registered nurses in the United States. The majority of these nurses were educated in the Philippines, with a markedly increased number coming from Asia and the British Commonwealth countries, the United Kingdom, Ireland, Australia, New Zealand and Canada in recent years (1992–1997). Similar trends prevail for foreign-educated physicians, laboratory technicians, and other health care providers.

Role is defined as the set of expectations and behaviors associated with a specific position. Considerable research has been conducted on the patient sick role and on roles of nurses, physicians and other health care providers. Furthermore, it is suggested that persons entering the United States from a similar culture (e.g., Canada, England, Ireland) with English as the primary language may experience a lesser degree of culture shock than someone from a more diverse culture. For example, it is suggested that staff from Canada, Australia, or the United Kingdom will experience less difficulty with cultural adjustment to the U.S. than persons from the Near and Middle East, Asia or Africa in which language, religion, dress, and many other components of culture may be markedly different. Although social scientists speculate that people from similar cultures are more readily able to relate to one another, health care providers must be able to transcend cultural differences and to recognize that there are differences in role expectations.

Discrepancies in role expectations tend to create intrapersonal and interpersonal conflict. For example, nurses in Taiwan, the Philippines, and many African nations, expect the families of patients to participate significantly in caregiving during the patient's hospitalization. All aspects of personal hygiene are provided by family members, who may be encouraged to remain with the patient around the clock, often sleeping on the floor or in uncomfortable lounge chairs.

In many countries nurses have considerably expanded roles and their scope of practice is correspondingly broader. For example, in Nigeria it is clearly stated by the Board of Nursing and Midwifery that nurses diagnose and treat common illnesses such as malaria, typhoid, cholera, tetanus and similar maladies. In order to graduate from a nursing program in the Philippines, nursing students must deliver a minimum of 25 babies unassisted and also assist at major and minor surgeries. In Haiti, nurses routinely start intravenous lines, perform episiotomies, and repair lacerations. In terms of the mastery of technical skills, recent graduates of many foreign nursing programs have logged a considerable number of hours of clinical experience, often as apprentices who are mentored by experienced nurses who serve as their clinical faculty.

Some British and Irish nurses perceive U.S. nurses as "junior physicians," second-guessing and anticipating therapy. It is the perception of many that in Britain and Ireland nurses have greater freedom in ordering nursing modalities without physician's orders. For example, decubitus care, ambulation, dressings and nutritional therapy are all nurse-initiated activities based on nursing assessment. British and Irish nurses also expect that the nursing role includes activities that are defined by U.S. nurses as non-nursing. For example, in many British hospitals nurses are expected to clean patients' units after discharge and prepare for the next admission.

In many nations nurse midwives are primarily responsible for obstetric care. In some ways the U.S. is anomalous with its emphasis on the medically dominated specialty of obstetric medicine. Viewing childbirth as a medical problem (versus a normal physiologic process) reveals an underlying philosophical difference between the U.S. health care delivery system and that in other nations. Some nurses who have been educated abroad are both nurses and midwives, thus the transition to the medically dominated model in the U.S. may leave them feeling underutilized and confused about the roles of the obstetrician and the maternal–child nurse or nurse midwife.

Due to the shortage of qualified health care providers in many less developed countries, there usually are fewer interdisciplinary differences about the nature and scope of practice for various health care disciplines. There are also various categories of licensed and unlicensed health care providers that contribute to the overall health and well being of people in countries around the world. For example, there are feldshers in the former Soviet Union, bare foot doctors in China and herbalists in nearly every nation.

Cultural Assessment in the Multicultural Workplace

Individual Cultural Self-Assessment

As indicated in Chapter 1, it is important for nurses to be aware of their own *ethnocentric* tendencies, which is best accomplished when individuals review their cultural attitudes, values, beliefs and practices. Figure 14-3 explains the importance of cultural values in the workplace, and Table 14-4 contains the Diversity in the Workplace survey form, which is one instrument used for gathering cultural data about staff and their beliefs about multiculturalism in the workplace. By gathering responses to the Diversity in the Workplace instrument, nurse managers can identify staff perceptions about diversity issues and determine what management strategies might be useful. A culturally diverse workforce should be a strength in meeting the needs of culturally diverse clients/patients and should be viewed as an asset. Nurse managers, however, need to release the cultural talents of this workforce.

Diversity in the Workplace

What Do You Think?

Please read the following statements on the left and record your perceptions about each statement using the numeric ranking scale to the right. Circle only one numeric response for each question. On the odd-numbered questions, you are evaluating the frequency with which specific actions/activities occur in your work setting. On the even-numbered questions, you are ranking the importance of managers' action/activities on an intensity scale (1 to 5) of importance.

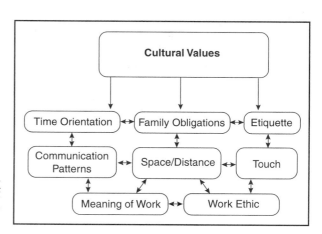

FIGURE 14-3. Influence of cultural values in the multicultural workplace.

After responding to the questions on the individual cultural assessment instrument, read Research Application 14-1, which summarizes a study in which the instrument was administered to staff nurses. Note that there are differences in responses given by white, black, Hispanic and Asian nurses who participated in the study, which indicates that perceptions of effective management actions vary according to the nurse's ethnic heritage.

Health care managers have a responsibility to create harmony within the multicultural workforce at their institutions. Suggestions in the literature for manager actions to deal effectively with cultural diversity may not agree with staff members' perspectives on the issue. The investigator introduced a quasi-experimental evaluation method that may be used as introductory work for research in multicultural workforce management. Using recommendations from the literature, the researcher asked 100 health care workers of various ethnic backgrounds, experience, and age to complete a 20-item Likert-type instrument concerning management actions that create multicultural harmony in a hospital setting. Results indicate that staff members perceive equal growth opportunity, achievable standards, understanding and respecting values, and striving to eliminate barriers as important actions. Concrete issues of equity and fairness are more significant to the workers than awareness education and opportunities for social activities among staff from various cultural backgrounds. The researcher concludes by indicating that staff are looking for actions by managers, not rhetoric.

Research Application 14-1	*Research on Actions by Nurse Managers that Enhance Multicultural Harmony*

Davis, P. D. (1995). Enhancing multicultural harmony. Ten actions for managers. *Nursing Management* 2(7), 32A–32H.

Health care managers have a responsibility to create harmony within the multicultural workforce at their institutions. Suggestions in the literature for manager actions to deal effectively with cultural diversity may not agree with staff members' perspectives on the issue. The investigator introduced a quasiexperimental evaluation method that may be used as introductory work for research in multicultural workforce management. Using recommendations from the literature, the researcher asked 100 health care workers of various ethnic backgrounds, experience, and age to complete a 20-item Likert-type instrument concerning management actions that create multicultural harmony in a hospital setting.

Clinical Application:
The study findings indicate that staff members perceive equal growth opportunity, achievable standards, respecting values, and striving to eliminate barriers as important actions. Nurses will find that concrete issues of equity and fairness are more significant to members of the staff than awareness education and opportunities for social activities among staff from various cultural backgrounds. The researcher indicates that staff are looking for actions by managers, not rhetoric.

TABLE 14-4

Individual Cultural Assessment Instrument

	Strongly Agree	Agree	No Opinion	Disagree	Strongly Disagree
1. Open acknowledgment and/or general discussion of cultural diversity occurs in my work environment.	1	2	3	4	5
3. Multicultural education or awareness programs are emphasizes in my work environment.	1	2	3	4	5
5. I have personally experienced communication or interaction difficulties with a manager because of my ethnic, cultural, gender, or racial values	1	2	3	4	5
7. Coworkers in my work environment tend to "hang out" during lunch or breaks with workers from the same cultural background.	1	2	3	4	5
9. Members of my own culture are participants on existing work committees or task forces that help set direction for the work environment.	1	2	3	4	5
11. In my work environment, I have access to work-related growth and development opportunities like my coworkers.	1	2	3	4	5
13. In my work environment, coworkers communicate verbally and/or through body language in ways that demean my culture or race.	1	2	3	4	5
15. All workers in my work environment are held to the same standards of job performance, regardless of gender, race, or cultural background.	1	2	3	4	5
17. Staff in my work environment are more successful if they share the same cultural values and ancestry as the manager.	1	2	3	4	5
19. When bicultural or multicultural conflict occurs in my work area, cultural, gender, and racial influences are openly discussed as part of the conflict resolution steps.	1	2	3	4	5
2. It is important that openness and general discussion of cultural diversity takes place in my work setting.	1	2	3	4	5
4. Multicultural education and awareness program emphasis is important in my work environment.	1	2	3	4	5
6. It is important that various cultural values are understood and respected by all managers working in a multicultural environment.	1	2	3	4	5
8. It is important for management to facilitate work and to plan culturally mixed social activity for the workers and my work environment.	1	2	3	4	5

(continued)

TABLE 14-4 (Continued)
Individual Cultural Assessment Instrument

	Strongly Agree	Agree	No Opinion	Disagree	Strongly Disagree
10. It is important for management to ensure that the cultures of all workers in my work environment are represented on work committees.	1	2	3	4	5
12. It is important for managers to recognize and encourage growth opportunities equally for all workers.	1	2	3	4	5
14. It is important for managers to work with staff to increase sensitivity to cultural values and perceptions that will help to reduce or eliminate racial and cultural barriers.	1	2	3	4	5
16. It is important for managers to have systems to identify and analyze which employees receive promotions and growth experiences, and to consider biases that influence performance standards so that they are achievable for all groups of staff.	1	2	3	4	5
18. It is important for the administration to recognize, reward, and value those managers who successfully promote, manage, and retain a harmonious multicultural work force.	1	2	3	4	5
20. It is important for managers to facilitate, promote, and participate in open dialogue about cultural influences and diverse perceptions that occur because of differences in ethnicity or gender.	1	2	3	4	5

Modified and used with permission. From Davis, P. D. (1995). Enhancing multicultural harmony. *Nursing Management 26*(7), 32D–32E © Springhouse Corporation.

Cultural Self-Assessment of Health Care Organizations, Institutions and Agencies

Before engaging in a cultural self-assessment of a health care organization, institution or agency, it is necessary to consider both *content* and *process*. Box 14-3 illustrates recommended *content* in a sample instrument. The instrument may be used to assess an *entire organization* such as a hospital, long-term care facility, home health agency, or other institution, organization or agency, or it may be modified for assessment of a *particular unit or division*. For example, staff in the operating room, specialty units, home health care division, ambulatory care area and so forth might perceive a need to engage in an *institutional self-assessment* due to changing demographics in populations served or concerns with quality of care for diverse clients/patients.

Figure 14-4 provides a schematic representation of the cultural self-assessment of a health care organization, institution, or agency. As with any assessment, begin

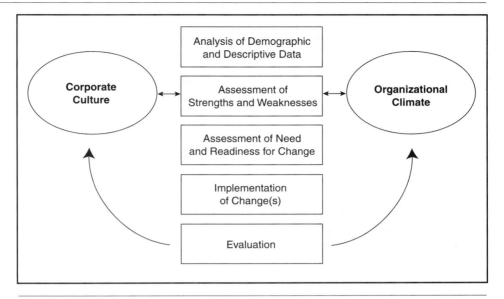

FIGURE 14-4.   Cultural self-assessment of health care organization, institution, or agency.

by gathering *demographic and descriptive data*. It is highly likely that some of these data already are collected and stored centrally. If reports containing the necessary data are available, they should be reviewed and discussed by the group as part of the cultural assessment process. Data such as types and numbers of diverse patients/clients and staff should be determined. There should be an assessment of the predominant languages spoken and effectiveness of the system being used for translation/interpretation.

The organizational *strengths and limitations* as they relate to multiculturalism should be assessed from an emic (insider) and etic (outsider) perspective, i.e., from the view point of health care providers (insiders) and clients/patients, those significant to them and visitors (outsiders). From the client/patient perspective, for example, examine the ways in which cultural aspects are part of the care provided. From the institutional perspective, critically examine the infastructure for philosophical, fiscal, and human resources that reflect a commitment—or lack of one—to promoting harmony in the multicultural workplace.

After completing the cultural self-assessment, determine the *need and readiness for change*. Be sure to anticipate staff *resistance to change*. Although most staff will support the change, it is insufficient for nurse managers and supervisors to say, "A new law has been passed mandating diversity" or "Hospital policy requires diversity." Different people will see different meanings in activities by organizations to become more culturally diverse. Members of the federal minority groups may see job opportunities, whereas white males may complain of "reverse discrimination." Resistance can be expected to increase to the degree that staff influenced by the changes have pressure on them to change and it will decrease to the degree they are actively involved in planning diversity activities. Resistance can be expected if the changes are made on personal grounds rather than as requirements, sanctions, or policies. Finally, resistance can be expected if the organization culture is ignored. There are informal as well as formal norms within every organization. An effective change will neither ignore old customs nor abruptly create new ones. As with most change, timing is important.

In developing an action plan for change, be sure to assess *community resources* available to assist with goal achievement. For example, it may be possible to mobilize human resources from the local ethnic community or to invite clergy to discuss health-related religious beliefs and practices. If organizational resources are limited, it may be possible to identify community-based resources available at low cost.

Process of Cultural Self-Assessment by Organizations, Institutions and Agencies

Although the manner in which the Cultural Self-Assessment is carried out will vary for each institution, organization and agency and for different units or divisions within it, the process remains fundamentally the same. After identifying key staff to lead the institutional cultural self-assessment process, the leaders should communicate the purpose of the cultural self-assessment to those who will be participating in it. It is important to involve grassroots members of the staff and to solicit input from the patient/client population served through interviews, focus groups, written surveys or other methods. Rather than reinventing the proverbial wheel, it is important to review existing databases to determine if demographic data already have been gathered. If so, review the information and include it with other data gathered during the assessment phase of the process.

After data have been gathered, a team of key leaders should convene to critically review and analyze it. Because this will be an active working group, membership should be limited to approximately 12 people. If the group size is larger, there should be consideration given to dividing into smaller sub-groups. The purpose of the review is to assess strengths and limitations/areas for continued growth in terms of promoting a harmonious multicultural environment for patients/clients and staff of diverse backgrounds. It is important to identify strengths and limitations from both an *emic* (insider) and *etic* (outsider) perspective. For example, although the staff may believe the system is structured adequately to meet the needs of linguistically diverse persons, it would be important to compare that perception with the patient/client point of view. Throughout the process, comparative analyses are being made between staff and patient/client input in order to identify strengths and limitations.

Once the strengths and limitations have been identified, there should be an assessment of the need and readiness for change. If changes are needed, it is important to identify why, who, what, when, where, and how. Determine who is likely to favor and oppose the proposed change, anticipate obstacles to it, and develop contingency plans. Identify fiscal and human resources that will be needed to bring about the recommended change(s). Depending on the nature of the recommendation and the corporate culture of the organization, an action plan should accompany the recommendation, i.e., specifically what does the group believe ought to be done? Be sure to include community resources that may be available to assist in implementing the recommendations. For example, it may be possible to involve foreign languages faculty and students from area colleges and universities to assist with translation for linguistically diverse patients/clients or to invite leaders from ethnic communities to provide staff inservices aimed at increasing understanding of the health care needs of persons from diverse backgrounds.

After the recommended change(s) have been implemented, there should be an evaluation of their effectiveness and revisions should be made as needed. Recognizing the rapid pace of change in contemporary health care, the process of institutional cultural self-assessment should be repeated at periodic intervals.

Promoting Harmony in the Multicultural Workplace

After conducting a cultural assessment of the health care organization, institution, or agency, the nurse will have data about the strengths and weaknesses, fiscal, human and community resources, areas in which to pursue change, and readiness of the staff to engage in change.

As indicated in Box 14-2, there are *facilitators* and *barriers* to promoting harmony in the multicultural workplace. Facilitators include identification of the cultural values of the organization, institution or agency, clear articulation of the mission statement and policies about diversity, zero tolerance for discrimination, effective cross-cultural

---

Box 14-2 *Promoting Harmony in the Multicultural Workplace*

Facilitators

Identification of cultural values of the organization, institution, or agency
Mission statement and policies about diversity
Zero tolerance for discrimination
Effective cross-cultural communication
Skill with conflict resolution involving diversity
Commitment to multiculturalism at all levels of management

Barriers

Hatred
Prejudice
Bigotry
Racism
Discrimination

(negative attitudes or behaviors based on race, ethnicity, religion, gender, sexual orientation, national origin, class, handicap/disability)

communication, skill with conflict resolution involving diversity, and commitment to multiculturalism at all levels of management. The barriers that must be overcome include hatred, prejudice, bigotry, racism, discrimination, and ethnoviolence. Negative behaviors aimed at employees, clients/patients, their families, others significant to them and other visitors, based on race, ethnicity, religion, gender, sexual orientation, national origin, class, or handicap/disability, should not be tolerated. All employees should be apprised that there will be zero tolerance for those who engage in negative behaviors, and management staff at all levels should be given the authority to impose sanctions when violations occur.

Summary

Given the demographic composition of contemporary society, nurses in the next decade will continue to find both challenges and opportunities as they practice nursing in multicultural health care settings. Microcosms of society at large, health care organizations, institutions and agencies will consist of staff from increasingly diverse backgrounds. It is important to remember that culture influences the manner in which people perceive, identify, define and solve problems in the workplace. Among the complex and interrelated factors that must be considered when addressing workplace diversity are cultural perspectives on values, the meaning of work, interpersonal relationships, cross-cultural communication patterns (including etiquette, touch, space/distance), gender and sexual orientation, moral and religious beliefs, hygiene and clothing. Characteristics of the staff member such as individual preferences, biases and prejudices for and against certain groups, educational background, and prior experiences living and working in culturally diverse settings also must be considered.

Understanding cultural differences in the workplace and developing skill in conflict resolution will continue to be needed in transcultural nursing administration as the next millennium approaches. The successful transcultural nurse administrator will behave respectfully toward others from diverse backgrounds and will implement policies that promote cultural understanding, knowledge and skill in the workplace. Nurses in leadership and management positions will apply the principles of transcultural nursing to the multicultural workplace just as they have done in the past to provide culturally competent and congruent care for clients and patients.

Review Questions

1. Compare and contrast the concepts *hatred, prejudice, racism, discrimination* and *ethnoviolence.* Critically examine the manner in which they may manifest themselves in the health care workplace.
2. What is meant by *transcultural nursing administration*? How is transcultural nursing administration useful for nurses who hold leadership positions in multicultural health care settings?

3. How does the cultural meaning of work embraced by staff from diverse cultures influence the corporate culture and organizational climate of contemporary health care institutions, organizations and agencies?
4. Identify strategies to promote effective cross-cultural communication in the multicultural workplace.
5. Critically analyze the cultural origins of conflict that may arise in the health care workplace.
6. Review the process and content of cultural self-assessment by organizations, institutions and agencies. What aspects of the change process must be considered when engaging in cultural self-assessment?
7. Identify facilitators and barriers to promoting harmony in the multicultural workplace.

Learning Activities to Promote Critical Thinking

1. Using the guidelines in Box 14-3, conduct a cultural assessment of a health care organization, institution or agency. Alternatively, you may use the guidelines to gather assessment data on a unit or department within a larger facility.
2. Ask at least 10 nurses working at a health care organization, institution or agency (hospital, long-term care facility, prison, home health care agency or related facility) if they would be willing to respond to the items found in the instrument in Table 14-4, Diversity in the Workplace. Average the numeric responses for each of the 20 items to identify trends. Write a one-page summary of your findings that includes a critical analysis of the results. What do the responses tell you about the organizational climate and corporate culture that prevail within the health care facility?
3. Reflect on your personal experience with hatred, prejudice, bigotry, racism, discrimination, and/or ethnoviolence. Were you the victim or the perpetrator? How did you feel during the incident(s)? Discuss your responses with another member of the class, preferably someone from a different cultural background from your own.
4. From a cultural perspective, critically examine the dress code or policy statement about clothing and accessories that are permitted for staff at a health care organization, agency or institution. How effectively does the code or policy address the widespread diversity that characterizes our contemporary health care workforce? Identify the strengths and limitations of the dress code or policy statement. What modifications or changes would you recommend to accommodate the attire worn by staff from diverse cultures?
5. Choose two of the six case studies presented at the beginning of the chapter and analyze them from the perspective of a nurse manager. For the purpose of analysis, assume the role of nurse manager and critically examine approaches you might use to change the negative attitudes and behaviors of those mentioned in the case studies.

Box 14-3 *Cultural Assessment of an Organization, Institution, or Agency*

Demographics/Descriptive Data

- What types of cultural diversity are represented by clients, families, visitors, and others significant to the clients? Indicate approximate numbers and percentages according to the conventional system already used for reporting census data.
- What types of cultural diversity are represented? What types of diversity are present among patients, physicians, nurses, x-ray technicians, and other staff? Indicate approximate numbers and percentages by department/discipline.
- How is the organization, institution, or agency structured? Who is in charge? How do you assess the administrators in terms of support for cultural diversity and interventions to foster multiculturalism?
- How many key leaders/decision makers within the organization, institution, or agency come from culturally diverse backgrounds?
- What languages are spoken by patients, family members/significant others, and staff?

Assessment of Strengths

- What are the cultural strengths or positive characteristics and qualities?
- What institutional resources (fiscal, human) are available to support multiculturalism?
- What goals and needs related to cultural diversity already have been expressed? What successes in making services accessible and culturally appropriate have occurred to date? Highlight goals, programs, and activities that have been successful.
- What positive comments have been given by clients and significant others from culturally diverse backgrounds about their experiences with the organization, institution, or agency?

Assessment of Community Resources

- What efforts are made to use multicultural community-based resources (e.g., anthropology and foreign languages faculty and students from area colleges and universities; community organizations for ethnic or religious groups; and similar resources)?
- To what extent are leaders from racial, ethnic, and religious communities involved with the institution (e.g., invited to serve on boards and advisory committees)?
- To what extent is there political and economic support for multicultural programs and projects?

Assessment of Weakness/Areas for Continued Growth

- What are cultural weaknesses, limitations, and areas for continued growth?
- What could be done to better promote multiculturalism?

Assessment From the Perspective of Clients and Families:

- How do clients (and families/significant others) evaluate the multicultural aspects of the organization, institution, or agency? Do quality assurance data indicate the clients from various cultural backgrounds are satisfied/dissatisfied with care? Be specific.
- How adequate is the system for translation and interpretation? What materials are available in the client's primary language (in written and other forms such as audiocassettes, videotapes, computer programs, etc.)?
  NOTE: the literacy level of clients must be assessed.
- Are educational programs available in the languages spoken by clients?
- Are cultural and religious calendars used in determining scheduling for preadmission testing, procedures, educational programs, follow-up visits, or other appointments?

Box 14-3. *(Continued)*

- Are cultural considerations given to the acceptability of certain medical and surgical procedures (e.g., amputations, blood transfusions, disposal of body parts, and handling various types of human tissue)?
- Are cultural considerations a factor in administering medicines? How familiar are nurses, physicians, and pharmacists with current research in ethnopharmacology?
- If a client dies, what cultural considerations are given during postmortem care? How are cultural needs associated with dying addressed with the family and others significant to the deceased? Does the roster of religious representatives available to nursing staff include traditional spiritual healers such as shamans and medicine men/women, as well as rabbis, priests, elders, and others?

Assessment From an Institutional Perspective:

- To what extent does the philosophy and mission statement support, foster, and promote multiculturalism and respect for cultural diversity? Is there congruence between philosophy/mission statement and reality? How is this evident?
- To what extent is there administrative support for multiculturalism? In what ways is support present or absent? Provide evidence to support this.
- Are data being gathered to provide documentation concerning multicultural issues? Are there missing data? Are data disseminated to appropriate decision makers and leaders within the institution? How are these data used?
- Are opportunities for continuing professional education and development in topics pertaining to multiculturalism provided for nurses and other staff?
- Are there racial, ethnic, religious, or other tensions? If so, try to objectively and nonjudgmentally assess their origins and nature in as much detail as possible.
- Are adequate resources being allocated for the purpose of promoting a harmonious multicultural health care environment? If not, indicate areas in which additional resources are needed.
- What multicultural library resources and audiovisual and computer software are available for use by nurses and other staff?
- What efforts are made to recruit and retain nurses and other staff from racially, ethnically, and religiously diverse backgrounds? What other types of diversity (e.g., sexual orientation) are fostered or discouraged?
- How would you describe the cultural climate of the institution? Are ethnic/racial/religious jokes prevalent? Are negative remarks or comments about certain cultural groups permitted? Who is doing the talking and who is listening to negative comments/jokes?
- Are human resources initiatives pertaining to advertising, hiring, promotion, and performance evaluations free from discrimination?
- Are cultural and religious considerations reflected in staff scheduling policies for nursing and other departments?
- Are policies and procedures appropriate from a multicultural perspective? What process is used for reviewing them for cultural appropriateness and relevance?

Assessment of Need and Readiness for Change

- Is there a need for change? If so, indicate who, what, when, where, why, and how.
- Who is in favor of change? Who is against it?
- What are the anticipated obstacles to change?
- What financial and human resources would be necessary to bring about the recommended changes?

References

Birdwhistell, R. L. (1970). *Kinetics and Content*. Philadelphia: University of Pennsylvania Press.

Brown, I. C. (1973). *Understanding Race Relations*. Englewood Cliffs, NJ: Prentice-Hall.

Davis, P. D. (1995). Enhancing multicultural harmony. *Nursing Management 26*(7), 32A–32H.

Flarey, D. L. (1993). The social climate of work environments. *Journal of Nursing Administration 23*(6), 9–15.

Henderson, G. (1994). *Cultural Diversity in the Workplace*. Westport, CT: Praeger.

Holmes, S. A. (1994, March 3). Survey finds minorities resent each other almost as much as they do whites. *New York Times*, A9.

Jezewski, M. A. (1993). Acting as a culture broker for culturally diverse staff. *Advisor for Nurse Executives 8*(10), 6–8.

Josselson, R. (1992). *The Space Between Us: Exploring Dimensions of Human Relationships*. San Francisco: Jossey-Bass.

Jung, C. A. (1968). In G. Adler. *The Collected Works of Carl Jung*. Vol. 10. Princeton, NJ: University Press.

Leininger, M. M. (1996). Founder's focus. Transcultural nursing administration: An imperative worldwide. *Journal of Transcultural Nursing 8*(1), 28–33.

Morgan, G. (1997). *Images of Organization*. Thousand Oaks, CA: Sage Publications.

Personal correspondence (1997, March 18). From Dr C. R. Davis, Director of Research and Evaluation/Director of Operations, Commission on Graduates of Foreign Nursing Schools: Philadelphia, PA.

Schwartz, R. H., & Sullivan, D. B. (1993). Managing diversity in hospitals. *Health Care Management Review 18*(2), 51–56.

Scrivastava, R., & Wong, K. (1992). Promoting cultural sensitivity in the workplace. *ANNA Journal 19*(4), 419.

Tulmann, D. F. (1992). Cultural diversity in nursing education: Does it affect racism in the nursing profession? *Journal of Nursing Education 31*(7), 321–324.

U.S. Bureau of the Census (1993). Place of birth of foreign-born persons: 1990. *1990 Census of Population, Social and Economic Characteristics United States*. Series 1990. CP-2–1. Washington, DC: U.S. Government Printing Office, p. 12.

U.S. Department of Health and Human Services, Bureau of Health Professions (1993). *Fact Sheet. Selected Facts About Minority Registered Nurses*. Washington, DC: U.S.

International Nursing and Health

Margaret M. Andrews

KEY TERMS

International Nursing
International Health
Primary Health Care
World Health Organization
 (WHO)
International Council of Nurses
National Health Care
Health For All by the Year 2000

Less Developed Countries
 (LDCs)
More Developed Countries
 (MDCs)
Infant Mortality
Child Mortality
Emerging Infectious Diseases
Immunization

Chronic Illnesses
Epidemiologic Transition
Occupational Prestige
Cultural Adjustment
Culture Shock
Refugees
International Sending Agency

OBJECTIVES

1. Discuss international nursing as a clinical specialty within the profession.

2. Examine the past and present role of nurses in meeting global health needs.

3. Provide an overview of the world's state of health, including the major causes of morbidity and mortality in various parts of the world.

4. Identify ways that nurses can prepare for international nursing.

5. Explore criteria for nurses to consider when choosing an international sending agency.

6. Identify selected health care agencies that send U.S. and Canadian nurses abroad.

Throughout this text the emphasis has been largely on U.S. and Canadian cultures and subcultures. This chapter will provide an overview of *international nursing*, a term that is sometimes used interchangeably with *transnational nursing*.

> International health is like a distant exotic place: difficult to reach, replete with unfamiliar tribal customs, strangely alluring, perhaps a bit dangerous; but with the prospect that the journey there would be immensely worthwhile (Basch, 1990).

There are many reasons for incorporating international nursing content into the curriculum and providing clinical learning opportunities whereby other parts of the

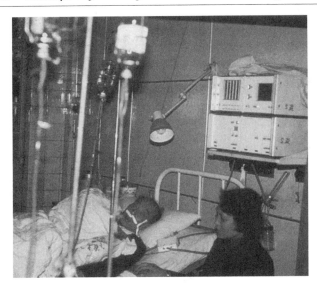

Intensive care unit in the People's Republic of China.

world can be experienced by nurses and nursing students. According to Styles (1993), when the year 2000 arrives, it will mark the beginning of the "International Century." This new century will be a time when political alignments and technology combine to encourage mobility and interchange and an era when national borders are less obvious and obstructive. Nurses must increasingly see themselves as part of a global community in which problems, solutions, resources, and opportunities are shared.

Historical Overview

Nursing is indisputably among the oldest and most universal human activities. Until the 19th century, nursing was carried on by families for their own members, by religious orders committed to the care of the sick, and in the large public institutions built for the care of the sick poor, by untrained persons from the lower socioeconomic class. As a result of the contributions of Florence Nightingale during the 19th century, modern nursing was born, and an era in which highly trained nurses traveled to all parts of the globe to practice their profession began.

Florence Nightingale and International Nursing

By age 29, Florence Nightingale had begun her nursing-related foreign travels as she journeyed to the Institution of Deaconesses at Kaiserwerth, Germany, a trip that she subsequently would make many times. Critical of the English hospital system, Nightingale encouraged international nursing education by targeting farmers' daughters to become trained as nurses using the Kaiserwerth model. Many young English women heeded the call and traveled to Germany for formal educational preparation in the art and science of nursing.

As English fatalities in the Crimean War escalated, military leaders agreed to allow Nightingale and her companions to travel to Scutari, which is located on the southwest border of the Black and Aegean seas. In Scutari, Nightingale organized the Barrack Hospital for casualties of the battles of Balaclava, Sebastopol, and Inkerman, as well as for those soldiers who fell victim to cholera. Following the Crimean War, the 36-year-old Nightingale rested briefly in Paris before returning to England, where she received a heroine's welcome for her wartime efforts to save the lives of wounded and sick soldiers. Shortly after her return to England, Nightingale again traveled and studied hospitals throughout Europe, where she was recognized as an expert on primary prevention and hospital procedures. Nightingale's hospital reforms reached beyond Europe to India, where she concluded that healthier living would result in increased longevity (Nightingale, 1859; Uhl, 1992).

At age 39, Nightingale published *Her Notes on Hospitals* (1859), in which she advocated improved hospital construction and physical maintenance to reduce deaths during hospitalization. In 1860, Nightingale founded a school of nursing at London's Saint Thomas Hospital, thus marking the beginning of both modern professional nursing and nursing education. Virtually all nursing education programs in the world today are modeled on the English pattern or one of two others that evolved from it: the French and the U.S. patterns.

Graduates of the Saint Thomas Hospital Nursing School were known as "Nightingale Nurses" and were prepared to train others. Nightingale nurses accepted positions where they could teach and promote the high standards of nursing care advocated by Nightingale, and hospitals from all over the world sought Nightingale nurses to start new schools of nursing. As early as 1867, Nightingale nurses were found in Australia, and throughout the 1880s, they were at work in Canada, Sweden, Germany, and most of the large hospitals in the United Kingdom and the United States.

North American Nurses Abroad

Early in the development of U.S. and Canadian nursing history, nurses prepared in the Nightingale tradition traveled abroad, often motivated by religious and/or moral convictions. In 1885, Linda Richards became the first U.S. nurse on record to engage in international nursing when she went to Japan under the auspices of the American Board of Missions to establish a school of nursing. Records from the Presbyterian Mission Board of Canada indicate that nurses were sent abroad more than 100 years ago, mainly to Taiwan, China, and India.

Nurses in both the U.S. and Canada served in World Wars I and II. The United Nations Relief and Rehabilitation Administration was established immediately after World War II to assist in repatriating the millions of displaced persons in Europe. By November 1945, there were 211 nurses in service, many of whom were from the U.S. and Canada.

The Red Cross Society, or Red Crescent as it is known in Muslim countries, responds to disasters worldwide, and nurses have been embers of its relief teams for many years. In 1946, Canadian Helen McArthur became director of nursing services of the Canadian Red Cross. McArthur was posted to Korea as associate coordinator of the League of Red Cross Societies. Her major concern was the care of 100,000 war orphans, many suffering from tuberculosis. For her contributions to nursing she was awarded the Coronation Medal honoring Queen Elizabeth's coronation in 1953 and the Florence Nightingale Medal from the International Red Cross in 1957, to name a few of her honors (Dier, 1988).

Initiated in 1950, the Colombo Plan offered scholarships to foreign nurses studying at Canadian universities and sent Canadian nurses overseas. With the establishment of the Canadian International Development Agency (CIDA) in 1968, more funds became available for development, which expanded the number of health-related projects. The demand for international nurses increased dramatically as agencies responded to the urgent health needs around the world.

With the creation of the World Health Organization in 1948 and the proliferation of technical assistance programs, nurses have become increasingly involved in international health. Today, nurses have many opportunities to go abroad for the purposes of travel, research, education, consultation, and service in virtually all clinical practice specialty areas.

Access to Health Care Services

In analyzing the overall status of the world's health, the nurse rapidly realizes that there is wide variation in the quality of health care and in access to services for many of the world's people. There are substantive differences between and within countries, and socioeconomic status is among the major factors in determining an individual's health and his or her access to health care services. At the 1978 International Conference on Primary Health Care held in Alma-Ata (in the former Union of Soviet Socialist Republics), leaders from 134 World Health Organization member nations declared that the health status of hundreds of millions of people in the world was unacceptable. In 1981, the Thirty-Fourth World Health Assembly adopted the global strategy of "Health for All by the Year 2000" and identified *primary health care* as keystone in improving global health.

Primary Health Care

Both the World Health Organization (WHO), and the International Council of Nurses (ICN) state that

> . . . primary health care is essential to health care made universally acceptable to individuals and families in the community by means acceptable to them, through their full participation and at costs the community and country can afford. It forms an integral part both of the country's health system, of which it is the nucleus, and of the overall social and economic development of the community (WHO, 1978, p. 2).

As conceived by the World Health Organization, *primary health care* includes five basic principles. The first is universal coverage, with care provided according to need. The second advocates a range of services—promotive, preventive, curative, rehabilitative, and terminal—that are provided in community-based settings as well as in hospitals. The third principle addresses the need for services to be effective, culturally acceptable, affordable, and manageable. The fourth principle advocates that communities be involved in primary health care and that self-reliance be encouraged while dependence is reduced. The fifth principle reaffirms that health must be related to other sectors of development. Comprising the largest sector of the global health care work force are nurses and midwives, whose role in primary health care is crucial.

The Primary Health Care movement has been responsible for a tremendous ideological shift: from curative to preventive care, from hospital care to community care and public health, and from urban to rural health care. Beyond the scope of this chapter is a review of the many primary health care programs that have been established by United Nations member countries and an evaluation of the effectiveness of the *Health for All by the Year 2000* program. In general, however, the outcomes have been quite favorable. The reader is encouraged to visit WHO's internet site (www.who.org) for further information on its programs and the contributions they have made to improving global health.

National Health Care

To ensure universal access to health care for its citizens, many countries have a national health program. Table 15-1 identifies the industrialized countries with a national health program. Notably absent from the table is the U.S., which spends in excess of $1 trillion a year on health-related services and products. Despite this large expenditure, the U.S. currently has more than 40 million citizens under 65 years of age with no health insurance (National Center for Health Statistics, 1995).

Global Health Care Problems

According to WHO (1997), each year approximately 52 million people die throughout the world, with 46.5 million deaths due to illness and disease. Of the 140 million babies born each year, almost 4 million die within hours or days from perinatal causes. More than 500,000 women die each year from causes related to pregnancy and childbirth.

On the positive side, some childhood diseases—measles, poliomyelitis, pertussis (whooping cough), and neonatal tetanus—are decreasing as a result of immunization programs. It should be noted that the cost of vaccines to accomplish this was less than $1 per child. The incidence of cardiovascular diseases in most developed countries

---

TABLE 15-1
Industrialized Countries with a National Health Program

Australia	Germany	Norway
Austria	Great Britain	Poland
Belgium	Greece	Portugal
Boznia-Herzegovina	Hungary	Romania
Bulgaria	Ireland	Russia
Canada	Italy	Spain
Denmark	Japan	Sweden
Finland	The Netherlands	Switzerland
France	New Zealand	

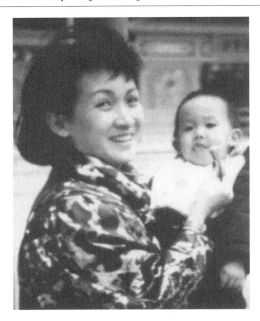

Life expectancy for women, infants, and children is significantly increased as a result of improved standards of living and immunization programs.

(except those in eastern Europe) has decreased in recent years due to health education and promotion efforts around the world. Infant and child mortality rates and the overall death rate are continuing to decrease globally, and life expectancy is increasing worldwide.

In analyzing global health, nations are frequently categorized as *Less Developed Countries* (LDCs, or agricultural, nonindustrialized nations) or *More Developed Countries* (MDCs, or industrialized nations), terms that are admittedly subjective and relative. For example, although the United States and Canada are categorized as MDCs, there are underdeveloped sections in which poverty-stricken people live in substandard housing with poor or absent sanitary facilities. Conversely, China, Mexico, and other nations classified as LDCs have rich cultural histories that predate the founding of the United States and Canada by many centuries. In all LDCs there is a small segment of the population that is very affluent. Recognizing these paradoxes, the categorization is still useful in examining *general patterns* of global health care.

Major Health Problems in Less Developed Countries

WHO estimates that 80 percent of illness in LDCs could be avoided if safe drinking water were available. As a result of unsafe water and other environmental conditions, *infectious* and *parasitic diseases* account for almost one-half of all deaths in LDCs. Tuberculosis, acute respiratory infections, diarrheal diseases (e.g., cholera, amebic dysentery), malaria, and sexually transmitted diseases are prevalent in most LDCs. Although not necessarily life-threatening, the most common infections in the LDCs are roundworm (*Ascaris*), hookworm (*Ancylostoma*), and whipworm (*Trichuris*). The protozoan *Giardia lamblia* is distributed worldwide, affecting almost 1 in every 3 people.

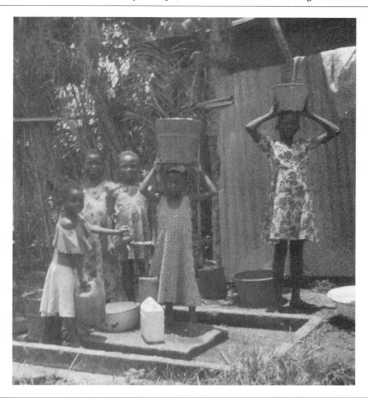

According to the World Health Organization, 80 percent of disease in less developed countries could be eradicated if people had clean water to drink. Many families rely on children to transport (carry) water from public water sources to their homes.

Every year, about 3.5 million new cases of *cancer* occur in LDCs, making it the second leading cause of death. Two-thirds of all cancers are attributable to lifestyle and environment, and at least one-third are preventable. As the life expectancy continues to increase and the chronic conditions associated with increasing life expectancy are manifested, cancer incidence rises. Although worldwide life expectancy is 65 years, the majority of LDCs still have a life expectancy below 50 years (notable exceptions are Argentina, Cuba, Singapore, and Sri Lanka, where a life expectancy of 70 or more years is enjoyed).

Ranked *third* as a cause of mortality in LDCs are *circulatory diseases* (including heart attack and stroke). One of the most prevalent risk factors associated with circulatory diseases is diabetes mellitus, a condition that is increasing everywhere in the world.

The *fourth* leading cause of death in LDCs is *perinatal problems*, largely due to (1) lack of prenatal health care resulting from inadequate access to maternal–child health care; (2) insufficient numbers of obstetricians, nurse-midwives, and trained lay birth attendants; and (3) cultural beliefs and practices about childbearing (e.g., cultural prohibitions against blood transfusions) and child rearing (e.g., ritual circum-

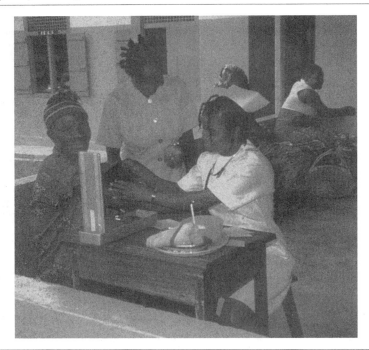

Despite primary prevention programs, such as blood pressure screening, vascular diseases are a leading cause of death in many countries of the world.

cision with nonsterile instruments for both males and females). In a regional analysis of global health care trends, sub-Saharan Africa has the highest birth and death rates, 45 births and 14 deaths per 1,000 population.

The *fifth* leading cause of mortality in LDCs is *accidents*. Interrelated with over-population and crowding in large urban centers, motor vehicle accidents, often involving pedestrians or bicycle riders, are growing at alarming rates. In some countries, the government's lack of involvement in establishing and monitoring motor vehicle safety standards, testing and licensing operators of motor vehicles, developing and enforcing traffic regulations, and maintaining safe roadways has been a contributing factor. Drownings, burns, industrial mishaps, and household accidents also claim large numbers of victims (Badran, 1993; WHO, 1996).

Major Health Problems in More Developed Countries

In many MDCs, the trend for noncommunicable diseases is generally downward, but *cancer, cardiovascular diseases, chronic bronchitis,* and *diabetes* are increasing. Antismoking campaigns in many MDCs are bringing positive results in the fight against lung cancer but for men only. Among women, death rates from lung cancer are increasing rapidly and are now three times greater than they were 35 years ago. Vascular disease (including heart attacks and strokes) and motor vehicle accidents, although declining, are still major causes of death. Suicide in MDCs has increased

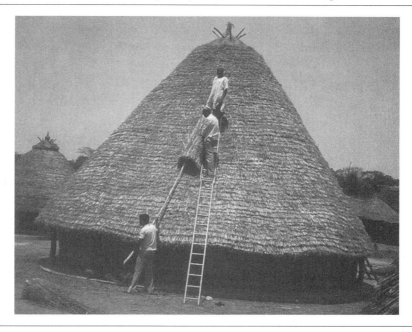

Occupational hazards are often responsible for the high incidence of accidental injuries in many parts of the world.

steadily and is 50 percent higher than it was 35 years ago. Japan leads the world with the highest life expectancy at 79 years and the lowest infant mortality rate at 4 per 1,000 live births (WHO, 1997).

Infant and Children's Health

The term *child mortality* is defined as the probability of dying by the age of 5 years. In 1995, the global average was 81.7 per 1,000 live births, with the MDCs reporting an average 8.5 per 1,000 live births, whereas the LDCs averaged 90.6 deaths birth 1,000 live births. Of more than 11 million child deaths in the developing world, nine million have been attributed to infectious diseases, about 25 percent preventable by immunization (WHO, 1996). Summarized in Table 15-2 are the infant mortality rates for the top 25 MDCs. As indicated in the table, Canada ranks sixth, whereas the U.S. is 24th on the list.

Infectious Diseases: Global Health Threat

According to WHO (1996), 17 million people are killed each year by infectious diseases. Summarized in Table 15-3 are the leading 10 causes of fatal infections.

The emergence or reemergence of infectious diseases is the result of multiple factors. It is partly the result of a shift of resources away from infectious disease control, public health and sanitation. In part, the global problem with infectious

TABLE 15-2
Infant Mortality Rates: Ranking the More Developed Countries

Rank	Country	Infant Mortality Rate (Number of Infant Deaths per 100,000 Live Births)
1	Japan	4.60
2	Finland	5.64
3	Sweden	5.96
4	Hong Kong*	6.13
5	Singapore	6.67
6	Canada	6.82
7	Switzerland	6.83
8	Federal Republic of Germany**	6.98
9	Norway	7.02
10	The Netherlands	7.06
11	France	7.33
12	German Democratic Republic**	7.33
13	Denmark	7.39
14	Northern Ireland	7.47
15	Scotland	7.73
16	Austria	7.84
17	England and Wales	7.88
18	Belgium	7.94
19	Spain	8.07
20	Australia	8.17
21	Ireland	8.20
22	New Zealand	8.31
23	Italy	8.53
24	United States	9.22
25	Greece	9.32

*Now part of People's Republic of China

**Now united as a single nation

Source: National Center for Health Statistics (1994). *Health, United States. 1993.* Hyattsville, MD: U.S. Public Health Service, p. 12.

diseases is caused by changes in the environment that have brought animals and insects that carry disease into closer contact with humans. The combination of populations growth (especially in large urban areas), international air travel, incessant migration, and the movement of refugees means that peoples of the world are more intermingled now than at any time in history. Human transmission is rapidly becoming the primary way in which diseases are spread, not just from person to person but from continent to continent—by airborne and droplet spread, sexual transmission, blood borne transmission, or direct contact.

The risk of foodborne diseases has been heightened by the globalization of trade and changes in the production, handling and processing of food. Despite Food and Drug Administration inspection, for example, authorities frequently alert the public

TABLE 15-3
Ten Leading Causes of Fatal Infections in the World

Disease	Number of Deaths
Acute lower respiratory tract infections (e.g., pneumonia)	4.4 million
Diarrheal diseases (e.g., cholera, typhoid, dysentery)	3.1 million
Tuberculosis	3.1 million
Malaria	2.1 million
Aquired immune deficiency syndrome (AIDS)	>2 million
Hepatitis B infections	1.1 million
Measles	>1 million
Neonatal tetanus	460,000
Whooping cough (pertussis)	350,000
Intestional worm diseases	135,000

Table based on data from: World Health Organization (1996). *The World Health Report 1996: Fighting Disease, Fostering Development.* Geneva: World Health Organization.

via media announcements to the dangers of contaminated meat and vegetables sold to unsuspecting victims in fast food restaurants or grocery stores. Environmental factors can lead to the exposure of humans to previously unknown diseases. For example, the destruction of forests has resulted in movement of animal and insect habitats that carry high risks of exposure to disease.

The problem is compounded by the fact that antimicrobial drugs, which were once effective against some of the most common infections have gradually become ineffective. The blame for the growing ineffectiveness of antimicrobial drugs may be traced to the following: (1) health care providers who prescribe antibiotics inappropriately (e.g., use wide-spectrum antibiotics rather than base treatment on culture and sensitivity results or give in to patient requests for unnecessary antibiotic treatment); (2) patients who take the antimicrobials incorrectly (usually by those who stop taking the drug as soon as symptoms diminish rather than finishing the prescribed course of treatment) or self-treat without knowing the diagnosis or recommended treatment (e.g., take penicillin for colds); (3) tenacious, microbes that mutate so rapidly that the development of new antimicrobials cannot keep pace; and (4) widespread non-prescription availability of antimicrobial drugs, especially in many LDCs where regulation of drugs is lax.

Emerging Infectious Diseases

The term *emerging infections* refers to those whose incidence in humans has increased during the last two decades or that threaten to increase in the near future. The term includes previously unknown infectious diseases or those spreading to new geographic areas. During the past 20 years, more than 30 new microorganisms have emerged, some of which cause lethal disease in localized outbreaks or over great distances, at a cost of enormous suffering and expense to society. The term infectious also refers to conditions that were easily controlled by antibiotics or chemotherapy but have developed antimicrobial resistance (Heyman, 1997; WHO, 1996).

The most dramatic example of a new disease is acquired immunodeficiency syndrome (AIDS), caused by the human immunodeficiency virus (HIV). WHO (1996) estimates that 20 million adults worldwide have become infected with the *human immune virus* (HIV) since the start of the pandemic. Approximately 2 million of those have developed AIDS, a condition that afflicts people in both MDCs and LDCs. In the world as a whole, heterosexual intercourse has rapidly become the dominant mode of transmission of the virus. As a result, the LDCs already hold as many newly infected women as men, and the MDCs are approaching equal incidence in men and women. Homosexual transmission has remained significant in North America, Australia, Asia, and Northern Europe, although even in these areas heterosexual transmission is showing the fastest rate of increase. WHO (1997) estimates that by the year 2000, cumulative totals of 30 to 40 million men, women, and children will have been infected and 12 to 18 million will have developed AIDS.

Nearly 90 percent of the projected HIV infections and AIDS cases for this decade will occur in the LDCs. In sub-Saharan Africa, where more than 6 million adults already are infected, the situation is critical. Research Application 15-1 summarizes a study of AIDS patients who are cared for at home by women of the Bagandan tribe in Uganda. As many as one-third of pregnant women attending some urban antenatal clinics are HIV-infected. As a result, WHO estimates that 5 to 10 million HIV-infected children will have been born by the year 2000 (WHO, 1996).

In 1995, there were at least 333 million new cases of sexually transmitted diseases worldwide, excluding HIV infections. Sexually transmitted infectious diseases are sometimes interconnected with cancer. For example, sexually transmitted human papilloma viruses are responsible for most of the 520,000 cases of cervical cancer a year, 65 percent of the cases in MDCs and 87 percent of those developing in LDCs (WHO, 1996).

| Research Application **15-1** | *AIDS Caregivers in Uganda* |

MacNeil, J. M. (1996). Use of culture care theory with Bagandan women as AIDS caregivers. *Journal of Transcultural Nursing,* 7(2), 14–20.

Although many countries in sub-Saharan Africa are experiencing the effects of AIDS, Uganda, with its estimated 18 million population, has the highest rates of HIV infection in the region, sometimes affecting 25 to 40 percent of people in the sexually active age group. The highest incidence is found in the central and southern parts of Uganda near Kampala, Masaka, and Rakai, where the Bagandans are the largest cultural group.

Ethnonursing, supported by life history and Leininger's sunrise model, was used to discover care among 12 key and 25 general Bagandan informants providing AIDS caregiving to family members at home. In-depth interviews were conducted with informants from home-based nursing care programs. Data were analyzed and revealed six major themes. The findings highlighted the struggle of Baganda women to provide care for family members with AIDS; identified intergenerational care as essential for survival and prevention of HIV infection; and offered insight into improving the quality of life for those are HIV positive.

For Bagandan women, culture care means survival to help secure a future for the next generation and is interrelated with education and land claims. Disputes over ownership of land upon the death of a husband were common, often resulting in violence against the widow and challenges to the legal system. Care also meant continuing in the face of adversity and despite the burden of caring over time. Some informants learned that they also were HIV positive at the same time they had to accept their husband's illness. Acceptance led to acknowledgement of the loss of one's long-term future, and in many cases, the loss of young children who were also HIV positive. Although Bagandan women are traditionally subservient to their husbands, death of spouses and adult children from AIDS often resulted in women assuming traditional male authority over financial decisions. Surviving widows often rejected traditional customs such as a brother-in-law's obligation to marry a widow, thus causing change in family and social relationships.

Clinical Application:
This study revealed new insights into specific cultural beliefs, values and care modalities that can be used to provide nursing care for Bagandan women. Nurses, in turn, can use these cultural insights to help meet the challenge of this global illness and to fulfill their caring mandate to society.

According to Dr. Hiroshi Nakajima, Director-General of WHO, until recently there was a widespread feeling that the struggle against infectious diseases was almost won. Diseases such as plague, diphtheria, dengue, meningococcal meningitis, yellow fever, and cholera have reappeared as public health threats in many countries, after years of decline (Nakajima, 1997).

A new breed of deadly hemorrhagic fevers, of which Ebola is the most notorious, have struck in Africa, Asia, Latin America, and the United States. Ebola made its initial appearances in Zaire and the Sudan in 1976 and has emerged several times since, most notably in Zaire in 1995, where the 80 percent fatality rate caused worldwide alarm (Nakajima, 1997; WHO, 1996).

Since the hantavirus pulmonary syndrome was first recognized in the southwestern United States in 1993, it has been detected in more than 20 states. Cases have also occurred in Canada, Argentina, Brazil, and Paraguay. Caused by contact with infected mouse feces, the reported fatality rate for hantavirus pulmonary syndrome is 50 percent (Centers for Disease Control, 1996).

Epidemics of foodborne and waterborne infections due to new organisms such as crytosporidium or new strains of bacteria such as *Escherichia coli* 0157:H7 have affected MDCs and LDCs. A completely new strain of *Vibrio cholera* 0139 that appeared in Southeast India in 1992 has spread to other areas of India and parts of Southeast Asia. Tuberculosis, once regarded as virtually under control, is making a deadly comeback, killing about 3.1 million people annually. Drug-resistant tuberculosis is spreading in many countries, including the United States and Canada.

Despite the emergence of these deadly emerging infectious diseases, there is still a lack of national and international political will and resources to develop the systems necessary to detect them and stop their spread. According to WHO (1996), "Without doubt, diseases as yet unknown but that have the potential to be the AIDS of tomorrow, lurk in the shadows" (p. 4).

Antimicrobial Resistance

Resistance of diseases to antimicrobial drugs has increased significantly in the last decade, resulting in decreased ability to control diseases such as tuberculosis, malaria, cholera, dysentery, and pneumonia. Consequently, people with infections are ill for longer periods of time and are at greater risk of dying while epidemics are prolonged.

Resistant organisms have no natural barriers. International air travel has facilitated the transmission of diseases from remote locations to more populated areas and from continent to continent. As resistance spreads, the effective life span of drugs decreases. With stronger controls on the manufacturers of pharmaceuticals, the length of time needed to develop new antimicrobials has increased significantly, further widening the gulf between infection and control. Resistant strains of the tuberculosis bacilli are widespread, with alarming outbreaks of the largely caused by multi–drug-resistant strains in the U.S. and Canada. Both of the organisms that cause pneumonia are rapidly becoming resistant to drugs. The same is true of salmonellae, the leading cause of foodborne infections, and enterococci bacteria, which cause complications in many hospitalized patients. A large global problem, hospital or nosocomial infections are responsible for 70,000 deaths a year in the U.S. alone (WHO, 1996).

Immunization of Children

The global eradication of smallpox was officially declared by WHO in 1980, with the last reported case occurring in Somalia in 1977. May 1996 marked the 200th anniversary of the first successful immunization, by Dr. Edward Jenner in England, who protected a child against smallpox by inoculating him with cowpox virus. Currently, 80 percent of the world's children have been immunized against six diseases—diphtheria, measles, pertussis (whooping cough), poliomyelitis, tetanus and tuberculosis.

There are, however, national differences in policies governing the immunization of children. In the United States, for example, routine immunization of children against tuberculosis has not been recommended, whereas immunization against mumps, rubella, hepatitis B, *Hemophilus influenza* type b, and varicella zoster virus (chicken pox) is urged by the American Academy of Pediatrics and the U.S. Public Health Service. American children also are immunized against polio, diphtheria, tetanus, pertussis, and measles, as recommended by the World Health Organization (Centers for Disease Control, 1996; WHO, 1996). Compliance with vaccination schedules remains one of the greatest problems for global immunization programs. High dropout rates leave many children only partially protected and reduce the overall benefit that immunization of children provides to society.

Chronic Illnesses

According to WHO (1997), dramatic increases in life expectancy and changes in lifestyle will be responsible for global epidemics of cancer and other chronic diseases in the next two decades. In 1996, the global average life expectancy reached 65 years compared with a half a century ago, when most people died before the age of 50. Between 1990 and 1995 the number of people aged 65 and older increased to 380 million, reflecting a 14 percent global increase. Increased longevity is frequently accompanied by chronic illness or premature disability. Chronic diseases are responsible for more than 24 million deaths a year, with the leading causes being circulatory diseases (including heart disease and stroke), cancer, and chronic obstructive pulmonary disease. Many people become disabled or die from musculoskeletal disorders such as arthritis and osteoporosis.

As life expectancy increases, so does the certainty that people will become increasingly prone to develop diseases that are more common among older age groups. People living in LDCs face the challenge of surviving infectious diseases and other conditions associated with their social and economic circumstances plus the burden of chronic illness associated with an aging population This situation is known as the *epidemiologic transition*, the changing pattern of health in which poor countries inherit the problems of the rich, including illness and the harmful effects of tobacco, alcohol and drug use, and of accidents, suicide and violence. Because the LDCs continue to bear the weight of endemic infectious diseases, this is referred to as the *double burden* (WHO, 1997).

The development of chronic diseases is seldom due to a single cause. In addition to inherited vulnerability, many lifestyle factors, such as smoking, heavy alcohol consumption, inappropriate diet, and inadequate physical activity, are known to increase the health risks. Whereas the previously mentioned factors are, to some extent, within the control of the well-informed individual, factors such as poverty, poor reproductive and maternal health, genetic predisposition, occupational hazards, and stressful working conditions may not be so easily controlled. Many people are suffering and dying prematurely from chronic diseases. This trend is linked to lifestyles that have undergone radical changes in recent years, from physical outdoor labor to sedentary work, from rural life to urban existence, from traditional diet to unhealthy foods, from negligible consumption of alcohol and/or tobacco to daily or heavy consumption of one or both.

Although the concepts of mental health and mental illness are culturally constructed, hundreds of millions of adults are known to suffer from mental illnesses ranging from chronic depression to dementia. Whereas mood disorders afflict an estimated 340 million people at any given time, dementia (including Alzheimer's Disease) affects an estimated 29 million globally. Although the manner in which mental illnesses are diagnosed and treated varies widely throughout the world, they require each nation to respond with appropriate programs. For further information on global issues in mental and emotional health, the reader is encouraged to visit the internet site of the World Federation for Mental Health (www.wfmh.com).

To meet the global health challenges, WHO (1997) has identified six areas for international action:

1. Integration of disease-specific interventions in both physical and mental health into a comprehensive chronic disease control package that incorporates prevention, diagnosis, treatment and rehabilitation and improved training of health professionals.
2. Wider application of existing cost-effective methods of disease detection and management.
3. Global campaign to encourage healthy lifestyles, with an emphasis on the development of children and adolescents in relation to risk factors such as diet, exercise and smoking.
4. Healthy public policies that support disease prevention programs.

5. Acceleration of research into new drugs and vaccines and into the genetic determinants of diseases.
6. Alleviation of pain, reduction of suffering and provision of palliative care for those who cannot be cured.

The World's Nurses

Although there is no valid statistical information on nursing or midwifery personnel because of classification problems and lack of established information systems, it is estimated that there are 40 million nurses available to care for the world's estimated 5.7 billion people. Although the population of the United States accounts for approximately 5 percent of the world population, one-quarter of the world's nurses are in the United States. Two-thirds of the world's nurses and midwives live in the MDCs (5 million in Europe; 2.5 million in the United States and Canada). Table 15-4 summarizes the number of physicians and nurses/midwives in selected regions of the world. During the past decade, there has been a steady increase in international exchanges by U.S. and Canadian nurses, a trend that is likely to continue.

In addition to a lack of uniformity in classifying nursing and midwifery personnel, there are significant discrepancies in roles and functions, standards of performance, and quality of care by nurses in various parts of the world. In the eastern Mediterranean region, for example, there are 22 different categories of nurses, many having the same functions and responsibilities, though they come from widely different educational backgrounds. The scope of practice for nurses varies widely from country to country. In parts of Africa and Asia, nurses may prescribe medications, perform some surgeries, suture wounds, and set fractured bones. In some cases, apprenticeship training occurs, with on-the-job skill development and clinical instruction being supervised by staff

TABLE 15-4
Number of Physicians and Nurses in Selected Parts of the World

World Region	Total (Thousands)			
	Physicians	Nurses*	Physicians	Nurses*
Africa	0,109	0,448	2.4	9.9
Latin America	0,234	0,294	7.3	9.7
North America	0,458	1,164	18.2	51.1
East Asia	0,749	1,545	6.3	13.2
South Asia	0,445	0,871	3.2	6.2
Europe	1,021	2,025	21.1	54.8
Oceania	0,032	0,153	14.2	67.6
Former USSR	0,996	NA	36.5	NA
World total	4,044	6,501	9.1	14.8

*And midwives.

NA = not available.

Table based on data from Basch, P. (1990). *Textbook of International Health.* New York: Oxford University Press, p. 316.

Research Application 15-2

Occupational Prestige for Registered Nurses in the Asia-Pacific Region

Johnson, M., & Bowman, C. C. (1997). Occupational prestige for registered nurses in the Asia-Pacific region: Status consensus. *International Journal of Nursing Studies, 34*(3), 201–207.

Occupational prestige for registered nurses, associated with professional recognition, has its origins in intricate social class and status issues. The type of work an individual performs, or occupation, defines the individual's location within an industrialized society's social class system. Occupations requiring greater skill, longer training, and higher education receive greater rewards and prestige.

Regional consensus in the ascription of professional occupational status and consequent prestige between health workers and registered nurses in the Asia-Pacific region were studied. The purposes of the study were to (1) determine and compare the occupational status of registered nurses and medical officers within the Asia-Pacific region and other countries; (2) determine the educational level required for entry to practice as a registered nurse within the Asia-Pacific region and other countries; and (3) describe the educational levels of registered nurses within the Asia-Pacific region and other countries.

The countries included in the sample were those with membership in the Asia-Pacific Economic Cooperation (APEC) plus other nations in the region having similar occupational status of health professionals. Data also were gathered from published census data pertaining to Australia, Canada, Singapore, the United Kingdom, and the United States. In this descriptive study, a questionnaire was mailed to the individual country representative of ICN (N = 24) and published census data were gathered for countries in the study.

The findings reveal consensus that registered nurses and medical officers are regarded at the level of professional in 66 percent (N = 16) of the countries. Nursing in Australia, although rapid and complete in its transition to degree-level education, still reflects a paraprofessional status compared with the professional status of medical officers. Registered nurses from Thailand and the Philippines led the region in within-group consensus, with 80 percent of registered nurses holding a baccalaureate degree as their minimum educational qualification.

Clinical Application:

Occupational prestige for nurses may result in improved job satisfaction, enhanced abilities in health promotion activities, and autonomy in decision making related to patient care. Findings highlight the need to promote professional status for all registered nurses within the Asia-Pacific region and outline areas for potential disjuncture between status and prestige achievement. Because nursing is a global profession, nurses need to know about social, economic, and status differences in various countries around the world as they engage in international activities.

---

nurses working in the unit. As indicated in Research Application 15-2, occupational prestige for registered nurses varies in different regions of the world.

Educational Preparation for Nurses

Each country has special educational programs, and curricula vary widely in content, length, standards, and evaluation criteria. General education required to enter the nursing program ranges from 6 to 13 years, and the length of the nursing program varies from 1 to 4 years. There are general and specialty programs at the basic level of education. Post-basic educational programs in nursing vary widely in length and usually prepare nurses as specialists in clinical practice, education, or administration. In some nations, post-basic education prepares nurses in specialties not recognized in North America, such as dental and veterinary nursing.

International Council of Nurses (ICN)

The International Council of Nurses (ICN) is an independent, non-governmental federation of 112 national nurses associations, including the American Nurses Association and the Canadian Nurses Association. ICN represents more than 1.4 million nurses and is the leading voice on ethics for nurses worldwide.

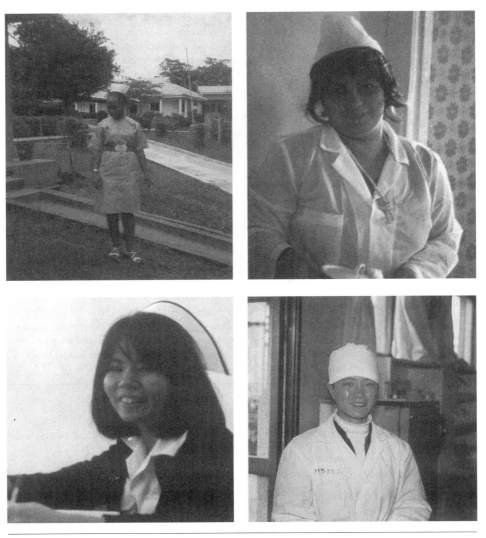

The world's nurses (clockwise from top left): Nigeria, Russia, China, and Hong Kong.

Founded in 1899, ICN is the oldest international professional organization in the health care field. The ICN works either through its own projects or in collaboration with other international organizations to promote health services. It encourages efforts by national nurses' associations to develop nursing standards and advance the economic position of nurses. ICN is currently testing a unifying framework called the International Classification for Nursing Practice (ICNP), which is intended to establish a common language about nursing care that can be compared across borders, populations, settings and time (Clark, 1996; Nielsen & Mortensen, 1996). ICN promotes its objectives through standard-setting programs, seminars, publications, and meetings. The official publication of the ICN is the *International Nursing Review*.

International organizations, notably WHO and the United Nations Children's Fund (UNICEF), work closely with the ICN on matters affecting health in all parts of the world. For example, ICN and WHO have issued a joint declaration on AIDS, dealing with the rights and responsibilities of nurses worldwide in caring for people infected with this disease. ICN also has worked with WHO to increase nurses' awareness and knowledge of the problems related to substance abuse and help nurses provide care for patients with addictions. The organization is active in such United Nations initiatives as Safe Motherhood, Health for All by the Year 2000, and Occupational Health.

ICN administers the Florence Nightingale International Foundation, which focuses on educational activities in nursing and serves as a permanent memorial to the founder of modern nursing. Every year International Nurses Day is celebrated on Florence Nightingale's birthday, May 12th.

Since 1991, ICN has administered a biennial questionnaire to determine how members ranked nursing issues worldwide. In 1993–94, ICN elicited responses from representatives of 46 of its 112 member countries for a response rate of 46 percent. Although there were regional differences, nursing education was ranked a top priority by national nurses associations (NNAs). With the trend toward health sector restructuring, nursing curricula must coincide with changes in health systems and must prepare nurses for community-oriented care. Curricula must also reflect contemporary health problems such as HIV/AIDS, mental health issues, and lifestyle disease issues. Nursing practice and standards of care tied for second place. In the wake of restructuring of health services and cuts in nursing staff in many countries, nurses are being challenged to provide high quality care with limited resources (ICN, 1995).

Sixty-seven percent of responding nurses' associations reported a nursing shortage in their country, with the greatest shortages occurring in Africa, the East Mediterranean, and European regions. To fill the unfilled, budgeted positions for nurses, 45 percent of respondents indicated that their government was recruiting nurses from abroad. Third and fourth on the priority list, respectively, were nursing legislation and work conditions for nurses. Seventy-four percent of responding NNAs have a nursing practice law in their country. The lowest priorities have been assigned to nursing specialties and administration/management (ICN, 1995).

International Nursing as a Specialty

There has been a spirited professional debate about whether *international nursing*, a term that is sometimes used interchangeably with *transnational nursing*, is a specialty, a framework through which some aspect of nursing is delivered, or transcultural

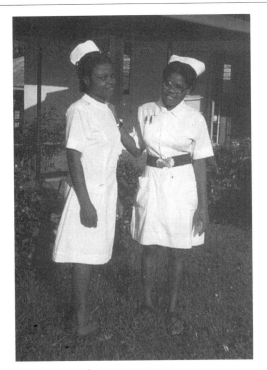

In many African nations, a staff nurse (right, wearing a belt) provides clinical instruction for nursing students (left).

nursing practiced across international boundaries. In referring to specialization within nursing, Peplau (1965) states that at first, particular nurses move in a direction of special interest, which presents as an immediate opportunity or need. Their focus becomes narrowed to one part of a larger field, thus allowing for greater depth in developing that part. In general, a specialty has three characteristics: (1) There is a unique body of knowledge and skills specific to a particular field; (2) This body of knowledge and skills is built on a theoretical base; and (3) This body of knowledge and skills can be identified and taught to professionals who possess a broad knowledge and skill base in nursing.

The most closely related specialty is transcultural nursing, a term which is sometimes used synonymously with cross-cultural, intercultural, or multicultural nursing. It is the opinion of this author, however, that the focus of international (or transnational) nursing extends beyond those areas of concern in transcultural nursing or the recognized nursing specialties and subspecialties.

International nursing is a specialty because it consists of a unique body of knowledge with specific problems and domains of practice not shared by other recognized nursing specialties (Andrews, 1985, 1986, 1992; DeSantis, 1998; Devereaux, 1993). The following are some of the unique characteristics of international nursing not shared by other recognized nursing specialties:

1.   Challenges related to understanding health care delivery systems and nurse practice regulations in other countries.

2. Learning about the nursing role and clients' expectations of nurses.
3. Working with counterparts who ultimately bear responsibility for nursing practice, education, and research in their nations.
4. Functioning safely with unfamiliar equipment, supplies, and medications.
5. Confronting ethical dilemmas having complex transnational components.
6. Working with limited health care resources (in some LDCs).
7. Collaborating with health care team members representing categories that may not exist in the United States or Canada.
8. Learning about tropical illnesses and other health care problems unfamiliar in the nurse's country of origin (including cultural definitions of health and illness, culture-bound syndromes).
9. Understanding and effectively working with political, social, economic, and cultural systems unlike those in the nurse's homeland.
10. Identifying and effectively using health care resources in the host country.
11. Solving problems related to visas, immunizations, licenses, insurance, and other necessities in a foreign country.

Instead of expending energy on debating whether international nursing is a specialty, the time has come to explore ways in which curricularly sound educational programs can prepare nurses to practice in the "International Century."

International Nursing as a Career

As with other careers, international nursing has benefits and drawbacks. Travel is stimulating, but living abroad has many challenges. For example, many health projects have multi-national teams, with nurses, physicians and other health care providers coming from dozens of different countries. In Sweden and Denmark, nurses care for many political refugees from countries about which they often have little knowledge. In many parts of the world, nurses find themselves providing care for refugees whose culture and language are often unfamiliar. In order to be successful in the international arena, the nurse needs a high degree of dedication, exceptional technical knowledge, and facility in informal diplomacy.

The total number of persons whose primary professional focus is international health is unknown, despite efforts by nurses and others to gather the data. An estimated 9000 U.S. health professionals are working in the international health field. Of these, 3800 are considered "long term," i.e., employed for 1 year or more; 1700 are short term, usually consultants; and 3200 are volunteers. Of the total, the largest category is nurses, followed by physicians and administrators. Most professionals do not follow lifelong careers in international health care but devote an average of about 12 years beyond professional education (Baker, Weisman, & Piwoz, 1984; Basch, 1990; Devereaux, 1993).

International Nursing: A Two-Way Street

When reflecting on their international experiences, most nurses who have spent substantial periods of time abroad indicate that they have learned *from* the exchange

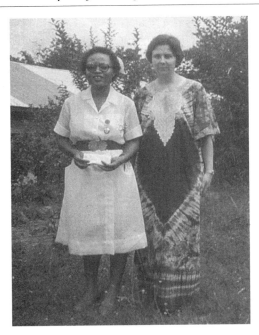

International nursing is a two-way street in which the U.S. or Canadian nurse both learns from and contributes to the health care of the people in other countries. Author (right) with Nigerian counterpart in a school of nursing.

as well as contributed to improved health for the people in the host country. Research on this subject reveals that nurses identify gaining increased knowledge in the following areas: cultural awareness, alternative health care delivery models (e.g., England's hospice care, elder care in Scandinavian countries), ways to include family members in nursing care, conservation of resources, nonbiomedical nursing interventions (e.g., therapeutic use of music, therapeutic massage, meditation to reduce anxiety and pain), and increased political awareness.

Preparation for International Nursing

Nurses often ask about academic qualifications and experience necessary for international health work. There is, in fact, no identified international health career pattern for U.S. or Canadian nurses in the sense that such a career existed (and to some degree still exists) in the colonial powers (England, France, Germany, the Netherlands, and other European nations) that have had vast overseas administrative responsibilities.

How do U.S. and Canadian nurses prepare to go abroad? What types of formal academic and continuing education are appropriate, useful, and helpful?

Academic Preparation

Addressing the need for formal educational preparation for international nursing, Leininger captures the urgency of the task (1981, p. 371):

Time is running out to help nurses in international consultations and work without having transcultural knowledge and skills....Tourism and television are not enough.

Formal education, by well-prepared educators, and application of the principles of transcultural nursing in the health care setting are indeed the ultimate goal; culturally sensitive caring to promote health and well-being.

With increasing frequency, U.S. and Canadian nurse-educators are recognizing the importance of incorporating international nursing into the curriculum of baccalaureate, master's, and doctoral programs and in providing continuing education courses with an international focus. Nurses and nursing students are expressing an increased interest in international nursing and are traveling, studying, and working abroad in greater numbers each year. Nursing students are seeking information about the appropriate ways in which to become prepared for the practice of nursing in other countries and are choosing programs that have internationalized their curriculum.

As the nurse prepares for international/transnational health care, he or she may wonder, "How can I ever learn all I need to know about a culture so I won't appear foolish or alienate clients?" First of all, recognize that it is impossible to learn all there is to know about another culture, regardless of how many years spent living in the country. By definition, the nurse will always be perceived as an outsider, stranger, or foreigner.

Research on international health care indicates that most U.S. and Canadian nurses work with more than one culture, often rotating back and forth between an international assignment and a position in the United States or Canada. Nonetheless, there are still skills and attitudes that nurses can develop. The following is a list of attributes that the Peace Corps seeks in its volunteers (and it has been widely adopted by corporations, hospitals, and other groups sending their staff overseas):

1. Listening skills, including listening for the nonverbal
2. Careful observation
3. Patience, not always expecting "them" to do the adjusting
4. Flexibility, openness to change and to learn from others
5. Ability to take risks, try new things, development of "emotional muscle"
6. Awareness of one's own values and cultural assumptions
7. Sense of humor
8. Ability to identify cultural resources in the community
9. Recognition that the reasons for one's feelings of frustration (or noncompliance on the part of clients) may be cultural in origin.

Summarized in Box 15-1 are the ways in which U.S. and Canadian nurses can prepare for international nursing, in addition to formal academic coursework.

Patterns of Cultural Adjustment

Whenever people are immersed in another culture, they will go through a period of *cultural adjustment*. One of the more well known patterns of cultural adjustment is the W model. Many variations on this theory exist, but the general pattern has been well documented in intercultural communications research. It is one of the few concepts agreed on by most professionals involved in cross-cultural education. Figure 15-1 illustrates the theory.

> **Box 15-1** *Preparation for International Nursing*
>
> - Reading about the culture, politics, economics, religions, and health care of the country
> - Reviewing scholarly and popular literature about the culture
> - Talking with host nationals living in the United States or Canada
> - Eating foods from the country (ethnic restaurants, practicing with chopsticks)
> - Contacting consulate or embassy of country to be visited
> - Contacting U.S. or Canadian government offices for information
> - Language studies
> - Watching documentaries/travel films
> - Visiting the country as a tourist prior to taking a professional position

Cultural Adjustment

There are five stages of cultural adaptation illustrated as the points on a W; this pattern may depend on the length of stay and the purpose of being in the other culture. The five stages are

1. *Excitement*, or the *honeymoon period*, which is characterized by enthusiasm resulting from the newness and sense of adventure.
2. *Culture shock.* The excitement is gone. Things are not "like back home"; social cues and relationships are difficult; there are feelings of alienation and homesickness and a temporary dislike of the host culture.
3. *Surface adjustment.* During this stage, the nurse is beginning to catch on; things are starting to make sense; rudimentary language (more accurate communication) skills are acquired, and the nurse is able to communicate some basic ideas and feelings, making some relationships in the local culture; the nurse begins to feel more comfortable.

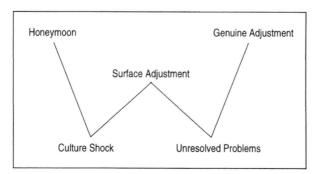

FIGURE 15-1. The W model of cultural adjustment.

4. *Frustration* and a deeper level of *unresolved problems* arise; the assignment period in the culture may seem very long, and the nurse may experience feelings of boredom, frustration, and isolation.
5. *Genuine adjustment* is characterized by acceptance of the new culture as just another way of living; the nurse may not always approve of cultural practices but understands the differences and begins to peel back some of the rich layers of the culture. The nurse has established genuine, real relationships with people in the host country.

All nurses experience the components identified in the cultural pattern when living in an unfamiliar culture. Some may decide that trying to adjust is too difficult and return home at the early "cultural shock" stage. Being aware that there is a pattern to feelings and reactions to the new culture is one step in making the nurse more effective in the international setting. Clients from other nations experience similar cultural patterns when they enter the United States or Canada. Shorter in duration, a phenomenon known as *reentry shock* can be expected when the nurse returns home. Reentry shock consists of feelings of general dissatisfaction, criticism for lifeways of his or her home country, and free-floating anxiety.

Refugees

Although most nurses visit another culture with the knowledge that they will, at some point, return home, some refugees can never return home. Therefore, what nurses may see in these people is not only culture shock but a genuine process of grieving over the loss of their homeland, for these clients may be suffering the permanent loss of an integral part of their being, their physical culture (Muecke, 1992). In addition, migration and resettlement require psychological adaptation. In a study by Aroian (1990), loss and disruption, novelty, occupational adjustment, language accommodation, and subordination were described as predominant aspects of migration and resettlement.

Going Abroad

In the next section, you will be given guidelines for making decisions about going abroad and choosing sending agencies that are congruent with your philosophical beliefs.

Motivation

Before choosing a sending agency, it is essential to examine one's motivation for going abroad. In studies of U.S. nurses engaging in international consultation, several reasons motivating nurses have been identified, including enjoyment of people from other cultures, interest in travel, moral convictions, religious beliefs, financial rewards, personal invitation by host country counterparts, cross-cultural exchange of ideas, professional commitment, and service to those in need. Identifying motivation and determining the goal(s) and purpose(s) for the international experience will facilitate selection of the appropriate type of position and sending agency (Andrews, 1985, 1986, 1988, 1992; Horsley, 1991).

Length of Time Abroad

Related to the motivation for going abroad is the length of time that you plan to spend overseas. Before contacting potential sending agencies, it is important to determine a time commitment, stated in terms of days, weeks, months, or years. Opportunities for short-term international experiences (less than 6 months) vary widely and are likely to require tradeoffs in benefits provided by the agency. Travel/study programs usually assume that the applicant is willing to pay part or all of the expenses for the trip. Long-term international experiences offer a wide variety of opportunities, with contracts varying according to the agency's needs and resources.

Geographic Region

If a particular region is preferred, this must be matched with the sending agency's activities and projects. Some agencies specialize in a particular region, whereas others have programs on virtually every continent. The following reasons may motivate the nurse to choose a particular region or country: (1) political stability of the country; (2) personal/emotional reasons such as a significant other living in the area; and/or (3) matching host country needs with the expertise of the nurse.

Although global politics may shift rapidly, the Middle East, South Africa, and certain parts of Central and South America have a reputation for volatile politics, including anti-American demonstrations. Personal safety is of concern, and careful research should be conducted before accepting an assignment in a politically unstable area. State Department reports, information provided by the sending agency, informal discussions with recently returned visitors to the country, and current news sources may provide the necessary information to determine the safety of the area.

Reasonable Expectations of Sending Agencies

Although specific details will vary according to the sending agency, Box 15-2 is intended to provide guidelines for asking questions. Sending agencies expect questions and recognize that interviewing is a two-way process.

Negotiating a Contract

The preceding discussion has focused on some aspects that are reasonable to expect in a contractual agreement with a sending agency. Before signing the contract, it is important to study the details carefully and to discuss any unclear matters with the agency representative. A written job description should accompany the contract along with a statement detailing the conditions surrounding contract termination by either the nurse or the sending agency.

Box 15-2 *Guidelines for Choosing an International Sending Agency*

Salary/stipend:

- What is the salary/stipend in U.S. or Canadian dollars?
- If any portion is paid in local currency, what is the exchange rate?
- What has been the history of fluctuation in the exchange rate during the past 2 years?
- What is the cost of living compared with the salary/stipend?
- What is the average cost for housing, food, transportation, and utilities in the host country?
- Can local currency be exchanged for U.S. dollars? Can U.S. or Canadian dollars be used to purchase local currency?
- Can salary earned in the country be taken out of the country? If so, by what means? Bank transfer? Cashier's check?
- What length of time is usually required for bank transactions? International transfers? Local banking needs?
- To which government(s) are taxes owed? What is the rate of taxation? How, when, and where should tax statements be processed/filed?

Travel to host country assignment:

- Is round-trip airfare paid by agency? Are spouse and/or dependents sent or eligible for discounted fares?
- Is there a payback clause for early contract termination?
- Who makes travel arrangements? Is a confirmation by the ticket holder required?
- How frequently are return trips to the United States or Canada allowed/paid for by the agency?

Housing and moving:

- Does the agency provide housing? In an expatriate community or in a neighborhood inhabited by host country nationals?
- What is the type of housing provided? Is there central heating and/or air conditioning, running water, toilet and bathing facilities, window screens?
- What type of energy is used? What is the average monthly cost?
- Is there a reliable source of electricity available? If not, is there a generator?
- Is the housing furnished or unfurnished?
- What are the conditions of the move? By what means (air, surface, sea)? Is travel and household insurance included? Amount of coverage provided? Who is responsible for packing?
- What household goods and commodities are reasonable to expect locally? At what cost?
- Does the agency have special arrangements for shipping items such as regular mail pouch service, agency deliveries, etc?
- If housing allowance is given, are family members included?

Local transportation:

- Are vehicles available to staff for job-related travel? For personal use after hours and on weekends?
- What is the cost of gasoline? Maintenance of a vehicle? Does the agency employ a mechanic? Are reliable local mechanics available? Are replacement parts for vehicles available?
- Does the agency provide car loans? What are the terms? Is there a waiting list for vehicle purchases? If so, how long? What is the average price for a vehicle?
- What are local regulations on drivers' licenses, automobile insurance?
- If vehicles are not available, what methods of local transportation are used by agency staff? Cost? Availability? Safety?
- Are women permitted to drive vehicles? If not, is a driver provided by the agency? During what hours/times?

Box 15-2. *(Continued)*

Insurance benefits:

- What type of health, life, disability, and retirement insurance is available? Are family members included?
- In case of illness, what is the agency policy concerning treatment? What health care facilities may be accessed for personal and family health care?
- If local hospitals are used, what is the quality of care compared with the United States? What type of pediatric care is available locally for dependent children?
- Is paid leave and/or airfare to the United States granted for health care emergencies? For compassionate leave?

Vacations and holidays:

- What U.S., Canadian, and local holidays does the agency recognize?
- What is the length and frequency of vacation/holiday absences? Are there limitations to travel during vacations?
- In politically volatile areas, are more frequent vacations permitted/encouraged?
- Does the agency have an informal or formal network allowing for staff to vacation at reduced cost?
- Do staff offer hospitality to other agency members while traveling? Is it expected that all staff reciprocate by housing agency members during vacations and/or job-related travel?

Orientation program:

- What is the length, location, and nature of the agency orientation?
- Are language studies required? Where do language studies occur? Who pays for classes?
- Are local interpreters available? Are there any gender-related or age-related factors to consider when using an interpreter?
- Does the orientation include study of the political, economic, social, cultural, religious, and health-related aspects of the host country?
- Who is the U.S./Canadian ambassador to the host country? Where is the U.S./Canadian embassy located?
- In case of natural disaster or political unrest, what is the emergency evacuation plan for expatriates?

Choosing an International Sending Agency

Because there are many agencies that send nurses abroad, it is beyond the scope of this chapter to provide an exhaustive list. Appendix D lists the names and addresses of selected agencies that engage the services of nurses for health-related projects. Not included in the listing are a wide variety of church-related organizations, universities, foundations, private industries, study/travel groups, professional nursing associations and the U.S. and Canadian militaries.

Nurses may affiliate with a variety of sponsoring agencies. Sponsorship may be through a U.S. or Canadian organization or through the host country (ministry of health, university, hospital, school of nursing, public health agency, or other). International agencies, such as WHO, also engage the services of nurses for consultation and clinical practice. Joint sponsorship, though relatively uncommon, also may occur. For example, some religious groups have both international and national organizations that may elect joint sponsorship.

Summary

With increasing frequency, U.S. and Canadian nurses are traveling, studying, researching, consulting, teaching, administering, and practicing nursing abroad. The decision to engage in an international interchange requires much thought and planning. Philosophical congruence with the sending agency or organization, selection of geographic area of interest, length of time available, and matching background with host-country needs are factors that interplay with the desire to go abroad.

Many U.S. and Canadian nurses are relatively naïve about negotiating a contract with a sending agency. An overview of reasonable questions to pursue with the agency has been provided, including discussions of salary/stipend, travel to the assignment site, housing and moving expenses, local transportation, insurance coverage, vacation and holiday leave, and orientation policies. The names and addresses of selected health-related sending agencies are listed.

Review Questions

1. Critically analyze the state of the world's health. What are the major diseases that threaten the health of people globally?
2. What economic, social, and cultural factors influence the health and well-being of people in various parts of the world? How do these factors affect life expectancy, morbidity and mortality?
3. What factors influence whether a nation is categorized as a More Developed Country (MDC) or a Less Developed Country (LDC)? Do you think this categorization is useful in understanding patterns of health and illness globally? Be sure to explain the reasons for your answer.
4. Explain what is meant by the term *emerging infectious diseases* and discuss why these diseases pose such a serious threat to the health of people around the world. Identify one emerging infectious disease and explore what can be done to curb its spread.
5. Discuss the past and present role of nurses in meeting global health challenges. Identify nurses who have made historic contributions in international nursing and health.
6. If you were planning to work as a nurse in another country, what activities would enable you to prepare for your new position? What resources are available to assist you?

Learning Activities to Promote Critical Thinking

1. Identify someone who has recently moved to the United States or Canada from another country. After reviewing the section of the chapter dealing with cultural adjustment, ask the person to tell you about his or her experiences since arriving. How does the response compare with the W model? What is your assessment of the stage of cultural adjustment the person is experiencing?

2. Identify a foreign-born nurse and ask him or her to describe the health care delivery system in his or her country of origin. Compare and contrast the U.S./Canadian health care delivery system with that of the country you have chosen.

3. Select a country (other than your own), and examine the professional and lay health care systems. You may find it helpful to conduct a library search to identify relevant articles, books, and audiovisual materials available on the topic.

4. Watch your local television guide for programs on international health. Choose one program and critically review its contents in terms of accuracy, caliber of sources used, presence/absence of reporting biases, clarity of presentation, effectiveness in conveying the message(s), and identification of intended audience (e.g., adults, high school students, etc.).

5. If you learned that you would be leaving next month for Kenya to work as a staff nurse in the outpatient department of a clinic, how would you prepare yourself?

6. If the opportunity presents itself, participate in a travel/study abroad program at your college/university. What information will you need to plan for your trip? Where will you go to obtain the necessary information?

References

Andrews, M. M. (1985). International consultation by United States nurses. *International Nursing Review 32*(1), 50–54.

Andrews, M. M. (1986). U.S. nurse consultants in the international marketplace. *International Nursing Review 33*(2), 50–55.

Andrews, M. M. (1988). Educational preparation for international nursing. *Journal of Professional Nursing 4*(6), 430–435.

Andrews, M. M. (1992). Cultural perspectives on nursing in the 21st century. *Journal of Professional Nursing 8*(1), 7–15.

Aroian, K. J. (1990). A model of psychological adaptation to migration and resettlement. *Nursing Research 39*(1), 5–10.

Badran, I. G. (1993). Accidents in the developing world. *World Health Organization 46*(1), 14–15.

Baker, T. D., Weisman, C., & Piwoz, E. (1984). United States health professionals in international health work. *American Journal of Public Health 74*(5), 438–441.

Basch, P. F. (1990). *Textbook of International Health*. New York: Oxford Press.

Brown, P. (1988). *People Who Have Helped the World: Florence Nightingale*. Waterford, Herts, UK: Exley.

Centers for Disease Control and Prevention (1996). Recommended childhood immunization schedule: United States. *Immunization Action News 3*(5), 1.

DeSantis, L. (1988). The relevance of transcultural nursing to international nursing. *International Nursing Review 35*(4), 110–112, 116.

Devereaux, G. (1993). Making the most of things . . . nursing overseas. *Nursing Times 89*(1), 44–46.

Dier, K. A. (1988). International nursing: The global approach. *Recent Advances in Nursing 20*, 39–60.

Heyman, D. (1997). Emerging infectious diseases. *World Health 50*(1), 3–5.

Horsley, M. R. (1991). Transcultural travel tips for the nurse abroad. *Imprint 38*(2), 107–112.

International Council of Nurses (1995). Worldwide survey of nursing issues. *International Nursing Review 42*(4), 125–127.

Leininger, M. (1981). Transcultural nursing: Its progress and its future. *Nursing and Health Care 9*, 365–371.

Leininger, M. M. (1992). Editorial. Globalization of transcultural nursing: A worldwide imperative. *Journal of Transcultural Nursing 4*(2), 2–3.

Leininger, M. M. (1993). Editorial. International Council of Nursing and Transcultural Nursing Society: Alike or different? *Journal of Transcultural Nursing 5*(1), 2–3.

Leininger, M. (1995). *Transcultural Nursing: Concepts, Theories, Research and Practices*. New York: McGraw-Hill, Inc.

Muecke, M. (1992). Nursing research with refugees. *Western Journal of Nursing Research 14*(6), 703–720.

Nakajima, H. (1997). Let's work together to control infectious diseases. *World Health 50*(1), 3.

National Center for Health Statistics (1995). *Health United States, 1994*. Washington, DC: U.S. Government Printing Office.

Nightingale, F. (1859). *Her Notes on Hospitals*. London: Parker.

Peplau, H. (1965). Specialization in professional nursing. *Nursing Science 8*, 24–27.

Styles, M. M. (1993). The world as classroom. *Nursing and Health Care 14*(10), 507.

Uhl, J. E. (1992). International affairs: Nightingale—The international nurse. *Journal of Professional Nursing 8*(1), 5.

Upvall, M. J. (1993a). HIV/AIDS prevention in Zanzibar: The role of nursing education. *Nursing and Health Care 14*(10), 524–527.

Upvall, M. J. (1993b). Therapeutic syncretism: A conceptual framework of persistence and change for international nursing. *Journal of Professional Nursing 9*(1), 56–62.

World Health Organization (1978). *Primary Health Care: Report of the International Conference on Primary Health Care.* Geneva: World Health Organization.

World Health Organization (1992). *Eighth Report on the World Health Situation.* Geneva: World Health Organization.

World Health Organization (1996). *The World Health Report 1996: Fighting Disease, Fostering Development.* Geneva: World Health Organization.

World Health Organization (1997). *The World Health Report 1997: Conquering Suffering, Enriching Humanity.* Geneva: World Health Organization.

Appendix A
. . . .
Andrews/Boyle Transcultural Assessment Guide

Cultural Affiliations

With what cultural group(s) does the client report affiliation (e.g., American, Hispanic, Navajo, or combination)? To what degree does the client identify with the cultural group (e.g., "we" concept of solidarity or as a fringe member)?

Where was the client born?

Where has the client lived (country, city) and when (during what years)? *Note:* If a recent relocation to the United States, knowledge of prevalent diseases in country of origin may be helpful. Current residence? Occupation?

Values Orientation

What are the client's attitudes, values, and beliefs about developmental life events such as birth and death, health, illness, and health care providers?

Does culture affect the manner in which the client relates to body image change resulting from illness or surgery (e.g., importance of appearance, beauty, strength, and roles in cultural group)? Is there a cultural stigma associated with the client's illness (i.e., how is the illness or client condition viewed by the larger culture)?

How does the client view work, leisure, education?

How does the client perceive change?

How does the client perceive changes in lifestyle relating to current illness or surgery?

How does the client value privacy, courtesy, touch, and relationships with individuals of different ages, social class (or caste), and gender?

How does the client view biomedical/scientific health care (e.g., suspiciously, fearfully, acceptingly)? How does the client relate to persons outside of his or her cultural group (e.g., withdrawal, verbally or nonverbally expressive, negatively or positively)?

Cultural Sanctions and Restrictions

How does the client's cultural group regard expression of emotion and feelings, spirituality, and religious beliefs? How are dying, death, and grieving expressed in a culturally appropriate manner?

How is modesty expressed by men and women? Are there culturally defined expectations about male-female relationships, including the nurse–client relationship?

Does the client have any restrictions related to sexuality, exposure of body parts, certain types of surgery (e.g., amputation, vasectomy, hysterectomy)?

Are there any restrictions against discussion of dead relatives or fears related to the unknown?

Communication

What language does the client speak at home? What other languages does the client speak or read? In what language would the client prefer to communicate with you?

What is the fluency level of the client in English—both written and spoken use of the language? Remember that the stress of illness may cause clients to use a more familiar language and to temporarily forget some English.

Does the client need an interpreter? If so, is there a relative or friend whom the client would like to interpret? Is there anyone whom the client would prefer did not serve as an interpreter (e.g., member of the opposite sex, a person younger/older than the client, member of a rival tribe or nation)?

What are the rules (linguistics) and modes (style) of communication? How does the client prefer to be addressed?

Is it necessary to vary the technique of communication during the interview and examination to accommodate the client's cultural background (e.g., tempo of conversation, eye contact, sensitivity to topical taboos, norms of confidentiality, and style of explanation)?

How does the client's nonverbal communication compare with that of individuals from other cultural backgrounds? How does it affect the client's relationship with you and with other members of the health care team?

How does the client feel about health care providers who are not of the same cultural background (e.g., black, middle-class nurse and Hispanic of a different social class)? Does the client prefer to receive care from a nurse of the same cultural background, gender, and/or age?

What are the overall cultural characteristics of the client's language and communication processes?

Health-Related Beliefs and Practices

To what cause(s) does the client attribute illness and disease (e.g., divine wrath, imbalance in hot/cold or yin/yang, punishment for moral transgressions, hex, soul loss, pathogenic organism)?

What are the client's cultural beliefs about ideal body size and shape? What is the client's self-image vis-à-vis the ideal?

What name does the client give to his or her health-related condition?

What does the client believe promotes health (eating certain foods, wearing amulets to bring good luck, sleep, rest, good nutrition, reducing stress, exercise, prayer, rituals to ancestors, saints, or intermediate deities)?

What is the client's religious affiliation (e.g., Judaism, Islam, Pentacostalism, West African voodooism, Seventh-Day Adventism, Catholicism, Mormonism)? How actively involved in the practice of this religion is the client?

Does the client rely on cultural healers (e.g., curandero, shaman, spiritualist, priest, minister, monk?) Who determines when the client is sick and when he or she is healthy? Who influences the choice/type of healer and treatment that should be sought?

In what types of cultural healing practices does the client engage (use of herbal remedies, potions, massage, wearing of talismans, copper bracelets or charms to discourage evil spirits, healing rituals, incantations, prayers)?

How are biomedical/scientific health care providers perceived? How does the client and his or her family perceive nurses? What are the expectations of nurses and nursing care?

What comprises appropriate "sick role" behavior? Who determines what symptoms constitute disease/illness? Who decides when the client is no longer sick? Who cares for the client at home?

How does the client's cultural group view mental disorders? Are there differences in acceptable behaviors for physical versus psychological illnesses?

Nutrition

What nutritional factors are influenced by the client's cultural background? What is the meaning of food and eating to the client?

With whom does the client usually eat? What types of foods are eaten? What is the timing and sequencing of meals?

What does the client define as food? What does the client believe comprises a "healthy" versus an "unhealthy" diet?

Who shops for food? Where are groceries purchased (e.g., special markets or ethnic grocery stores)? Who prepares the client's meals?

How are foods prepared at home [type of food preparation, cooking oil(s) used, length of time foods are cooked, especially vegetables, amount and type of seasoning added to various foods during preparation]?

Has the client chosen a particular nutritional practice such as vegetarianism or abstinence from alcoholic or fermented beverages?

Do religious beliefs and practices influence the client's diet (e.g., amount, type, preparation, or delineation of acceptable food combinations, e.g., kosher diets)? Does the client abstain from certain foods at regular intervals, on specific dates determined by the religious calendar, or at other times?

If the client's religion mandates or encourages fasting, what does the term *fast* mean (e.g., refraining from certain types or quantities of foods, eating only during certain times of the day)? For what period of time is the client expected to fast?

During fasting, does the client refrain from liquids/beverages? Does the religion allow exemption from fasting during illness? If so, does the client believe that an exemption applies to him or her?

Socioeconomic Considerations

Who comprises the client's social network (family, friends, peers, and cultural healers)? How do they influence the client's health or illness status?

How do members of the client's social support network define caring (e.g., being continuously present, doing things for the client, providing material support, looking after the client's family)? What is the role of various family members during health and illness?

How does the client's family participate in the promotion of health (e.g., lifestyle changes in diet, activity level, etc.) and nursing care (e.g., bathing, feeding, touching, being present) of the client?

Does the cultural family structure influence the client's response to health or illness (e.g., beliefs, strengths, weaknesses, and social class)? Is there a key family member whose role is significant in health-related decisions (e.g., grandmother in many African American families or eldest adult son in Asian families)?

Who is the principal wage earner in the client's family? What is the total annual income? (*Note*: this is a potentially sensitive question.) Is there more than one wage earner? Are there other sources of financial support (extended family, investments)?

What insurance coverage (health, dental, vision, pregnancy) does the client have?

What impact does economic status have on lifestyle, place of residence, living conditions, ability to obtain health care? How does the client's home environment (e.g., presence of indoor plumbing, handicap access) influence nursing care?

Organizations Providing Cultural Support

What influence do ethnic/cultural organizations have on the client's receiving health care (e.g., Organization of Migrant Workers, National Association for the Advancement of Color People [NAACP], Black Political Caucus, churches such as African American, Muslim, Jewish, and others, schools including those which are church-related, Urban League, community-based health care programs and clinics).

Educational Background

What is the client's highest educational level obtained?

Does the client's educational background affect his or her knowledge level concerning the health care delivery system, how to obtain the needed care, teaching-learning, and any written material that he or she is given in the health care setting (e.g., insurance forms, educational literature, information about diagnostic procedures and laboratory tests, admissions forms)?

Can the client read and write English, or is another language preferred? If English is the client's second language, are materials available in the client's primary language?

What learning style is most comfortable/familiar? Does the client prefer to learn through written materials, oral explanation, or demonstration?

Religious Affiliation

How does the client's religious affiliation affect health and illness (e.g., life events such as death, chronic illness, body image alteration, cause and effect of illness)?

What is the role of religious beliefs and practices during health and illness? Are there special rites or blessings for those with serious or terminal illnesses?

Are there healing rituals or practices that the client believes can promote well-being or hasten recovery from illness? If so, who performs these?

What is the role of significant religious representatives during health and illness? Are there recognized religious healers (e.g., Islamic imams, Christian Scientist practitioners or nurses, Catholic priests, Mormon elders, Buddhist monks)?

Cultural Aspects of Disease Incidence

Are there any specific genetic or acquired conditions that are more prevalent for a specific cultural group (e.g., hypertension, sickle cell anemia, Tay Sachs, G6PD, lactose intolerance)?

Are there socioenvironmental diseases more prevalent among a specific cultural group (e.g., lead poisoning, alcoholism, HIV/AIDS, drug abuse, ear infections, family violence)?

Are there any diseases against which the client has an increased resistance (e.g., skin cancer in darkly pigmented individuals, malaria for those with sickle cell anemia)?

Biocultural Variations

Does the client have distinctive physical features characteristic of a particular ethnic or cultural group (e.g., skin color, hair texture)? Does the client have any variations in anatomy characteristic of a particular ethnic or cultural group (e.g., body structure, height, weight, facial shape and structure [nose, eye shape, facial contour], upper and lower extremities)?

How do anatomic, racial and ethnic variations affect the physical examination?

Developmental Considerations

Are there any distinct growth and development characteristics that vary with the client's cultural background (e.g., bone density, psychomotor patterns of development, fat-folds)?

What factors are significant in assessing children of various ages from the newborn period through adolescence (e.g., expected growth on standard grid, culturally acceptable age for toilet training, introducing various types of foods, gender differences, discipline, socialization to adult roles)?

What is the cultural perception of aging (e.g., is youthfulness or the wisdom of old age more highly valued)?

How are elderly persons handled culturally (e.g., cared for in the home of adult children, placed in institutions for care)? What are culturally acceptable roles for the elderly?

Does the elderly person expect family members to provide care, including nurturance and other humanistic aspects of care?

Is the elderly person isolated from culturally relevant supportive persons or enmeshed in a caring network of relatives and friends?

Has a culturally appropriate network replaced family members in performing some caring functions for the elderly person?

Resources in Transcultural Health and Nursing

American Nurses Association
600 Maryland Avenue, S.W.
Suite 100 West
Washington, DC 20024-2571
(202) 651-7000

Asian-Pacific Islander Nurses Association
C/O College of Mount Saint Vincent
6301 Riverdale Avenue
Riverdale, NY 10471
(718) 405-3351

Association of Black Nursing Faculty in Higher
Education
5823 Queens Cove
Lisle, IL 60532
(708) 969-3809

Canadian Nurses Association
50 Driveway
Ottawa, Ontario K2P 1E2
(613) 236-4547

Centers for Disease Control and Prevention (CDC)
Associate Director for Minority Health
Centers for Disease Control
1600 Clifton Road, N.E.—Mailstop D39
Atlanta, GA 30333
(404) 639-7210

Chi Eta Phi Sorority, Inc.
3029 13th Street, N.W.
Washington, DC 20036
(202) 232-3858

Council on Nursing and Anthropology Association
(CONAA)
C/O Dr. Eileen M. Jackson
Department of Anthropology
University of North Carolina at Greensboro
900 Englewood Street
Greensboro, NC 27403
(336) 274-0026

National Association of Hispanic Nurses
1501 16th Street, N.W.
Washington, DC 20036
(202) 387-5000

National Black Nurses Association
1511 K Street, N.W.
Washington, DC 20005
(202) 393-6870

National Institutes of Health (NIH)
Office of Research on Minority Health
National Institutes of Health
Building 1, Room 260
9000 Rockville Pike
Bethesda, MD 20892
(301) 402-1366

National Resource Center on Minority Aging
Populations
University Center on Aging
San Diego University
College of Human Services
San Diego, CA 92182-0273
(619) 594-6765

Native American Nurses Association
927 Treadale Lane
Cloquet, MN 55720
(218) 879-1227

rica, Inc.

ıth Services

for Minority

D-18

Rockvı...
(301) 443-03b>

Transcultural Nursing Society
c/o Madonna University
College of Nursing and Health
36600 Schoolcraft Road
Livonia, MI 48150-1173
(303) 432-5470 or toll free (888) 432-5470

U.S. Department of Health and Human Services
U.S. Public Health Service
Indian Health Service
Parklawn Building
5600 Fishers Lane
Rockville, MD 20852-9788
(301) 443-4242

U.S. Department of Health and Human Services
U.S. Public Health Service
Office of Minority Health
P.O. Box 37337
Washington, DC 20013-7337
(800) 444-6472

Internet Sites (or Resources)

Government Web Sites

U.S. Department of Health and Human Services
http://www.dhhs.gov

Office of Minority Health, U.S. Department of Health
and Human Services
http://www.omhrc.gov

Indian Health Service
http://www.ihs.gov

Center for Disease Control & Prevention
http://www.cdc.gov

National Center for Health Statistics
http://www.cdc.gov/nchswww/nchshome.html

Morbidity & Mortality Weekly Report
http://www.cdc.gov/epo/mmwr/mmwr.html

National Institutes of Health
http://www.nih.gov

Private Foundations, Organizations, and Universities

Commonwealth Fund of New York
http://www.cmwf.org

Native American Web Sites
http://www.pitt.edu%7Elmitten/indians.html

Minority Health Network (MHNet)
http://www.pitt.edu/~ejb4/min/desc.html

Global Health Network (GHNet)
http://www.pitt.edu/HOME/GHNet/Towards/
02-Define.html

AJNOnline
http://www.ajn.org

World Health Organization (WHO)
http://who.ch

WHO links include

National Council for International Health
http://www.who.ch/programmes/ina/ngo/ngo144.html

International Council of Nurses
http://www.who.ch/programmes/ina/ngo/ngo-51.html

Interactive HealthCare Directories
http://www.erols.com/stewpub

Miscellaneous
Ethnic NewsWatch is a full text database of the newspapers, magazines and journal of the ethnic, minority and native press. Coverage is local, national and global.

Appendix C

· ·

Selected Agencies Sending
Nurses Abroad

U.S. Government Agencies

Action/Peace Corps
Recruiting Office
P-301
Washington, DC 20526

U.S. Agency for International Development (USAID)
Recruitment Branch, Room 111SA2
515 22nd Street, NW
Washington, DC 20523

U.S. Department of Defense
The Pentagon
Washington, DC 20330

U.S. Department of State
General Recruitment Division
Recruitment Branch
2201 C Street N.W.
Washington, DC 20520

Canadian Government Agency

Canadian Council for International Development
(CETA)
170 Laurier Avenue West
Suite 900
Ottawa, Ontario K1P 5V5
(819) 997-5456

U.S. Private Agencies

American Red Cross
17th and D Streets, NW
Washington, DC 20006

Amdoc/Option Agency
3550 Afton Road
San Diego, CA 92702

American Medical International
9465 Wilshire Boulevard, Suite 307
Beverly Hills, CA 90212

Care
151 Ellis Street, N.E.
Atlanta, GA 30303-2349

Concern
P.O. Box 1790
Santa Ana, CA 92702

Direct Relief International
P.O. Box 30820
Santa Barbara, CA 93130

HCA International Company
P.O. Box 550
Department N87-887
Nashville, TN 37202

International Voluntary Services, Inc.
1901 Pennsylvania Ave., N.W.
Suite 501
Washington, DC 20006

Medicine and Public Health: Develop Assistance
Abroad
200 Park Avenue
New York, NY 10003

Project HOPE
The People-to-People Health Foundation, Inc.
Division of Nursing
Education and Personnel Department
Carter Hall
Millwood, VA 22646

Thomas Dooley Foundation
442 Post Street
San Francisco, CA 94102

548

Westinghouse Health Systems
P.O. Box 866
Columbia, MD 21044

Whittaker International Services Company
Medical Careers Center
P.O. Box 12029
Arlington, VA 22209

Canadian Nongovernment Agency

Canadian Council for International Cooperation
1 Nichols Street, Third Floor
Ottawa, Ontario K1N 7B7
(613) 236-4547

Provides a listing of 130 nongovernment agencies in a directory called *ID Profiles*

International Organizations

International Council of Nurses (ICN)
Box 42
1211 Geneva 20
Switzerland

Pan American Health Organization
Nursing Section, Health Services Division
525 23rd Street, NW
Washington, DC 20037

World Health Organization (WHO)
Avenue Appia
1211 Geneva, 27
Switzerland

Information Clearinghouses

An information clearinghouse has current reports on the types of nurses that are needed for specific countries but does not usually provide placement services.

American Council of Voluntary Agencies for Foreign Service, Inc.
Technical Assistance Clearinghouse
200 Park Avenue
New York, NY 10003

American Nurses' Association*
600 Maryland Ave., S.W.
Suite 100 West
Washington, D.C. 20024-2571
(202) 651-7000

Canadian Nurses Association*
50 Driveway
Ottawa, Ontario K2P 1E2
(613) 236-4547

National Council for International Health (NCIH)†
1701 K Street, NW, Suite 600
Washington, DC 20006
(202) 833-5900

The ANA and CNA will send a letter of introduction to the national nurses association of any country the nurse plans to visit.

†*NCIH is a membership organization that provides a computerized listing of health-related international employment opportunities and a directory of U.S.-based agencies involved in international health assistance.*

Index